AF894673

Cartilage Imaging

Thomas M. Link
Editor

Cartilage Imaging

Significance, Techniques, and New Developments

Springer

Editor
Thomas M. Link
Department of Radiology and Biomedical Imaging
University of California at San Francisco
San Francisco, CA
USA
thomas.link@ucsf.edu

ISBN 978-1-4419-8437-1 ISBN 978-1-4419-8438-8 (eBook)
DOI 10.1007/978-1-4419-8438-8
Springer New York Dordrecht Heidelberg London

Library of Congress Control Number: 2011924334

© Springer Science+Business Media, LLC 2011
All rights reserved. This work may not be translated or copied in whole or in part without the written permission of the publisher (Springer Science+Business Media, LLC, 233 Spring Street, New York, NY 10013, USA), except for brief excerpts in connection with reviews or scholarly analysis. Use in connection with any form of information storage and retrieval, electronic adaptation, computer software, or by similar or dissimilar methodology now known or hereafter developed is forbidden.
The use in this publication of trade names, trademarks, service marks, and similar terms, even if they are not identified as such, is not to be taken as an expression of opinion as to whether or not they are subject to proprietary rights.
While the advice and information in this book are believed to be true and accurate at the date of going to press, neither the authors nor the editors nor the publisher can accept any legal responsibility for any errors or omissions that may be made. The publisher makes no warranty, express or implied, with respect to the material contained herein.

Printed on acid-free paper

Springer is part of Springer Science+Business Media (www.springer.com)

Preface

One of the first systematic histological evaluations of the role of joint cartilage was published in 1843 by Ecker and was entitled "Ueber Abnuetzung und Zerstoerung des Gelenkknorpels" [1]. In 1942, Bennett et al. stated that degeneration of articular cartilage is the origin of osteoarthritis and that the degeneration is an inherent senescence of the cartilaginous tissue [2]. For many years, cartilage loss and degeneration were considered as inevitable, eventually leading to decrease in joint function, osteoarthritis, and immobility, with limited therapeutic options.

Cartilage degeneration has been identified as a major threat to our aging society with substantial implications for health care and as a major socio-economic burden. Hence today, there is tremendous activity in developing strategies and treatments to prevent cartilage "Abnuetzung" (loss). These include injury prevention programs, cartilage repair, as well as oral and local treatments. While these therapies are clearly in their infancy, their development requires sensitive and reliable cartilage imaging and quantification techniques; these are indispensible to monitor the effects of new therapies and prevention strategies. Thus *cartilage imaging* gains a major and central role in the management of degenerative joint disease.

The goal of this book was not simply to summarize currently available imaging techniques to assess cartilage, but also to provide clinical perspectives and an outlook on future developments. Major experts in this growing field contributed to this book, which is geared to radiologists, orthopedic surgeons, rheumatologists, and clinical and basic researchers. We believe that cartilage imaging and noninvasive quantification will be essential tools in preserving joint function and tackling the ever-increasing challenge of osteoarthritis in our society.

I would finally like to acknowledge our developmental editor Michael Griffin's hard work and support during the preparation of this book.

San Francisco, CA, USA — Thomas M. Link, MD

References

1. Ecker A. Ueber Abnuetzung und Zerstoerung der Gelenkknorpel. Arch Physiol Heilk. 1843;2:235–48.
2. Bennett G, Waine H, Bauer W. Changes in the knee joint at various ages. New York: Commonwealth Fund; 1942.

Preface

Contents

Contributors

Thomas Baum, MD
Department of Radiology and Biomedical Imaging, Musculoskeletal and Quantitative Imaging Research Group, University of California, San Francisco, CA, USA
and
Department of Radiology, Technische Universität München, Ismaninger Str. 22, 81675 Munich, Germany

Arijitt Borthakur, PhD
Department of Radiology, Center for Magnetic Resonance and Optical Imaging, School of Medicine, University of Pennsylvania, Philadelphia, PA, USA

Deborah Burstein, PhD
Department of Radiology, Beth Israel Deaconess Medical Center, Boston, MA, USA

Julio Carballido-Gamio, PhD
Grupo Tecnológico Santa Fe, S.A. de C.V., Mexico City, Mexico
and
Department of Radiology and Biomedical Imaging, University of California at San Francisco, San Francisco, CA, USA

Sunny Cheung, MD
Division of Orthopedic Sports Surgery, Mission Bay Orthopedic Institute, University of California, San Francisco, CA, USA

Bernard J. Dardzinski, PhD
Exploratory and Translational Sciences – Imaging, University of Pennsylvania, Merck & Co., Inc., Children's Hospital of Pennsylvania, West Point, PA, USA

Stephan Domayer, MD
Department of Orthopaedics, Medical University of Vienna, Vienna, Austria

Jeffrey Duryea, PhD
Department of Radiology, Brigham and Women's Hospital, Boston, MA, USA

Felix Eckstein, MD
Institute of Anatomy & Musculoskeletal Research, Paracelsus Medical University, Salzburg, Austria
and
Chondrometrics GmbH, Ainring, Germany

Martha L. Gray, PhD
Department of Electrical Engineering and Computer Science, MIT, Harvard-MIT Division of Health Sciences and Technology (HST), New England Baptist (NEB) Bone and Joint Center, BIDMC, Cambridge, MA, USA

Ali Guermazi, MD
Department of Radiology, Boston University, Quantitative Imaging Center (QIC), Boston, MA, USA

Daichi Hayashi, MBBS, BSc
Department of Radiology, Boston University School of Medicine, Boston, MA, USA

Andrew Horvai, MD, PhD
Department of Pathology, University of California, San Francisco, CA, USA

Martin Hudelmaier, MD
Paracelsus Medical University, Institute of Anatomy and Musculoskeletal Research, Salzburg, Austria

David J. Hunter, MBBS, PhD, FRACP
Division of Research, New England Baptist Hospital, Boston, MA, USA
and
Rheumatology Department, Royal North Shore Hospital, University of Sydney, Australia

Vladimir Juras, PhD
Department of Radiology, MR Center, General Hospital of Vienna, Medical University of Vienna, Vienna, Austria

J. Bruce Kneeland, MD
Department of Radiology, Center for Magnetic Resonance and Optical Imaging, School of Medicine, University of Pennsylvania, Philadelphia, PA, USA

Frédéric E. Lecouvet, MD, PhD
Department of Radiology and Medical Imaging, Cliniques Universitaires Saint-Luc – UC Louvain, Brussels, Belgium

Xiaojuan Li, PhD
Department of Radiology and Biomedical Imaging, University of California, San Francisco, CA, USA

Hans Liebl
Medical School, Technical University of Munich, Munich, Germany

Thomas M. Link, MD
Department of Radiology and Biomedical Imaging, University of California at San Francisco, San Francisco, CA, USA

C. Benjamin Ma, PhD
Sports Medicine and Shoulder Service, Department of Orthopedic Surgery, University of California, San Francisco, San Francisco, CA, USA

Sharmila Majumdar, PhD
Department of Radiology and Biomedical Imaging, University of California at San Francisco, San Francisco, CA, USA

Tallal C. Mamisch, MD
Department of Orthopaedic Surgery, University of Bern, Bern, Switzerland
and
Department of Radiology, MR Center, General Hospital of Vienna, Medical University of Vienna, Vienna, Austria

Patrick Omoumi, MD
Department of Radiology and Medical Imaging, Saint-Luc University Hospital – UC Louvain, Brussels, Belgium

Ravinder Reddy, PhD
Department of Radiology, School of Medicine, University of Pennsylvania, Philadelphia, PA, USA

Frank W. Roemer, MD
Department of Radiology, Klinikum Augsburg, Augsburg, Germany;
Department of Radiology, Boston University, Quantitative Imaging Center (QIC), Boston, MA, USA

Christoph Stehling, MD
Department of Clinical Radiology, University of Muenster, Muenster, Germany

Siegfried Trattnig, MD
Department of Radiology, MR Center, Medical University of Vienna, General Hospital of Vienna, Vienna, Austria

Bruno C. Vande Berg, MD, PhD
Department of Radiology and Medical Imaging, Saint-Luc University Hospital – UC Louvain, Brussels, Belgium

Goetz H. Welsch, MD
Department of Radiology, MR Center, General Hospital of Vienna, Medical University of Vienna, Vienna, Austria
and
Department of Trauma Surgery, University of Erlangen-Nuremberg, Erlangen, Germany

Wolfgang Wirth, PhD
Institute of Anatomy and Musculoskeletal Research, Paracelsus Medical University, Salzburg, Austria

Walter R.T. Witschey, PhD
Department of Radiology, Center for Magnetic Resonance and Optical Imaging, School of Medicine, University of Pennsylvania, Philadelphia, PA, USA

Chapter 1
Anatomy and Histology of Cartilage

Andrew Horvai

Keywords Anatomy • Histology • Cartilage • Matrix composition • Osteoarthritis • Neoplasia • Fibrocartilage

Introduction

Cartilage is a connective tissue structure that is composed of a collagen and proteoglycan-rich matrix and a single cell type: the chondrocyte. Cartilage is unique among connective tissues in that it lacks blood vessels and nerves and receives its nutrition solely by diffusion [1]. In fetal life, cartilage forms the template for the majority of the skeleton but persists in selected locations into adulthood including articular surfaces, ribs, ears, and the tracheobronchial tree. Structurally, cartilage provides a firm material which, depending on subtype, is adapted to resist and damp compressive and tensile forces. Functionally, it plays important roles in skeletal development, growth and repair, joint articulation, lubrication, and patency of the respiratory tract. Although the mechanical properties of cartilage are functions of the extracellular matrix, it is the chondrocyte that directs the synthesis and composition of the matrix. Though few in number, chondrocytes also mediate critical pathways of regeneration and growth by highly regulated signal transduction pathways that are now becoming better understood [2, 3].

Most pathology of cartilage involves degenerative diseases, particularly osteoarthritis. However, cartilage neoplasms, especially the benign forms, are among the most common primary tumors of bone and illustrate the close association between radiologic and pathologic findings.

A. Horvai (✉)
Department of Pathology, University of California, 1600 Divisadero Street, B220, San Francisco, CA 94115, USA
e-mail: andrew.horvai@ucsf.edu

Anatomy

Grossly, cartilage consists of a translucent pale-blue to yellow-white (depending on subtype and collagen content) rubbery tissue (Fig. 1.1). Perichondrium is a layer of dense fibrous tissue that covers cartilage in most locations except the articular surfaces. No neurovascular structures penetrate beyond the perichondrium. Consequently, all nutrition arrives by diffusion, limiting the thickness of cartilage surfaces to a few centimeters - a rule that manifests in even the largest animals. As cartilage ages, it transforms from blue-white to yellowish and opaque, which may be related to dehydration and age-related pigment deposits [4]. Cartilage is attached to the underlying bone by means of radial collagen fibers that penetrate from bone into the cartilage over a complex three-dimensional interface. However, the specialized collagen fibers of cartilage do not extend into subchondral bone.

Hyaline (from the Greek *hyalos* meaning "glass or transparent stone") cartilage is the predominant type in the human body and forms all diarthrotic articular surfaces, the most peripheral part of the nucleus pulposus of the intervertebral disk, portions of the ribs, and tracheobronchial tree. A specialized type of hyaline cartilage is also present in the epiphyseal plate (growth plate). Fibrocartilage is present in the temporomandibular and sternoclavicular joints and the annulus fibrosus of the intervertebral disk as well as the meniscus at the knee and the labrum of the shoulder. Finally, elastic cartilage is largely restricted to the external ear and a few other sites. All cartilage is ideally suited to resist compressive forces. However, the presence of type I collagen and elastin in fibrocartilage and elastocartilage, respectively, also allows these tissues to resist tension. The anatomic and functional differences of the three major cartilage subtypes are summarized in Table 1.1. Although the anatomy of cartilage differs somewhat depending on subtype, articular cartilage is the most common and best studied in terms of biochemical and histologic features.

T.M. Link (ed.), *Cartilage Imaging: Significance, Techniques, and New Developments*,
DOI 10.1007/978-1-4419-8438-8_1, © Springer Science+Business Media, LLC 2011

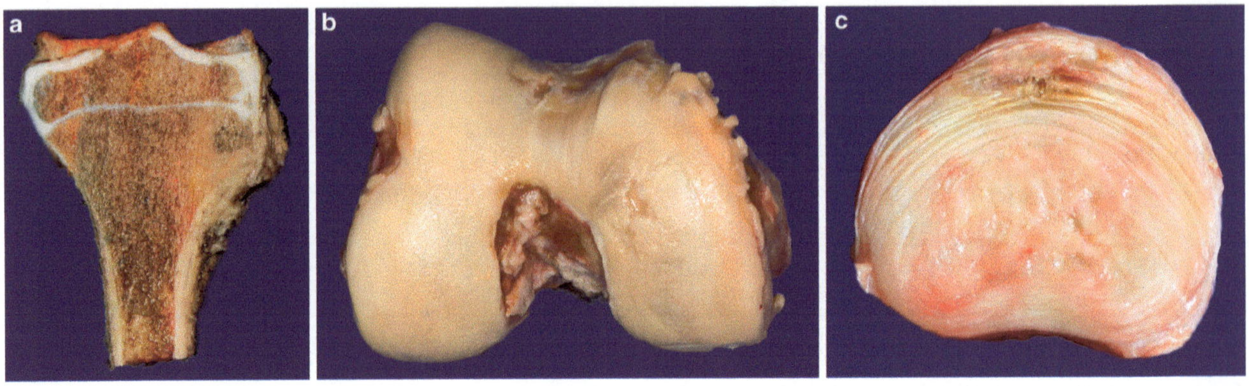

Fig. 1.1 Gross appearance of cartilage. Hyaline cartilage, in young patients, can be seen in the articular surface and growth plate (**a**) and is usually a translucent *blue-white* rubbery material (**a**). With aging, the articular surface becomes more opaque and *yellow-white* (**b**). Fibrocartilage of the intervertebral disk (**c**) has a dense, fibrous off-white appearance with concentric layers of fibers in the annulus fibrosus

Table 1.1 Summary of three main cartilage types

Type	Mechanical function	Locations	Unique components
Hyaline	Compression	Articular, growth plate	
Fibro	Tension	Temporomandibular joint, sternoclavicular joint, annulus fibrosus, meniscus, labrum	Collagen type I
Elasto	Tension	External ear, ligamentum flavum, epiglottis	Elastin

Matrix Composition

The cartilage matrix consists predominantly of extracellular water (66–78%) with the remaining (dry) weight composed of proteoglycans, collagen, and additional specialized proteins [5]. The approximate distribution of components of hyaline cartilage is outlined in Table 1.2. In articular cartilage, water is unevenly distributed such that the highest concentration is present at the articular surface [6]. The constant diffusion and tidal movement of water in and out of the cartilage matrix with joint compression allow nutrients to reach the chondrocytes. Proteoglycans, discussed in more detail below, are directly responsible for the high water content of cartilage. Proteoglycans are composed of high molecular weight proteins with carbohydrate side chains resulting in large, charged molecules that attract water thereby increasing their volume dramatically.

Collagen represents ~50% of the dry weight of the matrix. In cartilage, type II collagen (encoded by the *COL2A1* gene) predominates and confers the tensile stiffness and strength to the matrix [7, 8]. The expansive pressure of water within the matrix is opposed by the collagen cross-links that restrict expansion and result in a steady-state turgor pressure. This turgor pressure is critical to maintain the viscoelastic properties of the matrix. Type II collagen is composed of three identical αI polypeptide chains to form a triple helix. The αI monomer is produced as a propeptide with large N- and C-terminal regions that are required for assembly in the chondrocyte. Specific proteases in the extracellular matrix, ADAMTS-3 and BMPI, cleave the N- and C-terminal domains, respectively [9, 10]. The αI trimers then associate in a staggered array via covalent cross-links that continue to accumulate over time with a concomitant increase in fiber strength. Type II collagen is relatively resistant to degradation by most proteases; therefore, little collagen turnover is observed under normal circumstances, but specialized matrix metalloproteases (MMPs) are able to selectively target a single site on the αI helix [11]. MMPs, specifically MMP-13, play a significant role in degenerative joint disease, as discussed in greater detail below.

Table 1.2 Approximate fractional composition of hyaline cartilage

Component	Fraction (%)
Water	80
Collagen type II	10
Proteoglycans	8
Other cartilage-specific collagens (IX, X, XI)	<1
Other proteins	<1
Inorganic salts	<1

Fibrocartilage is distinguished by the presence of smaller amounts of type I collagen, while all three types of cartilage also contain small amounts of other cartilage-specific collagens: collagen IX (anchorin), collagen X (chondrocalcin), and collagen XI. Types IX and XI appear to play roles during fetal development [7, 8], decreasing in abundance during adult life. Types IX and XI collagens are present on the surface of chondrocytes and bind the cells to the surrounding matrix. Type X collagen is most prevalent in the growth plate and is necessary for endochondral ossification [5]. It is not typically found in articular cartilage except in osteoarthritis.

In addition to the above cartilage-specific collagens, scant amounts of collagen VI, a relatively ubiquitous type found in various mesenchymal tissues, are also present.

Proteoglycans account for ~40% of the dry weight of cartilage and demonstrate a remarkable structural hierarchy. At the highest level of organization, multiple proteoglycans are non-covalently attached to a central hyaluronic acid moiety, stabilized by a small protein known as link protein. A proteoglycan is composed of a protein backbone to which long, sulfated, carbohydrate side chains are covalently attached at approximate right angles to the backbone. A single proteoglycan may be glycosylated with 100–150 such side chains. The resulting organization is similar to a bottle brush. The predominant proteoglycan in cartilage is Aggrecan, a 2316 amino acid protein with globular domains at the N- and C-terminal ends and a large intervening sequence that is densely glycosylated. Chondrotoin sulfate and keratan sulfate are the most common carbohydrate side chains [12]. Chondrotoin sulfate is a glycosaminoglycan relatively specific to cartilage and is composed of approximately 25–30 sugar dimers (N-acetylgalactosamine and glucuronic acid). Keratan sulfate is a repeating disaccharide of N-acetylglucosamine and galactose that is smaller (5–6 dimers) and more widely distributed in the body than chondrotoin sulfate. As a result of the sulfated carbohydrate side chains, proteoglycans are highly charged, thereby attracting water and expanding in volume. Proteoglycans are vital in cartilage's ability to resist compression by extruding and re-imbibing water in response to load.

Unlike the more stable collagens, proteoglycans undergo continuous proteolytic cleavage during life with release of small fragments into the synovial fluid [5]. Chondrocyte-derived MMPs are responsible for this degradation. In the case of aggrecan, at least, the resulting shorter molecule becomes relatively more resistant to degredation so the process is somewhat self-limited. Chondrocytes also maintain a steady-state equilibrium by the synthesis of new aggrecan molecules, but this equilibrium is disturbed under pathologic conditions.

In addition to the above primary structural components, cartilage contains numerous other minor proteins that serve both structural and regulatory roles including other proteoglycans, fibronectin, galectin, as well as growth promoting and catabolic factors [5].

Normal Histology

Articular Cartilage

The hyaline cartilage of diarthrotic articular surfaces is the most prevalent and best characterized of the cartilage subtypes. Microscopically, joint cartilage is composed of large amounts of smooth-appearing extracellular matrix within which are distributed a relatively scant population of chondrocytes within circumscribed *lacunae* (the pericellular spaces devoid of chondroid matrix) (Fig. 1.2).

The articular cartilage may be divided into four zones (superficial, transitional, deep, and calcified; Fig. 1.3) [13]. The transition among the first three zones is somewhat arbitrary, but the deep and calcified zones are separated by a distinct front of mineralization known as the *tidemark*. The tidemark is a unique histologic feature of articular cartilage and is not present in other hyaline cartilage. The organization

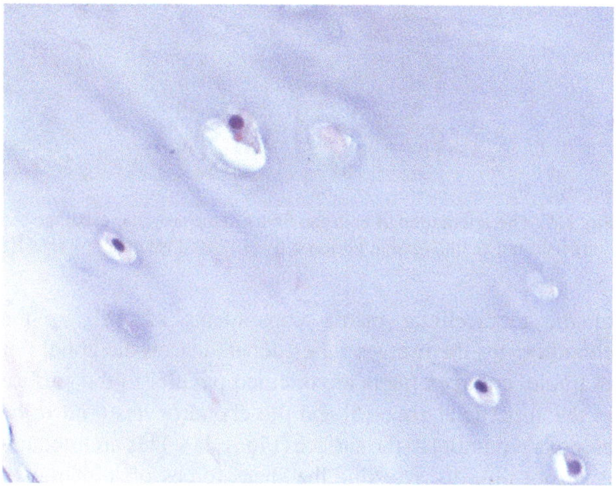

Fig. 1.2 Hyaline cartilage has a pale-blue, smooth "glassy" quality using the standard hematoxylin and eosin (H&E) stain. Note the relative paucity of chondrocytes, typically with only a single cell in a lacuna

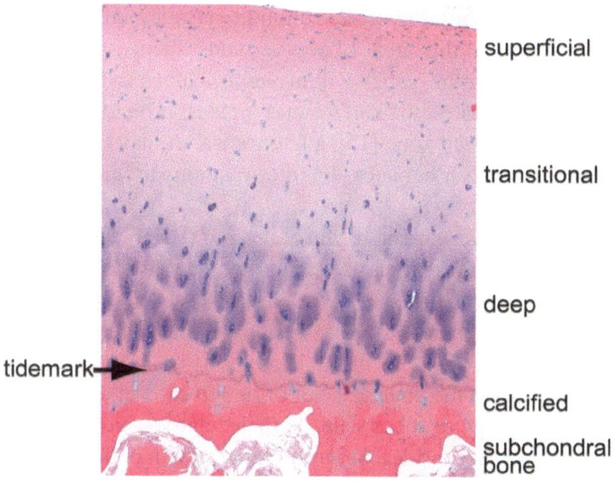

Fig. 1.3 Microarchitecture of articular cartilage. The tidemark is a distinguishing feature of articular cartilage separating calcified from noncalcified zones. Note that the distribution of proteoglycans, as illustrated by the blue, hematoxylin staining, is nonuniform and tends to be highest surrounding chondrocytes in the deep zone (H&E stain)

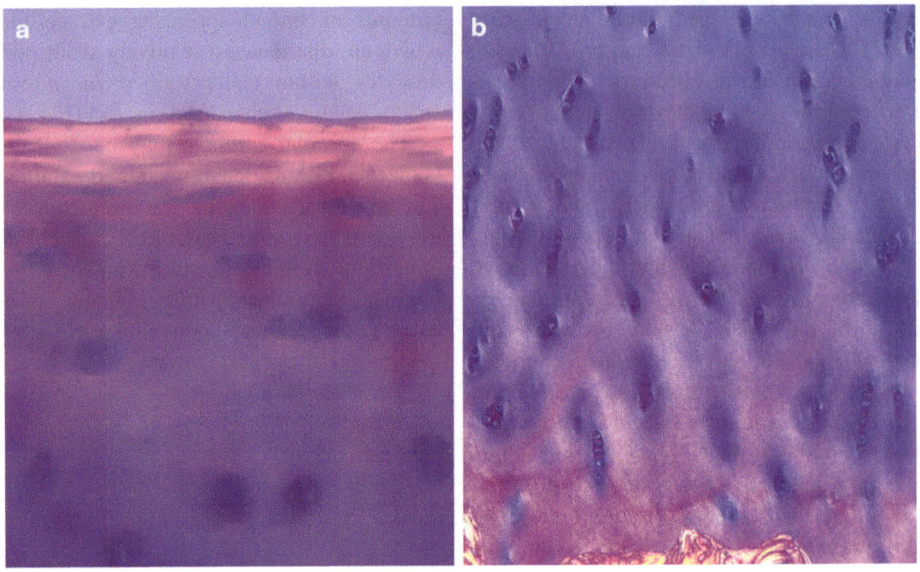

Fig. 1.4 The orientation of collagen fibers in the articular cartilage changes from parallel on the surface (**a**) to more radial (**b**) in the deeper zones demonstrated as fine orange fibrils on by polarized microscopy (H&E stains)

of the extracellular matrix constituents as well as the chondrocytes themselves varies depending on the zone. For example, collagen fibers are oriented parallel to the surface in the superficial zone [6] and the chondrocytes tend to be elongated parallel to the surface (Fig. 1.4a). This architecture is responsible for resisting the shear forces of joint movement at the surface. The transitional and deep zones show a radial arrangement of collagen fibers (Fig. 1.4b) and the chondrocytes tend to be arrayed perpendicular to the articular surface. The latter areas are responsible for resistance to compressive forces. The calcified zone forms the attachment to the subchondral bone, and chondrocytes are enlarged but very sparse in this area. Like other constituents, proteoglycan concentration varies within the articular cartilage such that it is lowest at the surface and greatest around chondrocytes in the deep zone [14], a feature which may be demonstrated by denser hematoxylin (blue) staining around lacunae (Fig. 1.3).

In most cases, hematoxylin and eosin (H&E) histology is adequate to interpret cartilage pathology and is sufficient for routine clinical use. However, under some circumstances, special histochemical stains, such as the cationic dyes Safrarin-O (Fig. 1.5a) or Alcian blue (Fig. 1.5b), may be used to assess the abundance of proteoglycans in the matrix. The advantage of these stains is their relative selectivity for acidic polysaccharides. Safrarin-O reacts with both carboxylated and sulfated polysaccharides, while Alcian blue can be used selectively to stain both types (pH 2.5) or just sulfated polysaccharides (pH 1.0). Although these dyes do offer increased specificity and likely stoichiometric binding to sulfate groups on chondrotoin sulfate or keratan sulfate [15], it should be remembered that histochemical methods are seldom strictly quantitative given variability in section thickness, inhomogeneous matrix concentrations in a single joint and the reagents themselves.

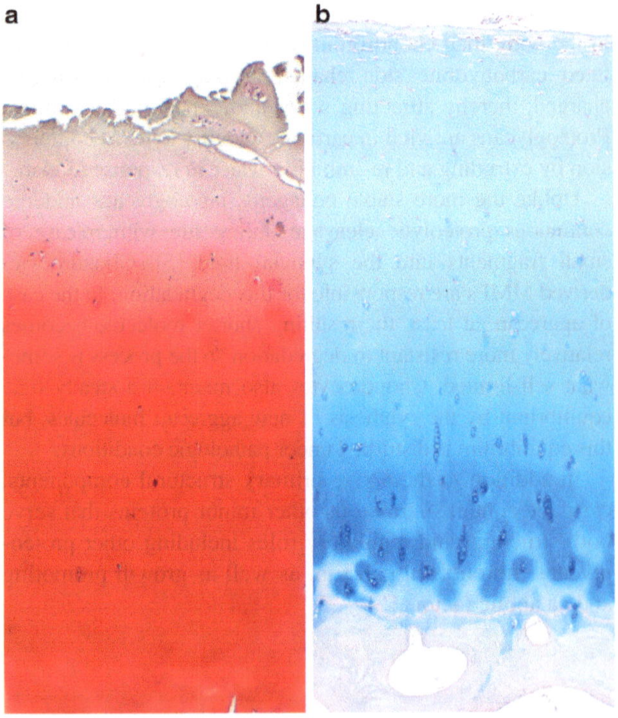

Fig. 1.5 Special histochemical stains may be used to determine the distribution and quantity of proteoglycan components. Safrarin-O (**a**) stains acid polysaccharides (both carboxylated and sulfated) orange, while Alcian blue at pH 1.0 (**b**) is relatively specific for sulfated polysaccharides including chondrotoin sulfate, producing a turquoise color

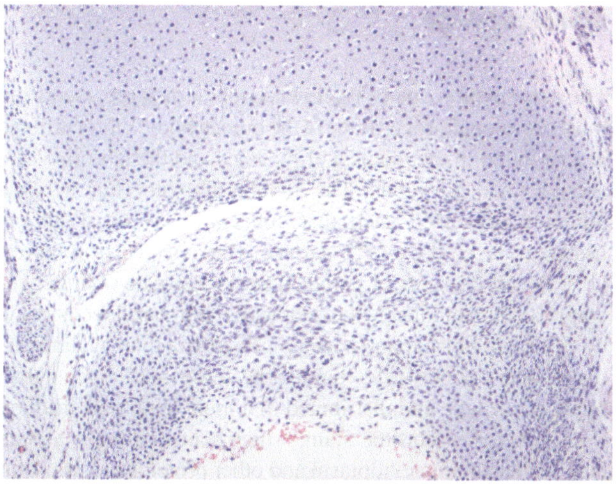

Fig. 1.6 The condensation of mesenchymal cells at the sites of future bones in the embryo gives rise to a cartilage anlage. Chondrocytes continue to differentiate from the perichondrium. By 10 weeks gestation, as seen here, the chondrocytes have secreted extracellular matrix (H&E stain)

Normal articular cartilage contains only a single cell type, the chondrocyte [16]. Unlike other types of connective tissue, cartilage is remarkable for its lack of blood vessels, nerves, inflammatory cells, or fibroblasts. Chondrocytes are derived from immature mesenchymal cells that differentiate from somatic or visceral mesoderm during early fetal life (Fig. 1.6) and are responsible for the synthesis and maintenance of the matrix components and regulatory molecules. Studies suggest that osteoblasts arise from the same precursor stem cell, but the hypovascular matrix of cartilage favors the differentiation of a chondrocyte [17]. Importantly, chondrocytes may also differentiate from adult mesenchymal stem cells, at least in vitro [18], a finding that has received much attention as a possible treatment for degenerative joint disease. Mesenchymal stem cells treated with a cocktail of transforming growth factor beta (TGF-β), dexamethasone, and bone morphogenetic proteins (BMPs) result in cells that produce type II and type X collagen, although they do not completely recapitulate chondrogenesis during development [19, 20]. Nevertheless, the ability of mesenchymal stem cells to undergo chondrogenic differentiation *in vitro* is a crucial step to establish the optimal conditions for therapeutic approaches [21].

At the molecular level, several key regulatory proteins play roles in chondrocyte differentiation. The transcription factor Sox-9 appears to be a master regulator of chondrocyte differentiation from precursor cells. However, Sox-9 may not be lineage-specific, also driving the differentiation of osteoprogenitor cells [22]. Along with Sox-9, the transcription factors, RunX2 and Indian hedgehog (Ihh), contribute to the regulation of chondrocyte maturation, and abnormal expression of all three proteins is thought to be important in the pathogenesis of some cartilage neoplasms [23].

Classically, chondrocytes have a round, pale eosinophilic cytoplasm and a small, hyperchromatic, central nucleus. The characteristic clear space (*lacuna*) identified on routine hematoxylin and eosin stained slides surrounding a chondrocyte is actually an artifact of processing. The clearing results from retraction of the matrix and cell away from one another during formalin fixation. In vivo, the chondrocyte actually makes contact with a specialized layer of collagen-poor matrix. Unlike other mesenchymal cells, chondrocytes make few intercellular contacts. Cells in separate lacunae make no contact, but occasionally multiple cells may be present within a lacuna (a finding referred to as *cloning* or *nesting*), and their cytoplasmic processes in such lacuna do form cell–cell contacts. Ultrastructurally, chondrocytes have abundant endoplasmic reticulum and Golgi but sparse mitochondria (Fig. 1.7). Not only does the orientation of the chondrocytes

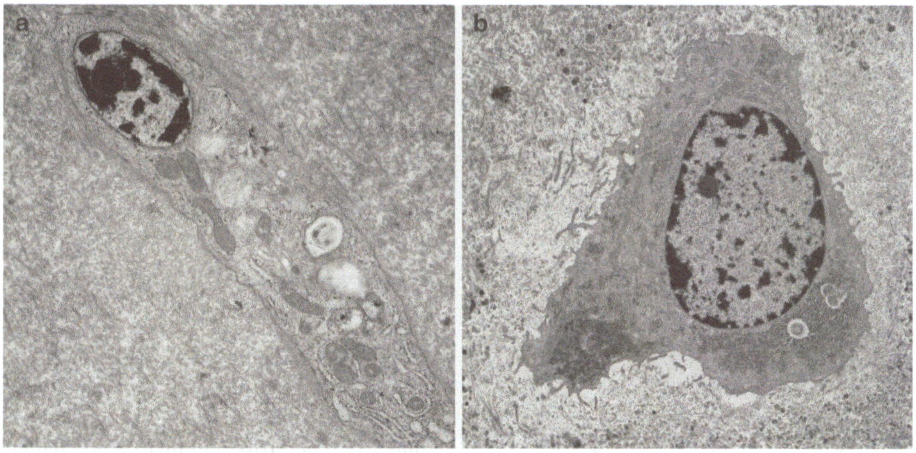

Fig. 1.7 Ultrastructure of chondrocytes in articular cartilage. Superficial cells near articular surface (**a**) tend to have a fusiform spindled shape, while deeper chondrocytes (**b**) are round to polygonal with obvious cell processes

vary across zones of the articular surface (described above), but superficial chondrocytes have more basal cell processes while deeper cells have more abundant endoplasmic reticulum and Golgi. These differences may be related to the organization of collagen fibers in the different layers.

Growth Plate

In long bones, longitudinal growth is achieved by a primary ossification center known as the growth plate or physis (Fig. 1.1a). In the functional growth plate, a specialized type of hyaline cartilage, which undergoes a highly regulated process of proliferation, mineralization, and apoptosis, is responsible for the growth. The maturing epiphyseal plate can be divided into zones (*reserve*, *proliferating*, *hypertrophied*, and *mineralization*) that correspond to stages of maturation of chondrocytes (Fig. 1.8) [24]. The chondrocytes do not literally move through the matrix. Rather, they proliferate, hypertrophy, and undergo apoptosis in place while cartilage matrix is added and ultimately replaced by osteoid at the metaphyseal aspect of the growth plate. The net effect is longitudinal growth. The chondrocytes of the growth plate have abundant cytoplasm and prominent nuclei. In the proliferating zone, they are arrayed in regular, linear nests, a pattern that is pathognomonic of growth plate cartilage. As mentioned above, the cartilage contains collagen X (chondrocalcin) in a pericellular distribution, especially in the zone of mineralization.

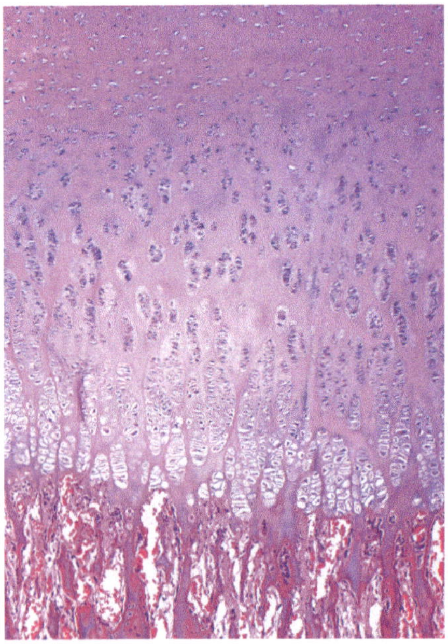

Fig. 1.8 Microarchitecture of the maturing growth plate demonstrating the morphologic features of chondrocytes in the zones of endochondral ossification

Fibrocartilage

The annulus fibrosus of the intervertebral disk represents the most prevalent fibrocartilage in the human body. Fibrocartilage is also found in the menisci of the knee and the labrum of the shoulder and hip joints. The annulus fibrosus (Fig. 1.1c) is uniquely organized such that concentric layers of fibrous tissue are layered over the surface when viewed from above [13]. Broad fascicles of collagen fibers alternate obliquely to compose the annulus. Microscopically, fibrocartilage is made up of a more fibrillar and eosinophilic matrix than hyaline cartilage. The chondrocytes tend to be fewer and smaller than hyaline cartilage and distributed in a more haphazard fashion (Fig. 1.9a). A trichrome stain, which stains collagen a deep blue while staining cytoplasm and other proteins red, is useful to demonstrate the extensive unidirectional arrangement of collagen (Fig. 1.9b) that imparts resistance to tensile forces.

Elastic Cartilage

The cartilage of the external ear (pinna), ligamentum flavum, and epiglottis are composed of elastic cartilage (or *elastocartilage*). Elastic cartilage is typically more cellular than hyaline cartilage and the cells are haphazardly distributed, although the chondrocytes are similar in cytomorphology [13]. On routine H&E histology, the abundant elastin fibers impart an amorphous blue hue that is distinct from the glassy appearance of hyaline cartilage although the distinction can be subtle. These fibers are best demonstrated using special histochemistry using sliver-based stains (Fig. 1.10).

Pathology

The pathology of cartilage includes congenital-developmental, degenerative, and neoplastic processes. A complete discussion of these entities is beyond the scope of this chapter, but selected entities that illustrate characteristic features, particularly as they relate to radiographic findings, are described below.

Osteoarthritis

Osteoarthritis (degenerative joint disease) is a common disorder affecting the majority of adults and includes a variety of etiologies that result in similar pathology of diarthrotic joints [5]. The gross and histologic changes in osteoarthritis consist of a *noninflammatory* disorganization and destruction

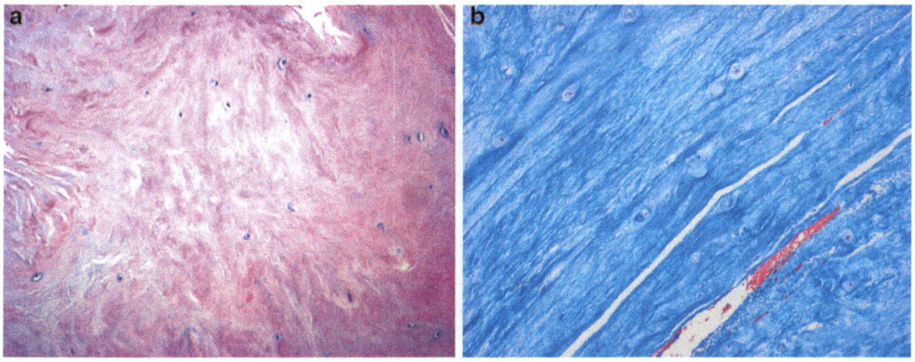

Fig. 1.9 Fibrocartilage of the annulus fibrosus has a pinker (eosinophilic) staining quality than hyaline cartilage and a somewhat haphazard arrangement of chondrocytes (**a**, H&E stain). A Gomori trichrome stain highlights the abundant, directional collagen fibers with bright blue staining (**b**)

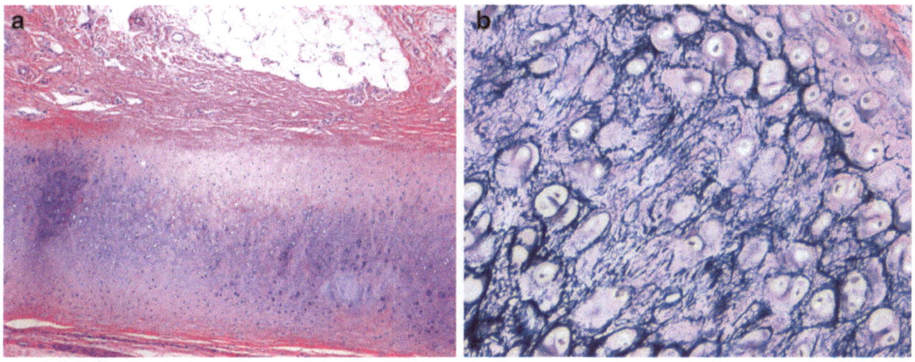

Fig. 1.10 On routine hematoxylin and eosin histology, elastic cartilage is similar to hyaline cartilage as in this example from the external ear (**a**). However, the presence of abundant elastin fibers can be demonstrated by the black filaments using Verhoeff stain (**b**)

of the articular cartilage with associated subchondral bone changes. Briefly, the articular surface shows cracks and fissures of the cartilage, ultimately leading to cartilage loss and exposure of the underlying subchondral bone. Over time, this bone becomes polished to a smooth surface, a process known as *eburnation* (from the Latin *ebus* meaning: "of ivory") (Fig. 1.11a). Microscopically, depending on severity, the cartilage shows fissures and clefts, thinning, a decrease in proteoglycans, *cloning* of chondrocytes, and duplication of the tidemark (Fig. 1.11b) [13]. A histologic grading system, initially established by Mankin [25], based on four categories of structural integrity, cellularity, proteoglycan abundance, and tidemark integrity is still in use (Table 1.3). The severity score (ranging from 0 to 14) correlates reasonably well with biochemical metrics of osteoarthritis severity.

The morphologic changes described and illustrated above represent changes to the matrix and chondrocytes at the cellular and molecular level. Virtually every component of articular cartilage is somehow affected during the process. The major change in collagen is the degradation of type II collagen fibers by MMPs synthesized by the chondrocytes. The normally horizontally arranged fibers in the superficial zone are cleaved as a relatively early step in the process resulting in the fissures and clefts seen histologically. As previously mentioned, the collagen normally resists the swelling capacity of the water-rich proteoglycans, and destruction of the collagen network accounts for the increased hydration and hypertrophy of the articular cartilage early in the course of the disease.

Although proteoglycans are continuously synthesized and secreted by chondrocytes, the loss of aggrecan in osteoarthritis eventually exceeds the chondrocyte's capacity and the matrix becomes depleted in proportion to the severity of the disease. Furthermore, the chondrocytes produce a different balance of proteoglycans that recapitulates immature cartilage rich in chondrotoin sulfate with decreased keratan sulfate [26]. It is not entirely clear whether the altered composition contributes significantly to the mechanical changes in the matrix or if the net loss of proteoglycans is sufficient to account for the changes.

Matrix metalloproteases (MMPs), also synthesized by chondrocytes, play critical roles in the osteoarthritis phenotype.

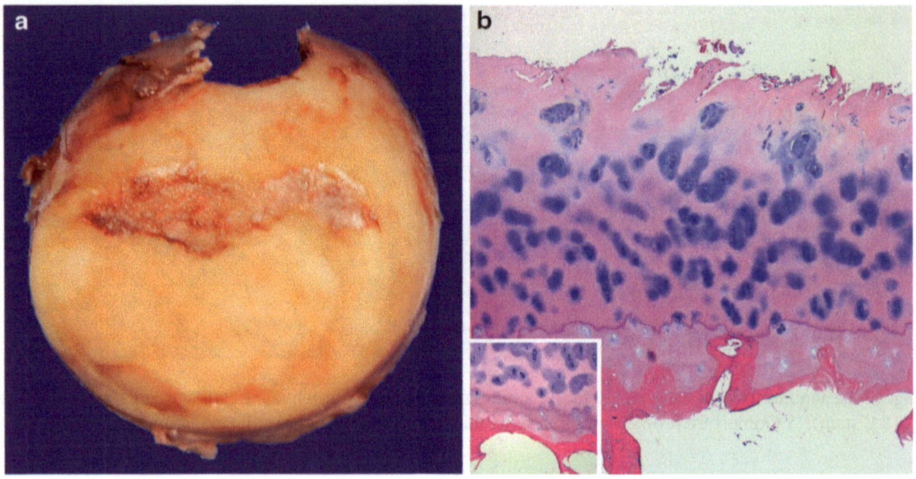

Fig. 1.11 Gross and microscopic features of osteoarthritis. Grossly, clefts and destruction of the articular cartilage with exposed subchondral bone are hallmarks (**a**). Microscopic features of osteoarthritis include fissures, cloning of chondrocytes, and a reduction of proteoglycan and duplication of the tidemark (**b**) (*inset*)

Table 1.3 Histologic grading of osteoarthritis specimens (Mankin score)

Structure	Score
Normal	0
Surface irregularities	1
Pannus	2
Clefts to transitional zone	3
Clefts to radial zone	4
Clefts to calcified zone	5
Complete disorganization	6
Cells	Score
Normal	0
Diffuse hypercellularity	1
Cloning	2
Hypocellularity	3
Proteoglycans (Safranin-O staining)	Score
Normal	0
Slight reduction	1
Moderate reduction	2
Severe reduction	3
No staining	4
Tidemark integrity	Score
Intact	0
Crossed by blood vessels	1

Source: Mankin et al. [25]

MMP-13, mentioned above, and a second enzyme, aggrecanase, are responsible for the cleavage of aggrecan at the interglobular domain liberating soluble fragments that are no longer anchored to the matrix and thus dissolve into the synovial fluid [27]. MMP-13 is found in highest concentration in the deep zone while aggrecanase is more widely distributed. To a lesser extent, MMP-9 and MMP-1 also contribute to the destruction of matrix.

Osteoarthritis, despite the suffix, is technically an inaccurate term since the inflammatory component is minimal in most cases. Nevertheless, certain cytokines and diffusible factors associated with other inflammatory conditions do exist in low concentrations within cartilage matrix possibly through diffusion from synovial or bone marrow origins. Although initially thought to be an impermeable barrier, the osteochondral junction contains channels that allow the diffusion of materials. TGF-β, for example, induces MMP-13 and ADAMTS potentially leading to matrix destruction. BMPs represent a second class of diffusible signals that stimulate chondrocytes to produce various matrix components. BMPs are regulated by a set of specific antagonists, which are often elevated at different stages of osteoarthritis further disturbing the balance of matrix production and destruction [28]. A number of interleukins, TNF-α, prostaglandins, and nitric oxide have been implicated in osteoarthritis pathogenesis [5].

Neoplasia

Cartilage neoplasms are relatively rare and consist of a variety of intraosseous, extraosseous, and surface proliferations of chondrocytes and matrix. With rare exceptions, the matrix of cartilage tumors is hyaline type. Most notably, neoplastic cartilage usually lacks the linear, zonal architecture of articular cartilage. Instead, most benign cartilage neoplasms grow as an aggregate of multiple tumor lobules. Individual lobules may have a peripheral zone of endochondral ossification producing a “ring” of mineralization (Fig. 1.12) that is an important

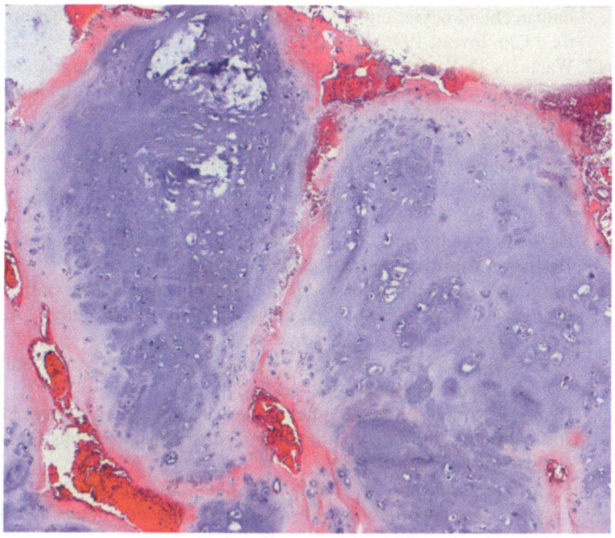

Fig. 1.12 A characteristic feature of cartilage neoplasms is a thin shell of peripheral osteoid (pink) around individual tumor lobules (pale-blue). If mineralized, the osteoid corresponds to the ring-like calcifications seen radiographically

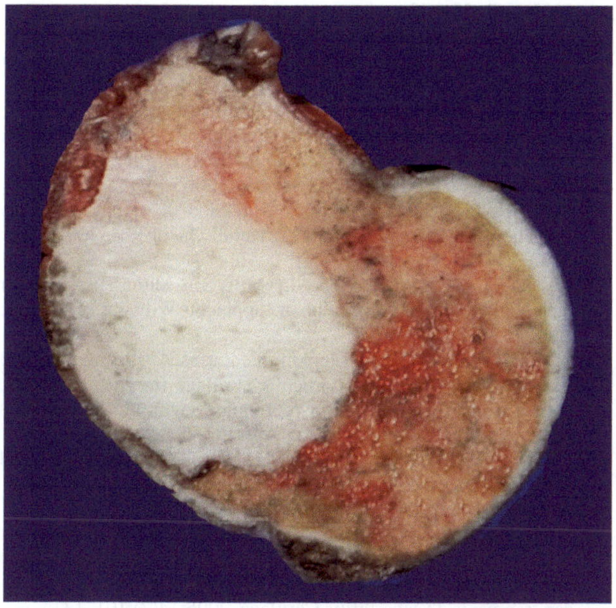

Fig. 1.13 An enchondroma, as seen in this example in the distal femur, consists of a sharply demarcated, *blue-white* translucent tumor

correlate with the rings often seen radiographically in cartilage tumors.

The prototypical benign cartilage neoplasm is the *enchondroma* (or simply *chondroma*). Grossly, an enchondroma consists of a well-circumscribed ovoid nodule of pale blue translucent cartilage, typically <5 cm (Fig. 1.13) [29].

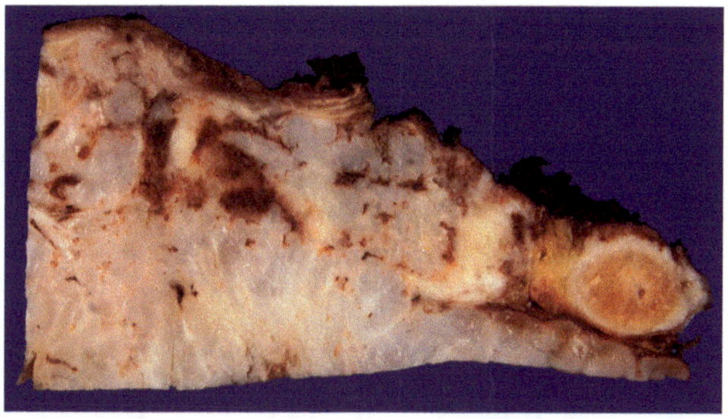

Fig. 1.14 Chondrosarcoma arising from rib consists of a large, confluent mass of cartilage with cortical destruction and a prominent soft tissue component

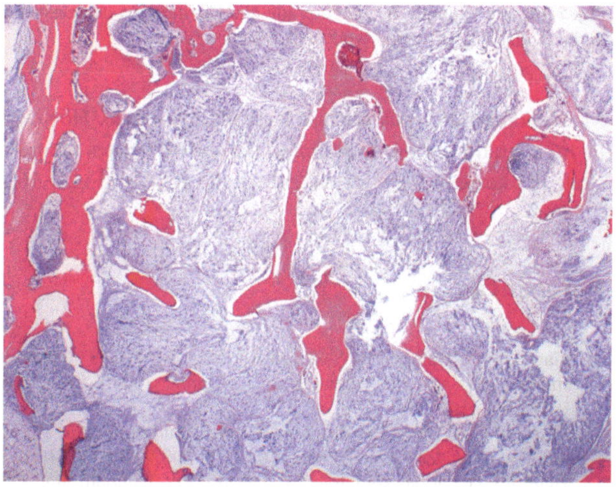

Fig. 1.15 A characteristic microscopic feature of chondrosarcoma is the presence of permeation: a spread of tumor matrix and cells around viable, lamellar bone

Depending on site, enchondromas may be quite cellular and even demonstrate atypia [30]. However, the most important finding supporting a benign diagnosis is a sharp margination between the tumor and the surrounding bone. Enchondromas may expand the cortex but spread *through* the cortex into soft tissues is incompatible with the diagnosis.

The single most important pathologic feature that distinguishes chondrosarcoma from enchondroma is the presence of a permeative or infiltrative pattern in the former [30]. Grossly, this may be evidenced by a single, large confluent intraosseous mass with ill-defined margins or soft tissue extension (Fig. 1.14). The hallmark, microscopically, is a demonstration of a tumor "spilling" between trabeculae of viable lamellar bone (Fig. 1.15). The matrix may be a gelatinous, viscid liquid (*myxoid*) rather than hyaline, likely due to abnormalities in matrix components and composition.

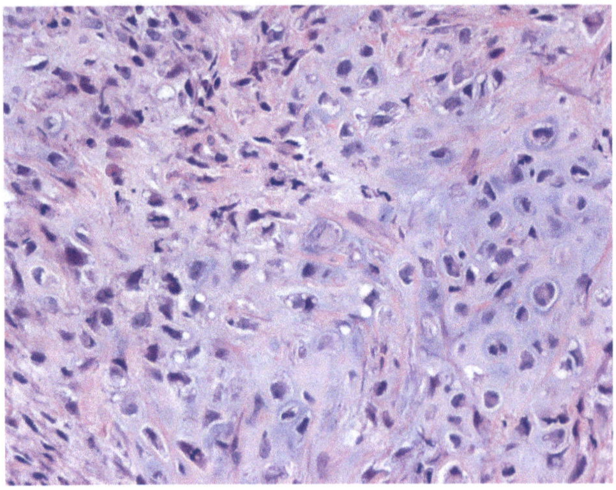

Fig. 1.16 An example of a high-grade chondrosarcoma demonstrates high cellularity, cytologic atypia, and mitotic figures

Most chondrosarcomas are histologically low-grade. However, in high grade chondrosarcomas, the chondrocytes demonstrate marked cytologic atypia and mitotic activity (Fig. 1.16).

References

1. Maroudas A, Bullough P, Swanson SA, Freeman MA. The permeability of articular cartilage. J Bone Joint Surg Br. 1968;50(1):166–77.
2. Karsenty G, Wagner EF. Reaching a genetic and molecular understanding of skeletal development. Dev Cell. 2002;2(4):389–406.
3. Tuan RS. Cellular signaling in developmental chondrogenesis: N-cadherin, Wnts, and BMP-2. J Bone Joint Surg Am. 2003;85-A Suppl 2:137–41.
4. Van der Korst JK, Skoloff L, Miller EJ. Senescent pigmentation of cartilage and degenerative joint disease. Arch Pathol. 1968;86(1):40–7.
5. Martel-Pelletier J, Boileau C, Pelletier JP, Roughley PJ. Cartilage in normal and osteoarthritis conditions. Best Pract Res Clin Rheumatol. 2008;22(2):351–84.
6. Venn MF. Chemical composition of human femoral and head cartilage: influence of topographical position and fibrillation. Ann Rheum Dis. 1979;38(1):57–62.
7. Eyre DR. The collagens of articular cartilage. Semin Arthritis Rheum. 1991;21(3 Suppl 2):2–11.
8. Eyre DR, Weis MA, Wu JJ. Articular cartilage collagen: an irreplaceable framework? Eur Cell Mater. 2006;12:57–63.
9. Jones GC, Riley GP. ADAMTS proteinases: a multi-domain, multi-functional family with roles in extracellular matrix turnover and arthritis. Arthritis Res Ther. 2005;7(4):160–9.
10. Prockop DJ, Sieron AL, Li SW. Procollagen N-proteinase and procollagen C-proteinase. Two unusual metalloproteinases that are essential for procollagen processing probably have important roles in development and cell signaling. Matrix Biol. 1998;16(7):399–408.
11. Reboul P, Pelletier JP, Tardif G, Cloutier JM, Martel-Pelletier J. The new collagenase, collagenase-3, is expressed and synthesized by human chondrocytes but not by synoviocytes. A role in osteoarthritis. J Clin Invest. 1996;97(9):2011–9.
12. Watanabe H, Yamada Y, Kimata K. Roles of aggrecan, a large chondroitin sulfate proteoglycan, in cartilage structure and function. J Biochem. 1998;124(4):687–93.
13. Bullough PG. Joints. In: Mills SE, editor. Histology for pathologists. 3rd ed. Philadelphia: Lippincott Williams & Wilkins; 2007. p. 97–122.
14. Roughley PJ. Articular cartilage and changes in arthritis: noncollagenous proteins and proteoglycans in the extracellular matrix of cartilage. Arthritis Res. 2001;3(6):342–7.
15. Rosenberg L. Chemical basis for the histological use of safranin O in the study of articular cartilage. J Bone Joint Surg Am. 1971;53(1):69–82.
16. Stockwell R, Meachim G. The chondrocytes. In: Freeman MA, editor. Adult articular cartilage. London: Pitman Medical; 1973.
17. Bianco P, Riminucci M, Gronthos S, Gehron-Robey P. Bone marrow stromal stem cells: nature, biology, and potential applications. Stem Cells. 2001;19(3):180–92.
18. Johnstone B, Hering TM, Caplan AI, Goldberg VM, Yoo JU. In vitro chondrogenesis of bone marrow-derived mesenchymal progenitor cells. Exp Cell Res. 1998;238(1):265–72.
19. Barry F, Boynton RE, Liu B, Murphy JM. Chondrogenic differentiation of mesenchymal stem cells from bone marrow: differentiation-dependent gene expression of matrix components. Exp Cell Res. 2001;268(2):189–200.
20. Ichinose S, Yamagata K, Sekiya I, Muneta T, Tagami M. Detailed examination of cartilage formation and endochondral ossification using human mesenchymal stem cells. Clin Exp Pharmacol Physiol. 2005;32(7):561–70.
21. Henning TD, Sutton EJ, Kim A, Golovko D D, Horvai A, Ackerman L, et al. The influence of ferucarbotran on the chondrogenesis of human mesenchymal stem cells. Contrast Media Mol Imaging. 2009;4(4):165–73.
22. Akiyama H, Kim JE, Nakashima K, Balmes G, Iwai N, Deng JM, et al. Osteo-chondroprogenitor cells are derived from Sox9 expressing precursors. Proc Natl Acad Sci USA. 2005;102(41):14665–70.
23. Park HR, Park YK. Differential expression of runx2 and Indian hedgehog in cartilaginous tumors. Pathol Oncol Res. 2007;13(1):32–7.
24. Rosenberg AE, Roth SI. Bone. In: Mills SE, editor. Histology for pathologists. 3rd ed. Philadelphia: Lippincott Williams & Wilkins; 2006. p. 75–95.
25. Mankin HJ, Dorfman H, Lippiello L, Zarins A. Biochemical and metabolic abnormalities in articular cartilage from osteo-arthritic human hips. II. Correlation of morphology with biochemical and metabolic data. J Bone Joint Surg Am. 1971;53(3):523–37.
26. Cs-Szabo G, Roughley PJ, Plaas AH, Glant TT. Large and small proteoglycans of osteoarthritic and rheumatoid articular cartilage. Arthritis Rheum. 1995;38(5):660–8.
27. Struglics A, Larsson S, Pratta MA, Kumar S, Lark MW, Lohmander LS. Human osteoarthritis synovial fluid and joint cartilage contain both aggrecanase- and matrix metalloproteinase-generated aggrecan fragments. Osteoarthritis Cartilage. 2006;14(2):101–13.
28. Tardif G, Hum D, Pelletier JP, Boileau C, Ranger P, Martel-Pelletier J. Differential gene expression and regulation of the bone morphogenetic protein antagonists follistatin and gremlin in normal and osteoarthritic human chondrocytes and synovial fibroblasts. Arthritis Rheum. 2004;50(8):2521–30.
29. Unni KK. Cartilaginous lesions of bone. J Orthop Sci. 2001;6(5):457–72.
30. Horvai A. Cartilage-forming tumors. In: Folpe AL, Inwards C, editors. Bone and soft tissue pathology. Philadelphia: Saunders; 2010. p. 333–54.

Chapter 2
Clinical Aspects: A Rheumatologist's Perspective

David J. Hunter

Keywords Clinical aspects • Rheumatologist • Perspective • Symptomatic osteoarthritis • Diagnosis • Synovial joints • Synovitis • Effusion

Introduction

From a rheumatologist's perspective, cartilage imaging is most significant in the setting of osteoarthritis. Symptomatic osteoarthritis (OA) causes substantial physical and psychosocial disability [1]. In the early 1990s, over 7 million Americans were limited in their ability to participate in their main daily activities, such as going to school or work or maintaining their independence – simply because of their arthritis [2]. Interestingly, the risk for disability (defined as needing help walking or climbing stairs) attributable to knee OA is as great as that attributable to cardiovascular disease and greater than that due to any other medical condition in elderly persons [1]. Like arthritis prevalence, the prevalence of arthritis-related disability is also expected to rise by the year 2020, when an estimated 11.6 million people will be affected [2].

Compounding this picture are the enormous financial costs that our nation bears for treating arthritis, its complications, and the disability that results from uncontrolled disease. The total annual cost in the United States is almost $65 billion – a figure equivalent to a moderate national recession [3]. This amount includes an estimated medical bill of $15 billion each year for such expenses as 39 million physician visits and more than half a million hospitalizations (CDC, 1999, unpublished data). OA accounts for 90% of hip and knee replacements [4]. The balance is largely due to indirect costs such as those from wage losses [3]. Thus, arthritis has become one of our most pressing public health problems – a problem that is expected to worsen in the next millennium with the increasing prevalence of this disease.

This chapter delineates the characteristic symptoms and signs associated with cartilage loss and OA and how they can be used to make the clinical diagnosis with discussion of the role of imaging. The predominant symptom in most patients presenting with OA is pain. Over recent years a number of imaging-based studies have narrowed the discord between knowledge about structural findings on imaging and symptoms. The remainder of the chapter focuses on what we know causes pain in OA and contributes to its severity, with a predominant focus on imaging findings.

What Is OA?

OA can be viewed as the clinical and pathological outcome of a range of disorders that result in structural and functional failure of synovial joints [5]. This highly prevalent disease occurs when the dynamic equilibrium between the breakdown and repair of joint tissues is overwhelmed [6]. The resulting progressive joint failure may cause pain, physical disability, and psychological distress [1], although many persons with structural changes consistent with OA are asymptomatic [7]. The reasons why there is this disconnect between disease severity and the level of reported pain and disability are largely unknown, although recent imaging studies are beginning to shed light on this.

Typically OA presents as joint pain. During a 1-year period, 25% of people over 55 years have a persistent episode of knee pain, of whom about one in six consult their general practitioner about it [8]. Symptomatic knee OA (pain on most days and radiographic features consistent with OA) occurs in approximately 12% of those aged over 55 [8].

While OA is common in the knee, it is even more prevalent in the hands, especially the distal (DIP) and proximal (PIP) interphalangeal joints and the base of the thumb (CMC). When symptomatic, especially so for the base of thumb joint,

D.J. Hunter (✉)
Division of Research, New England Baptist Hospital, 125 Parker Hill Ave, Boston, MA 02120, USA
and
Rheumatology Department, Royal North Shore Hospital, University of Sydney, Pacific Highway, St. Leonards, NSW 2065, Australia
e-mail: david.hunter@sydney.edu.au

T.M. Link (ed.), *Cartilage Imaging: Significance, Techniques, and New Developments*,
DOI 10.1007/978-1-4419-8438-8_2, © Springer Science+Business Media, LLC 2011

hand OA is associated with functional impairment [9, 10]. OA of the thumb carpo-metacarpal joint is a common condition that can lead to substantial pain, instability, deformity, and loss of motion [11]. Over the age of 70 years, approximately 5% of women and 3% of men have symptomatic OA affecting this joint with impairment of hand function [9].

The prevalence of hip OA is about 9% in Caucasian populations [12]. In contrast, studies in Asian, black, and East Indian populations indicate a very low prevalence of hip OA [13]. The prevalence of symptomatic hip OA is approximately 4% [14].

What Are the Characteristic Symptoms of OA?

The joint pain of OA is typically described as mechanical; that is, exacerbated by activity and relieved by rest. More advanced OA can cause rest and night pain leading to loss of sleep which further exacerbates pain. The cardinal symptoms that suggest a diagnosis of OA include:

- Pain (typically described as activity-related or mechanical, may occur with rest in advanced disease; often deep, aching and not well localized; usually of insidious onset)
- Reduced function
- Stiffness (of short duration, also termed "gelling," i.e., short-lived stiffness after inactivity)
- Joint instability, buckling or giving way
- Patients may also complain of reduced movement, deformity, swelling, crepitus, and increased age (OA is unusual before age 40) in the absence of systemic features (such as fever)
- When pain persists pain-related psychological distress

Tailoring the Physical Exam: What Signs Are Associated with OA?

Physical examination should include an assessment of body weight and body mass index, joint range of motion, the location of tenderness, muscle strength, and ligament stability. For lower limb joint involvement, this should include assessment of body mass and postural alignment in both standing and walking [15]. The features on physical examination that suggest a diagnosis of OA include:

- Tenderness, usually located over the joint line
- Crepitus with movement of the joint
- Bony enlargement of the joint, e.g., Heberden's and Bouchard's nodes, squaring of the first CMC, typically along the affected joint line in the knee
- Restricted joint range of motion
- Pain on passive range of motion
- Deformity, e.g., angulation of the DIP and PIP joints, varus (bowed legs) deformity of the knees
- Instability of the joint
- Altered gait
- Muscle atrophy or weakness
- Joint effusion

The Diagnosis of OA

Bearing in mind that radiographs are notoriously insensitive to the earliest pathological features of OA, the absence of positive radiographic findings should not be interpreted as confirming the complete absence of symptomatic disease. Conversely, the presence of positive radiographic findings does not guarantee that an osteoarthritic joint is also the active source of the patient's current knee or hip symptoms, where other sources of pain including periarticular sources, such as pes anserine bursitis at the knee and trochanteric bursitis at the hip, often contribute [7]. According to the ACR criteria for classification of hand OA (unlike the hip and knee where radiographs enhance the sensitivity and specificity), X-rays are less sensitive and specific than physical examination in the diagnosis of symptomatic hand OA [16]. The usefulness of X-rays relates more importantly to the exclusion of other diagnostic possibilities rather than confirmation of osteoarthritic disease [17].

> In clinical practice, the diagnosis of OA should be made on the basis of the medical history and physical examination, and the role of radiography is to confirm this clinical suspicion and rule out other conditions.

When disease is advanced, it is visible on plain radiographs, which show narrowing of joint space, osteophytes, and sometimes changes in the subchondral bone. MRI can be used in infrequent circumstances to facilitate the diagnosis of other causes of joint pain that can be confused with OA (osteochondritis dissecans, avascular necrosis). Laboratory testing has little role in establishing the diagnosis of OA. Because OA is a noninflammatory arthritis, laboratory findings are expected to be normal.

What Are the Diagnostic Criteria for Osteoarthritis?

When making the diagnosis of OA, consider using the criteria of the American College of Rheumatology for diagnostic purposes and classification of OA of the hip, knee, and hands in patients with pain in these joints [16, 18]. These are the criteria that are used in research studies and should be used to inform the diagnosis of OA in individuals, but not limiting the information gathering to these criteria and considering the wealth of other information that patients with OA may provide, which can help to either confirm or refute an OA diagnosis.

In the process of taking a history, it is important to ask how the pain has affected the person's function at home, work, and in recreational activities. Also, ask about how the person is coping with pain and how well that is going. It is important to look for signs of psychological distress, e.g., signs of anxiety such as excessive pain avoidant posturing, sleep onset insomnia, or signs of depression such as early morning wakening, weight loss, irritability, or a marked in increase in memory/concentration problems.

Factors That Contribute to Pain

The source of pain is not particularly well understood and is best framed in a biopsychosocial framework (posits that biological, psychological, and social factors all play a significant role in pain in OA) [19, 20].

From a biological perspective, neuronal activity in the pain pathway is responsible for the generation and ultimate exacerbation of the feeling of joint pain. During inflammation, chemical mediators are released into the joint, which sensitize primary afferent nerves such that normally innocuous joint movements (such as increased physical activity, high heeled shoes, and weather changes) now elicit a painful response. This is the neurophysiological basis of allodynia, i.e., the sensation of pain in response to a normally nonpainful stimulus such as walking. Over time this increased neuronal activity from the periphery can cause plasticity changes in the central nervous system by a process termed "wind-up." In this instance, second order neurones in the spinal cord increase their firing rate such that the transmission of pain information to the somatosensory cortex is enhanced. This central sensitization phenomenon intensifies pain sensation and can even lead to pain responses from regions of the body remote from the inflamed joint, i.e., referred pain.

Pain has long been recognized as a complex sensory and emotional experience [21]. Each individual has a unique experience of pain influenced by their life experience and genotypic profile. An individual's stable psychological characteristics (trait) and the immediate psychological context in which pain is experienced (state) both influence perception of pain. A full understanding of pain requires consideration of psychological and social environmental processes mediating a patient's response to their disease [22]. The biopsychosocial model is a very useful approach to understanding and assessing the experience of pain in persons with OA [23]. Constitutional factors that can predispose to symptoms include self-efficacy, pain catastrophizing, and the social context of arthritis (social support, pain communication) are all important considerations in understanding the pain experience.

Local Tissue Pathology

The structural determinants of pain and mechanical dysfunction in OA are also not well understood but are believed to involve multiple interactive pathways. In broad terms, there are a number of tissues within the joint that contain nociceptive fibers, and these are the likely sources of pain in osteoarthritis. The subchondral bone, periosteum, periarticular ligaments, periarticular muscle spasm, synovium, and joint capsule are all richly innervated and are the likely source of nociception in OA. In population studies, there is a significant discordance between radiographically diagnosed OA and knee pain [7]. While radiographic evidence of joint damage predisposes to joint pain, it is clear that the severity of the joint damage on the radiograph bears little relation to the severity of the pain experienced.

However, utilizing other imaging modalities such as magnetic resonance imaging (MRI), significant structural associations, such as bone marrow lesions [24, 25], subarticular bone attrition [26], synovitis, and effusion [27, 28], have been related to knee pain. It remains unclear which of these local tissue factors predominate as until recently these analyses did not account for the fact that much of the structural change is collinear (a person who has more severe disease will have worse structural change in multiple tissues including the bone, synovium, etc.) and were not adjusting for other tissue changes. A recent analysis confirmed most beliefs that it is likely that changes in the subchondral bone and synovial activation/effusion predominate [29].

The different tissues within the joint and their respective contribution to symptoms are discussed below.

Hyaline Articular Cartilage

Articular cartilage is both aneural and avascular. As such, cartilage is incapable of directly generating pain, inflammation, stiffness, or any of the symptoms that patients with OA typically describe [30]. Given its relative unimportance to OA's symptomatic presentation, it is ironic that articular cartilage has received so much attention while other common symptom sources in the joint are ignored. Some studies have suggested a relation between cartilage morphometry and lesions and the symptoms of OA [31]. It is important to note that this disease of the whole joint concurrently affects other tissues that do contain nociceptors. The studies that have demonstrated a relation of cartilage damage to pain have traditionally investigated the role of cartilage in predisposing to symptoms in isolation from other tissues and as such are fundamentally flawed. A recent study suggested that areas of denuded cartilage are related to symptoms [32]. Again, the likely mechanism for symptom genesis is through secondary mechanisms such as: (1) exposing the underlying subchondral bone and the inherent symptom genesis from this structural alteration, (2) vascular congestion of subchondral bone leading to increased intraosseous pressure, and (3) synovitis secondary to articular cartilage damage with activation of synovial membrane nociceptors.

Subchondral Bone

Periarticular bone changes associated with OA can be segregated into distinct patterns based on the anatomic location and pathogenic mechanisms. These alterations include progressive increase in subchondral plate thickness, alterations in the architecture of subchondral trabecular bone, formation of new bone at the joint margins (osteophytes), development of subchondral bone cysts, and advancement of the tidemark associated with vascular invasion of the calcified cartilage.

Of these lesions that which has the most supportive evidence for a role in symptom genesis is the bone marrow lesion (Fig. 2.1). Lesions in the bone marrow play an integral if not pivotal role in the symptoms that emanate from knee OA and its structural progression [24]. Bone marrow lesions were found in 272 of 351 (77.5%) persons with painful knees compared with 15 of 50 (30%) persons with no knee pain ($P<0.001$). Large lesions were present almost exclusively in persons with knee pain (35.9% vs. 2%; $P<0.001$). After adjustment for severity of radiographic disease, effusion, age, and sex, all lesions and in particular large lesions remained associated with the occurrence of knee pain. More recently, their relation to pain severity [25] and incident pain [33] was also demonstrated. There is conflicting data albeit from smaller studies with different methods suggesting no relation of bone marrow lesions to pain [34, 35]; however, the balance of data would support a strong relation of bone marrow lesions to pain.

Other bone-related causes of pain include periostitis associated with osteophyte formation [36], subchondral microfractures [37], bone attrition [26], and bone angina due to decreased blood flow and elevated intraosseous pressure [38].

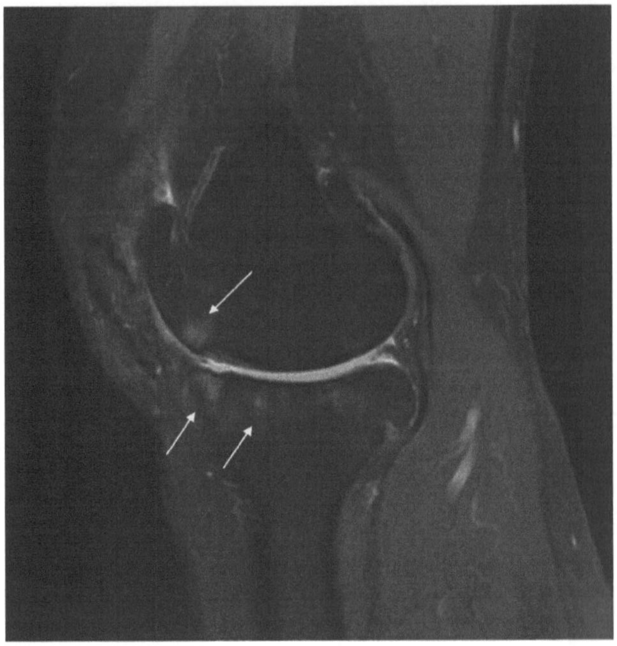

Fig. 2.1 T2 weighted fat suppressed sagittal sequence depicting multiple diffuse hyperintensities (*arrows*) abutting the subchondral plate in the weight-bearing proximal tibia and trochlea characteristic of bone marrow lesions

The particular bone pathology most responsible for pain remains elusive; however, identifying this would be a major advance in delineating appropriate therapeutic targets. One likely source that remains underexplored is that of intraosseous hypertension. The pathophysiology remains unclear, although phlebographic studies in OA indicate impaired vascular clearance from bone and raised intraosseous pressure in the bone marrow near the painful joint [38–41]. What may subsequently cause pain is as yet unknown. Increased trabecular bone pressure, ischemia, and inflammation are all possible stimuli.

Synovitis, Effusion

The synovial reaction in OA includes synovial hyperplasia, fibrosis, thickening of synovial capsule, activated synoviocytes, and in some cases lymphocytic infiltrate (B- and T-cells as well as plasma cells) [42]. The site of infiltration of the synovium is of obvious relevance as one of the most densely innervated structures of the joint is the white adipose tissue of the fat pad, which also shows evidence of inflammation and can act as a rich source of inflammatory adipokines [43]. Synovial causes of pain include irritation of sensory nerve endings within the synovium from osteophytes and synovial inflammation that is due, at least in part, to the

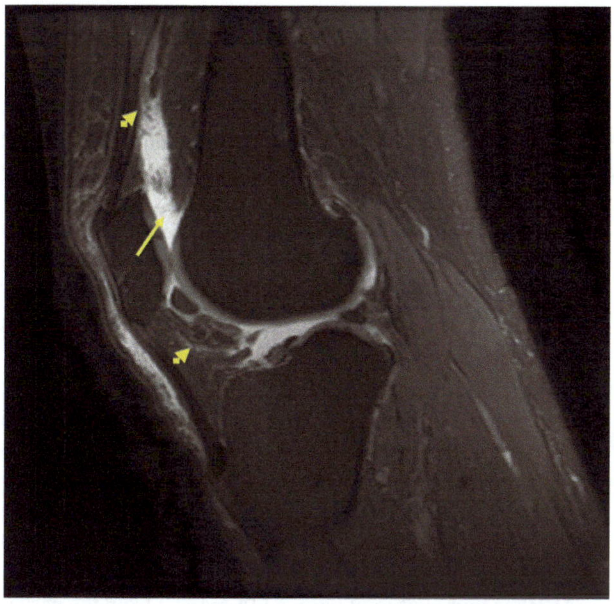

Fig. 2.2 Effusion (*arrow*) and peripatellar synovitis (*arrowhead*) on T2 weighted fat suppressed sagittal sequence. On noncontrast sequences such as this, the magnitude of synovitis is difficult to determine

release of prostaglandins, leukotrienes, proteinases, neuropeptides, and cytokines [20, 44].

Synovitis and effusion are frequently present in osteoarthritis and correlate with pain and other clinical outcomes (Fig. 2.2) [27]. Synovial thickening around the infrapatellar fat pad using noncontrast MRI has been shown on biopsy to represent mild chronic synovitis [45]. A semiquantitative measure of synovitis from the infrapatellar fat pad is associated with pain severity, and similarly change in synovitis is associated with change in pain severity [28]. This study assessed 270 subjects (158 male, 112 female) with at least one follow-up MRI. Mean synovitis score at baseline was 3.3 (1.9) with an average change of 0.15 (1.5). There was a correlation of baseline synovitis with baseline pain score (Pearson correlation coefficient $r=0.20, p=0.0005$). Changes in summary synovitis score were associated with changes in pain over time ($p=0.005$). An increase of one unit in summary synovitis score resulted in a 3.11 mm increase in VAS pain score (0–100 scale). Of the three locations for synovitis, changes in the infrapatellar fat pad were most strongly related to pain change (4.2 mm increase in pain per unit increase in synovitis).

In an important caveat to this analysis, a recent study compared nonenhanced proton-density-weighted fat-suppressed (PDFS) sequences with T1-weighted (T1w) fat-suppressed (FS) contrast-enhanced (CE) sequences for semiquantitative assessment of peripatellar synovitis in OA [46]. This data suggested that signal alterations in Hoffa's fat pad on nonenhanced images do not always represent synovitis as seen on T1w CE images but are a rather nonspecific albeit sensitive finding. Semiquantitative scoring of peripatellar synovitis in OA ideally should be performed using T1w CE sequences and should include scoring of synovial thickness.

Meniscus

The meniscus has many functions in the knee, including loadbearing, shock absorption, stability enhancement, and lubrication [47, 48]. The menisci transmit anywhere from 45% to 60% of the compressive loads in the knee [47]. If the meniscus does not cover the articular surface that it is designed to protect due to change in position, or if a tear leaves it unable to resist axial loading, it will not perform this role. The absence of a functioning meniscus increases peak and average contact stresses in the medial compartment of the knee in a range of 40–700% [49–51].

Knee OA after meniscectomy/meniscal repair is traditionally considered a result of the joint injury that leads to the meniscectomy in the first instance and the increased cartilage contact stress due to the loss of meniscal tissue [52–54]. Meniscectomy is often accompanied by the onset of OA because of the high focal stresses imposed on articular cartilage and subchondral bone subsequent to excision of the meniscus. The studies that have explored the relationship between the meniscus and risk of disease progression in OA provide a clear indication of the risk inherent with damage to this vital tissue [55–57]. Each aspect of meniscal abnormality (whether change in position or damage) (Fig. 2.3) had a major effect on risk of cartilage loss in osteoarthritis.

Thus, the intact and functional meniscus is clearly important to the preservation of joint integrity and prevention of further joint damage. In contrast the meniscus plays a much smaller role in symptom genesis. An unfortunate consequence of the frequent use of MRI in clinical practice is the frequent detection of meniscal tears [58]. Degenerative lesions, described as horizontal cleavages, flap (oblique), or complex tears or meniscal maceration or destruction are associated with older age and are almost universal in persons with osteoarthritis [58]. In asymptomatic subjects with a mean age of 65 years, a tear was found in 67% using magnetic resonance imaging (MRI), whereas in patients with symptomatic knee OA, a meniscal tear was found in 91% [59]. In the interests of preserving menisci, an important cautionary note: meniscal tears are nearly universal in persons with knee OA and are unlikely to be a cause of increased symptoms [59, 60]. The penchant to remove menisci is to be avoided, unless there are symptoms of locking or extension blockade, at which point surgical treatment often becomes necessary [61].

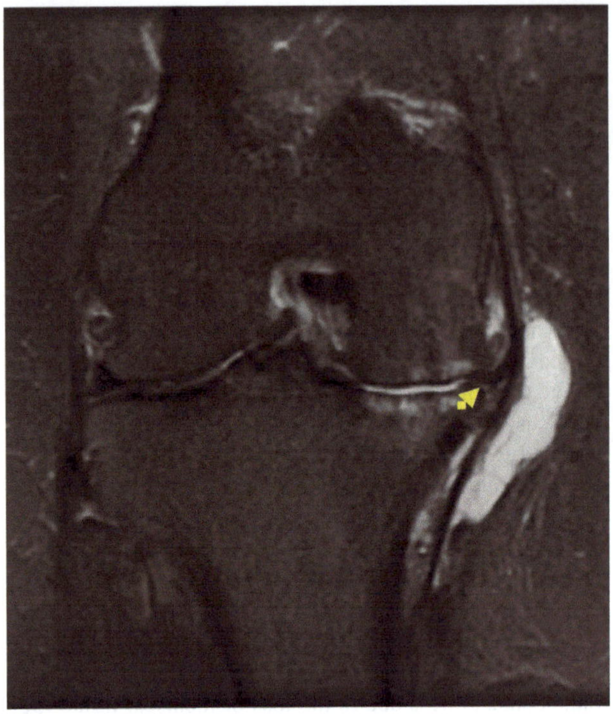

Fig. 2.3 Medial tibiofemoral osteoarthritis with extensive bone marrow lesions, attrition of the opposing articular surfaces and cartilage loss. In addition, a macerated meniscus has been extruded out of the medial compartment (*arrowhead*)

The Role of Other Tissues

Periarticular muscles influence joint loading, and impairments in muscle function have been observed in people with OA [62]. Various studies have investigated the role of muscle strength on joint integrity, and some have explored the impact on physical functioning. Sharma et al. [63] conducted a 3-year longitudinal cohort study investigating factors contributing to poor physical functioning in 257 patients with knee OA. They found that in addition to factors such as age, reduced absolute quadriceps and hamstrings strength and poor proprioceptive acuity increased the likelihood of poor physical functioning as measured by the time to perform five repetitions of rising and sitting in a chair. In addition to their exploration in observational studies, there is ample evidence from clinical trials demonstrating that muscle strengthening exercises result in improvements in pain, physical function, and quality of life in people with knee OA [64, 65].

Obesity is the single most important risk factor for development of severe OA of the knee and more so than other potentially damaging factors including heredity [66]. Even if it is usually accepted that mechanical loading contributes to joint destruction in overweight patients, recent advances in the physiology of adipose tissue add further insights in understanding the relationship between obesity and osteoarthritis. Indeed, the positive association between overweight or obesity and osteoarthritis is observed not only for knee joints but also for nonweight-bearing joints, such as hands [67, 68]. Furthermore, if weight loss may prevent the onset of osteoarthritis, the loss of body fat is more closely related to symptomatic benefit than is the loss of body weight [69]. Local fat depots may play an important role in disease and symptoms genesis. Among these tissues, the synovium and infrapatellar fat pad appear to produce large amounts of adipokines [70]. Until recently, the fat pad, which is an extrasynovial but an intra-articular tissue, had been neglected. However, this adipose tissue is able to release growth factors, cytokines and adipokines [43]. Since obese individuals have higher concentrations of inflammatory markers, inflammation may contribute to functional limitation and disease progression in those with OA [71]. Besides direct effects on the joint, inflammatory mediators can affect muscle function and lower the pain threshold.

Another source of joint pain in OA may be from the nerves themselves. Following joint injury in which there is ligamentous rupture, the nerves which reinnervate the healing soft tissues contain an overabundance of algesic chemicals such as substance P and calcitonin gene-related peptide. An interesting observation of these new nerves was that their overall morphology was abnormal with fibers appearing punctate and disorganized [72, 73]. Since these phenomena are consistent with the innervation profiles described in nerve injury models, we speculate that injured joints may develop neuropathic pain post-trauma. Indeed, treatment of inflamed joints with the neuropathic pain analgesic gabapentin can also relieve arthritis pain [74].

Conclusion

Though cartilage is aneural and avascular, it plays a central role in the pathophysiology of symptomatic OA, and cartilage abnormalities are directly associated with damage to other tissues within the joint that contain nociceptors. The pathophysiology of pain in OA is complex and similarly the symptomatic presentation in OA diverse and heterogeneous. Recent studies, particularly those with an emphasis on MRI, are providing unique insights into the relation between structure and symptom genesis. The traditional predominant focus of imaging studies and preclinical investigation is cartilage. However, the subchondral bone, periosteum, periarticular ligaments, periarticular muscle spasm, synovium, and joint capsule are all richly innervated and are the likely source of nociception in OA. Attention to the many modulating factors that alter the experience of pain may improve the way we treat this disease.

References

1. Guccione AA, Felson DT, Anderson JJ, Anthony JM, Zhang Y, Wilson PW, et al. The effects of specific medical conditions on the functional limitations of elders in the Framingham Study. Am J Public Health. 1994;84:351–8.
2. Arthritis prevalence and activity limitations – United States, 1990. MMWR – Morbidity & Mortality Weekly Report. 1994;43:433–8.
3. Yelin E, Callahan LF. The economic cost and social and psychological impact of musculoskeletal conditions. National Arthritis Data Work Groups [see comments]. [Review] [68 refs]. Arthritis Rheum. 1995;38:1351–62.
4. Segal L, Day SE, Chapman AB, Osborne RH. Can we reduce disease burden from osteoarthritis? [see comment]. Med J Aust. 2004;180:S11–7.
5. Nuki G. Osteoarthritis: a problem of joint failure [Review] [55 refs]. Z Rheumatol. 1999;58:142–7.
6. Eyre DR. Collagens and cartilage matrix homeostasis [Review] [37 refs]. Clin Orthop Relat Res. 2004;427:S118–22.
7. Hannan MT, Felson DT, Pincus T. Analysis of the discordance between radiographic changes and knee pain in osteoarthritis of the knee. J Rheumatol. 2000;27:1513–7.
8. Peat G, McCarney R, Croft P. Knee pain and osteoarthritis in older adults: a review of community burden and current use of primary health care [see comments] [Review] [45 refs]. Ann Rheum Dis. 2001;60:91–7.
9. Zhang Y, Niu J, Kelly-Hayes M, Chaisson CE, Aliabadi P, Felson DT. Prevalence of symptomatic hand osteoarthritis and its impact on functional status among the elderly: The Framingham Study. Am J Epidemiol. 2002;156:1021–7.
10. Cunningham LS, Kelsey JL. Epidemiology of musculoskeletal impairments and associated disability. Am J Public Health. 1984;74:574–9.
11. Armstrong AL, Hunter JB, Davis TR. The prevalence of degenerative arthritis of the base of the thumb in post-menopausal women. J Hand Surg Br. 1994;19:340–1.
12. Felson DT, Zhang Y. An update on the epidemiology of knee and hip osteoarthritis with a view to prevention [Review] [116 refs]. Arthritis Rheum. 1998;41:1343–55.
13. Nevitt MC, Xu L, Zhang Y, Lui LY, Yu W, Lane NE, et al. Very low prevalence of hip osteoarthritis among Chinese elderly in Beijing, China, compared with whites in the United States: the Beijing osteoarthritis study. Arthritis Rheum. 2002;46:1773–9.
14. Lawrence RC, Helmick CG, Arnett FC, Deyo RA, Felson DT, Giannini EH, et al. Estimates of the prevalence of arthritis and selected musculoskeletal disorders in the United States [see comments]. Arthritis Rheum. 1998;41:778–99.
15. Kraus VB, Vail TP, Worrell T, McDaniel G, Kraus VB, Vail TP, et al. A comparative assessment of alignment angle of the knee by radiographic and physical examination methods. Arthritis Rheum. 2005;52:1730–5.
16. Altman RD. Classification of disease: osteoarthritis [Review] [38 refs]. Semin Arthritis Rheum. 1991;20:40–7.
17. Cibere J. Do we need radiographs to diagnose osteoarthritis? [Review] [60 refs]. Best Pract Res Clin Rheumatol. 2006; 20:27–38.
18. Altman R, Asch E, Bloch D, Bole G, Borenstein D, Brandt K, et al. Development of criteria for the classification and reporting of osteoarthritis. Classification of osteoarthritis of the knee. Diagnostic and Therapeutic Criteria Committee of the American Rheumatism Association. Arthritis Rheum. 1986;29:1039–49.
19. Dieppe PA, Lohmander LS. Pathogenesis and management of pain in osteoarthritis [Review] [100 refs]. Lancet. 2005;365:965–73.
20. Hunter DJ, McDougall JJ, Keefe FJ. The symptoms of osteoarthritis and the genesis of pain. Rheum Dis Clin North Am. 2008;34:623+.
21. Kane RL, Bershadsky B, Lin WC, Rockwood T, Wood K, Kane RL, et al. Efforts to standardize the reporting of pain. J Clin Epidemiol. 2002;55:105–10.
22. Orbell S, Johnston M, Rowley D, Espley A, Davey P. Cognitive representations of illness and functional and affective adjustment following surgery for osteoarthritis. Soc Sci Med. 1998;47:93–102.
23. Keefe FJ, Smith SJ, Buffington AL, Gibson J, Studts JL, Caldwell DS. Recent advances and future directions in the biopsychosocial assessment and treatment of arthritis [Review] [126 refs]. J Consult Clin Psychol. 2002;70:640–55.
24. Felson DT, Chaisson CE, Hill CL, Totterman SM, Gale ME, Skinner KM, et al. The association of bone marrow lesions with pain in knee osteoarthritis [see comments]. Ann Intern Med. 2001;134:541–9.
25. Hunter D, Gale D, Grainger G, Lo G, Conaghan P. The reliability of a new scoring system for knee osteoarthritis MRI and the validity of bone marrow lesion assessment: BLOKS (Boston Leeds Osteoarthritis Knee Score). Ann Rheum Dis. 2008;67:206–11.
26. Torres L, Dunlop DD, Peterfy C, Guermazi A, Prasad P, Hayes KW, et al. The relationship between specific tissue lesions and pain severity in persons with knee osteoarthritis. Osteoarthritis Cartilage. 2006;14:1033–40.
27. Hill CL, Gale DG, Chaisson CE, Skinner K, Kazis L, Gale ME, et al. Knee effusions, popliteal cysts, and synovial thickening: association with knee pain in osteoarthritis. J Rheumatol. 2001;28:1330–7.
28. Hill CL, Hunter DJ, Niu J, Clancy M, Guermazi A, Genant H, et al. Synovitis detected on magnetic resonance imaging and its relation to pain and cartilage loss in knee osteoarthritis. Ann Rheum Dis. 2007;66:1599–603.
29. Lo G, McAlindon T, Niu J, Zhang Y, Beals C, Dabrowski C, et al. Strong association of bone marrow lesions and effusion with pain in osteoarthritis. Arthritis Rheum. 2008;56(9):S790. Ref Type: Abstract.
30. Felson D. The sources of pain in knee osteoarthritis [Review] [34 refs]. Curr Opin Rheumatol. 2005;17:624–8.
31. Hunter DJ, March L, Sambrook PN. The association of cartilage volume with knee pain. Osteoarthritis Cartilage. 2003;11:725–9.
32. Moisio K, Eckstein F, Song J, Cahue S, Marshall M, Dunlop D, et al. The relationship of denuded subchondral bone area to knee pain severity and incident frequent knee pain. Arthritis Rheum. 2008;58(9):S237–8. Ref Type: Abstract.
33. Felson DT, Niu J, Guermazi A, Roemer F, Aliabadi P, Clancy M, et al. Correlation of the development of knee pain with enlarging bone marrow lesions on magnetic resonance imaging. Arthritis Rheum. 2007;56:2986–92.
34. Link TM, Steinbach LS, Ghosh S, Ries M, Lu Y, Lane N, et al. Osteoarthritis: MR imaging findings in different stages of disease and correlation with clinical findings. Radiology. 2003;226:373–81.
35. Kornaat PR, Bloem JL, Ceulemans RY, Riyazi N, Rosendaal FR, Nelissen RG, et al. Osteoarthritis of the knee: association between clinical features and MR imaging findings. Radiology. 2006;239: 811–7.
36. Cicuttini FM, Baker J, Hart DJ, Spector TD. Association of pain with radiological changes in different compartments and views of the knee joint. Osteoarthritis Cartilage. 1996;4:143–7.
37. Burr DB. The importance of subchondral bone in the progression of osteoarthritis [Review] [13 refs]. J Rheumatol Suppl. 2004;70: 77–80.
38. Simkin P. Bone pain and pressure in osteoarthritic joints [Review] [34 refs]. Novartis Found Symp. 2004;260:179–86.
39. Arnoldi CC, Lemperg K, Linderholm H. Intraosseous hypertension and pain in the knee. J Bone Joint Surg Br. 1975;57:360–3.
40. Arnoldi CC, Djurhuus JC, Heerfordt J, Karle A. Intraosseous phlebography, intraosseous pressure measurements and 99mTC-polyphosphate scintigraphy in patients with various painful conditions in the hip and knee. Acta Orthop Scand. 1980;51:19–28.

41. Arnoldi CC. Vascular aspects of degenerative joint disorders. A synthesis. [Review] [270 refs]. Acta Orthopaedica Scand Suppl. 1994;261:1–82.
42. Roach HI, Aigner T, Soder S, Haag J, Welkerling H, Roach HI, et al. Pathobiology of osteoarthritis: pathomechanisms and potential therapeutic targets [Review] [138 refs]. Curr Drug Targets. 2007;8:271–82.
43. Ushiyama T, Chano T, Inoue K, Matsusue Y, Ushiyama T, Chano T, et al. Cytokine production in the infrapatellar fat pad: another source of cytokines in knee synovial fluids. Ann Rheum Dis. 2003;62:108–12.
44. McDougall J. Arthritis and pain. Neurogenic origin of joint pain [Review] [138 refs]. Arthritis Res Ther. 2006;8:220.
45. Fernandez-Madrid F, Karvonen RL, Teitge RA, Miller PR, An T, Negendank WG. Synovial thickening detected by MR imaging in osteoarthritis of the knee confirmed by biopsy as synovitis. Magn Reson Imaging. 1995;13:177–83.
46. Roemer F, Hunter D, Guermazi A, Zhang Y, Bohndorf K. Semiquantitative assessment of peripatellar synovitis in osteoarthritis: a comparative study of non-enhanced vs. contrast-enhanced MRI. AJR Am J Roentgenol. 2009; 192:1696–700.
47. Seedhom BB, Dowson D, Wright V. Proceedings: functions of the menisci. A preliminary study. Ann Rheum Dis. 1974;33:111.
48. Verstraete KL, Verdonk R, Lootens T, Verstraete P, De Rooy J, Kunnen M. Current status and imaging of allograft meniscal transplantation [Review] [32 refs]. Eur J Radiol. 1997;26:16–22.
49. Baratz ME, Fu FH, Mengato R. Meniscal tears: the effect of meniscectomy and of repair on intraarticular contact areas and stress in the human knee. A preliminary report. Am J Sports Med. 1986;14(4):270–5.
50. Fukubayashi T, Kurosawa H. The contact area and pressure distribution pattern of the knee. A study of normal and osteoarthrotic knee joints. Acta Orthop Scand. 1980;51(6):871–9.
51. Kurosawa H, Fukubayashi T, Nakajima H. Load-bearing mode of the knee joint: physical behavior of the knee joint with or without menisci. Clin Orthop Relat Res. 1980;149:283–90.
52. Tapper EM, Hoover NW. Late results after meniscectomy. J Bone Joint Surg Am. 1969;51:517–26.
53. Johnson RJ, Kettelkamp DB, Clark W, Leaverton P. Factors effecting late results after meniscectomy. J Bone Joint Surg Am. 1974;56:719–29.
54. Englund M, Roos EM, Lohmander LS. Impact of type of meniscal tear on radiographic and symptomatic knee osteoarthritis: a sixteen-year followup of meniscectomy with matched controls. Arthritis Rheum. 2003;48:2178–87.
55. Biswal S, Hastie T, Andriacchi TP, Bergman GA, Dillingham MF, Lang P. Risk factors for progressive cartilage loss in the knee: a longitudinal magnetic resonance imaging study in forty-three patients. Arthritis Rheum. 2002;46:2884–92.
56. Berthiaume MJ, Raynauld JP, Martel-Pelletier J, Labonte F, Beaudoin G, Bloch DA, et al. Meniscal tear and extrusion are strongly associated with progression of symptomatic knee osteoarthritis as assessed by quantitative magnetic resonance imaging. Ann Rheum Dis. 2005;64:556–63.
57. Hunter DJ, Zhang YQ, Niu JB, Tu X, Amin S, Clancy M, et al. The association of meniscal pathologic changes with cartilage loss in symptomatic knee osteoarthritis. Arthritis Rheum. 2006;54:795–801.
58. Englund M, Guermazi A, Gale D, Hunter DJ, Aliabadi P, Clancy M, et al. Incidental meniscal findings on knee MRI in middle-aged and elderly persons. N Engl J Med. 2008;359:1108–15.
59. Bhattacharyya T, Gale D, Dewire P, Totterman S, Gale ME, McLaughlin S, et al. The clinical importance of meniscal tears demonstrated by magnetic resonance imaging in osteoarthritis of the knee [comment]. J Bone Joint Surg Am. 2003;85-A:4–9.
60. Englund M, Niu J, Guermazi A, Roemer FW, Hunter DJ, Lynch JA, et al. Effect of meniscal damage on the development of frequent knee pain, aching, or stiffness. Arthritis Rheum. 2007;56:4048–54.
61. Englund M, Lohmander LS. Risk factors for symptomatic knee osteoarthritis fifteen to twenty-two years after meniscectomy. Arthritis Rheum. 2004;50:2811–9.
62. Hurley MV. The role of muscle weakness in the pathogenesis of osteoarthritis [Review] [125 refs]. Rheum Dis Clin North Am. 1999;25:283–98.
63. Sharma L, Cahue S, Song J, Hayes K, Pai YC, Dunlop D. Physical functioning over three years in knee osteoarthritis: role of psychosocial, local mechanical, and neuromuscular factors. Arthritis Rheum. 2003;48:3359–70.
64. Roddy E, Zhang W, Doherty M, Roddy E, Zhang W, Doherty M. Aerobic walking or strengthening exercise for osteoarthritis of the knee? A systematic review [see comment] [Review] [44 refs]. Ann Rheum Dis. 2005;64:544–8.
65. Roddy E, Zhang W, Doherty M, Arden NK, Barlow J, Birrell F, et al. Evidence-based recommendations for the role of exercise in the management of osteoarthritis of the hip or knee – the MOVE consensus [see comment] [Review] [65 refs]. Rheumatology. 2005;44:67–73.
66. Coggon D, Reading I, Croft P, McLaren M, Barrett D, Cooper C, et al. Knee osteoarthritis and obesity. Int J Obes Related Metab Disord J Int Assoc Study Obes. 2001;25:622–7.
67. Cicuttini FM, Baker JR, Spector TD. The association of obesity with osteoarthritis of the hand and knee in women: a twin study. J Rheumatol. 1996;23:1221–6.
68. Sayer AA, Poole J, Cox V, Kuh D, Hardy R, Wadsworth M, et al. Weight from birth to 53 years: a longitudinal study of the influence on clinical hand osteoarthritis. Arthritis Rheum. 2003;48:1030–3.
69. Toda Y, Toda T, Takemura S, Wada T, Morimoto T, Ogawa R. Change in body fat, but not body weight or metabolic correlates of obesity, is related to symptomatic relief of obese patients with knee osteoarthritis after a weight control program. J Rheumatol. 1998;25:2181–6.
70. Presle N, Pottie P, Dumond H, Guillaume C, Lapicque F, Pallu S, et al. Differential distribution of adipokines between serum and synovial fluid in patients with osteoarthritis. Contribution of joint tissues to their articular production. Osteoarthritis Cartilage. 2006;14:690–5.
71. Spector TD, Hart DJ, Nandra D, Doyle DV, Mackillop N, Gallimore JR, et al. Low-level increases in serum C-reactive protein are present in early osteoarthritis of the knee and predict progressive disease. Arthritis Rheum. 1997;40:723–7.
72. McDougall JJ, Bray RC, Sharkey KA. Morphological and immunohistochemical examination of nerves in normal and injured collateral ligaments of rat, rabbit, and human knee joints. Anat Rec. 1997;248:29–39.
73. McDougall JJ, Yeung G, Leonard CA, Bray RC. A role for calcitonin gene-related peptide in rabbit knee joint ligament healing. Can J Physiol Pharmacol. 2000;78:535–40.
74. Hanesch U, Pawlak M, McDougall JJ, Hanesch U, Pawlak M, McDougall JJ. Gabapentin reduces the mechanosensitivity of fine afferent nerve fibres in normal and inflamed rat knee joints. Pain. 2003;104:363–6.

Chapter 3
Clinical Aspects: An Orthopedic Surgeon's Perspective

Sunny Cheung and C. Benjamin Ma

Keywords Clinical aspects • Orthopedic • Surgeon • Perspective • Chondral defects • Bone contusion • Chondral damage • Chondroplasty • Arthroplasty • Osteotomy

Introduction

Improvements in musculoskeletal imaging in the past decade have allowed orthopedic surgeons to make great advances in the diagnosis and management of soft tissue pathologies in the musculoskeletal system. As the technology for MRI has enhanced the resolution for visualizing cartilage and other soft tissues, this has improved the orthopedic surgeons' ability to plan preoperatively the treatment of cartilage lesions, and, in selected circumstances, to also monitor the subsequent postoperative course for efficacy. In particular, articular damage of the knee joint is one of the most common reasons for both younger and older patients to seek an orthopedic consultation. While MRIs are helpful in diagnosing focal cartilage defects, diffuse cartilage damage in the setting of osteoarthritis often does not require advanced imaging modalities such as an MRI for diagnosis and treatment. In most cases, plain radiography in the weight-bearing setting provides adequate information to the orthopedic surgeon for both the conservative and surgical management of osteoarthritis. As osteoarthritis has been covered extensively in the previous chapter, this chapter will focus on chondral lesions in the knee of a younger, more active population as a model for how orthopedic surgeons approach many of the pathologies that affect cartilage.

C. Benjamin Ma (✉)
Sports Medicine and Shoulder Service,
Department of Orthopedic Surgery,
University of California, San Franciso,
1500 Owens Street, San Francisco, CA 94158, USA
e-mail: maben@orthosurg.ucsf.edu

Classification of Chondral Defects

There is some confusion in the literature as there are numerous reported classifications for cartilage defects, some of which are based on arthroscopic inspection and others which are based on imaging [1, 2]. The first classification system used by orthopedic surgeons in describing the extent of cartilage lesions was the Outerbridge classification [3] Originally used for patella chondral defects, it has since been modified and extrapolated for use in other joints and remains the most widely used classification system due to its ease of use and acceptable rates of reproducibility and accuracy (Fig. 3.1) [4]. This is an arthroscopic classification based on visual inspection and probing of the cartilage (Table 3.1). Thus, when discussing chondral defects, it is important to realize that most orthopedic surgeons refer to this grading system and thus should not be confused with radiologic classifications that often appear on an MRI report.

The Relationship of Bone Contusion to Chondral Damage

Acute knee trauma often leads to injury not only of the soft tissue but also to the bony structures. Bone contusion or bruising appears as high signal on T2-weighted sequences with decreased intensity on T1-weighted sequences. This represents bone marrow edema and microfractures of the cancellous bone. Further, the initial concussive blow from acute trauma might exceed a supraphysiological threshold, altering the load-bearing properties of subchondral bone and leading to changes in the overlying cartilage. While many bone bruises resolve over time, the articular cartilage may suffer irreversible damage, with persistent changes seen even at 6 years after initial injury [5]. Histologic studies have associated the presence of bone bruising with the loss of proteoglycans and necrosis of chondrocytes in the subchondral bone after an ACL rupture [6]. A follow-up study revealed

T.M. Link (ed.), *Cartilage Imaging: Significance, Techniques, and New Developments*,
DOI 10.1007/978-1-4419-8438-8_3, © Springer Science+Business Media, LLC 2011

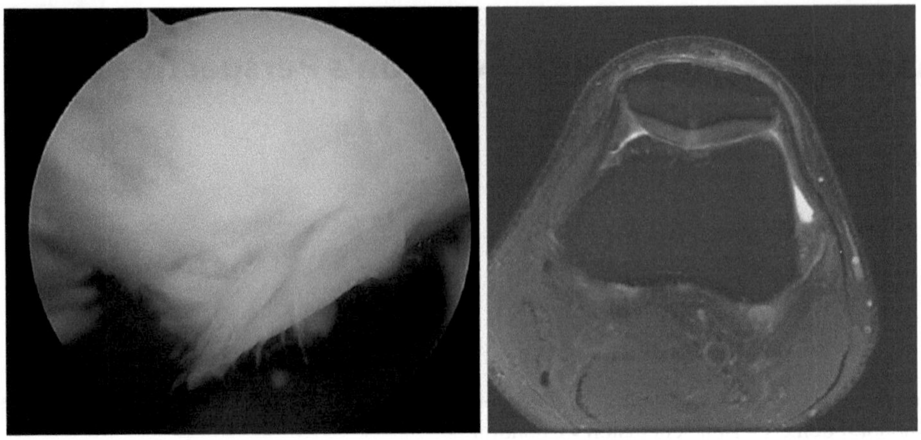

Fig. 3.1 Grade 2 Outerbridge defect of the patella apex. *Left*: Arthroscopic view. *Right*: Corresponding axial T2-weighted MRI sequence

Table 3.1 Description of the modified Outerbridge classfication

Grade	Description
0	Normal cartilage
1	Softening and swelling
2	Partial-thickness defect with fissures that do not reach subchondral bone, or exceed 1.5 cm diameter
3	Fissures that reach subchondral bone and diameter greater than 1.5 cm
4	Exposed subchondral bone

a significant correlation of bone bruises with increased pain as well as duration of joint effusion and antalgic gait [7].

More evidence linking bone contusions with chondral injuries are seen in repeat MRIs of patients at 12–14 weeks after acute knee injuries. While 80% had a greater than 50% reduction in bone bruise volume, two types of resolution for bone bruising were seen: one from the periphery and one towards the joint margin. All cases with resolution towards the joint margin had associated osteochondral injuries, suggesting that a bone bruise may indicate overlying osteochondral injury [8]. A separate case series of acute knee injuries demonstrated normal cartilage on initial arthroscopy, but a repeat MRI at 6–12 months after injury showed 67% with persistent osteochondral changes such as cartilage thinning, osteochondral defects, and cortical impaction [9]. However, multiple other studies attempting to correlate the location of bone bruises with cartilage damage at the corresponding area have yielded inconsistent findings [10]. Nevertheless, a natural history study of bone marrow edema on MRI demonstrated that medial lesions were associated with a 5.6 higher risk for medial arthritis and lateral lesions with a 2.8 higher risk for lateral arthritis, even when adjusted for varus or valgus limb alignment. This data suggests that the presence of bone bruising is a risk factor for structural deterioration of the knee in osteoarthritis [11].

Clinical Presentation

Injuries to the articular cartilage often occur in the setting of an acute traumatic injury. While there can be various causes for knee pain, one of the symptoms of articular pathology is the presence of an effusion. Unlike rupture of the anterior cruciate ligament, which leads to a joint effusion almost immediately, in the case of cartilage injury, patients often describe swelling which occurs a few hours or the next day following an acute injury or an overload activity to the knee, such as a prolonged hike or marathon. Patients may also feel a sensation of catching, which suggests either meniscal injury or the presence of loose bodies (from detached fragments of cartilage) or loose chondral flaps. A history of previous injury such as a meniscal tear will also place a patient at risk for subsequent cartilage injury. As the weight-bearing load across the knee joint is altered from the loss of meniscal integrity, abnormal articular contact stresses occur, causing increased peak local contact stresses on the chondral surface [12]. Other injuries to the knee, such as a ligamentous rupture leading instability, may also place the articular surface at risk for further injury. Finally, unlike osteoarthritis, focal chondral defects do not usually elicit night pain.

Physical examination of the knee typically begins with inspection of the lower limb alignment. A valgus knee may indicate lateral-sided osteoarthritis, while varus alignment may indicate medial-sided osteoarthritis. A varus thrust during gait is also a sign of medial osteoarthritis. Increased warmth and effusion compared to the contralateral side indicates an irritated knee joint in general. A decreased range of motion or flexion contracture may indicate the presence osteophytes from osteoarthritis. Painful crepitus often occurs with advanced chondral wear. A thorough ligamentous exam may reveal pseudolaxity under varus or valgus stress; this does not reflect actual laxity to the medial or lateral collateral ligaments, but rather the loss of cartilage on either the medial or lateral side allows the joint space to "open up" more than normal. As the most common focal cartilage lesions are located on the patella and the medial femoral condyle [13], a patellofemoral grind test or palpation of the undersurface medial or lateral facet of the patella often elicits pain. Occasionally, palpation of the medial femoral condyle articular surface with the knee slightly flexed may also elicit pain if a cartilage lesion is present.

Once a diagnosis of chondral injury is suspected based on the initial history and examination, further imaging is ordered based on the location of the suspected lesion. For example, if a patellofemoral lesion is suspected, then merchant views of the patellofemoral joint with the knee flexed at 45° would be included in the plain radiography series. Weight-bearing posterior–anterior 30° views are very helpful in evaluating the extent of medial or lateral compartment osteoarthritis. If limb malalignment is suspected as an underlying contributing factor, then full-length lower extremity standing views are helpful to quantify the amount of malalignment and the angle of correction that would be required for an osteotomy, if warranted.

While plain radiography is adequate for the evaluation and treatment of diffuse osteoarthritis, MRI is the best modality to confirm the diagnosis of focal chondral defect and to rule out any associated internal derangements such as meniscal tears or ligamentous injury. MRI will help orthopedic surgeons not only in the diagnosis of cartilage injury, but it also provides invaluable information for preoperative planning. Characteristics of the chondral defect such as size, depth, and location are very important in formulating surgical treatment options. Partial thickness lesions or torn flaps of cartilage may be amenable to simple chondroplasty (debridement to a smoother surface with arthroscopic shavers). Small contained lesions may do well with marrow stimulation techniques such as microfracture. Larger lesions on the femoral condyle may require osteochondral autograft transplantation or autologous chondrocyte implantation (ACI). Very large focal lesions may require osteochondral allograft transplantation. The location of the lesion may influence the treatment; for example, the results of microfracture in patella lesions are not as good as in the femoral condyle. Accessibility considerations may limit lesions of the tibial plateau or the posterior femoral condyle to just microfracture procedures. Finally, the presence of concomitant meniscal or ligamentous injury will need to be addressed in order to provide a stable, optimal environment for cartilage healing.

Surgical Management of Chondral Defects

Chondroplasty Debridement

Arthroscopic debridement and lavage has a palliative role in the treatment of small or partial thickness chondral lesions in which the goal is preservation of the remaining intact surrounding cartilage. Loose chondral fragments causing mechanical symptoms, pain, and inflammation are removed with a combination of shavers and biters. It is most often used in the patellofemoral joint where other surgical options are limited. Patients are counseled that the outcomes are not predictable but may ameliorate their symptoms [14]. In the treatment of osteoarthritis, arthroscopic debridement has not been shown to be better than placebo [15, 16].

Microfracture and Marrow Stimulation Techniques

Marrow stimulation procedures include osteochondral drilling, abrasion, arthroplasty, and microfracture. The goal of these procedures is to facilitate the delivery of progenitor cells from the marrow to form a fibrocartilage scar tissue over the defect. Indications include Outerbridge grade 3 or 4 defects spanning 2–3 cm^2. An intact cartilage edge is essential in order to contain the healing clot [17]. The exposed bone is debrided of all unstable cartilage and the calcified cartilage cap. Perforations are made about 3 mm apart and 2–4 mm deep into the subchondral bone (Fig. 3.2) [18]. Best results are seen in age younger than 35 years and lesions less than 400 mm^2. Most improvement occurs within the first year, although maximum improvement may not occur until 2–3 years postoperatively. Following the operation, patients are on a continuous passive motion machine and crutch-assisted touch-down weight bearing for 6–8 weeks [19].

Osteochondral Autograft Transfer/ Mosaicplasty

This procedure involves harvesting osteochondral plugs from a nonweight-bearing region (usually the trochlea or the perimeter around the intercondylar notch) and transferring them to an affected lesion on the femoral condyle that is not suitable for microfracture. The lesion is prepared by drilling and debridement to leave a clean cylindrical recipient site without any loose fragments. Each donor plug is then inserted into the recipient site, perpendicular to the articular contour, and in a press-fit fashion. Typically, multiple plugs of 6–8 mm diameter are used to fill the lesion in a "cobblestone" fashion (Fig. 3.3). The availability of donor site dictates the maximum size of the lesion that can be treated with this technique, usually up to 2.5 cm^2 [20]. The donor sites fill in with fibrocartilage over time, while the graft site forms a congruent gliding surface with the transplanted hyaline cartilage. The donor sites are usually the

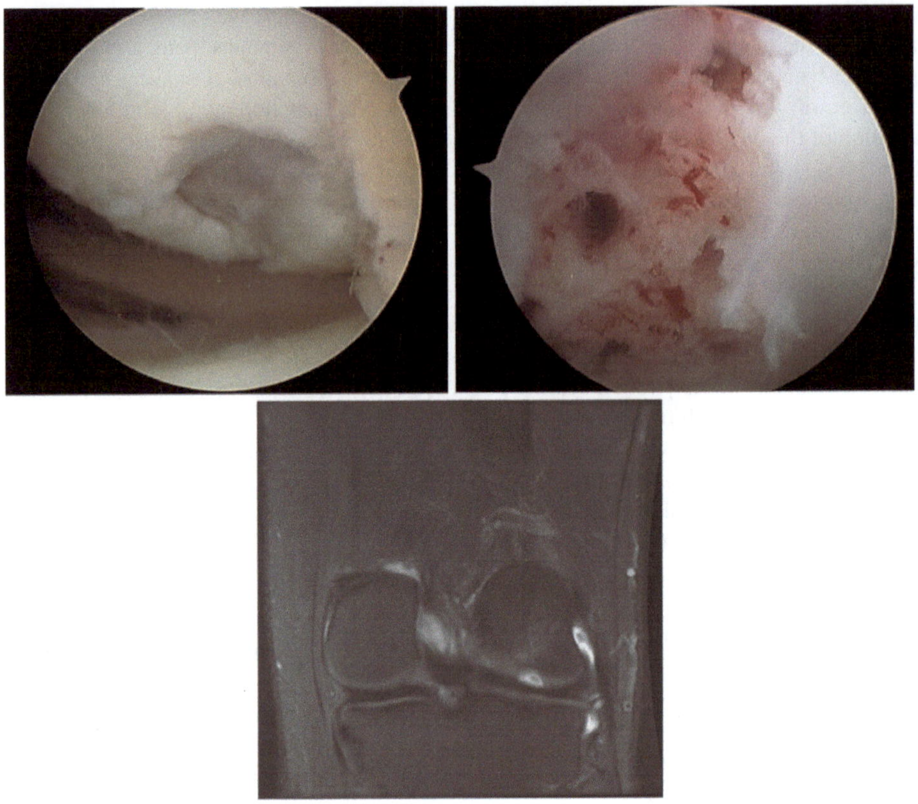

Fig. 3.2 Grade 4 lesion on the medial femoral condyle. *Left*: Lesion prior to preparation. *Right*: Lesion after debridement and microfracture. Note the presence of bleeding from the marrow surface. *Bottom*: Coronal T2-weighted sequence illustrating the lesion

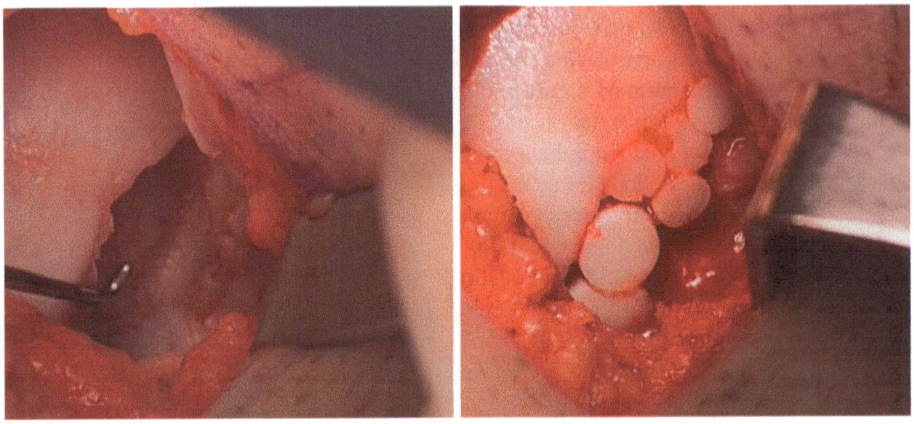

Fig. 3.3 *Left*: Large cartilage defect on the femoral condyle prior to preparation. *Right*: Mosaicplasty of plugs obtained from the trochlea

medial and lateral trochlea and around the intercondylar notch. At 10-year follow-up, 92% good/excellent results are achieved in the femoral condyle, while results in the patella/trochlea are not as good with only 79% good/excellent results [21].

Osteochondral Allograft

Similar to osteochondral autograft transfer, this technique uses size-matched fresh cadaver donor plugs instead. This procedure is reserved for chondral defects greater than

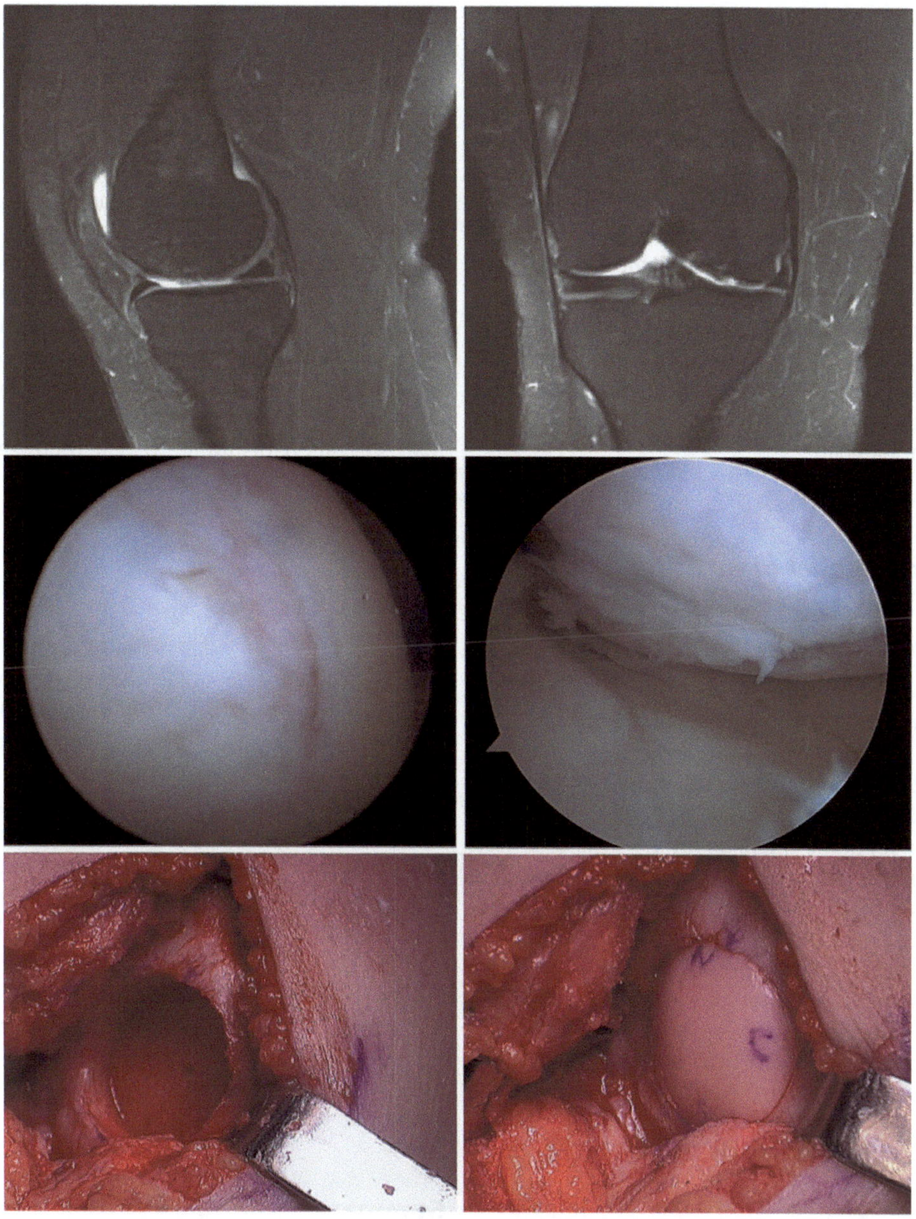

Fig. 3.4 Sagittal (*upper left*) and coronal (*upper right*) T2-weighted sequence of showing a large medial femoral condyle chondral defect. Arthroscopic views of the lesion in flexion (*middle left*) and extension (*middle right*). An arthrotomy showing the prepared recipient site (*lower left*) and the transferred osteochondral allograft (*lower right*)

2.5 cm^2 and requires the availability of a fresh or cold-stored allograft for maximum chondrocyte viability (Fig. 3.4). Timing is also important as the viability of the chondrocytes diminishes significantly 14 days after storage [22]. This technique is usually indicated for larger lesions. It is not uncommon that realignment procedures, such as high tibial osteotomy (HTO), will need to be performed at the same time to protect the affected compartment.

Autologous Chondrocyte Implantation

This technique is a two-stage procedure in which cartilage fragments are first harvested arthroscopically; this is usually taken from the intercondylar notch. The cartilage fragments are then processed and chondrocytes are isolated. The cells are then cultured and allowed to expand over the next 6–8 weeks. Once the donor cells are ready, they are reimplanted into the defect and covered by a periosteal or synthetic patch. This procedure theoretically can be used on Outerbridge grade 3–4 lesions ranging from 2 to 10 cm^2, but because it is a costlier two-stage procedure, it is most often reserved as a second-line treatment when the patient has failed debridement, microfracture, or osteochondral autograft transfer [23]. Bipolar "kissing" lesions are contraindicated (such as lesions on both the patella and the opposing trochlea). A randomized trial comparing ACI vs. microfracture showed that both techniques achieved similar results (77% satisfaction) at 5 years [24]. One of the complications of this procedure is graft hypertrophy where the resurfaced area has overgrowth of cartilaginous tissue. This is usually diagnosed with MRI and can be treated with arthroscopic debridement.

Surgical Management of Arthritis

Nonoperative Options

Patients presenting with significant knee pain and disability due to osteoarthritis should first be managed with nonsteroidal anti-inflamatories, activity modification, and unloader braces. The use of heel wedges (lateral posting for medial compartment arthritis and vice versa) is controversial as multiple studies have not demonstrated significant differences compared to placebo [25]. Intra-articular viscosupplementation and steroid injections offer a temporizing measure to alleviate the pain but does not alter the progression of disease. When patients have exhausted their conservative treatment modalities, surgical intervention, such as an osteotomy or arthroplasty, offers viable long-term pain relief.

Realignment Procedures/Osteotomy

Younger patients with advanced arthritis in either medial or lateral compartment may be candidates for a valgus-producing high tibial osteotomy (HTO) or a varus-producing distal femur osteotomy (DFO), respectively (Fig. 3.5). The goal is to shift the weight-bearing axis away from the affected arthritic compartment. Concurrent arthritis in the patellofemoral joint is not a contraindication, although the opposite tibio-femoral compartment should have relatively intact cartilage and a normal meniscus [26, 27]. If strict indications are followed, 74% good/excellent results are seen at 10-year follow-up [28].

Arthroplasty

Less active older patients with medial compartment osteoarthritis may be good candidates for unicompartmental knee arthroplasty. Indications include an intact ACL and PCL, correctable varus deformity to neutral, and less than 15° flexion contracture. Advances in technology have increased the durability of the implants. The Oxford Unicompartmental Knee (Biomet, Warsaw, IN) has a survivorship of 84–100% at 10-year follow-up and 93% at 15-year follow-up [29]. Patients with severe arthritis affecting both medial and lateral compartments or who do not meet criteria for a unicompartmental knee arthroplasty can benefit from a total knee arthroplasty. This is a predictable procedure yielding greater than 95% survivorship at 10-year follow-up using modern implants [30].

Future Directions

As MRI technology continues to evolve, new modalities and sequences have been developed that provide more information. Quantitative MRI collects information about the tissue rather than just an image, such as the amount and quality of the cartilage. This can allow objective evaluation of cartilage health. In addition, quantitative MRI is being used increasingly to stage disease and monitor the progress of disease or treatment (i.e., ongoing cartilage loss). T1ρ (rho) is one of the quantitative MR imaging sequence that have shown promises for clinical use. Early studies have shown it to be highly sensitive to molecular changes in cartilage degeneration compared to standard T2-weighted sequences, and it may become the modality of choice in evaluation of early arthritis [31, 32].

Summary

Orthopedic surgeons have traditionally relied on plain radiographs in the diagnosis and treatment of diffuse osteoarthritis. However, technological advances in the past decade, especially in MRI, have allowed significant improvements in the diagnosis and treatment of more focal cartilage disorders in a younger population. Our ability to interpret enhanced soft tissue data from MRI not only allows for a more accurate diagnosis, but also assists in the discussion with patients regarding their prognosis and surgical options. MRI is also an invaluable tool in preoperatively planning, allowing surgeons to pick the most appropriate procedure ranging from simple arthroscopic debridement to marrow

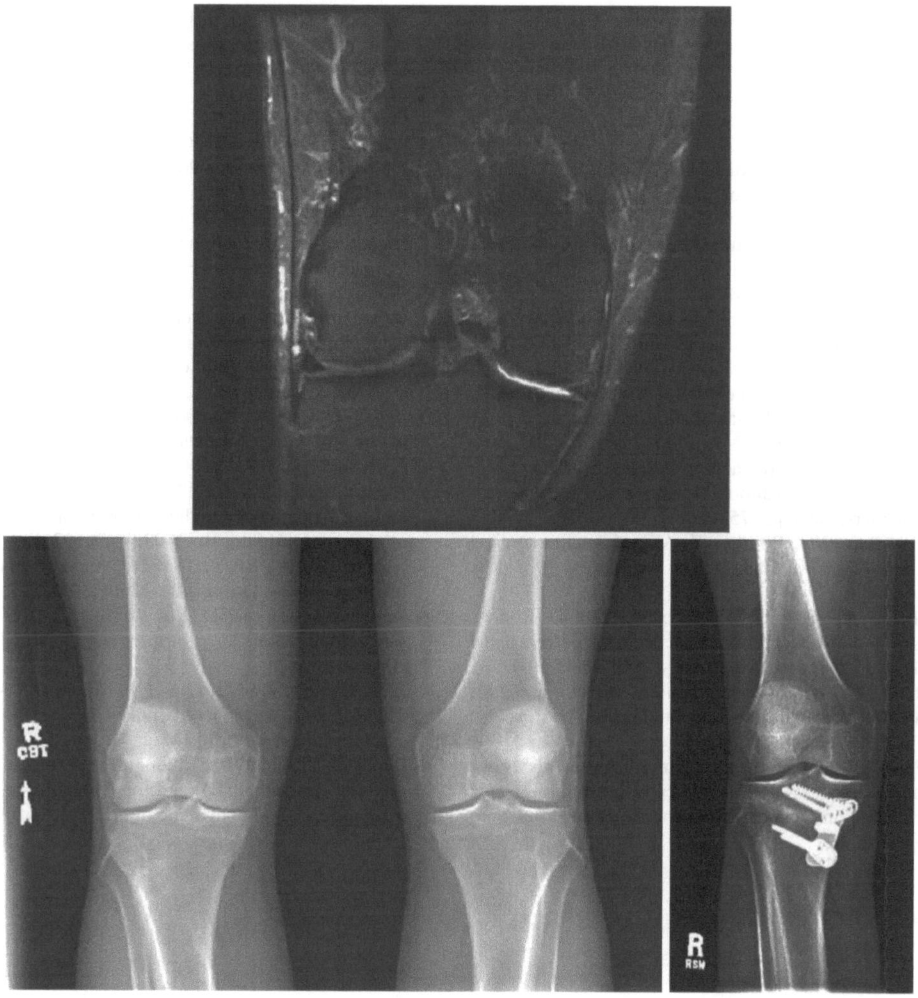

Fig. 3.5 T2-weighted coronal sequence showing right medial compartment arthritis in a 45-year-old male. Note the normal-appearing cartilage and meniscus in the lateral compartment (*top*). Preoperative weight-bearing radiographs (*left*). Postoperative radiographs at 3 months showing a healing opening wedge valgus tibial osteotomy (*right*)

stimulation, mosaicplasty, osteochondral allograft, osteotomy, or arthroplasty. Even more promising is quantitative MRI, which may eventually surpass conventional MRI in the diagnosis of subtle cartilage injuries.

References

1. Noyes FR, Stabler CL. A system for grading articular cartilage lesions at arthroscopy. Am J Sports Med. 1989;17:505–13.
2. Brittberg M, Winalski CS. Evaluation of cartilage injuries and repair. J Bone Joint Surg Am. 2003;85:58–69.
3. Outerbridge RE. The etiology of chondromalacia patella. J Bone Joint Surg Br. 1961;43-B:752–7.
4. Cameron ML, Briggs KK, Steadman JR. Reproducibility and reliability of the outerbridge classification for grading chondral lesions of the knee arthroscopically. Am J Sports Med. 2003;31: 83–6.
5. Faber KJ, Dill JR, Amendola A, Thain L, Spouge A, Fowler PJ. Occult osteochondral lesions after anterior cruciate ligament rupture: six year magnetic resonance imaging follow-up study. Am J Sports Med. 1999;27:489–94.
6. Johnson DL, Urban Jr WP, Caborn DNM, Vanarthos WJ, Carlson CS. Articular cartilage changes seen with magnetic resonance imaging-detected bone bruises associated with acute anterior cruciate ligament rupture. Am J Sports Med. 1998;26:409–14.
7. Johnson DL, Bealle DP, Brand Jr JC, Nyland J, Caborn DNM. The effect of a geographic lateral bone bruise on knee inflammation after acute anterior cruciate ligament rupture. Am J Sports Med. 2000;28:152–5.
8. Davies NH, Niall D, King LJ, Lavelle J, Healy JC. Magnetic resonance imaging of bone bruising in the acutely injured knee – short-term outcome. Clin Rad. 2004;59:439–45.
9. Vellet AD, Marks PH, Fowler PJ, Munro TG. Occult posttraumatic osteochondral lesions of the knee: prevalence, classification, and short-term sequelae evaluated with MR imaging. Radiology. 1991;178:271–6.
10. Mandalia V, Fogg AJB, Chari R, Murray J, Beale A, Henson JHL. Bone bruising of the knee. Clin Rad. 2005;60:627–36.

11. Felson DT, McLaughlin S, Goggins J, LaValley MP, Gale ME, Totterman S, et al. Bone marrow edema and its relation to progression of knee osteoarthritis. Ann Intern Med. 2003;139:330–6.
12. DiStefano VJ. Function, post-traumatic sequalae and current concepts of management of knee meniscus injuries: a review article. Clin Orthop Relat Res. 1980;151:143–6.
13. Curl WW, Krome J, Gordon ES, Rushing JR, Smith BP, Poehling GG. Cartilage injuries: a review of 31,516 knee arthroscopies. Arthroscopy. 1997;13:456–60.
14. Kwartowtiz MA, Reider B. Debridement of articular cartilage in the knee. In: Miller MD, Cole BJ, editors. Textbook of arthroscopy. Philadelphia: Saunders; 2004. p. 568–74.
15. Moseley JB, O'Malley K, Petersen NJ, Menke TJ, Brody BA, Kuykendall DH, et al. A controlled trial of arthroscopic surgery for osteoarthritis of the knee. N Engl J Med. 2002;347:81–8.
16. Kirkley A, Birmingham TB, Litchfield RB, Giffin JR, Willits KR, Wong CJ, et al. A randomized trial of arthroscopic surgery for osteoarthritis of the knee. N Engl J Med. 2008;359:1097–107.
17. Freedman KB, Cole BJ. Microfracture technique in the knee. In: Miller MD, Cole BJ, editors. Textbook of arthroscopy. Philadelphia: Saunders; 2004. p. 575–9.
18. Steadman JR, Rodkey WG, Rodrigo JJ. Microfracture: surgical technique and rehabilitation. Clin Orthop Relat Res. 2001;391: S362–9.
19. Steadman JR, Briggs KK, Rodrigo JJ, Kocher MS, Gill TJ, Rodkey WG. Outcomes of microfracture for traumatic chondral defects of the knee: average 11-year follow-up. Arthroscopy. 2003;19:477–84.
20. Barber FA, Chow JCY. Arthroscopic chondral osseous autograft transplantation (COR procedure) for femoral defects. Arthroscopy. 2006;22:10–6.
21. Hangody L, Füles P. Autologous osteochondral mosaicplasty for the treatment of full-thickness defects of weight-bearing joints: ten years of experimental and clinical experience. J Bone Joint Surg Am. 2003;Suppl 2:25–32.
22. Williams SK, Amiel D, Ball ST, Allen RT, Wong VW, Chen AC, et al. Prolonged storage effects on the articular cartilage of fresh human osteochondral allografts. J Bone Joint Surg Am. 2003; 85-A(11):2111–20.
23. Freedman KB, Cole BJ. Autologous chondrocyte implantation in the knee. In: Miller MD, Cole BJ, editors. Textbook of arthroscopy. Philadelphia: Saunders; 2004. p. 625–32.
24. Knutsen G, Drogset JO, Engebretsen L, Grontvedt T, Isaksen V, Ludvigsen TC, et al. A randomized trial comparing autologous chondrocyte implantation with microfracture: findings at five years. J Bone Joint Surg Am. 2007;89:2105–12.
25. Reilly KA, Barker KL, Shamley D. A systematic review of lateral wedge orthotics – how useful are they in the management of medial compartment osteoarthritis? Knee. 2006;13(3):177–83.
26. Morrey BF. Upper tibial osteotomy for secondary osteoarthritis of the knee. J Bone Joint Surg Br. 1989;71(4):554–9.
27. Wang JW, Hsu CC. Distal femoral varus osteotomy for osteoarthritis of the knee. Surgical technique. J Bone Joint Surg Am. 2006;88(Suppl 1 Pt 1):100–8.
28. Akizuki S, Shibakawa A, Takizawa T, Yamazaki I, Horiuchi H. The long-term outcome of high tibial osteotomy: a ten-to 20-year follow up. J Bone Joint Surg Br. 2008;90(5):592–6.
29. Khanna G, Levy BA. Oxford unicompartmental knee replacement: literature review. Orthopedics. 2007;30S:11–4.
30. Kelly MA, Clarke HD. Long-term results of posterior cruciate-substituting total knee arthroplasty. Clin Orthop Relat Res. 2002;404:51–7.
31. Li X, Han ET, Ma CB, Link TM, Newitt DC, Majumdar S. In vivo 3 T spiral imaging based multi-slice T(1rho) mapping of knee cartilage in osteoarthritis. Magn Reson Med. 2005;54(4):929–36.
32. Lejay H, Holland BA. Technical advances in musculoskeletal imaging. In: Stoller DW, editor. Magnetic resonance imaging in orthopaedics and sports medicine. Baltimore: Lippincott; 2007. p. 1–28.

Chapter 4
Conventional Radiography as an Indirect Measure for Cartilage Pathology

Daichi Hayashi, Jeffrey Duryea, Frank W. Roemer, and Ali Guermazi

Keywords Radiography • Cartilage • Pathology • Knee • Lyon-Schuss view • Fixed-flexion view • Kellgren–Lawrence

Introduction

Conventional radiography is the simplest and least expensive method for imaging joints affected by various joint pathologies. Radiographs have been widely used to assess structural changes associated with osteoarthritis (OA). Radiography is used in clinical practice in patients to establish the diagnosis of OA and to monitor the progression of the disease. Strengths of radiography include its ability to clearly visualize bony features, such as marginal osteophytes, subchondral sclerosis, and subchondral cysts that are associated with OA. Although direct visualization of cartilage is not possible, it can provide an indirect estimate of cartilage thickness and meniscal integrity by the interbone distance or joint space width (JSW). Assessment of OA severity mainly relies on joint space narrowing (JSN) and subchondral bone lesions. Increase in JSN is the most commonly used criterion for the longitudinal assessment of OA progression and the complete loss of JSW, characterized by bone-on-bone contact, is one of the factors considered in the decision for joint replacement [1].

In this chapter, we will describe the role of conventional radiography as a means of indirect assessment of cartilage thickness, using imaging of knee OA as an illustrative example. We will describe protocols for standardized radiographic examination of the knee, causes of JSN, and both semiquantitative and quantitative assessments of JSW in knee OA. Lastly, a brief discussion of radiographic assessment of the patellofemoral (PF) joint of the knee, the hip and ankle joints will be provided.

Protocols for Standardized Radiographic Assessment of the Knee

Traditionally, the extended-knee radiograph (i.e., a bilateral weight-bearing anteroposterior (AP) view of both knees in full extension) has been the technique employed to image the tibiofemoral joint [2, 3]. It was the procedure used to acquire reference images for contemporary pictorial atlases of the radiographic severity of tibiofemoral OA [4, 5] and remains an accepted radiographic technique for characterizing the bony changes of OA (e.g., marginal osteophytes and subchondral sclerosis). Although the diagnostic utility of the extended-knee radiograph is established, this technique is severely limited as a method to visualize reproducibly the radiographic joint space [6].

This limitation stems from numerous technical shortcomings of the examination with respect to variability in the positioning of the knee in serial examinations. For example, longitudinal changes in weight-bearing (e.g., due to weight gain or loss) may affect the extent of voluntary knee extension. Changes in the distance between the knee and radiographic cassette may alter the degree of radiographic magnification in the image. Whereas the above sources of variation in knee position are likely to contribute random measurement error to estimates of tibiofemoral JSW, changes in knee pain from examination to examination (as may occur in a clinical trial of a purported disease-modifying OA drug) may introduce systematic measurement errors [1]. This discrepancy was demonstrated by a previous study [7] in which significant increases in tibiofemoral JSW were detected in extended-knee radiographs taken 7–14 days apart of OA subjects who had undergone relief of an induced flare of knee OA pain. These sources of error seriously limit the utility of the extended-knee radiograph to detect true JSN, the cardinal indicator of progression of knee OA [4].

D. Hayashi (✉)
Department of Radiology, Boston University School of Medicine, FGH Building, 3rd Floor, Boston, MA 02118, USA
e-mail: Daichi.Hayashi@bmc.org

T.M. Link (ed.), *Cartilage Imaging: Significance, Techniques, and New Developments*,
DOI 10.1007/978-1-4419-8438-8_4, © Springer Science+Business Media, LLC 2011

Table 4.1 Comparison of technical specifications for standardized radiographic assessment using Lyon-Schuss (LS) view and fixed-flexion (FF) view

	Lyon-Schuss	Fixed flexion
Fluoroscopic assistance	Yes	No
Knee orientation	Posteroanterior	Posteroanterior
Degree of flexion	Fixed (20–35°)	Fixed (20–35°)
Standard for knee flexion	Schuss position	Schuss position
Standard for foot rotation	10°	10°
Standard for X-ray beam angulation	Adjust to bring the medial tibial plateau into sharpest focus	10° Caudal
Adjustment for radiographic magnification	Optional	Optional

Over the past 15 years, several groups of investigators have developed alternative protocols for standardized positioning of the knee for a radiographic assessment of the tibiofemoral joint. Common to all of the techniques described in this chapter is a standard for knee flexion, rather than extension, that provides contact between the tibia and the posterior aspect of the femoral condyle (i.e., the region in which cartilage damage in OA is often most marked) [8]. The protocols differ, however, with respect to the degree of flexion required, angulation of the X-ray beam, and the parameter that is adjusted to meet the examination's positioning standards (Table 4.1).

A key distinction among current positioning protocols is the use of fluoroscopy to confirm satisfactory radioanatomical positioning of the medial tibial plateau (i.e., parallel or near-parallel alignment with the central X-ray beam) before acquisition of the radiograph [1, 9, 10].

Lyon-Schuss View

The Lyon-Schuss (LS) radiographic view [9] uses a posteroanterior Schuss position of the subject (i.e., placement of the anterior aspect of the hip, the patella, and tip of the great toe against the radiographic cassette or surface of the vertical radiographic table). Coplanar alignment of the hip, patella, and great toe fixes the degree of flexion for repeat examinations (20–35°, depending on the relative lengths of the tibia and foot). To compensate for the effect of knee flexion on the orientation of the medial tibial plateau relative to the horizontal plane, fluoroscopy is used to adjust the angle of the X-ray beam caudally to bring the tibial plateau into sharpest focus. Early data derived from the LS radiograph confirmed that it afforded reproducibility of measurement of medial tibiofemoral JSW superior to that of the conventional extended-knee view [11].

A recent modification of the LS protocol has incorporated use of the SynaFlexer™ (Synarc, Inc., San Francisco, California), an acrylic positioning frame in which subjects stand and position themselves to fix knee flexion and external foot rotation in Schuss position [12]. Recent applications of the protocol have also adopted the intermargin distance as the standard for evaluating radioanatomic alignment of the medial tibial plateau [1, 10, 13, 14].

Fixed-Flexion View

Peterfy et al. have developed an empirically derived set of positioning standards for standardized knee radiography [15]. Based on fluoroscopically assisted measurements of beam angulation that produce parallel radioanatomic alignment of the medial tibial plateau in samples of normal and OA knees in Schuss position (9.0±3.6°), the authors designed position standards for the posteroanterior fixed-flexion (FF) view. As with the LS view, both knees are in contact with the cassette and coplanar with the hips, patellae, and tips of the great toes (Table 4.1). The FF view requires that the X-ray beam be directed 10° caudally, unlike the LS view in which the beam angle is varied with each examination in an attempt to align the beam with the medial tibial plateau. Positioning of the knee and foot for the FF view is facilitated by use of the SynaFlexer™ positioning frame [12, 15].

The FF view permits highly precise measurements of JSW [15]. However, because of biologic variability in the anatomy of the tibial plateau, the FF technique often produces radiographs with skewed radioanatomic alignment of the medial tibial plateau [16]. This problem has led investigators to explore a modification of the FF protocol that entails ascertainment of the quality of alignment produced by 10° caudal angulation and reacquisition of the radiograph with small adjustments of the angle (cranially or caudally) until satisfactory alignment is achieved [1, 13, 17].

Other Views

The semiflexed anteroposterior view uses fluoroscopy to guide knee flexion and rotation to achieve reproducible anatomic markers of parallel alignment of the medial tibial plateau relative to a horizontal X-ray beam [18]. Although this technique has been shown to afford estimates of JSW that are more precise than those obtained from the conventional extended-knee view, its accuracy of measurement is affected by the requirement for magnification correction [19].

In an effort to develop a more exportable, nonfluoroscopically assisted alternative to the semiflexed anteroposterior view, the same group of authors developed the semiflexed metatarsophalangeal (MTP) posteroanterior view [20]. This protocol does not require correction for radioanatomic alignment, but use of a foot map is necessary to facilitate reproducibility of foot rotation and placement of the first MTP joints beneath the front of the radiographic cassette. Several studies of the performance of this protocol have noted that as many as 70% of MTP radiographs exhibit skewed alignment of the medial tibial plateau [1, 16]. Additionally, alignment in MTP views is notably less reproducible over time than in the short term, resulting in lesser sensitivity to JSN than concurrent semiflexed AP radiographs [16].

Performance of Lyon-Schuss and Fixed-Flexion Views

The developers of the standardized knee radiographic protocols described above have each offered evidence to indicate that their protocol affords measurements of tibiofemoral JSW that are more precise and reproducible than those obtainable from the conventional extended-knee radiograph [11, 15, 18, 20]. Although measurement precision is an important theoretical determinant of sensitivity to the detection of change (e.g., thinning of articular cartilage), it is not a sufficient basis to conclude that one standardized technique is more advisable than another for use in longitudinal studies of OA progression. Such choices are best made on the basis of direct comparisons of alternative protocols in the same subjects. Head-to-head comparisons of alternative positioning protocols are rare in the OA literature [1]. Although studies have shown that the sensitivity to radiographic JSN is enhanced by fluoroscopically assisted joint positioning and/or beam angulation, it should be acknowledged that the nonfluoroscopically assisted methods can detect disease progression in knee OA with noteworthy sensitivity [21].

Joint Space on Radiographs as an Indirect Measure of Cartilage Thickness

JSW has been used as an indirect measure of hyaline articular cartilage thickness in the tibiofemoral joint. Buckland-Wright et al. measured JSW from weight-bearing plain-film macroradiographs obtained in the tunnel view and compared this with the sum of femoral and tibial cartilage thicknesses measured from double-contrast macroarthrograms of the same regions of the same knees, obtained in the nonweight-bearing lateral position in 20 subjects with knee OA. Comparison of JSW with the sum of the tibial and femoral cartilage thicknesses revealed a significant correlation between the two measurements in the medial, but not the lateral, compartment [18]. More recently, Amin et al. examined the relationship between progression of JSN on radiographic images and cartilage loss on MRI. While their results provided longitudinal evidence that radiographic progression of JSN was correlated with cartilage loss assessed on MRI, radiography was not a sensitive measure. The authors concluded that if radiography was used alone, a substantial proportion of knees with cartilage loss would be missed [22]. In particular, a focal cartilage defect in the weight-bearing compartment (Fig. 4.1) or a defect located in the nonweight-bearing portion of posterior femoral condyle (Fig. 4.2) may not be visible on radiography and can only be revealed by MRI. Moreover, in longitudinal studies, radiographic progression of JSN is not a sensitive or specific measure of OA disease progression when compared to MRI findings (Figs. 4.3–4.5).

Previously held beliefs that ascertainment of JSN and its changes are a reflection only of damage to articular cartilage were shown to be incorrect after recent studies demonstrated that alterations in the meniscus, such as meniscal extrusion or subluxation, also contributed to JSN [23–25]. A more recent cross-sectional and longitudinal study by Hunter et al. used both MRI and weight-bearing posteroanterior radiographs [12] to explore the relative contribution of semiquantitative cartilage morphologic features and the meniscus position to the ordinal radiographic JSN [25]. They found that features of the meniscus (position and degeneration) accounted for a substantial proportion of the explained variance in JSN, and change in meniscal position accounted for a substantial proportion of change in JSN.

The same group of authors also conducted a study using a quantitative approach to ascertain the contributions of cartilage (measured with a 3D morphometric approach) and meniscal position on MRI to JSW as measured in the LS radiographs of the knee [26]. Sixty-five percent of the variation in medial JSW was explained by regional cartilage thickness measures, different Kellgren–Lawrence (KL) grade (see the next section for explanations), and meniscal coverage. Of these measures, the medial tibial cartilage thickness measures and central region of the central medial femur (ccMF) played a consistent role in variations in medial JSW observed across all KL grades. Furthermore, ccMF and the addition of percent meniscal coverage to this model explained the remaining differences in mean medial JSW found between those subjects with definite JSN (KL grade 3) and those without OA.

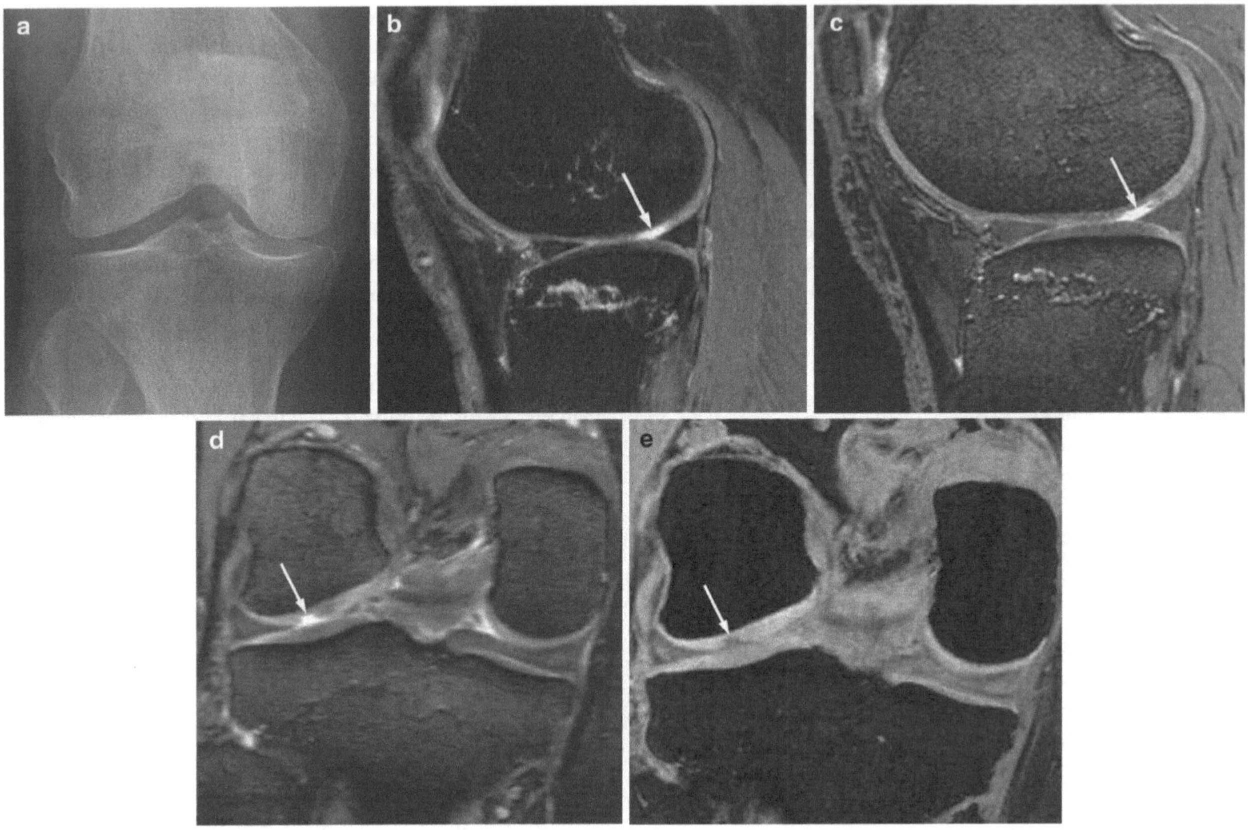

Fig. 4.1 Example of a case in which posteroanterior, fixed-flexion (FF) radiograph (**a**) does not show any joint space narrowing (Kellgren–Lawrence [KL] grade 0) in the right knee. MRI reveals a focal cartilage defect in the central portion of lateral femoral condyle (*arrows*). The lesion is better depicted in the sagittal fat-suppressed intermediate-weighted sequence (**b**) than sagittal (**c**) and coronal (**d**) DESS sequence. As expected, the focal defect appears less conspicuous and smaller on coronal FLASH sequence (**e**)

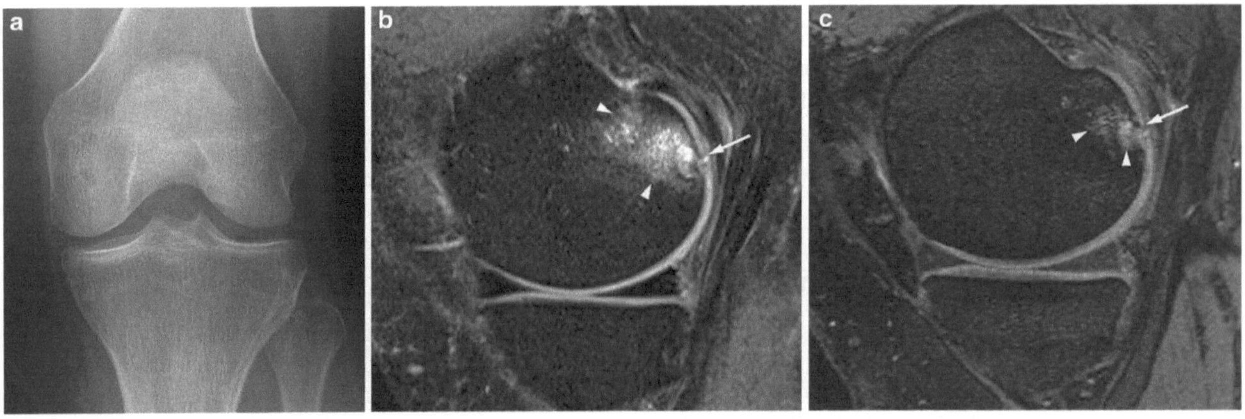

Fig. 4.2 Example of a case in which posteroanterior, fixed-flexion (FF) radiograph (**a**) does not show any joint space narrowing (Kellgren–Lawrence [KL] grade 0) in the left knee. MRI reveals a focal cartilage defect (*arrows*) in the posterior aspect of medial femoral condyle in the left knee. A subchondral bone marrow lesion is also present and is depicted to a fuller extent in the sagittal fat-suppressed intermediate-weighted sequence (**b**) compared to the DESS sequence (**c**). None of these changes can be visible on plain radiographs

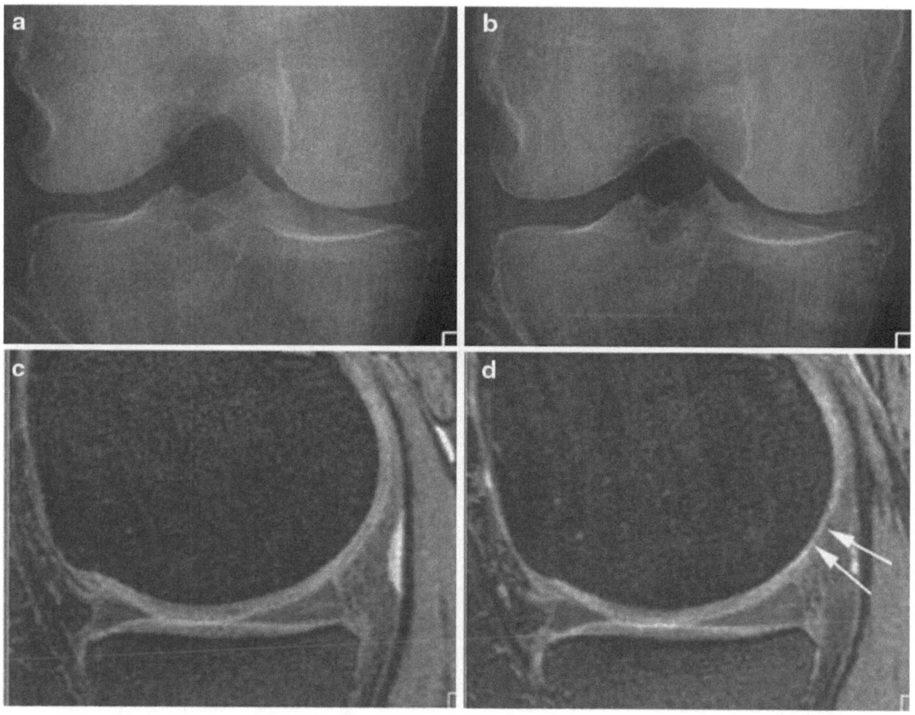

Fig. 4.3 Progressive MRI-detected cartilage loss. Baseline (**a**, **c**) and 24-months follow-up examinations (**b**, **d**). No radiographic progression is seen (**a**, **b**). On sagittal DESS MRI, progressive cartilage loss in the posterior medial femur is observed at follow-up (*arrows*, **c**, **d**)

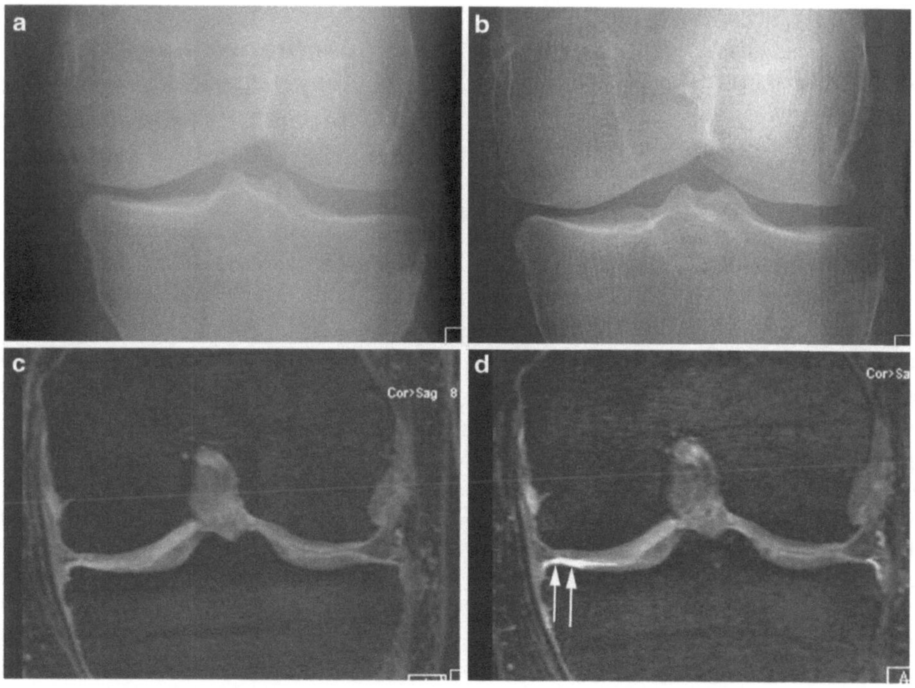

Fig. 4.4 Focal cartilage loss on MRI. Radiography does not show progressive joint space narrowing (JSN) (**a**, **b**), i.e., identical joint space width from baseline to follow-up. Coronal DESS MRI (**c**, **d**) shows incident focal cartilage defect in the central part of the medial tibial plateau at follow-up (*arrows*)

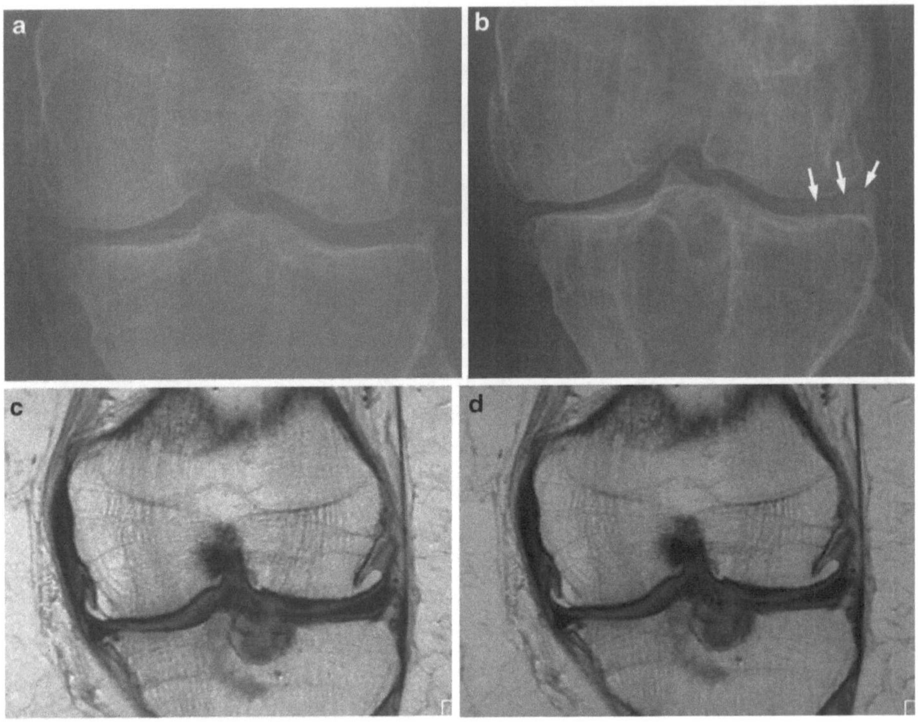

Fig. 4.5 Progressive joint space narrowing (JSN) (**a**, **b**) but no progression on coronal intermediate-weighted MRI (**c**, **d**). Positioning from baseline to follow-up is slightly discordant. Lateral osteophyte projected into joint space at follow-up (*arrows*) suggests slightly different degree of knee flexion at follow-up. No progression of MRI-detected cartilage loss or meniscal damage/extrusion is seen at follow-up

The structural alterations that form the OA disease process are markedly collinear, i.e., as hyaline articular cartilage becomes more morphologically abnormal, the other structural processes parallel these changes, with increasing degenerative findings in the meniscus and increasing meniscal displacement [25]. The causal process is therefore complex and JSN genuinely reflects changes in all of these structures, and in some knees cartilage loss is less important as a cause than meniscal variables. One should also note that the lateral joint space may become widened as a result of severe medial JSN. In such secondary widening of joint space, articular cartilage in the lateral compartment may be normal.

Relevance and importance of these findings have been described previously [26]. In clinical trials assessing disease-modifying osteoarthritis drugs (DMOADs), it is essential to know the selective target of the drug (e.g., cartilage or meniscus). If the meniscus is the drug's target tissue, radiographic changes in JSW are not to be expected (if the meniscus does not show extrusion). Likewise, if the drug target were cartilage at latter disease stages, the contribution of meniscal malposition may influence JSW measures substantively. These factors need to be considered in planning for both observational studies monitoring progression and clinical trials [26].

Semiquantitative Assessment of Joint-Space Narrowing Using Kellgren–Lawrence and Osteoarthrits Research Society International Grading Systems

The severity of OA can be estimated by semiquantitative radiographic scoring systems. Several grading scales incorporating combinations of features have been developed. The two most widely utilized systems are the KL grading [4] and the Osteoarthritis Research Society International (OARSI) grading system [27]. Both systems have been applied widely in clinical trials and epidemiologic studies. The KL grading is traditionally used to classify populations according to those who have OA with a grade of ≥2. The individual radiographic features of the OARSI grading system have been widely used both in cross-sectional and observational epidemiologic studies, with JSN as a surrogate measure of disease progression, although more recent studies have tended to use quantitative measures of JSW.

Published atlases provide image examples that represent the specific grades [27]. Modifications have been introduced to these scoring systems, adding either complexity or simplification [28]. Examples of KL grading and OARSI modifications are summarized in Tables 4.2 and 4.3, respectively.

Table 4.2 Description of Kellgren–Lawrence (KL) and modified Kellgren–Lawrence grading systems

	Kellgren–Lawrence	Modified Kellgren–Lawrence
Grade 0	No feature of osteoarthritis (OA)	No feature of osteoarthritis
Grade 1	Doubtful joint-space narrowing and possible osteophyte lipping	Equivocal osteophyte
Grade 2	Definite osteophytes and possible joint-space narrowing	Unequivocal osteophyte
Grade 3	Moderate multiple osteophytes, definite joint-space narrowing, and some sclerosis and possible deformity of bone ends	Joint-space narrowing
Grade 4	Large osteophytes, marked joint-space narrowing, severe sclerosis, and definite deformity of bone ends	Bone-to-bone appearance

Table 4.3 Original and Modified Osteoarthritis Research Society International (OARSI) grading system for medial and lateral tibiofemoral joint-space narrowing

Grading system	Grading
Original OARSI	Grade 0 (normal)–3 (severe)
Modified OARSI	Grade 0: Normal, OARSI grade 0
	Grade 1: Narrowed, OARSI grade 1–2
	Grade 2: Severe, OARSI grade 3 or joint space width (JSW) <0.5 mm

One of the major drawbacks of these grading systems is their lack of sensitivity to change [22]. JSW is a crude measure of indirect assessment of articular cartilage, and cartilage is only one contributor to physiologic JSW as described earlier. In addition, expected annual rates of cartilage loss are minimal, as has been shown by quantitative MRI morphometry [29]. Furthermore, visually detectable minor changes in JSW do not necessarily translate into a change in grading when radiographic grading systems are used. For this reason, some researchers have introduced half-grades to account for subtle longitudinal change [30]. When compared with MRI as the reference standard, radiography has shown an excellent specificity with regard to the detection of longitudinal cartilage loss. However, the reported sensitivity is low [22].

Quantitative Assessments of Joint Space

Although semiquantitative scoring is an accepted and widely used method to evaluate a knee radiograph for OA, it relies fundamentally on a qualitative and subjective assessment of the image. Quantitative measures of JSW use a "ruler," either a physical device or a software application, to measure the JSW as the distance between the projected femoral and tibial margins on the image.

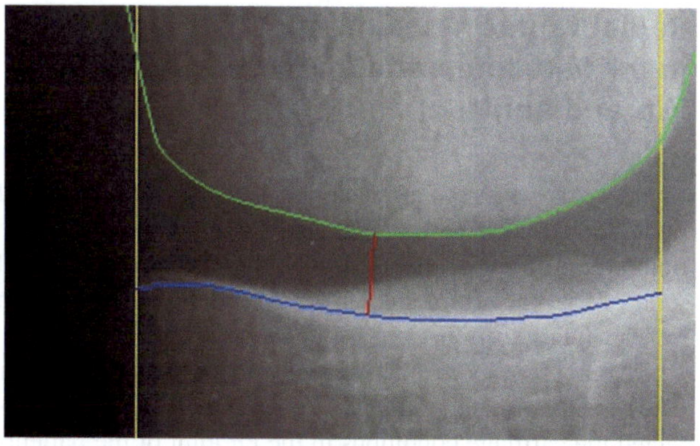

Fig. 4.6 Example of software joint delineation in the medial compartment of the tibiofemoral joint of the knee. The femoral margin (*green*) is defined as the projected edge of the bone, and the tibial margin (*blue*) is a bright band. The location of the minimum joint space width (JSW) is marked in *red*

Initially, quantitative measures of JSW were made by an observer viewing the radiograph over a light box [31, 32]. The reader determined the location of the minimum distance between the femoral and tibial margins and made a measurement of the distance with a graduated hand-held lens.

Later, software-based methods were developed to measure radiographic knee JSW [33–36] and generally function by delineating the margins of the femur and tibia as shown in Fig. 4.6. The femoral margin is defined as the projected edge of the bone, while the software determines the tibial margin as a bright band corresponding to the projection of the X-ray beam through the radio-dense cortical shell at the base of the tibial plateau.

The use of image processing software to quantify JSW offers several advantages over a manual reading. The method is fast and, in principle, more objective than hand-held lens technique and can provide measures of JSW at locations other than the minimum [37, 38], since the joint margins are delineated by the software. These methods do require a digital version of the image, which can be provided for plain films by a radiographic film digitizer, or files can be analyzed directly for fully digital modalities such as computed radiography (CR) and digital radiography (DR).

Studies using the software methods have demonstrated an improved precision over the manual method and semiquantitative scoring [34–36, 39]. More recently, these methods have been evaluated using longitudinal knee radiographs to quantify the responsiveness to change [10, 38]. Various degrees of responsiveness have been observed depending on the degree of OA severity, length of the follow-up, and knee positioning protocol used.

Radiographic Assessment of Cartilage in the Patellofemoral Joint of the Knee, Hip, and Ankle

Indirect assessment of articular cartilage using conventional radiography has been reported also for joints other than the tibiofemoral joint of the knee, including the patellofemoral joint of the knee, hip, and ankle. We briefly describe such reports in this section.

Chang et al. performed a study to determine whether assessments of patellofemoral (PF) joint space reliably predicted the cartilage conditions in the PF joint of the patients undergoing total knee arthroplasty for advanced knee OA [40]. The agreements between the radiographic assessments and the gross assessments on the lesion severities and locations were only fair. The cross-table analyses showed that approximately half of subjects with a normal radiographic joint space had moderate or severe cartilage degeneration of the PF joint identified with gross assessments. Thus, authors concluded that prediction of the cartilage conditions of the PF joint by the radiographic joint space could be inaccurate.

Plain radiographs have been used as the primary diagnostic method for hip OA for many decades. Cartilage degeneration can be demonstrated radiologically as JSN, i.e., decreased distance between opposing articular bony surfaces of the femoral head and the acetabulum, and asymmetric JSN is a highly reliable sign of OA [41]. However, this is again not a direct visualization of cartilage and JSN needs to be interpreted with caution. The presence of JSN may show discordance with the clinical picture and 29% of subjects with hip pain may show completely normal radiographs [42]. In other studies, JSN was a better predictor of hip pain compared to osteophytes [43, 44]. Hip OA is defined according to minimum joint spaces of <2.5 mm ("probable" OA) and <1.5 mm ("definite" OA) [43]. However, various studies have challenged the application of absolute measurements. One study showed that a wide JSW variation exists normally, ranging from 3 to 8 mm and from 2 to 6 mm at the superolateral and superomedial sites, respectively, with an associated right/left asymmetry in 5.9% of subjects [45]. In the same study, the JSW was related to acetabular anatomy, being larger in dysplasia and smaller in coxa profunda, regardless of the presence of OA. In another study, the minimum JSW decreased progressively with age in women, but it was unaltered in men [46]. A study on 78 normal radiographs showed that no difference exists between right and left sides, but women show a narrower mean JSW compared to men [47].

OA of the ankle joint is rarer than that of the knee or the hip. Reports of radiographic JSW assessment of the ankle have been limited, and most of those measurement techniques have not been well validated to date [48]. Recently, Moon et al. conducted a study to compare semiquantitative radiographic grading of ankle OA with cartilage damage observed during arthroscopy [49]. Ankles with medial JSN showed varying severity of cartilage damage. The positive predictive value of cartilage damage increased from 77% for medial JSN regardless of the presence of talar tilting to 98% for medial JSN with talar tilting. Their observations suggest the inclusion of talar tilting in grading schemes enhances the assessment of cartilage damage.

Conclusion

In summary, we have described the role of conventional radiography as a means of indirect assessment of cartilage thickness in knee OA. We also described protocols for standardized radiographic examination of the knee, causes of JSN, and both semiquantitative and quantitative assessments of JSW. Radiographically detected JSN is the only structural end point currently accepted by the regulatory bodies in the United States (U.S. Food and Drug Administration) and Europe (European Medicines Agency) to prove efficacy of DMOADs targeting OA in phase-III clinical trials. However, we need to be aware of several limitations characteristic to radiographic assessment of JSN. Exact reproducibility of positioning is challenging, which is of relevance especially in multicenter and longitudinal studies. The most important drawback of radiography, however, is its inability to directly visualize cartilage. Consequently, it is nonspecific and insensitive to change. Meniscal damage and subluxation contribute to radiographic JSW and may also account for longitudinal JSN. A large number of ongoing epidemiologic and clinical trials in OA use both plain radiographic and MRI data, and the most valid and responsive set of endpoints are being sought. Before recommending the widespread use of one particular imaging construct in structure modifying clinical trials, it is crucial that we have this information as well as an established relationship with clinical endpoints, such as pain, function, and need for arthroplasty.

References

1. Hellio Le Graverand M-P, Mazzuca S, Duryea J, Brett A. Radiographic-based grading methods and radiographic measurement of joint space width in osteoarthritis. Radiol Clin N Am. 2009;47:567–79.
2. Ahlback S. Osteoarthritis of the knee. A radiographic investigation. Acta Radiol Diagn (Stockh). 1968;Suppl 277:7–72.
3. Leach RE, Gregg T, Siber FJ. Weight bearing radiography in osteoarthritis of the knee. Radiology. 1970;97:265–8.
4. Kellgren JH, Lawrence JS. Radiological assessment of osteoarthritis. Ann Rheum Dis. 1957;16:494–502.

5. Altman RD, Hochberg M, Murphy WAJ, Wolfe F, Lequesne M. Atlas of individual radiographic features in osteoarthritis. Osteoarthritis Cartilage. 1995;3:3–70.
6. Mazzuca SA, Brandt KD, Katz BP. Is conventional radiography suitable for evaluation of a disease modifying drug in patients with knee osteoarthritis? Osteoarthritis Cartilage. 1997;5:217–26.
7. Mazzuca SA, Brandt KD, Lane KA, Katz BP. Knee pain reduces joint space width in conventional standing anteroposterior radiographs of osteoarthritic knees. Arthritis Rheum. 2002;46:1223–7.
8. Messieh SS, Fowler PJ, Munro T. Anteroposterior radiographs of the osteoarthritic knee. J Bone Joint Surg Br. 1990;72:639–40.
9. Conrozier T, Mathieu P, Piperno M, Favret H, Colson F, Vignon M, et al. Lyon Schuss radiographic view of the knee. Utility of fluoroscopy for the quality of tibial plateau alignment. J Rheumatol. 2004;31:584–90.
10. Hellio Le Graverand M-P, Vignon EP, Brandt KD, Mazzuca SA, Piperno M, Buck R, et al. Head-to-head comparison of the Lyon Schuss and fixed flexion radiographic techniques. Long-term reproducibility in normal knees and sensitivity to change in osteoarthritic knees. Ann Rheum Dis. 2008;67:1562–6.
11. Piperno M, Hellio Le Graverand MP, Conrozier T, Bochu M, Mathieu P, Vignon E, et al. Quantitative evaluation of joint space width in femorotibial osteoarthritis: comparison of three radiographic views. Osteoarthritis Cartilage. 1998;6:252–9.
12. Kothari M, Guermazi A, von Ingersleben G, Miaux Y, Sieffert M, Block JE, et al. Fixed-flexion radiography of the knee provides reproducible joint space width measurements in osteoarthritis. Eur Radiol. 2004;14:1568–73.
13. Mazzuca SA, Hellio Le Graverand MP, Vignon E, Hunter DJ, Jackson CG, Kraus VB, et al. Performance of a non-fluoroscopically assisted substitute for the Lyon schuss knee radiograph: quality and reproducibility of positioning and sensitivity to joint space narrowing in osteoarthritic knees. Osteoarthritis Cartilage. 2008;16:1555–9.
14. Hellio Le Graverand MP, Buck RJ, Wyman BT, Vignon E, Mazzuca SA, Brandt KD, et al. Change in regional cartilage morphology and joint space width in osteoarthritis participants versus healthy controls: a multicentre study using 3.0 Tesla MRI and Lyon-Schuss radiography. Ann Rheum Dis. 2010;69:155–62.
15. Peterfy C, Li J, Zaim S, Duryea J, Lynch J, Miaux Y, et al. Comparison of fixed-flexion positioning with fluoroscopic semi-flexed positioning for quantifying radiographic joint-space width in the knee: test-retest reproducibility. Skeletal Radiol. 2003;32: 128–32.
16. Mazzuca SA, Brandt KD, Buckwalter KA. Longitudinal comparison of the metatarsophalangeal and semiflexed anteroposterior views: detection of radiographic joint space narrowing in osteoarthritic knees. Arthritis Rheum. 2002;46 Suppl 9:S150.
17. Charles HC, Kraus VB, Ainslie M, Hellio Le Graverand MP. Optimization of the fixed-flexion knee radiograph. Osteoarthritis Cartilage. 2007;15:1221–4.
18. Buckland-Wright JC, Macfarlane DG, Lynch JA, Jasani MK, Bradshaw CR. Joint space width measures cartilage thickness in osteoarthritis of the knee: high resolution plain film and double contrast macroradiographic investigation. Ann Rheum Dis. 1995;54:263–8.
19. Mazzuca SA, Brandt KD, Buckwalter KA, Lequesne M. Pitfalls in the accurate measurement of joint space narrowing in semiflexed, anteroposterior radiographic imaging of the knee. Arthritis Rheum. 2004;50:2508–15.
20. Buckland-Wright JC, Wolfe F, Ward RJ, Flowers N, Hayne C. Substantial superiority of semiflexed (MTP) views in knee osteoarthritis: a comparative radiographic study, without fluoroscopy, of standing extended, semiflexed (MTP), and schuss views. J Rheumatol. 1999;26:2664–74.
21. Nevitt MC, Peterfy C, Guermazi A, Felson DT, Duryea J, Woodworth T, et al. Longitudinal performance evaluation and validation of fixed-flexion radiography of the knee for detection of joint space loss. Arthritis Rheum. 2007;56:1512–20.
22. Amin S, LaValley MP, Guermazi A, Grigoryan M, Hunter DJ, Clancy M, et al. The relationship between cartilage loss on magnetic resonance imaging and radiographic progression in men and women with knee osteoarthritis. Arthritis Rheum. 2005;52:3152–9.
23. Adams JG, McAlindon T, Dimasi M, Carey J, Eustace S. Contribution of meniscal extrusion and cartilage loss to joint space narrowing in osteoarthritis. Clin Radiol. 1999;54:502–6.
24. Gale DR, Chaisson CE, Totterman SM, Schwartz RK, Gale ME, Felson D. Meniscal subluxation: association with osteoarthritis and joint space narrowing. Osteoarthritis Cartilage. 1999;7:526–32.
25. Hunter DJ, Zhang YQ, Tu X, Lavalley M, Niu B, Amin S, et al. Change in joint space width: hyaline articular cartilage loss or alteration in meniscus? Arthritis Rheum. 2006;54:2488–95.
26. Hunter DJ, Buck R, Vignon E, Eckstein F, Brandt K, Mazzuca SA, et al. Relation of regional articular cartilage morphometry and meniscal position by MRI to joint space width in knee radiographs. Osteoarthritis Cartilage. 2009;17:1170–6.
27. Altman RD, Gold GE. Atlas of individual radiographic features in osteoarthritis, revised. Osteoarthritis Cartilage. 2007;15(Suppl A): A1–56.
28. Guermazi A, Hunter DJ, Roemer FW. Plain radiography and magnetic resonance imaging diagnostics in osteoarthritis: validated staging and scoring. Bone Joint Surg Am. 2009;91:54–62.
29. Eckstein F, Maschek S, Wirth W, Hudelmaier M, Hitzl W, Wyman B, et al. One year change of knee cartilage morphology in the first release of participants from the Osteoarthritis Initiative progression subcohort: association with sex, body mass index, symptoms and radiographic osteoarthritis status. Ann Rheum Dis. 2009;68:674–9.
30. Felson DT, Nevitt MC, Yang M, Clancy M, Niu J, Torner JC, et al. A new approach yields high rates of radiographic progression in knee osteoarthritis. J Rheumatol. 2008;35:2047–54.
31. Lequesne M, Brandt K, Bellamy N, Moskowitz R, Menkes CJ, Pelletier JP, et al. Guidelines for testing slow acting drugs in osteoarthritis. J Rheumatol Suppl. 1994;41:65–71; discussion 62–63.
32. Ravaud P, Chastang C, Auleley GR, Giraudeau B, Royant V, Amor B, et al. Assessment of joint space width in patients with osteoarthritis of the knee: a comparison of 4 measuring instruments. J Rheumatol. 1996;23:1749–55.
33. Dacre JE, Huskisson EC. The automatic assessment of knee radiographs in osteoarthritis using digital image analysis. Br J Rheumatol. 1989;28:506–10.
34. Lynch JA, Buckland-Wright JC, Macfarlane DG. Precision of joint space width measurement in knee osteoarthritis from digital image analysis of high definition macroradiographs. Osteoarthritis Cartilage. 1993;1:209–18.
35. Conrozier T, Vignon E. Quantitative radiography in osteoarthritis: computerized measurement of radiographic knee and hip joint space. Baillières Clin Rheumatol. 1996;10:429–33.
36. Duryea J, Li J, Peterfy CG, Gordon C, Genant HK. Trainable rule-based algorithm for the measurement of joint space width in digital radiographic images of the knee. Med Phys. 2000;27:580–91.
37. Conrozier T, Lequesne M, Favret H, Taccoen A, Mazières B, Dougados M. Measurement of the radiological hip joint space width. An evaluation of various methods of measurement. Osteoarthritis Cartilage. 2001;9:281–6.
38. Neumann G, Hunter D, Nevitt M, Chibnik LB, Kwoh K, Chen H, et al. Location specific radiographic joint space width for osteoarthritis progression. Osteoarthritis Cartilage. 2009;17:761–5.
39. Marijnissen AC, Vincken KL, Vos PA, Saris DB, Viergever MA, Bijlsma JW, et al. Knee Images Digital Analysis (KIDA): a novel method to quantify individual radiographic features of knee osteoarthritis in detail. Osteoarthritis Cartilage. 2008;16:234–43.
40. Chang CB, Seong SC, Kim TK. Evaluations of radiographic joint space – do they adequately predict cartilage conditions in the

patellofemoral joint of the patients undergoing total knee arthroplasty for advanced knee osteoarthritis? Osteoarthritis Cartilage. 2008; 16:1160–6.
41. Karachalios T, Karantanas AH, Malizos K. Hip osteoarthritis: what the radiologist wants to know. Eur J Radiol. 2007;63:36–48.
42. Birrell F, Lunt M, Macfarlane G, Silman A. Association between pain in the hip region and radiographic changes of osteoarthritis: results from a population-based study. Rheumatology (Oxford). 2005;44:337–41.
43. Croft P, Cooper C, Wickham C, Coggon D. Defining osteoarthritis of the hip for epidemiologic studies. Am J Epidemiol. 1990;132: 514–22.
44. Jacobsen S, Sonne-Holm S, Soballe K, Gebuhr P, Lund B. The relationship of hip joint space to self reported hip pain. A survey of 4.151 subjects of the Copenhagen City Heart Study: the Osteoarthritis Substudy. Osteoarthritis Cartilage. 2004;12:692–7.
45. Lequesne M, Malghem J, Dion E. The normal hip joint space: variations in width, shape, and architecture on 223 pelvic radiographs. Ann Rheum Dis. 2004;63:1145–51.
46. Jacobsen S, Sonne-Holm S, Soballe K, Gebuhr P, Lund B. Factors influencing hip joint space in asymptomatic subjects. A survey of 4151 subjects of the Copenhagen City Heart Study: the Osteoarthritis Substudy. Osteoarthritis Cartilage. 2004;12:698–703.
47. Goker B, Sancak A, Arac M, Shott S, Block JA. The radiographic joint space width in clinically normal hips: effects of age, gender and physical parameters. Osteoarthritis Cartilage. 2003;11:328–34.
48. Goker B, Gonen E, Demirag MD, Block JA. Quantification of the radiographic joint space width of the ankle. Cin Orthop Relat Res. 2009;467:2083–9.
49. Moon JS, Shim JC, Suh JS, Lee WC. Radiographic predictability of cartilage damage in medial ankle osteoarthritis. Cin Orthop Relat Res. 2010. doi:10.1007/s11999-010-1352-2.

Chapter 5
Value of CT Arthrography in the Assessment of Cartilage Pathology

Patrick Omoumi, Bruno C. Vande Berg, and Frédéric E. Lecouvet

Keywords CT arthrography • MR arthrography • Cartilage lesions • Osteochondral lesions • Chondral repair

Introduction

Intraarticular contrast material has long been used to delineate cartilage lesions with X-rays. The first reports of arthrography date back to 1905 [1]. Attempts were made to overcome the inherent limitations of arthrography (due to the projection of three-dimensional structures on a plane), using tomographic techniques [2] and various projections [3]. The advent of computed tomography (CT) enabled arthrography to develop further. First reported in 1979 for the study of cruciate ligaments [4], computed tomographic arthrography (CT arthrography) was very early proved to be useful for the study of cartilage [5–7]. Although magnetic resonance imaging (MRI) is now considered to be the technique of choice for the assessment of the structure of cartilage (including biochemical analysis) and intrachondral lesions [8, 9], CT arthrography gained new interest with the advent of multidetector computer tomography (MDCT). This technique provides true isotropic imaging, with the possibility of high-resolution multiplanar reformatting [10]. It thus allows the evaluation of the entire joint cartilage and not only of cartilage areas perpendicular to the acquisition plane as with conventional CT arthrography [11]. In comparison to magnetic resonance imaging arthrography (MR arthrography), studies have shown that CT arthrography is at least as accurate, sensitive, and specific for the evaluation of cartilage thickness [12, 13], surface cartilage lesions, and cartilage loss [14, 15].

F.E. Lecouvet (✉)
Department of Radiology and Medical Imaging, Cliniques Universitaires Saint-Luc – UCLouvain, Avenue Hippocrate 10/2942, B-1200, Brussels, Belgium
e-mail: frederic.lecouvet@uclouvain.be

CT arthrography is indicated for the study of joint surfaces whenever MR arthrography cannot be performed, either because it is less available as in some countries, or contraindicated, or technically impossible (e.g., with obese or claustrophobic patients; presence of metallic hardware) [16]. Its main drawbacks remain, however, the exposition to ionizing radiation and the need for a joint puncture.

In this chapter, the technical aspects of the CT arthrography examinations for various joints, including pitfalls and limitations, as well as its most common indications are reviewed.

Technical Considerations

Type of Contrast Material

CT arthrography can be performed either using a single-contrast or a double-contrast method (iodinated contrast material and air). Air was used in the past to distend the joint space at conventional arthrography. With the advent of CT, distension of the joint space is no longer necessary. Furthermore, air does not penetrate cartilage lesions as well as fluid does. Finally, the use of intraarticular air decreases the contrast between the injected joint cavity and the low attenuating cartilage in comparison to intraarticular iodine. Thus, the single-contrast method using iodine, easier to perform [16, 17] and less painful [18], is now favored in most institutions.

Once injected in the joint, the concentration of iodinated contrast material decreases within minutes by diffusion into the cartilage and synovium, by resorption, and by fluid influx into the joint [19]. Thus, the CT examination has to be performed preferably within 30 min after the injection. To slow down the concentration decrease of the contrast material and to gain some flexibility in patient management, it is possible to use dimeric contrast agents, which have a slower resorption rate than monomeric contrast agents [20]. Another possibility is to add epinephrine to the injected contrast material

T.M. Link (ed.), *Cartilage Imaging: Significance, Techniques, and New Developments*, DOI 10.1007/978-1-4419-8438-8_5, © Springer Science+Business Media, LLC 2011

(for instance, by mixing 1 ml of a 0.1% solution containing 1 mg of epinephrine with 10 ml of contrast material) [21–23]. However, the use of epinephrine may increase postarthrographic morbidity [18], and given that the examination time is much faster with MDCT arthrography, epinephrine is rarely used.

To avoid beam-hardening artifacts, dilution of the contrast material can be performed with local anesthetics or saline. However, there is no established consensus on the need for dilution, which mainly depends on the radiologist preferences [15, 24–29]. If joint effusion is present, it can be aspirated to avoid significant dilution of the contrast material. If the CT arthrography does not provide any evident "mechanical" explanation for the effusion, the aspirated fluid can be sent for laboratory analysis to search for articular infection or crystal deposition.

Injection Procedures

Prior to injection, contraindications such as history of allergic reactions to contrast material, surrounding soft tissue infections and coagulation problems have to be ruled out.

The volume of injected contrast material necessary for proper capsular distension varies according to the joint and is the same as for other arthrographic techniques. As a rule, adequate distension is indicated by increased resistance to injection or retrograde flow of contrast material into the needle after disconnection of the syringe [30]. The injection should also be stopped if pain is generated.

Fluoroscopy is the most widely used guidance modality for articular puncture [27, 30]. However, many other injection techniques have been described, either image-guided, using CT [27, 31] ultrasound [32–35], or MRI [36] or by using surface anatomical landmarks [37–39]. The efficacy of the various guidance modalities has rarely been compared in the literature [34], and the choice of the guidance modality mainly relies on the radiologist's preference and on the equipment available. The injection is performed under aseptic conditions, following standard approaches, which have been widely described in the literature [40–42].

Usefulness of Conventional Radiographs Performed After the Injection

Before the injection of the contrast material, conventional radiographs are obtained to identify calcific deposition and osteochondral loose bodies. Of course, these radiographs also provide a global assessment of the joint and can orient the diagnosis towards degenerative or inflammatory disorders.

It has been shown that conventional radiographs performed after the injection of contrast material are not necessary in adjunction to CT arthrography for the shoulder, even with single-slice CT [43]. After evaluating 102 double-contrast CT arthrography of the shoulder for cartilage, labral, and rotator cuff lesions, with long-term follow-up for 84 of them, and surgical correlation for 40 of them, these authors have found no findings on postcontrast conventional radiographs that were not visible on either scout radiographs or CT sections. To our knowledge, no study has assessed the added value of postcontrast conventional radiographs to CT arthrography for other joints. Some authors still advise to perform those conventional arthrograms as a diagnostic help in adjunction to the CT examination [16]. One of their theoretical advantages is to detect small loose bodies, which could later become invisible at the CT arthrogram because of their imbibition by the contrast material. However, in our experience, there is little usefulness to those postcontrast conventional radiographs, especially when new advanced post-processing tools are available, with two exceptions. The first is wrist arthrography, for which dynamic conventional radiographs performed on the fluoroscopic table are quite useful for the detection and localization of tears of carpal intrinsic ligaments. Another indication for postinjection radiographs is for regions not imaged at CT for radioprotection purposes, as developed below.

Exercise Prior to CT?

It has been shown for shoulder MR arthrography that exercise has no beneficial or detrimental effect [44]. However, in our practice, we perform active and passive full range articular motion following the injection to allow the contrast material to completely cover cartilage surfaces [45] and enter small cartilage lesions.

Risks

As with any other arthrographic procedure, CT arthrography presents risks linked to the puncture (mainly infectious risks) and to the injected contrast material (allergic reactions) [46]. However, the risk of infection is quite rare: 1 infection out of 25,000 arthrograms as reported by Berquist [47] and 3 cases of iatrogenic septic arthritis out of 126,000 arthrographic procedures according to Newberg et al. [46]. The risk of severe allergic reactions is also low, although minor reactions can occur [47].

Moreover, as with other arthrographic techniques, there is a risk for vasovagal reactions and pain. The best prevention for vasovagal reactions is good communication with the patient and preparation of the injection material out of the patient's sight. Postarthrographic pain typically lasts a few hours to a couple of days and its onset can be delayed [48, 49]. Its cause is not well understood and study results diverge [50]. It may depend on the choice of the iodinated contrast material (its frequency increases when intraarticular air is used [18], or with ionic contrast materials, probably due to a higher sodium content) [18, 20, 24]. It may also depend on the use of epinephrine [18, 51], which may increase synovial irritation and subsequent pain by prolonging the contact of the contrast material with the synovium [51]. In general, the arthrographic procedure is well tolerated by patients. In the case of MR arthrography, Blanchard et al. showed that patients did not prefer MR imaging alone to arthrography [52]. In another study on MR arthrography, Binkert et al. showed that the discomfort generated by the articular puncture was better tolerated than the discomfort generated by the MRI examination that followed [53]. However, CT examinations being much faster, these conclusions may not be applicable to CT arthrography.

Besides those risks, the main drawback of CT arthrography compared to MRI and MR arthrography is the exposure of patients to ionizing radiation.

Acquisition Parameters

Care has thus to be taken to keep the radiation doses as low as possible, especially when scanning areas are close to radiosensitive organs such as shoulders (thyroid) and hips (gonads). This is however at the expense of signal to noise ratio (SNR). The area covered must be minimized as for the knee, where the supra-patellar recess is usually not scanned. Synovial and intraarticular conditions in this region will be depicted on early lateral radiographs covering the areas not imaged by CT. These radiographs should be performed before the imbibition occurs, masking synovial masses.

CT acquisition parameters include a narrow collimation, low pitch values, and a high milliampere-second value to obtain high-resolution isotropic multiplanar reformats (MPR) [54]. The use of bone algorithms provides high spatial resolution reformats. Bone windows are used to view the images. Post-processing of these high-resolution isotropic images may include curved and maximum intensity projection reformatting. Signal to noise ratio can be increased by retrospectively increasing the thickness of the reformats and using soft tissue algorithms [55, 56], however, at the expense of spatial resolution.

Limitations

The main limitation of CT arthrography compared to MRI and MR arthrography is its inability to detect purely intrachondral lesions, which are lesions that do not communicate with the cartilage surface. In contrast, those lesions can be seen on the fluid sensitive sequences such as fast spin echo intermediate- and T2-weighted sequences that are usually performed during MR arthrography along with T1-weighted sequences.

Findings

Normal Aspect of Cartilage

At CT arthrography, normal hyaline cartilage appears as a low attenuating structure well delimited by the high attenuating subchondral bone plate on one side and the contrast material filling the joint on the other side.

The surface of cartilage is smooth, with some physiological defects, such as the glenoid central defect or "bare spot," the trochlear notch and the pseudodefect of the capitellum at the elbow (Fig. 5.1), and the stellate lesion in the acetabulum. It is important to know these defects in order to differentiate them from cartilage loss [57, 58]. Besides those focal physiological defects, some intraarticular epiphyseal areas are physiologically not covered by cartilage (bare areas).

The internal structure of cartilage does not present any variation in its density at CT arthrography, and purely intrachondral lesions cannot be detected [8].

Evaluation of Superficial Chondral Lesions

CT arthrography enables the analysis of focal cartilage lesions with great conspicuity, thanks to the high spatial resolution inherent to the technique and the high attenuation difference between the cartilage and the contrast material delineating the cartilage surface. Lesions can be described according to their appearance on "en face" views as "fissures" if one of the dimensions of the lesion is much higher (Fig. 5.2) or as "ulcers" if it they are more round shaped. The usefulness of this description has, however, not been evaluated. Most of the grading systems of cartilage lesions at CT arthrography are derived from the grading systems used at arthroscopy and are mainly based on the depth of cartilage loss [25, 59–62]. Table 5.1 reports the most widespread classification, which is based on a modified Outerbridge score [60] (Figs. 5.3–5.7).

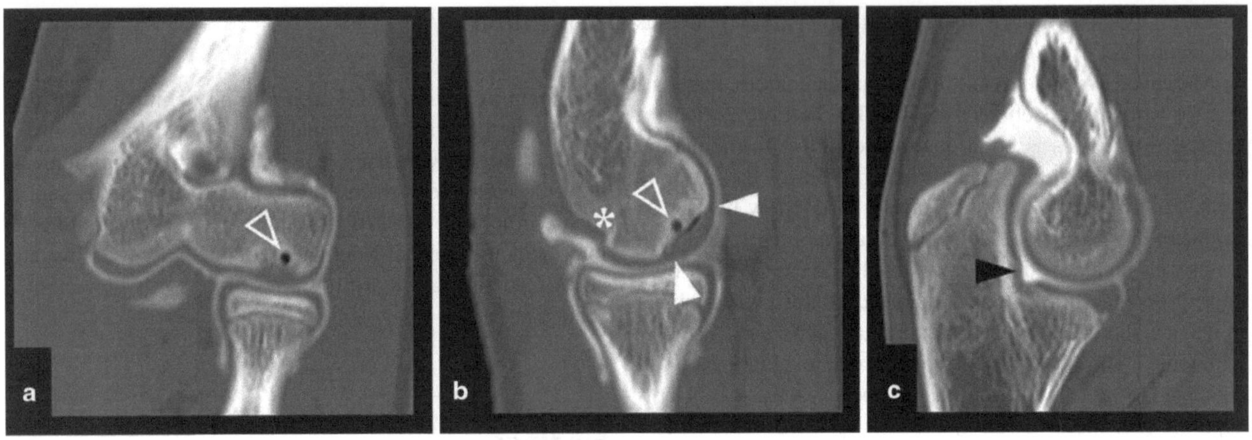

Fig. 5.1 (**a–c**) Computed tomographic (CT) arthrography of a 15-year-old boy presenting with left elbow pain. (**a**) Coronal and (**b**) sagittal reformats show an osteochondral lesion of the anterior aspect of the capitellum (*open arrowheads*), associating thickening and irregularity of cartilage (*white arrowheads*) with an underlying subchondral cyst containing gas (in relation to micromobility). This is suggestive of osteochondritis dissecans. No penetration of contrast material is visible, indicating the absence of extensive dissection (and limited risk of mobilization). The *asterisk* indicates the pseudodefect of the capitellum that should not be mistaken with an osteochondral lesion. (**c**) Sagittal image shows a trochlear notch (*black arrowhead*), another physiological defect

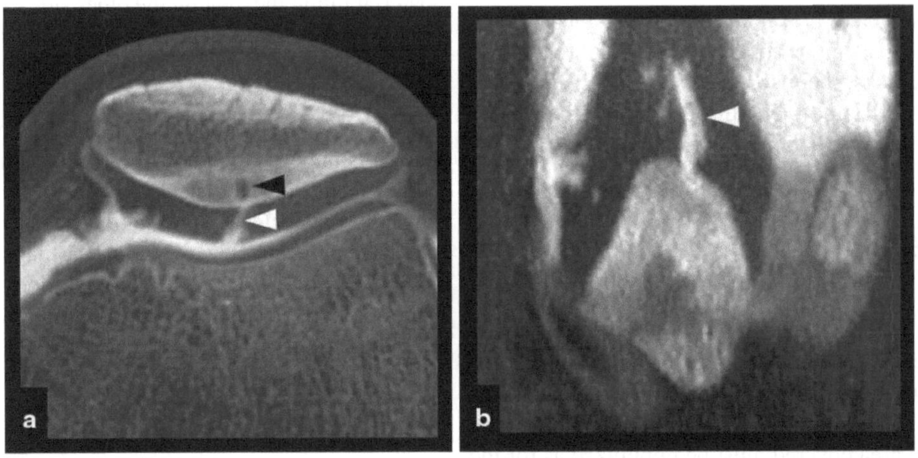

Fig. 5.2 (**a**, **b**) Computed tomographic (CT) arthrography of the knee in a 33-year-old man presenting with a grade 4 cartilage lesion (*white arrowhead*). (**a**) The axial reformat shows contrast product extending into the lesion to the subchondral bone, where an underlying cyst is visible (*black arrow*) (down-to-bone lesion). This lesion is described as a fissure, as seen on (**b**) the coronal multiplanar reformat (MPR) (longitudinal dimension much higher that the transverse dimension)

Table 5.1 Grading systems for cartilage lesions at anhroscoph and computed tomographic (CT) and MR arthrography/based on modified Outerbridge score

Grade	Arthroscopic findings	Computed tomographic (CT) and magnetic resonance (MR) arthrography
Grade 0	Normal	Smooth surface and normal thickness of cartilage
Grade 1	Fibrillation (without cartilage loss) and cartilage softening	Smooth surface and normal thickness of cartilage
Grade 2	Substance loss less than 50% of cartilage thickness	Penetration of contrast in cartilage to less than 50% in depth
Grade 3	Substance loss more than 50% of cartilage thickness but not down-to-bone	Penetration of contrast in cartilage to more than 50% in depth
Grade 4	Down to bone cartilage loss	Penetration of contrast down to subchondral bone

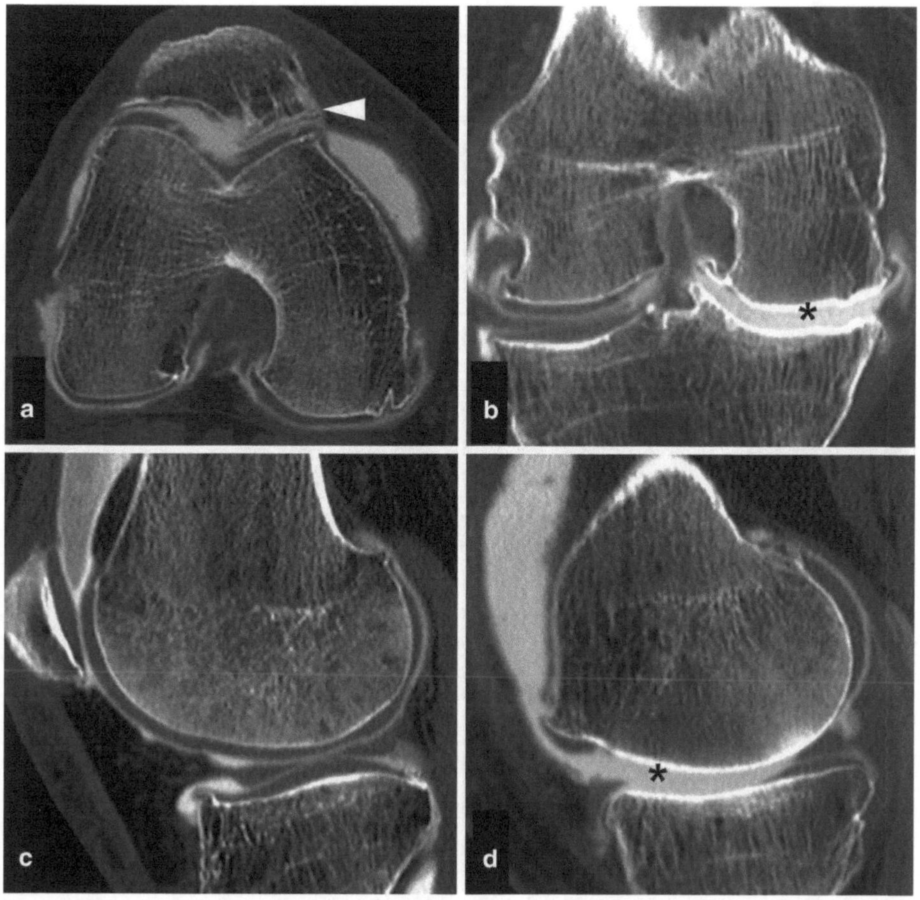

Fig. 5.3 (**a–d**) Preoperative computed tomographic (CT) arthrography of a 72-year-old woman with bi-compartmental osteoarthritis. (**a**) Axial reformat showing the femoro-patellar osteoarthritis, with cartilage loss and osteophytes (*arrowhead*). (**b**) Coronal and (**c, d**) sagittal reformats showing extensive grade 4 cartilage loss in the medial compartment (*asterisks*) associated with subchondral bone sclerosis, with relative sparing of the lateral compartment (**c**)

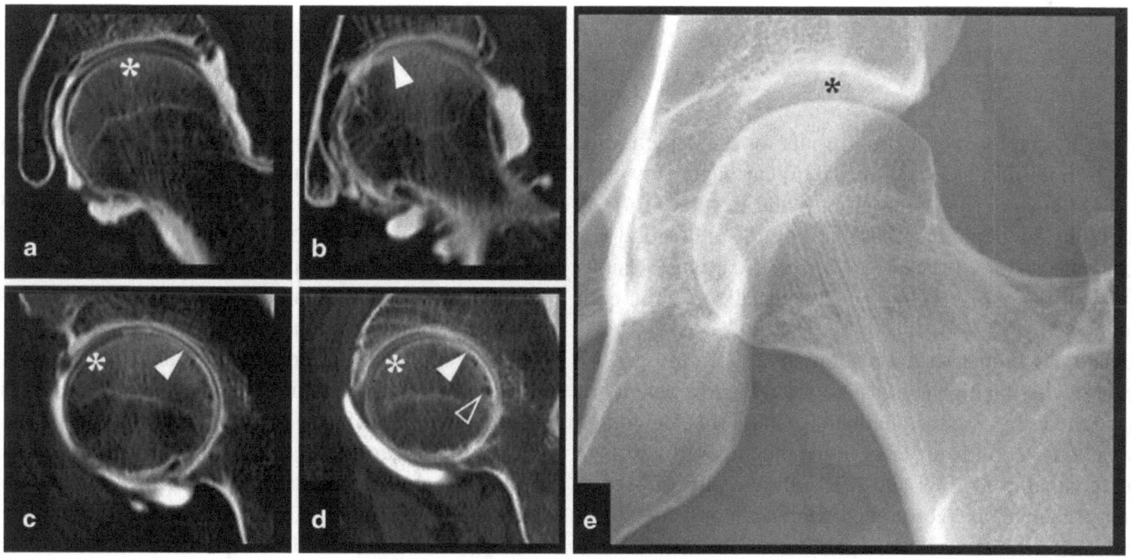

Fig. 5.4 (**a–e**): (**a–d**) Computed tomographic (CT) arthrography of a 69-year-old woman with left hip pain. (**a**) Anterior and (**b**) posterior coronal reformats and (**c, d**) sagittal reformats show no significant damage to the antero-superior portion of femoro-acetabular cartilage (*white asterisks*), where an increasing cartilage thickness gradient exists from the periphery to the center of the femoral head and from the medial to the lateral edge of the acetabulum. There is however an extensive grade 4 cartilage lesion on the posterior aspect of the joint (*arrowheads*). Note associated subchondral bone cysts (*open arrowhead*). (**e**) AP radiograph shows preserved joint space width (*black asterisk*)

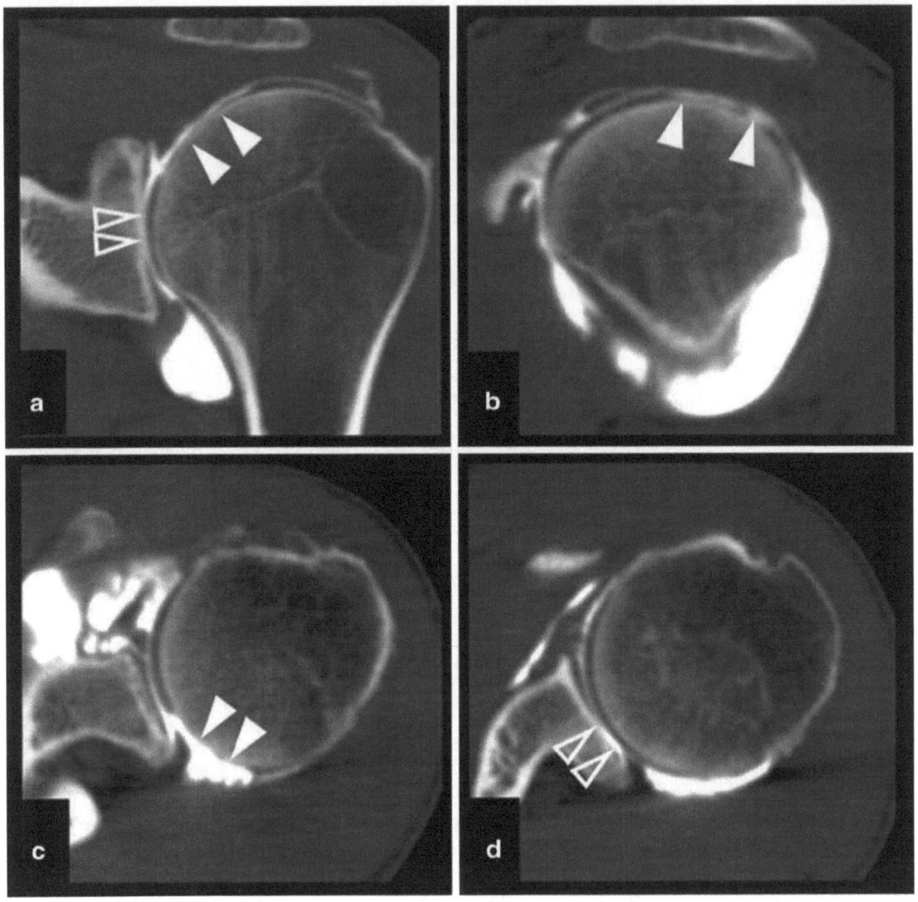

Fig. 5.5 (**a–d**) Computed tomographic (CT) arthrography of the shoulder in a 40-year-old man. (**a**) Coronal, (**b**) sagittal, and (**c**, **d**) axial reformats show extensive grade 4 cartilage lesions of the posterior aspect of humeral head (*arrowheads*) and glenoid cavity (*open arrowheads*)

CT arthrography shows good results for the depiction of lesions of both thin [15] and thick [26] cartilage. However, as with MRI and MR arthrography, the accuracy of CT arthrography at depicting those lesions is only good for higher-grade lesions (grade 2 and above, cartilage lesions without cartilage loss being poorly visualized with both techniques) [14, 15, 63].

To date, the higher spatial resolution of CT arthrography associated with the high contrast between the low density of cartilage and the highly attenuating intraarticular iodine allows a better confidence level in the diagnosis of cartilage lesions compared to MRI and MR arthrography. However, this may change as recent technical developments have contributed to increase the spatial resolution of MRI. A study by Li et al. compared the accuracy of CT arthrography (performed on a 64-slice scanner, with a resolution of $0.35 \times 0.35 \times 0.625\ mm^3$) to high-resolution MR arthrography (performed on a 3T scanner using a 3D sequence providing near isotropic images, with a resolution of $0.29 \times 0.29 \times 0.59\ mm^3$) [64] in assessing grade ≥2 cartilage lesions. This cadaveric study concludes that the two techniques are equally accurate, and no statistical difference in the subjective assessment between the two techniques was observed.

However, another parameter to take into account when comparing the two techniques is the acquisition time and the risk of motion artifacts. Most studies comparing the accuracy of CT arthrography and MR arthrography in assessing cartilage lesions are cadaveric studies. If acquisition times are much longer with MRI than with CT (particularly with the high-resolution 3D MRI sequences, i.e., 9 min 40 s in the study by Li et al.), those sequences might be prone to motion artifacts when applied to patients [8, 26, 28, 64–66].

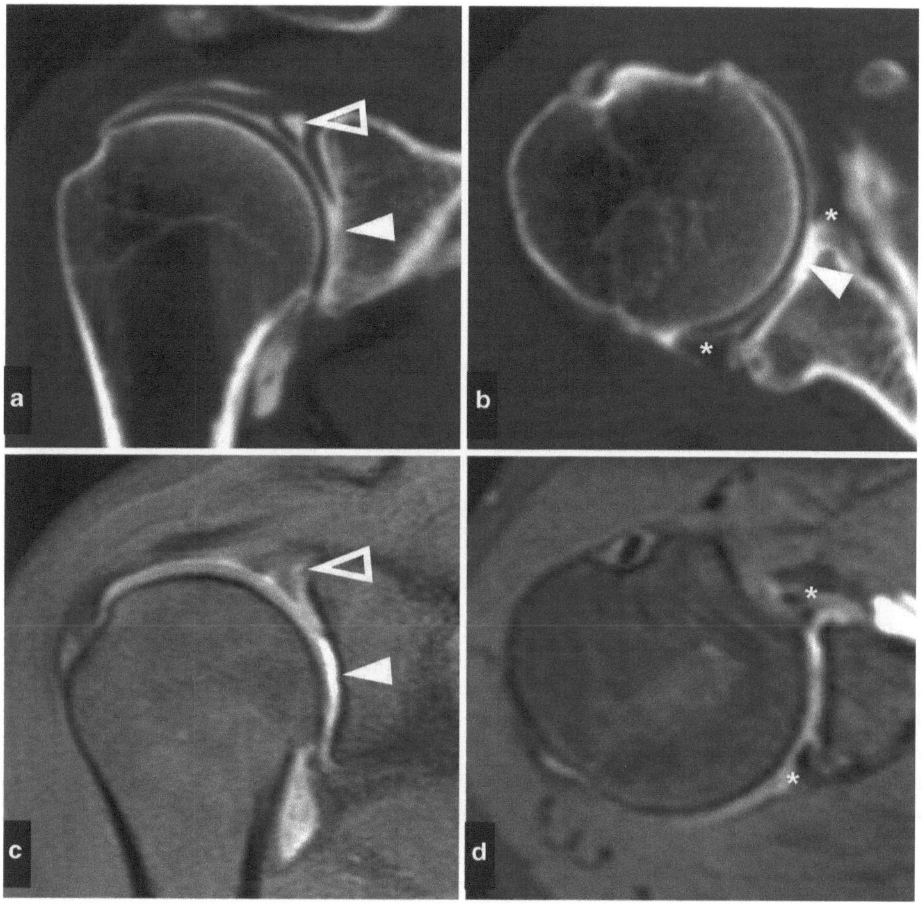

Fig. 5.6 (**a–d**): (**a**, **b**) Computed tomographic (CT) arthrography of the shoulder in a 48-year-old woman shows a grade 4 cartilage lesion of the antero-inferior aspect of the glenoid cavity (*arrowhead*). (**c**, **d**) MR arthrography performed the same day shows the same cartilage lesion (*arrowhead*). A SLAP II lesion (*open arrowhead*) is also visible on the coronal images, more evident on the coronal CT image (**a**), with extension of the tear to the anterior and posterior labrum (*asterisk*)

Evaluation of Cartilage Thickness

CT arthrography can be considered as the technique of choice for the assessment of cartilage thickness. It has been used as a reference in studies evaluating the accuracy of noninvasive MRI sequences to evaluate cartilage thickness [65]. In this regard, CT arthrography is more accurate than cartilage specific MRI sequences such as SPGR as well as MR arthrography, as shown by cadaveric studies on the ankle [12] and the hip [28], respectively. However, CT arthrography measurements can be influenced by some technical factors as recently shown by Anderson et al. in a phantom study [67]. The authors suggest the use of lower contrast material concentration and maximization of joint space by completely filling the joint capsule with diluted contrast material and/or by applying traction to the joint. It should also be stated that a more recent study concluded that multidetector-CT arthrography and MR arthrography are equally accurate in measuring cartilage thickness in the hip joint as far as the coronal plane is concerned [13].

Physiologically, the thickness of cartilage is highly variable from one individual to another, from one joint to another, and from one area of the joint to another. This is particularly true for the knee where the cartilage is usually thicker in areas with concave subchondral bone and thinner in areas adjacent to the menisci [68]. In the hip joint, an increasing cartilage thickness gradient exists from the periphery to the center of the femoral head and from the medial to the lateral edge of the acetabulum [28] (Fig. 5.4). Inversion of that thickness gradient is an early sign of degenerative osteoarthritis.

Evaluation of the Subchondral Bone

CT arthrography enables excellent analysis of subchondral bone changes associated with cartilage lesions and osteoarthritis, such as subchondral bone sclerosis, subchondral bone cysts, and osteophytes (Figs. 5.1–5.4). It can depict both marginal and central (nonmarginal) osteophytes, associated with more severe changes of osteoarthritis [69, 70]. However, contrary to MRI, it does not allow the assessment of bone marrow.

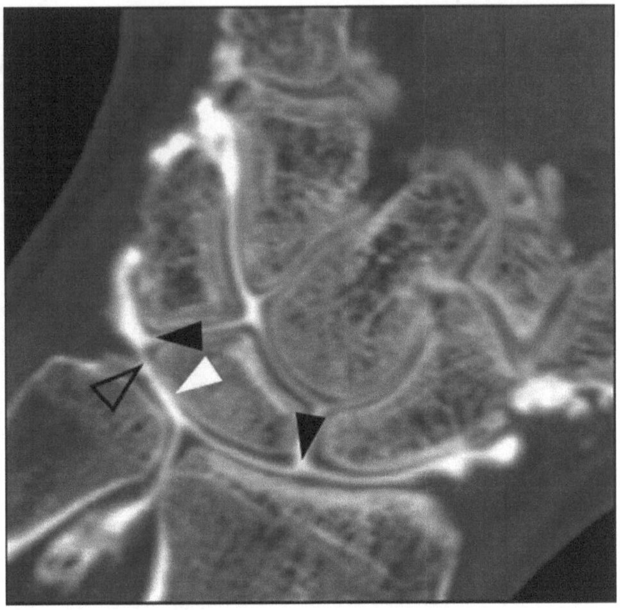

Fig. 5.7 Coronal reformat of a computed tomographic (CT) arthrography of the wrist in a 38-year-old man with a history of trauma shows a grade 4 cartilage lesion of the proximal surface of the lunate (*white arrowhead*). Tear of the interosseous ligaments of the proximal row (*black arrowheads*) and of the TFCC (*open arrowhead*) can also be delineated

Indications of CT Arthrography for the Study of Cartilage

Whenever MR Arthrography Is Not Possible

CT arthrography can be considered as an alternative to MRI whenever the latter technique is not possible or contraindicated. Claustrophobia, obesity, pacemakers, and ear implants represent such instances [16]. This also includes poor access to MRI scanners as in some European countries such as in the authors' countries, where CT arthrography often replaces MRI.

Evaluation of Internal Derangement of the Joints

Whenever MRI is not possible to perform, CT arthrography can be used as a first step for the assessment of causes of internal derangement of many joints. In the shoulder, CT arthrography is valuable in the assessment of rotator cuff lesions, causes of gleno-humeral instability, and isolated labral tears, including SLAP lesions (Fig. 5.6) [17]. For the knee, CT arthrography is valuable for meniscal injuries, as well as ligamental injuries, especially the ACL [14]. In the elbow, CT arthrography is as accurate as MRI in diagnosing complete tears of the ulnar collateral ligament preoperatively, and it is more accurate in evaluating partial undersurface tears [71]. In the wrist, CT arthrography has shown very good results for the study of interosseous carpal ligaments and the TFCC, in reference to arthroscopy [72] or visual inspection in cadavers [73]. As shown by Schmid et al., the performance of CT arthrography in detecting tears of the different segments of the scapholunate and lunotriquetral ligaments is at least equal or superior to MRI, wtj better interobserver reliability [73] (Fig. 5.7). Bony abnormalities of the wrist are also well visualized with CT arthrography [74]. In the hip, CT arthrography is accurate in detecting acetabular labral tears [75] in correlation to arthroscopy.

However, the main limitation of CT arthrography in comparison to MRI for the diagnosis of internal derangements of joints is in the assessment of lesions in soft tissues that do not communicate with the articular cavity, such as most tendinous lesions around the ankle [76].

When performed for these indications, CT arthrography can accurately diagnose cartilage lesions, sometimes as the only cause of the symptoms [77].

Preoperative Work-up of Osteoarthritis and Osteochondral Lesions, for Both Thick and Thin Cartilage

CT arthrography can accurately assess the extension and grade of cartilage lesions of both thick and thin cartilage. It is a valuable tool in the preoperative work-up of knee arthroplasty to diagnose the number of compartments that

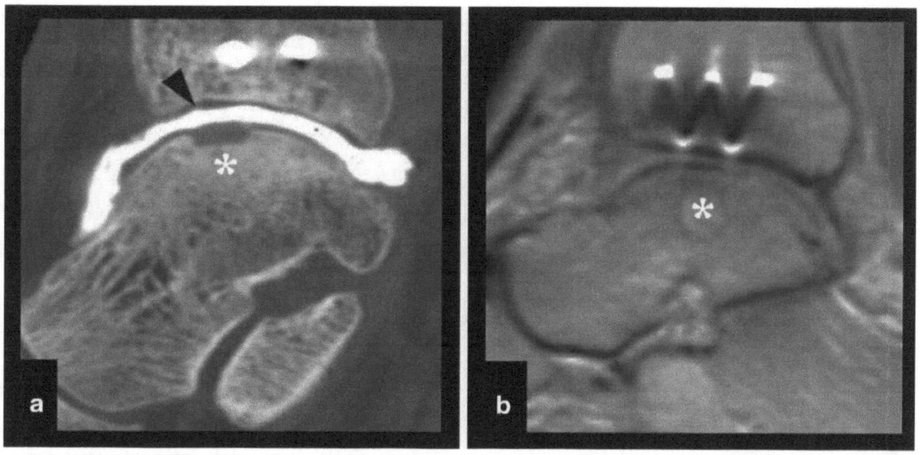

Fig. 5.8 (**a**, **b**) Forty-year-old man with a history of traumatic osteochondral lesion of the talus, treated with osteochondral graft. (**a**) The follow-up computed tomographic (CT) arthrography of the ankle shows the osteochondral graft (*asterisk*) covered by continuous fibrocartilaginous tissue. The tibial articular cartilage is irregular (*black arrowhead*). The metallic artifacts are much less prominent on the CT image compared to (**b**) the PD-weighted magnetic resonance imaging (MRI) image, where articular cartilage is difficult to evaluate

have to be replaced and to plan the type of the prosthesis (unicompartmental vs. total) (Fig. 5.3).

Postoperative Patients

One of the advantages of CT arthrography compared to MRI and MR arthrography is its lower sensitivity to metallic artifacts, which can be diminished using soft tissue reconstruction algorithms and multiplanar reformatting. This makes CT arthrography more suitable for postoperative patients who have metallic hardware near the joint [16, 78] (Fig. 5.8). For the knee, CT arthrography is also proved to accurately diagnose recurrent meniscal tears, a frequent cause of secondary osteoarthritis and frequent diagnostic issue [14, 21, 26].

Follow-up of Chondral Repair

Thanks to its ability to accurately assess the thickness of cartilage, delineate its surface, and visualize subchondral bony changes, CT arthrography is a technique of choice for the follow-up of cartilage repair techniques such as microfracture, chondral drilling, autologous chondrocyte implantation, and osteochondral grafting (Figs. 5.8 and 5.9). This is especially true for extremity joints, where radiation exposure of radiosensitive organs is less of a problem. However, there is little literature on the role of CT arthrography in the evaluation of cartilage repair.

Accurate Evaluation of Cartilage Thickness

As seen above, CT arthrography is considered the most accurate method in evaluating cartilage thickness, in the setting of research studies for instance [12, 13, 28].

Conclusion

CT arthrography allows good assessment of the cartilage surface and thickness. It allows accurate evaluation of cartilage loss for almost all joints, either with thick or thin cartilage.

CT arthrography can be used whenever MRI is not available or cannot be performed for the purpose of cartilage evaluation, either pre- or postoperatively. In addition to cartilage lesions, it has the potential to assess many other causes of internal derangement of joints. Its main limitation remains the inability to assess purely intrachondral lesions, while its weaknesses are radiation exposure and the need for joint puncture.

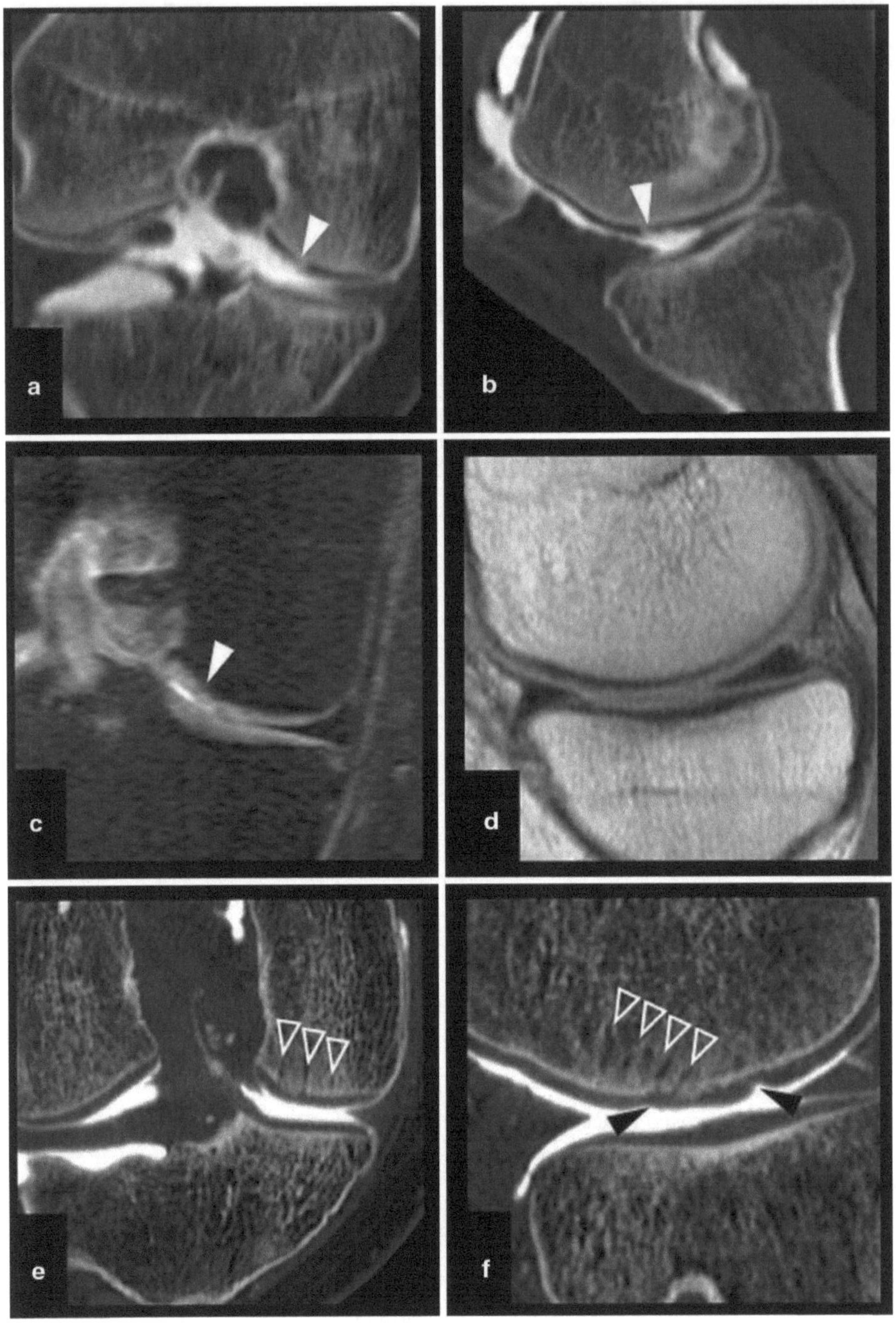

Fig. 5.9 (**a**–**f**) Thirty-five-year-old woman with a history of knee trauma. (**a**) Coronal and (**b**) sagittal reformats of computed tomographic (CT) arthrography show a grade 4 cartilage lesion of the medial femoral condyle. (**c**) Coronal DP-weighted fat-suppressed image and (**d**) sagittal DP-weighted magnetic resonance (MR) image shows signal abnormality of the femoral cartilage, but the grade of the lesion is difficult to define. (**e**) Coronal and (**f**) sagittal reformats from postoperative CT arthrography show signs of drilling in the subchondral bone, with overlying fibrocartilaginous repair tissue (*black arrowheads*)

References

1. Werndorff KR, Robinson I. Ueber intraarticulaere und interstitielle Sauerstoff – Insufflation zu radiologischen, diagnostischen und therapeutischen Zwecken. Verhandlungen der deutschen Roentgengesellschaft fuer orthopaedische Chirurgie (4th Congress) 1905.
2. Anderson PW, Maslin P. Tomography applied to knee arthrography. Radiology. 1974;110(2):271–5.
3. Maldague B, Malghem J. Le faux profil rotulien ou profil vrai des facettes rotuliennes. Ann Radiol. 1976;19:573–81.
4. Pavlov H, Hirschy JC, Torg JS. Computed tomography of the cruciate ligaments. Radiology. 1979;132(2):389–93.
5. Boven F, Bellemans MA, De Boeck H, Potvliege R. The value of computed tomography scanning in chondromalacia patellae. Skeletal Radiol. 1982;8(3):183–5.
6. Boven F, Bellemans MA, Geurts I, Potvliege R. A comparative study of the patello-femoral joint on axial roentgenogram, axial arthrogram, and computed tomography following arthrography. Skeletal Radiol. 1982;8(3):179–81.
7. Reiser M, Karpf PM, Bernett P. Diagnosis of chondromalacia patellae using CT arthrography. Eur J Radiol. 1982;2(3):181–6.
8. Rand T, Brossmann J, Pedowitz R, Ahn JM, Haghigi P, Resnick D. Analysis of patellar cartilage. Comparison of conventional MR imaging and MR and CT arthrography in cadavers. Acta Radiol (Stockholm, Sweden: 1987). 2000;41(5):492–7.
9. Link TM, Stahl R, Woertler K. Cartilage imaging: motivation, techniques, current and future significance. Eur Radiol. 2007; 17(5):1135–46.
10. Buckwalter K, Rydberg AJ, Kopecky KK, Crow K, Yang EL. Musculoskeletal imaging with multislice CT. Am J Roentgenol. 2001;176(4):979–86.
11. Vande B, Berg BV, Lecouvet FE, Malghem J. Frequency and topography of lesions of the femoro-tibial cartilage at spiral CT arthrography of the knee: a study in patients with normal knee radiographs and without history of trauma. Skeletal Radiol. 2002;31(11):643–9.
12. El-Khoury GY, Alliman KJ, Lundberg HJ, Rudert MJ, Brown TD, Saltzman CL. Cartilage thickness in cadaveric ankles: measurement with double-contrast multi-detector row CT arthrography versus MR imaging. Radiology. 2004;233(3):768–73.
13. Wyler A, Bousson V, Bergot C, Polivka M, Leveque E, Vicaut E, et al. Comparison of MR-arthrography and CT-arthrography in hyaline cartilage-thickness measurement in radiographically normal cadaver hips with anatomy as gold standard. Osteoarthritis Cartilage. 2009;17(1):19–25.
14. Vande Berg BC, Lecouvet FE, Poilvache P, Dubuc JE, Maldague B, Malghem J. Anterior cruciate ligament tears and associated meniscal lesions: assessment at dual-detector spiral CT arthrography. Radiology. 2002;223(2):403–9.
15. Lecouvet F, Dorzée B, Dubuc JE, Vande Berg BC, Jamart J, Malghem J. Cartilage lesions of the glenohumeral joint: diagnostic effectiveness of multidetector spiral CT arthrography and comparison with arthroscopy. Eur Radiol. 2007;17(7):1763–71.
16. Buckwalter KA. CT arthrography. Clin Sports Med. 2006;25(4): 899–915.
17. Lecouvet FE, Simoni P, Koutaïssoff S, Vande Berg BC, Malghem J, Dubuc JE. Multidetector spiral CT arthrography of the shoulder: clinical applications and limits, with MR arthrography and arthroscopic correlations. Eur J Radiol. 2008;68(1):120–36.
18. Hall FM, Goldberg RP, Wyshak G, Kilcoyne RF. Shoulder arthrography: comparison of morbidity after use of various contrast media. Radiology. 1985;154(2):339–41.
19. Obermann WR, Bloem JL, Hermans J. Knee arthrography: comparison of iotrolan and ioxaglate sodium meglumine. Radiology. 1989;173(1):197–201.
20. Blum AG, Simon JM, Cotten A, Quirin-Cosmidis I, Boyer B, Boutry N, et al. Comparison of double-contrast CT arthrography image quality with nonionic contrast agents: isotonic dimeric iodixanol 270 mg I/mL and monomeric iohexol 300 mg I/mL. Investig Radiol. 2000;35(5):304–10.
21. Mutschler C, Vande Berg BC, Lecouvet FE, Poilvache P, Dubuc J-E, Maldague B, et al. Postoperative meniscus: assessment at dual-detector row spiral CT arthrography of the knee. Radiology. 2003; 228(3):635–41.
22. Spataro RF, Katzberg RW, Burgener FA, Fischer HW. Epinephrine enhanced knee arthrography. Investig Radiol. 1978;13(4): 286–90.
23. Hall FM. Epinephrine-enhanced knee arthrography. Radiology. 1974;111(1):215–7.
24. Railhac JJ. Iopentol (Imagopaque® 300) compared with ioxaglate (Hexabrix® 320) in knee arthrography. A clinical trial assessing immediate and late adverse events and diagnostic information. Eur Radiol. 1997;7:S135–9.
25. Daenen BR, Ferrara MA, Marcelis S, Dondelinger RF. Evaluation of patellar cartilage surface lesions: comparison of CT arthrography and fat-suppressed FLASH 3D MR imaging. Eur Radiol. 1998;8(6):981–5.
26. Vande Berg BC, Lecouvet FE, Poilvache P, Jamart J, Materne R, Lengele B, et al. Assessment of knee cartilage in cadavers with dual-detector spiral CT arthrography and MR imaging. Radiology. 2002;222(2):430–6.
27. Binkert CA, Verdun FR, Zanetti M, Pfirrmann CW, Hodler J. CT arthrography of the glenohumeral joint: CT fluoroscopy versus conventional CT and fluoroscopy – comparison of image-guidance techniques. Radiology. 2003;229(1):153–8.
28. Wyler A, Bousson V, Bergot C, Polivka M, Leveque E, Vicaut E, et al. Hyaline cartilage thickness in radiographically normal cadaveric hips: comparison of spiral CT arthrographic and macroscopic measurements. Radiology. 2007;242(2):441–9.
29. Noël C, Campagna R, Minoui A, Thévenin F, Richarme D, Feydy A, et al. Fissures of the posterior labrum and associated lesions: CT arthrogram evaluation. J Radiol. 2008;89(4):487–93.
30. Jacobson JA, Lin J, Jamada DA, Hayes CW. Aids to successful shoulder arthrography performed with a fluoroscopically guided anterior approach. Radiographics. 2003;23(2):373–8.
31. Mulligan ME. CT-guided shoulder arthrography at the rotator cuff interval. Am J Roentgenol. 2008;191(2):W58–61.
32. Lohman M, Vasenius J. Ultrasound guidance for puncture and injection in the radiocarpal joint. Acta Radiol (Stockholm, Sweden: 1987). 2007;48(7):744–7.
33. Koivikko MP, Mustonen AOT. Shoulder magnetic resonance arthrography: a prospective randomized study of anterior and posterior ultrasonography-guided contrast injections. Acta Radiol (Stockholm, Sweden: 1987). 2008;49(8):912–7.
34. Rutten M, Collins J, Maresch B, Smeets J, Janssen C, Kiemeney L, et al. Glenohumeral joint injection: a comparative study of ultrasound and fluoroscopically guided techniques before MR arthrography. Eur Radiol. 2009;19(3):722–30.
35. Souza PM, Aguiar RO, Marchiori E, Bardoe SA. Arthrography of the shoulder: a modified ultrasound guided technique of joint injection at the rotator interval. Eur J Radiol. 2010;74(3):e29–32.
36. Petersilge CA, Lewin JS, Duerk JL, Hatem SF. MR arthrography of the shoulder: rethinking traditional imaging procedures to meet the technical requirements of MR imaging guidance. AJR Am J Roentgenol. 1997;169(5):1453–7.
37. DeMouy EH, Menendez CV, Bodin CJ. Palpation-directed (non-fluoroscopically guided) saline-enhanced MR arthrography of the shoulder. AJR Am J Roentgenol. 1997;169(1):229–31.
38. Berná-Serna JD, Redondo MV, Martínez F, Reus M, Alonso J, Parrilla A, et al. A simple technique for shoulder arthrography. Acta Radiol (Stockholm, Sweden: 1987). 2006;47(7):725–9.

39. Catalano OA, Manfredi R, Vanzulli A, Tomei E, Napolitano M, Esposito A, et al. MR arthrography of the glenohumeral joint: modified posterior approach without imaging guidance. Radiology. 2007;242(2):550–4.
40. Freiberger RH. Arthrography. Upper Saddle River: Prentice Hall; 1979.
41. Chevrot A, Pallardy G. Arthrographies opaques. Paris: Masson; 1988.
42. Crim J. Arthrography: principles and practice in radiology: published by Amirsys®. Philadelphia: Lippincott Williams & Wilkins; 2008.
43. Wilson AJ, Totty WG, Murphy WA, Hardy DC. Shoulder joint: arthrographic CT and long-term follow-up, with surgical correlation. Radiology. 1989;173(2):329–33.
44. Brenner ML, Morrison WB, Carrino JA, Nusser CA, Sanders TG, Howard RF, et al. Direct MR arthrography of the shoulder: is exercise prior to imaging beneficial or detrimental? Radiology. 2000;215(2):491–6.
45. Vande Berg BC, Lecouvet FE, Poilvache P, Maldague B, Malghem J. Spiral CT arthrography of the knee: technique and value in the assessment of internal derangement of the knee. Eur Radiol. 2002;12(7):1800–10.
46. Newberg AH, Munn CS, Robins AH. Complications of arthrography. Radiology. 1985;155(3):605–6.
47. Berquist TH. Imaging of articular pathology: MRI, CT, arthrography. Clin Anat (New York, NY). 1997;10(1):1–13.
48. Cerezal L, Abascal F, Garcia-Valtuille R, Canga A. Ankle MR arthrography: how, why, when. Radiol Clin North Am. 2005;43(4):693–707.
49. Saupe N, Zanetti M, Pfirrmann CW, Wels T, Schwenke C, Hodler J. Pain and other side effects after MR arthrography: prospective evaluation in 1085 patients. Radiology. 2009;250(3):830–8.
50. Binkert CA, Zanetti M, Gerber C, Hodler J. MR arthrography of the glenohumeral joint: two concentrations of gadoteridol versus ringer solution as the intraarticular contrast material. Radiology. 2001;220(1):219–24.
51. Corbetti F, Malatesta V, Camposampiero A, Mazzi A, Punzi L, Angelini F, et al. Knee arthrography: effects of various contrast media and epinephrine on synovial fluid. Radiology. 1986;161(1):195–8.
52. Blanchard TK, Bearcroft PW, Dixon AK, Lomas DJ, Teale A, Constant CR, et al. Magnetic resonance imaging or arthrography of the shoulder: which do patients prefer? Br J Radiol. 1997;70(836):786–90.
53. Binkert CA, Zanetti M, Hodler J. Patient's assessment of discomfort during MR arthrography of the shoulder. Radiology. 2001;221(3):775–8.
54. Rydberg J, Buckwalter KA, Caldemeyer KS, Phillips MD, Conces Jr DJ, Aisen AM, et al. Multisection CT: scanning techniques and clinical applications. Radiographics. 2000;20(6):1787–806.
55. Tack D, Genevois PA, Baert AL. Radiation dose from adult and pediatric multidetector computed tomography. Berlin: Springer; 2007.
56. Lee M-J, Kim S, Lee SA, Song HT, Huh YM, Kim DH, et al. Overcoming artifacts from metallic orthopedic implants at high-field-strength MR imaging and multi-detector CT. Radiographics. 2007;27(3):791–803.
57. Rosenberg Z, Beltran J, Cheung YY. Pseudodefect of the capitellum: potential MR imaging pitfall. Radiology. 1994;191(3):821–3.
58. Resnick D, Kang H, Pretterklieber ML. Internal derangements of joints, vol. 2. Amsterdam: Elsevier; 2007.
59. Noyes FR, Stabler CL. A system for grading articular cartilage lesions at arthroscopy. Am J Sports Med. 1989;17(4):505–13.
60. Outerbridge RE. The etiology of chondromalacia patellae. J Bone Joint Surg Br Vol. 1961;43-B:752–7.
61. Ihara H. Double-contrast CT arthrography of the cartilage of the patellofemoral joint. Clin Orthop Relat Res. 1985;198:50–5.
62. Kleemann RU, Krocker D, Cedraro A, Tuischer J, Duda GN. Altered cartilage mechanics and histology in knee osteoarthritis: relation to clinical assessment (ICRS Grade). Osteoarthritis Cartilage. 2005;13(11):958–63.
63. Waldt S, Bruegel M, Ganter K, Kuhn V, Link TM, Rummeny EJ, et al. Comparison of multislice CT arthrography and MR arthrography for the detection of articular cartilage lesions of the elbow. Eur Radiol. 2005;15(4):784–91.
64. Li J, Zheng ZZ, Li X, Yu Jk. Three dimensional assessment of knee cartilage in cadavers with high resolution MR-arthrography and MSCT-arthrography. Acad Radiol. 2009;16(9):1049–55.
65. Haubner M, Eckstein F, Schnier M, Lösch A, Sittek H, Becker C, et al. A non-invasive technique for 3-dimensional assessment of articular cartilage thickness based on MRI part 2: Validation using CT arthrography. Magn Reson Imaging. 1997;15(7): 805–13.
66. Berná-Serna JD, Martínez F, Reus M, Alonso J, Doménech GM, Campos M. Evaluation of the triangular fibrocartilage in cadaveric wrists by means of arthrography, magnetic resonance (MR) imaging, and MR arthrography. Acta Radiol (Stockholm, Sweden: 1987). 2007;48(1):96–103.
67. Anderson AE, Ellis BJ, Peters CA, Weiss JA. Cartilage thickness: factors influencing multidetector ct measurements in a phantom study. Radiology. 2008;246(1):133–41.
68. Vande Berg BC, Lecouvet FE, Poilvache P, Maldague B, Malghem J. Spiral CT arthrography of the postoperative knee. Semin Musculoskelet Radiol. 2002;6(1):47–55.
69. McCauley TR, Kornaat PR, Jee WH. Central osteophytes in the knee: prevalence and association with cartilage defects on MR imaging. Am J Roentgenol. 2001;176(2):359–64.
70. Guermazi A, Burstein D, Conaghan P, Eckstein F, Hellio Le Graverand-Gastineau MP, Keen H, et al. Imaging in osteoarthritis. Rheum Dis Clin North Am. 2008;34(3):645–87.
71. Timmerman LA, Schwartz ML, Andrews JR. Preoperative evaluation of the ulnar collateral ligament by magnetic resonance imaging and computed tomography arthrography. Evaluation in 25 baseball players with surgical confirmation. Am J Sports Med. 1994;22(1):26–31.
72. Theumann N, Favarger N, Schnyger P, Meuli R. Wrist ligament injuries: value of post-arthrography computed tomography. Skeletal Radiol. 2001;30(2):88–93.
73. Schmid MR, Schertler T, Pfirrmann CW, Saupe N, Manestar M, Wildermuth S, et al. Interosseous ligament tears of the wrist: comparison of multi-detector row CT arthrography and MR imaging. Radiology. 2005;237(3):1008–13.
74. Moser T, Dosch J-C, Moussaoui A, Buy X, Gangi A, Dietemann JL. Multidetector CT arthrography of the wrist joint: how to do it. Radiographics. 2008;28(3):787–800.
75. Nishii T, Tanaka H, Sugano N, Miki H, Takao M, Yoshikawa H. Disorders of acetabular labrum and articular cartilage in hip dysplasia: evaluation using isotropic high-resolutional CT arthrography with sequential radial reformation. Osteoarthritis Cartilage. 2007;15(3):251–7.
76. Schmid MR, Notzli HP, Zanetti M, Wyss TF, Hodler J. Cartilage lesions in the hip: diagnostic effectiveness of MR arthrography. Radiology. 2003;226(2):382–6.
77. Guntern DV, Pfirrmann CWA, Schmid MR, Zanetti M, Binkert CA, Schneeberger AG, et al. Articular cartilage lesions of the glenohumeral joint: diagnostic effectiveness of MR arthrography and prevalence in patients with subacromial impingement syndrome. Radiology. 2003;226(1):165–70.
78. Vande Berg B, Malghem J, Maldague B, Lecouvet FE. Multidetector CT imaging in the postoperative orthopedic patient with metal hardware. Eur J Radiol. 2006;60(3):470–9.

Chapter 6
MRI of Cartilage: Standard Techniques

Thomas M. Link

Keywords MRI • Cartilage • Standard techniques • MR arthrography • Field strength • dGEMRIC • Sequence protocol • T1rho quantification • T2 quantification • 3D SPGR • FLASH sequences

Magnetic resonance imaging (MRI) is the only imaging technique that allows direct visualization of cartilage with sufficient contrast. However, cartilage imaging is challenging and MRI needs to be tailored to best visualize cartilage morphology, which includes using scanners with adequate field strength, coils which allow high spatial resolution imaging, and optimized imaging sequences. Also MRI should not only allow to assess cartilage morphology but also abnormalities of tissues which are affected by cartilage damage or which may cause accelerated cartilage loss including abnormalities of the menisci, ligaments, and bone marrow. Among these tissues cartilage clearly has an outstanding role in joint degeneration and osteoarthritis; imaging is also most challenging in terms of required signal-to-noise ratio (SNR), spatial resolution, and contrast. Requirements for cartilage imaging therefore dictate overall requirements in terms of hardware and sequence profiles in degenerative joint disease, injury, and inflammatory arthropathies.

This chapter will focus on the required MR techniques for cartilage imaging, which include (i) field strength considerations, analyzing scanners with different field strengths from 0.2 to 7 T, (ii) review of coil technology, and (iii) analysis of sequence protocols and their role for imaging of cartilage and the tissues affected by cartilage damage.

Field Strength

Low-Field Scanners

Considerations concerning field strength should always take into account that cartilage imaging requires high signal-to-noise ratios and spatial resolution to adequately visualize focal cartilage pathology. Previous studies have shown that imaging with low-field strength clearly has limitations in assessing cartilage morphology and is therefore not recommended [1–3]. Woertler et al. [3] compared the diagnostic performance of a dedicated orthopedic MRI system (0.18 T) and a conventional MRI system (1.0 T) in the detection of articular cartilage lesions created in an animal model. Using receiver operating characteristics (ROC) analysis with three different radiologists these investigators found that the high-field system demonstrated a significantly better diagnostic performance than the low-field system in the detection of less than full thickness articular cartilage lesions ($P < 0.001$). Ahn et al. [4] studied cadaver patellae using a 0.2 T extremity-only magnet and found that high-grade cartilaginous lesions could be evaluated reliably with low-field-strength MRI by using a combination of imaging sequences. Limitations, however, were encountered analyzing less than full thickness cartilage lesions. Figure 6.1 shows a coronal T1-weighted image of the knee obtained at 0.2 T demonstrating limited spatial resolution and signal-to-noise ratio. Based on the results of these previous studies which indicate limitations of low-field MR scanners in visualizing less than full thickness cartilage lesions, it is therefore recommended to use MRI scanners with a minimum field strength of 1.0 T to image cartilage.

T.M. Link (✉)
Department of Radiology and Biomedical Imaging,
University of California at San Francisco, 400 Parnassus Avenue, A-367, San Francisco, CA 94131, USA
e-mail: tmlink@radiology.ucsf.edu; Thomas.Link@radiology.ucsf.edu

T.M. Link (ed.), *Cartilage Imaging: Significance, Techniques, and New Developments*,
DOI 10.1007/978-1-4419-8438-8_6, © Springer Science+Business Media, LLC 2011

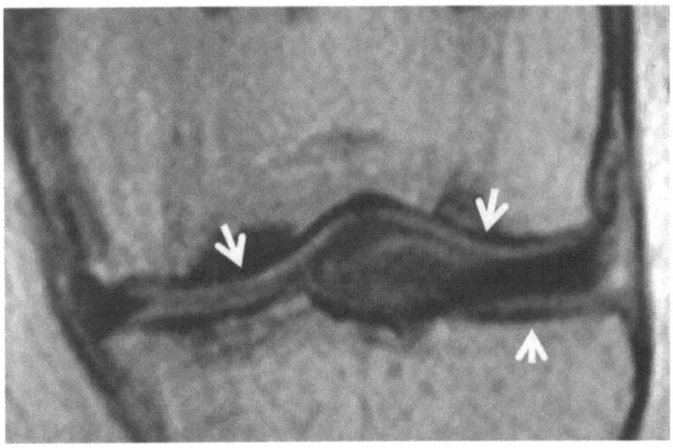

Fig. 6.1 Coronal T1-weighted SE sequence (520/24 ms) of the right knee obtained at 0.2 T with a dedicated extremity scanner in a patient with subchondral bone infarcts. Limitations of image SNR and spatial resolution are clearly demonstrated, which also limits visualization of cartilage abnormalities (*arrows*)

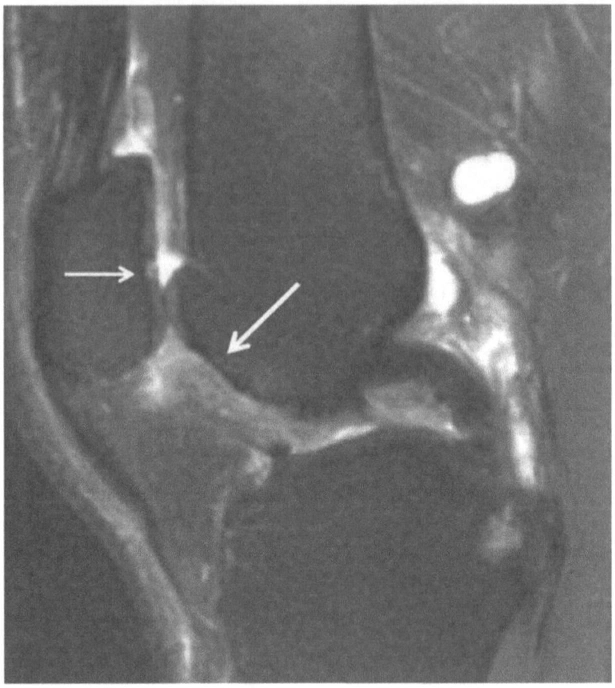

Fig. 6.2 Sagittal MR image (3,200/46 ms; TR/TE) of the knee obtained at 1.5 T in a patient with a focal patellar cartilage defect (*small arrow*) and more diffuse cartilage loss at the trochlea (*large arrow*) demonstrating potential of 1.5 T MRI to clearly depict cartilage lesions

1.5 T MRI

Current standard is 1.5 T imaging and most of the studies establishing MRI for assessment of OA were conducted at this field strength [5–8]. Semiquantitative scores to grade cartilage lesions and techniques to quantify cartilage volume were developed at 1.5 T [6, 9–11]. The early studies analyzing quantitative parameters to characterize the biochemical composition of cartilage such as T2 relaxation time and T1rho mapping as well as delayed Gadolinium-enhanced MRI of cartilage (dGEMRIC) were also performed at 1.5 T [12–14]. Figure 6.2 shows images of the knee with cartilage defects at the trochlea and patella obtained at 1.5 T, indicating the potential of this field strength to clearly visualize cartilage lesions.

3.0 T MRI

Though 1.5 T imaging is standard, a number of studies have demonstrated that 3.0 T MRI allows better visualization of cartilage lesions [15–20] and may therefore be better suited for the overall assessment of focal cartilage abnormalities. Link et al. showed in an animal model that cartilage lesions were better visualized and diagnostic performance improved at 3.0 T compared to 1.5 T using optimized high-resolution MRI sequences. Interestingly, however, standard lower spatial resolution intermediate-weighted fast spin-echo sequences did not improve diagnostic performance at 3.0 T. Figure 6.3 shows two corresponding intermediate-weighted fat-saturated MRI obtained at 1.5 and 3.0 T in a pig knee demonstrating a superficial cartilage defect at the patella, which is better visualized at 3.0 T. While this study was performed at the knee, additional studies performed at human cadaver ankles [15, 16] also showed improved diagnostic performance in assessing cartilage lesions as well as a higher sensitivity for assessing ligamentous and tendon pathology at 3.0 versus 1.5 T.

Recently Kijowski et al. [18, 21] performed a retrospective study to compare the diagnostic performance of 1.5 and 3.0 T MRI protocols for evaluating the articular cartilage of the knee joint in symptomatic patients. Analyzing 241 knee MRI's at 1.5 T and 226 MRI's at 3.0 T, these investigators found that sensitivity, specificity, and accuracy of MRI for detecting cartilage lesions were 69.3%, 78.0%, and 74.5% at 1.5 T and 70.5%, 85.9%, and 80.1% at 3.0 T. The MRI protocol had significantly higher specificity and accuracy ($P<0.05$) but not higher sensitivity ($P=0.73$) for detecting cartilage lesions at 3.0 than at 1.5 T. These investigators concluded that 3.0 T MRI protocols had improved diagnostic performance for evaluating the articular cartilage of the knee joint in symptomatic patients when compared with a 1.5 T protocol. In a similar study Wong et al. [22] compared clinical MR studies of the knee obtained at 1.5 and 3.0 T in the same patients. Four radiologists reviewed each study independently, scored image quality, and analyzed pathological

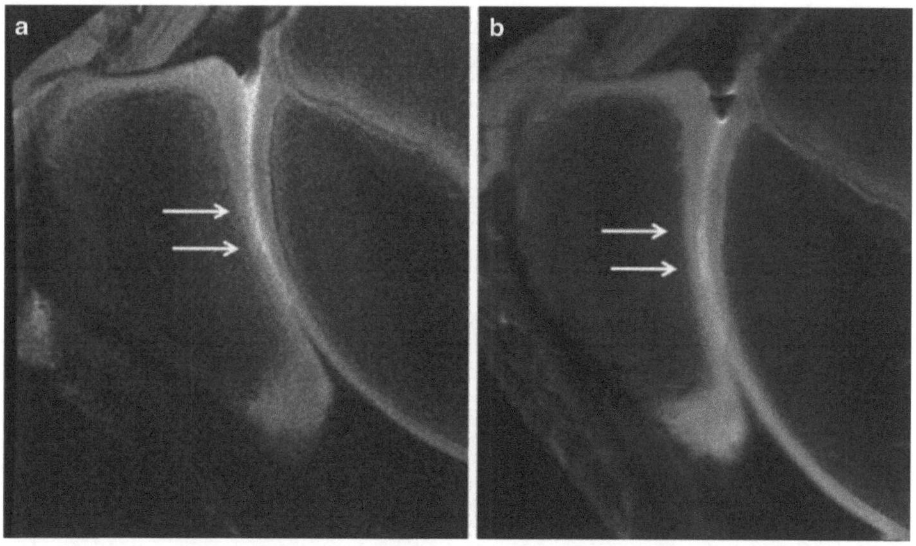

Fig. 6.3 Sagittal MR images of a pig knee with artificially created patellar cartilage defect obtained at 1.5 T (**a**) and 3.0 T (**b**) using fat-suppressed IM-weighted FSE sequences (4,000/35 ms; TR/TE for both 1.5 and 3.0 T). Superficial cartilage defect at the patella (*arrows*) is well shown on the 3.0 T image (**b**) but not well visualized on the 1.5 T image (**a**)

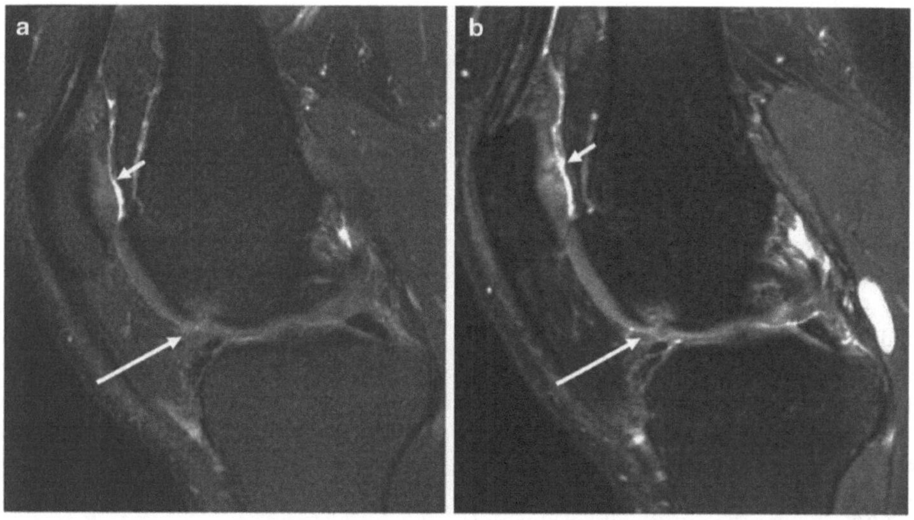

Fig. 6.4 Sagittal MRI of the knee obtained in a middle-aged runner with knee pain at 1.5 T (**a**) and 3.0 T (**b**) using fat-suppressed IM-weighted FSE sequences (3,200/46 and 4,300/51 ms). Cartilage defect at the patella (*small arrow*) and osteochondral lesion at the trochlea (*large arrow*) are better visualized at 3.0 T compared to 1.5 T

findings. Sensitivities, specificities, and accuracies in diagnosing cartilage lesions were calculated in the 19 patients with arthroscopy. Each radiologist scored the 3.0 T studies higher than those obtained at 1.5 T in visualizing anatomical structures and abnormalities ($p < 0.05$). Using arthroscopy as a standard of reference, diagnosis of cartilage abnormalities was improved at 3.0 T with higher sensitivity (75.7% versus 70.6%), accuracy (88.2% versus 86.4%), and correct grading of cartilage lesions (51.3% versus 42.9%). Also diagnostic confidence scores increased at 3.0 T compared to 1.5 T. Figures 6.4 and 6.5 show images obtained at 1.5 and 3.0 T clearly demonstrating improved visualization of cartilage lesions at 3.0 T. In summary these studies demonstrate that focal cartilage lesions are better visualized at 3.0 T though

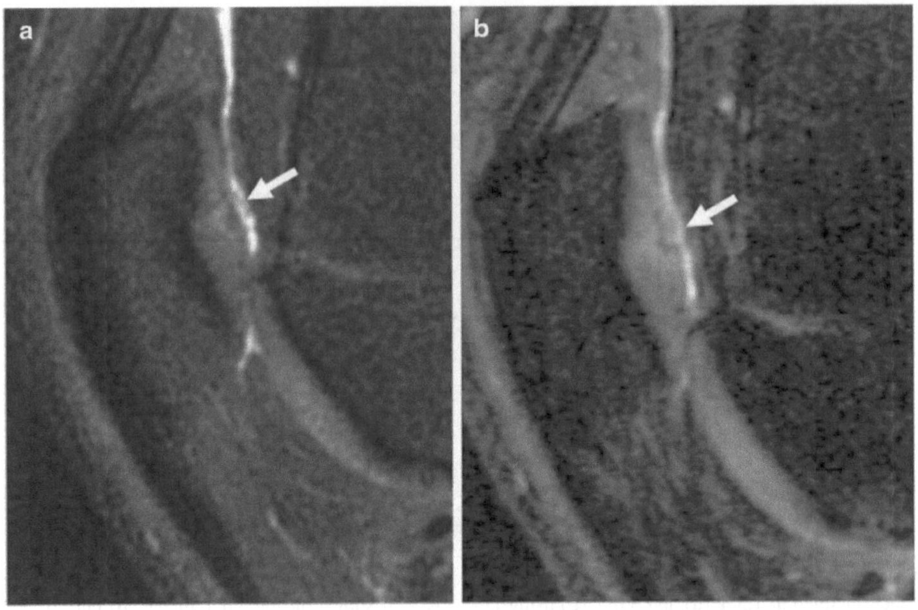

Fig. 6.5 1.5 T (**a**) and 3.0 T (**b**) sagittal fat-suppressed IM-weighted FSE MRI of the patella (3,200/46 and 4,300/51 ms). Fissures at the patella (*arrow*) are shown in greater detail at 3.0 T and the surface of the cartilage is substantially better evaluated at 3.0 T than at 1.5 T

differences in lesion detection between 3.0 and 1.5 T are not dramatic; yet grading of these lesions is substantially improved which may be of significance in preoperative planning of procedures or also eventually for pharmacological interventions.

Bauer et al. [17] compared the precision and accuracy of 3.0 and 1.5 T MRI in the quantification of cartilage volume by using direct volumetric measurements as a reference standard in a cadaver model. These investigators calculated an accuracy error for MRI-based volume calculation at the femur of 5.0% and 3.0% for water excitation and standard fat-suppressed SPGR sequences at 3.0 T versus 16% for the standard fat-suppressed SPGR sequence at 1.5 T. Effective signal-to-noise ratio (SNRE) and effective contrast-to-noise ratio (CNRE) were also substantially improved at 3.0 T. This study provides evidence that cartilage volumetric measurements obtained at 3.0 T are more accurate than those obtained at 1.5 T. Eckstein et al. [23] performed an in vivo study in patients with OA and normal volunteers to also evaluate the precision of quantitative MRI assessments of human cartilage morphology at 3.0 T and to correlate the measurements at 3.0 T with validated measurements at 1.5 T. They found that with a slice thickness of 1.5 mm, measurements at 3.0 T tended to be more reproducible than at 1.5 T and concluded that imaging at 3.0 T may provide superior ability to detect changes in cartilage status over time and to determine responses to treatment with structure-modifying drugs.

To achieve the best possible imaging technique for assessing cartilage and OA the National Institute of Health (NIH) sponsored Osteoarthritis Initiative (OAI) therefore adopted imaging at 3.0 T. The OAI is a nationwide, multicenter research study, which provides a large dataset of clinical information, questionnaires, radiographs, and MRI studies obtained from nearly 5,000 participants (4,796 participants at baseline), who are followed up every 12 months for a period of 48 months. The overall aim of the OAI is to develop a public domain research resource to facilitate the scientific evaluation of biomarkers for OA as potential surrogate endpoints for disease onset and progression. For the OAI, participants who have knee OA (*progression cohort*) and participants who have no symptoms of OA but risk factors (*incidence cohort*) were recruited. The imaging protocol includes morphological and quantitative MRI sequences performed at 3.0 T with five identical scanners from the same manufacturer [24].

7.0 T MRI

To date, MRI at 7.0 T is a research application and only limited studies were performed in human participants [25, 26]. Currently available sequence protocols have not been shown to be superior to 3.0 T in the assessment of cartilage. Future research work clearly will need to focus on developing adequate surface coils and optimized sequences for imaging at 7.0 T. Figure 6.6 shows images obtained at 3.0 and 7.0 T. Image quality is similar; however, increase in chemical shift artifacts and incomplete fat saturation are noted at 7.0 T.

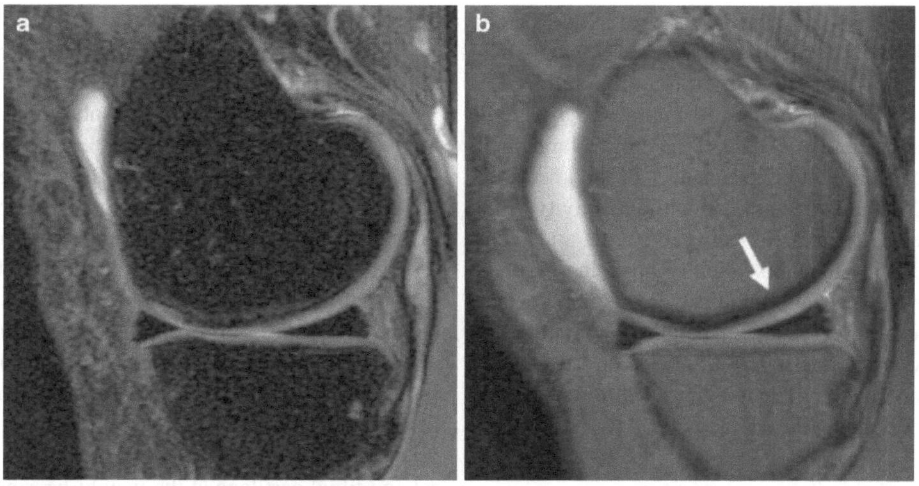

Fig. 6.6 Sagittal fast spin-echo MR images of the knee obtained at 3.0 T (**a**) and 7.0 T (**b**) (4,300/51 and 8,000/45 ms). Note increased chemical shift artifact at 7.0 T at the femur cartilage (*arrow*). SAR issues required multiple acquisitions at 7.0 T

Peripheral Extremity Magnets

Peripheral extremity magnets require lower installation, maintenance, and management costs than whole-body systems and these systems are beneficial for patients with claustrophobia. Moreover, they do not require the same amount of shielding necessary for a whole-body system and can potentially be used in private offices and thus made widely available. Since 0.2 T MRI scanners have limitations in visualizing cartilage and other anatomical structures such as ligaments (Fig. 6.1), dedicated extremity scanners operating at higher field strength were developed. Using a dedicated peripheral extremity-only MRI system operating at 1.0 T Roemer et al. [27] examined 34 knees using fat-suppressed fast spin-echo (FSE) proton density-weighted sequences. They found good to excellent interobserver performance for assessing OA associated abnormalities including cartilage lesions (Fig. 6.7). These high-field peripheral scanners may offer a low-cost alternative to obtain adequate image quality for assessing cartilage pathology. Currently, peripheral extremity scanners operating at 1.5 T field strength are also available.

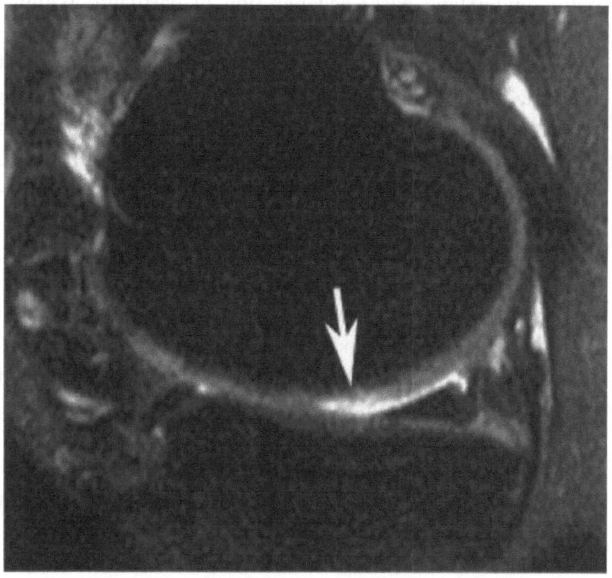

Fig. 6.7 Sagittal fat-suppressed PD-weighted MRI at 1.0 T depicts a focal cartilage defect (*arrow*) at the central weight-bearing medial femoral condyle (Courtesy Dr. Ali Guermazi, Boston University)

Depending on the *open MRI* configuration, patients can be placed either in a supine or weight-bearing position in the scanner. Open MRI scanners allow to assess functional aspects of joint function and may therefore be useful to investigate conditions associated with abnormal articulation in certain joint positions that may lead to accelerated OA. As an example, femoroacetabular impingement is a condition where labral and cartilage damage occurs due to an abnormal morphology of the head–neck junction (cam type impingement) or an abnormally deep acetabulum (pincer type impingement). This impingement typically occurs with flexion, abduction, and external rotation. Open MRI can be used to assess these functional aspects of the hip joint. Yamamura et al. [28] demonstrated in Japanese male and female participants that while impingement occurs frequently during daily activities, interestingly, it was not associated with accelerated OA of the hip in Japanese participants.

Open MRI scanners can also be used to assess patella kinematics and patellofemoral contact areas, which may play a role in the development of femoropatellar OA. Hinterwimmer et al. [29] studied a sample of 15 patients with genu varum and mild OA and 15 healthy volunteers in an open MRI scanner. 3D-GRE sequences of the knee were obtained in 0°, 30°, and 90° with and without activity of the extensor muscles. Contact areas between patella and femur cartilage were defined by intersection of opposing cartilage volumes. However, these investigators were not able to demonstrate significant differences in patella kinematics and patellofemoral contact areas ($P > 0.05$) between varus knees with mild OA and healthy knees either at different flexion angles or under extending muscle activity.

Weight-Bearing MRI

Recently there has been interest in weight-bearing MRI to better understand early degeneration of cartilage. Weight-bearing MRI can be performed using open MRI systems that have vertically orientated magnets such as the General Electric double-doughnut MRI system (SIGNA SP) or with whole-body MRI systems, which use special loading devices of the knee such as the one described by Nishii et al. [30]. While the vertical alignment of the magnets in a double-doughnut system allows true weight-bearing MRI studies, the field strength and image quality of these scanners are limited, affecting in particular cartilage imaging. Image quality in whole-body systems is generally superior and loading devices have also been successfully applied at 3.0 T scanners [30]. Static loading conditions are usually obtained by applying axial compression force of approximately 50% of body weight during imaging.

Anterior cruciate ligament (ACL) tears have been identified as an important factor in the pathogenesis of OA and it has also been found that patients with ACL repair experience accelerated OA [31]. Logan et al. [32] used a vertical open MRI system to study the tibiofemoral kinematics of the ACL-deficient weight bearing in ten patients. The tibiofemoral motion was assessed through the arc of flexion from 0° to 90° in the ACL-deficient and normal contralateral knees. These investigators found that ACL tears change tibiofemoral kinematics producing anterior subluxation of the lateral tibial plateau. This altered kinematics may explain, they hypothesized, at least in part, the increased incidence of secondary OA in patients with ACL tear. In another study, the same investigators [33] studied ten patients with isolated reconstruction of the ACL (hamstring autograft) in one knee and a normal contralateral knee using the same open MRI weight-bearing technique. They found that ACL reconstruction reduces sagittal laxity to within normal limits but does not restore normal tibiofemoral kinematics, which again may explain the relatively high rate of accelerated OA in this patient population.

Currently there has also been substantial interest in studying the cartilage response to load bearing in terms of volume and biochemical matrix change. It has been suggested that failure to respond to normal load bearing may occur due to disorder or degeneration of articular cartilage with collagen disorganization or abnormal water content [30]. Nishii et al. [30] used T2 relaxation time measurements to study the biochemical composition of the normal hyaline knee cartilage under loading. Sagittal T2 maps of the medial and lateral femorotibial joints of 22 healthy volunteers were obtained using 3.0 T MRI while applying axial compression force of 50% of body weight during imaging. T2 values of the femoral and tibial cartilage at the weight-bearing area were compared between unloading and loading conditions. These investigators found that under loading conditions, mean cartilage T2 values mostly decreased. At the medial joint compartment a significant decrease in T2 values with loading was observed at the femoral region in direct contact with the opposing tibial cartilage. A significant decrease in T2 values with loading was also observed at the medial and lateral tibia, at regions both covered and not covered by the meniscus.

In addition it has been found that the role of the meniscus during weight bearing is critical to prevent associated cartilage damage, and frequently meniscal damage and cartilage defects are associated. MRI directly visualizes changes of the meniscus, while applying axial compression forces, in terms of morphology, deformity, extrusion, and potentially biochemistry (Fig. 6.8). These findings may help in a better understanding of the evolution and pathophysiology of cartilage degeneration. Using weight-bearing MRI at 3.0 T Stehling et al. [34] found that the presence and grade of cartilage abnormalities in patients with OA was correlated with the degree of meniscal extrusion during loading, which indicates how abnormality of the meniscus during loading may potentially accelerate cartilage degeneration.

Surface Coils

In addition to adequate field strength, dedicated surface coils are very important prerequisites to achieve good image quality and visualization of cartilage. Surface coils for wrist, shoulder, knee, and ankle are currently standard; most of these coils are multichannel phased-array coils, which allow parallel imaging (PI) (Fig. 6.9). For visualization of smaller structures such as the fingers and toes, smaller so-called microscopy coils have been developed. These allow imaging with small field of views and high spatial resolution. The

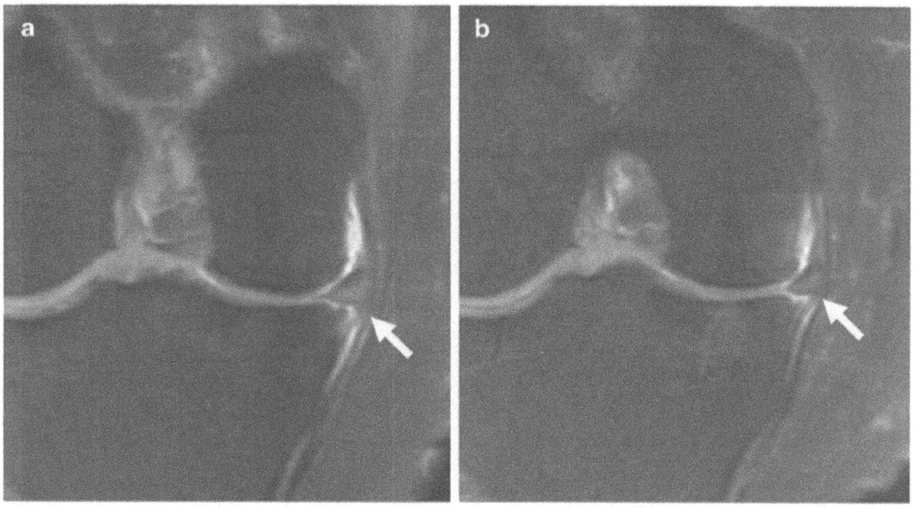

Fig. 6.8 Coronal MRI of the knee in patient with mild knee OA obtained using fat-suppressed proton density-weighted FSE sequences (3,000/10.3 ms) without (**a**) and with (**b**) loading (50% body weight) in a whole-body 3.0 T MR scanner. Note that the medial meniscal extrusion (*arrow*) is increased under loading conditions and shape of the meniscus also is mildly changed

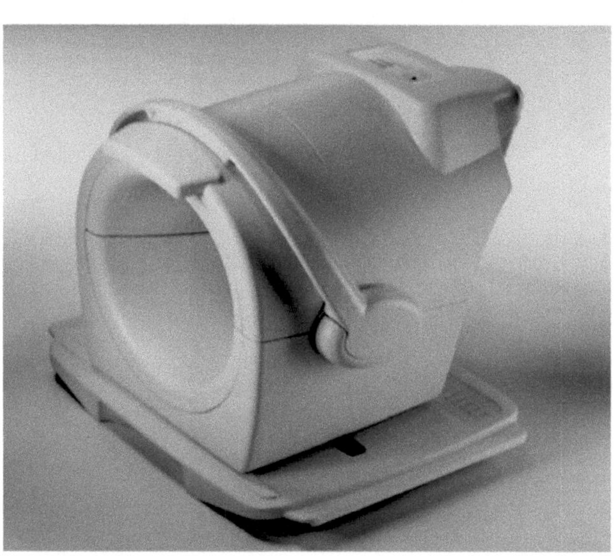

Fig. 6.9 Phased-array knee coil with eight channels

technical advancement of surface coils has substantially accelerated improvement of image quality with 3 T systems and currently one of the major limitations of 7 T imaging is the lack of adequate coil technology to make better use of the high field strength.

Figure 6.10 shows the effect of the coil on the image quality. While in (a) a nondedicated 2-element paddle coil was used, in (b) a dedicated 3-element shoulder coil was applied. The effect on visualization of the cartilage is evident. Even if a high-quality high-field scanner is used, inadequate coils will substantially limit image quality as shown by Lutterbey et al. [35]. These investigators used the standard body coil at 3.0 T for the imaging of the knee and found a substantially lower image performance than using a 1.5 T scanner with a dedicated knee coil.

Multichannel phased-array coils give high SNR and allow parallel imaging, which is very beneficial to increase image quality with the same acquisition time or allows shortening acquisition time by maintaining image quality. Parallel imaging means that each of the coils elements/channels provides image information separately, which is fused to obtain one image. Parallel imaging (PI) reduces scan time by increasing the sampling interval along the phase-encoding axis. When the MR signal is received by an array of coils, the scan can be accelerated by acquiring less phase-encoding data points and the missing data can be synthesized post-acquisition by using the spatial encoding information of all coil elements. Since scan time is directly proportional to number of phase-encodes, R-folds undersampling in the phase-encoding direction reduces scan time by the same factor, although penalty is paid in terms of signal-to-noise ratio (SNR). Especially in standard clinical musculoskeletal protocols, scan time reduction by employing parallel imaging can prevent motion artifacts as well as allow more flexibility in protocol design. Several different reconstruction algorithms have been proposed for parallel imaging, like sensitivity encoding (SENSE), simultaneous acquisition of spatial harmonics (SMASH), and more recently modified SENSE (mSENSE) and generalized autocalibrating partially parallel acquisition (GRAPPA).

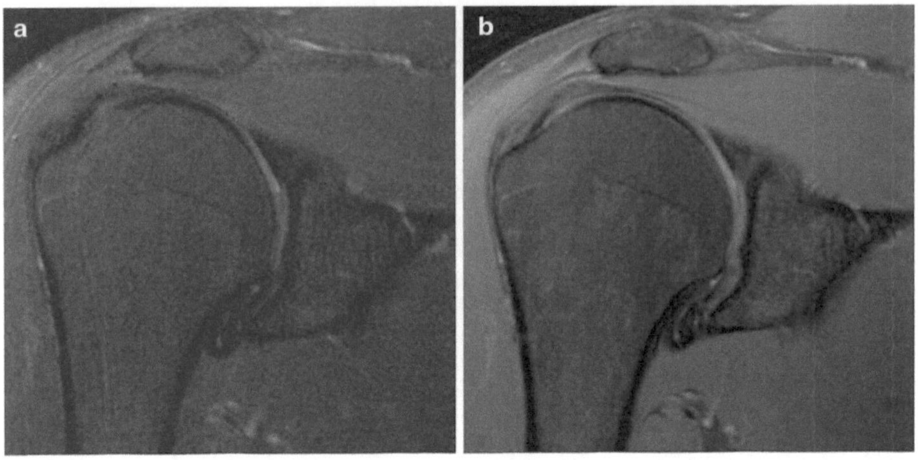

Fig. 6.10 Coronal MRI of the shoulder obtained at 3.0 T using fat-suppressed IM-weighted FSE sequences (3,300/51 ms) with (**a**) a nondedicated paddle coil and (**b**) a 3-element shoulder phased-array coil. Differences in image quality especially visualization of the cartilage and bone marrow are evident

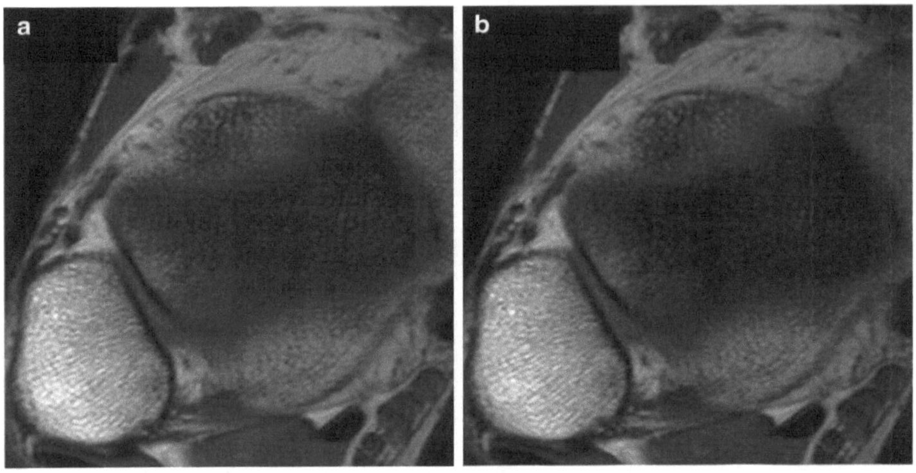

Fig. 6.11 Ankle MRI of a human cadaver ankle joint obtained at 3.0 T using a T1-weighted (675/15.7 ms) FSE sequence (**a**) without and (**b**) with parallel imaging. Images in (**b**) were obtained with a 44% shorter acquisition time. Note that no difference in image quality is observed, in particular in visualizing the ligaments

In an in vitro study performed in human cadaver specimens, Bauer et al. [36] compared an autocalibrating parallel imaging technique at 3.0 T with standard acquisitions at 3.0 T for small field-of-view imaging of the ankle. The scan time was reduced by 44% using parallel imaging techniques, compared to standard acquisitions, and images were analyzed for image quality by two radiologists. Macroscopic findings after dissection served as a reference for the pathologic evaluation. A significant difference in ligament and cartilage visualization or in image quality between standard and GeneRalized Autocalibrating Partially Parallel Acquisitions (GRAPPA) reconstruction at 3.0 T was not found in this study and the authors concluded that parallel imaging can provide more flexibility in protocol design by either shortening image acquisition time or improving image quality with the same acquisition time (Fig. 6.11).

Zuo et al. [37] evaluated the feasibility and reproducibility of quantitative cartilage imaging with parallel imaging at 3.0 T and determined the impact of the acceleration factor (AF) on morphological and relaxation measurements. They found that morphological parameters and relaxation time maps from parallel imaging showed comparable results with the conventional technique. Intraclass correlation coefficients (ICC) of the two methods for cartilage volume and mean cartilage thickness were very high both for T1rho, and T2 measurements and the reproducibility was excellent. In summary, for both quantitative and morphological OA imaging, multichannel phased-array coils with parallel imaging techniques are therefore recommended.

Sequence Protocols

Given the fact that both morphological and quantitative analyses are required to assess cartilage, a number of different sequences have been tailored and developed. In addition, as menisci, bone marrow, and ligaments are involved in cartilage disease processes, ideally a "whole-organ" assessment of the joint should be possible with these sequences.

Currently the workhorse sequences for morphological imaging of the joints are fast spin-echo (FSE) sequences. In particular, fluid-sensitive fat-suppressed sequences have been found useful to assess cartilage, bone marrow, ligaments, menisci, and tendons. Most experience and good results in morphological imaging of cartilage and subchondral pathology were gathered with (i) 2D proton density- (PD), intermediate- (IM) and T2-weighted FSE, (ii) 3D spoiled gradient-echo (SPGR) or fast low-angle shot (FLASH) gradient-echo sequences, and (iii) dual echo steady-state (DESS) sequences. Fat suppression in these sequences was found useful to better visualize cartilage pathology and reduce chemical shift artifacts. Table 6.1 gives an overview of currently used MR sequences with advantages and disadvantages.

IM- and T2-Weighted FSE Sequences

There is some controversy how exactly to define T2-, IM-, and PD-weighted sequences. General established terminology is the use of IM-weighted for sequences with echo times (TE) in the range of 30–60 ms, T2-weighted for TE's of 70–80 ms, and PD-weighted for TE's of 10–30 ms [20, 38]. In our experience, fat-suppressed, fluid-sensitive IM-weighted FSE sequences have been found most useful for standard imaging of cartilage as they are very versatile and in addition to good visualization of cartilage also allow evaluation of menisci, ligaments, and bone marrow. These sequences also provide better visualization of anatomic structures than T2-weighted FSE sequences. Proton density-weighted sequences with lower TE values may be helpful in better assessing the menisci and give additional information concerning tendons and ligaments but are less fluid sensitive (Fig. 6.12).

Standard parameters for FSE sequences used for cartilage imaging are as follows: Repetition time (TR): 3,000–4,000 ms, echo time (TE): 30–60 ms, and echo train length (ETL): 8. This TE range is chosen because it provides higher intrinsic contrast of the cartilage and is less prone to magic angle effects as compared with "true" PD-weighted pulse sequences obtained at shorter echo times. Slice thickness varies around 2–4 mm, but in a clinical setting usually 3 mm are used. In order to maintain an acceptable acquisition time and achieve a good SNR, the matrix size is in the order of 256×256 pixels but may be increased if imaging is performed at 3.0 T. Sequence parameters have to be adjusted to the joint with the parameter being most affected is the field of view. A clinically acceptable acquisition time is in the order of 3–6 min.

Table 6.1 MRI sequences used for cartilage imaging pros and cons

MR sequence	Pros	Cons
2D FSE (fast spin echo) with and without fat saturation	– Standard sequence – Used in clinical routine – Useful also for evaluation of menisci and ligaments – Evaluation of bone marrow if fat saturation is used	– Limited slice thickness – Cartilage signal changes do not correlate well with histology – Artifacts may obscure evaluation of cartilage
3D SPGR/FLASH (spoiled gradient-echo, fast low-angle shot) with fat saturation	– High spatial resolution with thin sections – Reformation in different planes – Well suited for cartilage volume assessment	– Cartilage is bright and focal signal abnormalities are not well demonstrated – Contrast between fluid and cartilage is limited
DESS (dual echo steady state) fluid sensitive	– High spatial resolution with thin sections – Reformation in different planes – Cartilage intermediate in signal – Good contrast between fluid and cartilage	– Limited for cartilage surface abnormalities
3D FSE (fast spin echo) with fat saturation (BLADE, CUBE)	– Thin sections and isotropic voxels – Reformation in different planes – Cartilage intermediate in signal – Good contrast between fluid and cartilage	– Substantial amount of noise – Not well suited for low-contrast lesions – Low in plane spatial resolution

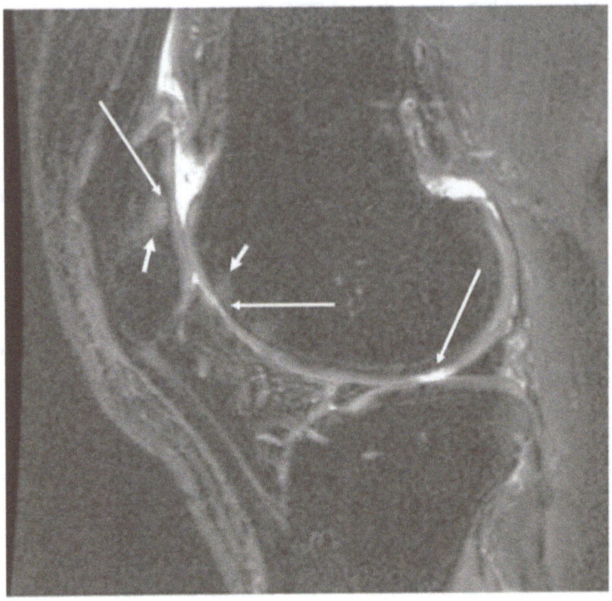

Fig. 6.12 Sagittal fat-suppressed IM-weighted FSE (3,200/30 ms) MRI of the knee obtained in a 54-year-old woman with advanced degenerative disease of the femoropatellar joint. Note that cartilage lesions (*long arrows*), bone marrow edema pattern (*short arrows*) at the trochlea and patella, tendons, menisci, ligaments are well visualized with this fluid-sensitive sequence

With IM- and T2-weighted FSE sequences, normal hyaline cartilage is intermediate in signal and fluid is bright, which allows good contrast to identify surface abnormalities as well as pathologies of the cartilage matrix. Sadaat et al. analyzed the performance of IM-weighted sequences in relation to histology in patients with advanced OA before undergoing total knee arthroplasty using 3.0 T MRI [39] (Fig. 6.13). Intraoperatively obtained specimens underwent histological analysis and sections were matched with preoperative MRIs. Preoperative MRI findings were compared to the corresponding region in histological sections. Parameters assessed included thinning of cartilage, differentiating <50%, >50%, and full thickness lesions, surface integrity including fissuring and fraying as well as signal pattern abnormalities of cartilage. Histological findings in areas of bone marrow edema pattern and cartilage swelling were also documented. The overall sensitivity, specificity, and accuracy were 72%, 69%, and 70% for cartilage thinning, 69%, 74%, and 73% for surface irregularities and 36%, 62%,and 45% for intracartilaginous signal abnormalities. The authors concluded that MRI using fat-suppressed IM-weighted FSE sequences showed good performance in assessing cartilage thickness and surface lesions, while cartilage signal changes were not well suited to characterize

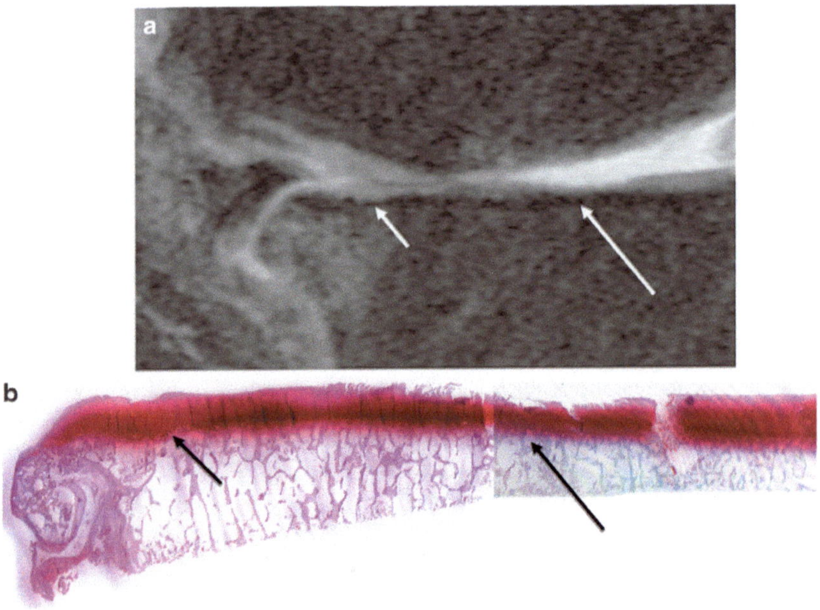

Fig. 6.13 Sagittal MRI of the knee obtained in a patient undergoing total knee replacement at 3.0 T using a fat-suppressed IM-weighted FSE sequence (4,300/51 ms) (**a**). (**b**) shows the corresponding histological slide (H&E) obtained after surgery. Cartilage degeneration with focal cartilage thinning and fraying on histological image and MRI (*arrows*) with additional abnormal signal of the cartilage and swelling (*small arrows*) on the MR image

the severity of cartilage degeneration as validated by histology. Thus signal abnormalities visualized on IM-weighted FSE sequences of the cartilage matrix may have limited value in characterizing cartilage degeneration and softening. In this study, areas of bone marrow edema pattern corresponded to fibrovascular tissue ingrowths.

Multiple clinical studies used IM- and T2-weighted FSE sequences with high sensitivity and specificity in assessing cartilage abnormalities [15, 40–43]. It should be noted that diagnostic performance for cartilage lesions is improved when different imaging planes are used. Bredella et al. [44] studied how detecting and grading articular cartilage defects in the knee are affected by using a combination of different imaging planes. They found that sensitivity for a sagittal T2-weighted FSE sequence was only 40%, and specificity was 100%. But sensitivity of a combination of axial and coronal fat-suppressed T2-weighted FSE sequences and sagittal T2-weighted FSE sequences was 94%, specificity was 99%, and accuracy was 98% using arthroscopy as a standard of reference.

However, it should also be considered that artifacts are not infrequently found in cartilage on FSE sequences, which demonstrate pattern that may mimic disease [45]. These patterns include pseudolaminar signal changes due to truncation artifacts, decreased signal intensity in the distal part of the trochlear cartilage, and apparent cartilage thinning of the cartilage adjacent to the anterior horn of the lateral meniscus. Given these patterns, limited specificity of FSE sequences in diagnosing cartilage lesions was found in a previous study (67.6%) [46]; in the same study, however, sensitivity and kappa values for analyzing cartilage lesions were high for fat-suppressed FSE sequences.

3D SPGR and FLASH Sequences

3D SPGR and FLASH sequences are well suited to depict cartilage volume and to some extent the cartilage surface. Sequence parameters used to visualize cartilage are in the range of TR: 20–35 ms, TE: 7–12 ms, and flip angle: 12–30°; parameters need to be optimized according to the field strength. The bright signal of cartilage in the SPGR and FLASH images limits visualization of internal cartilage pathology. Fissures may sometimes be not as well visualized given the low-intermediate signal of the surrounding fluid limiting cartilage-fluid contrast-to-noise ratio (Fig. 6.14). It should also be noted that these gradient-echo sequences are not suited to visualize bone marrow pathology and are very limited in assessing menisci, ligaments, and tendons. However, they have been found useful in segmenting cartilage for quantitative measurement of volume and thickness [10, 23, 47].

A number of studies have been performed comparing SPGR versus IM- or T2-weighted FSE sequences [19, 20, 46] and similar overall diagnostic performance in detecting focal cartilage lesions has been found for both sequences types. 3D SPGR and FLASH sequences provide high spatial resolution; however, imaging time with these sequences is usually fairly high and image quality can be degraded by motion artifacts. These gradient-echo sequences are also very sensitive to susceptibility artifacts, which should be considered after previous surgery, in particular after cartilage repair procedures. In our clinical practice we found IM-weighted FSE sequences easier to use and more practically applicable than SPGR or FLASH sequences. More recent studies also suggested that SPGR sequences may be

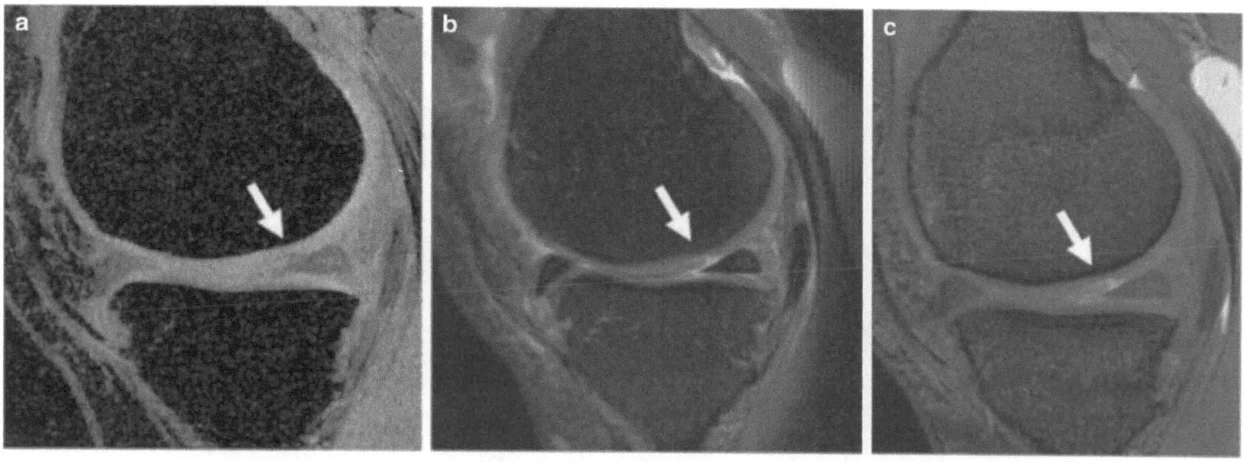

Fig. 6.14 Sagittal MR images of the knee obtained in a middle-aged runner using (**a**) a fat-suppressed SPGR (21/12.5 ms, flip angle: 15°), (**b**) an IM-weighted FSE (4,300/51 ms) and (**c**) a non-fat-suppressed fluid-sensitive fast imaging employing steady-state acquisition (FIESTA; 5.9/1.9 ms, flip angle: 15°) sequence. Cartilage fissure with delamination (*arrow*) is well visualized on the fluid-sensitive sequences (**b, c**) but not on the SPGR sequence where the cartilage appears uniformly bright (**a**)

less well suited to visualize subtle cartilage abnormalities compared to IM-weighted FSE sequences [15, 16]. Figure 6.14 illustrates well the limitations of the SPGR sequence in relation to the FSE sequence.

Other Sequences

In addition to FSE and SPGR/FLASH sequences, 3D double-echo steady-state sequences (DESS) have also shown good results in detecting cartilage lesions (Fig. 6.15). This mixed T1/T2*-weighted sequence provides high spatial resolutions with the cartilage appearing more intermediate in signal. In an experimental study, Woertler et al. [3] found a similar performance of fat-suppressed 3D FLASH and water-excited 3D DESS sequences in detecting cartilage surface lesions. Ruehm et al. analyzed patellar cartilage abnormalities in 58 consecutive patients using a 3D DESS and a T2-weighted FSE sequence. These authors concluded that the DESS sequence was less accurate in detecting cartilage surface abnormalities, yet more accurate in diagnosing cartilage softening [48]. It should be noted that 3D DESS sequences are usually obtained with thin sections, which allows for relatively high-quality reconstructions in additional imaging planes. In the "Osteoarthritis Initiative" sagittal thin section DESS sequences were implemented with reformations in the axial and coronal plane, in particular to better assess the patellar cartilage in the axial reformations.

A number of sequences have been developed to improve morphological depiction of cartilage. These include driven equilibrium Fourier transform (DEFT) and steady-state free precision (SSFP) imaging. DEFT imaging makes use of a much higher cartilage-to-fluid contrast; the signal of synovial fluid is higher than in SPGR sequences and the signal of cartilage is higher than in T2-weighted FSE sequences [49]. Yoshioka et al. used this sequence in 35 OA knees and correlated imaging findings with arthroscopy. In their study, the fat-suppressed 3D DEFT images showed results similar to SPGR and IM-weighted FSE sequences with high sensitivity yet relatively low specificity [46]. Gold et al. compared 3D DEFT and T2-weighted FSE sequences in 104 consecutive patients with knee pain and used arthroscopy in 24 patients as a standard of reference [50]. These investigators found that the 3D DEFT sequences provided excellent synovial fluid-to-cartilage contrast while preserving signal from cartilage, giving this method a high cartilage SNR. In addition 3D DEFT showed the full cartilage thickness better than T2-weighted FSE sequences, yet T2-weighted FSE sequences had superior fat suppression and fewer artifacts than 3D DEFT sequences.

SSFP imaging has been described as an efficient, high-signal method for obtaining 3D images and may be useful to depict cartilage since cartilage signal was found to be higher than in conventional sequences [51]. Kornaat et al. used this sequence in volunteers at 1.5 and 3 T and found that SSFP-based techniques showed higher increase in SNR and CNR efficiency at 3.0 T than SPGR sequences [52]. Figure 6.14 shows cartilage delamination at the medial femoral condyle of the knee imaged with a SSFP sequence (fast imaging employing steady-state acquisition, FIESTA) and compared to SPGR and IM-weighted FSE sequences. Bauer et al. compared

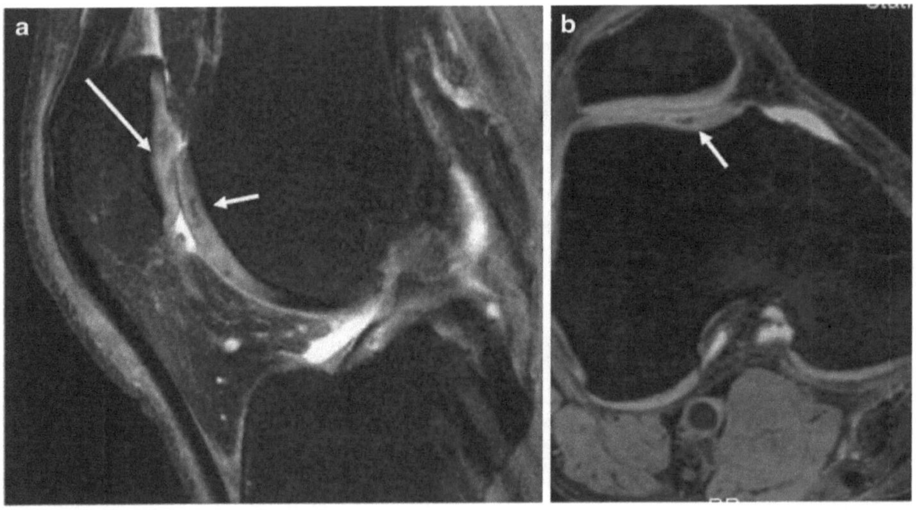

Fig. 6.15 Sagittal 3D DESS MRI (16.3/4.7 ms, flip angle: 25°) of the knee obtained in a 50-year-old man (**a**) and axial reconstruction from the image dataset (**b**). Note femoropatellar cartilage degeneration with surface irregularity (*long arrow*) and signal changes (*short arrow*). Low signal changes at the trochlea are consistent with chondrocalcinosis

SSFP, IM-weighted FSE, and SPGR sequences in their performance in assessing cartilage lesions at cadaver ankles and found the highest ROC (receiver operator characteristics) values for the IM-weighted FSE sequences at 3.0 T, yet IM-weighted FSE and SSFP sequences showed a similar performance at 1.5 T and both showed better results at 3.0 T and 1.5 T than the SPGR sequence [53]. To our knowledge, larger clinical studies, however, have not yet been performed using this sequence. It should be noted that the previously described DESS sequence is also a steady-state sequence and thus has similar cartilage signal features compared to the SSFP sequences, yet parameters are different to some extent.

Recently 3D FSE sequences have been applied for clinical imaging of the knee and ankle [54, 55]. These sequences generate isotropic voxels and allow high-quality reformations in any plane. Thus it may be possible to only obtain one sequence dataset and get the additional planes as reformations (Fig. 6.16). This would potentially save acquisition time and shorten patient examinations substantially. Ristow et al. [54] compared a fat-suppressed IM-weighted 3D FSE sequence with a standard 2D IM-weighted FSE sequence regarding image quality and diagnostic performance in assessing abnormal findings of the knee. These investigators found that isotropic 3D IM-weighted FSE imaging enhanced standard knee MRI by better visualizing high contrast lesions; however, 3D FSE image quality was lower and limitations with diagnostic performance were found compared to standard 2D FSE imaging. Clearly this technique, however, has future potential and with further improvements in the sequence design the sequence may replace 2D IM-weighted FSE sequences.

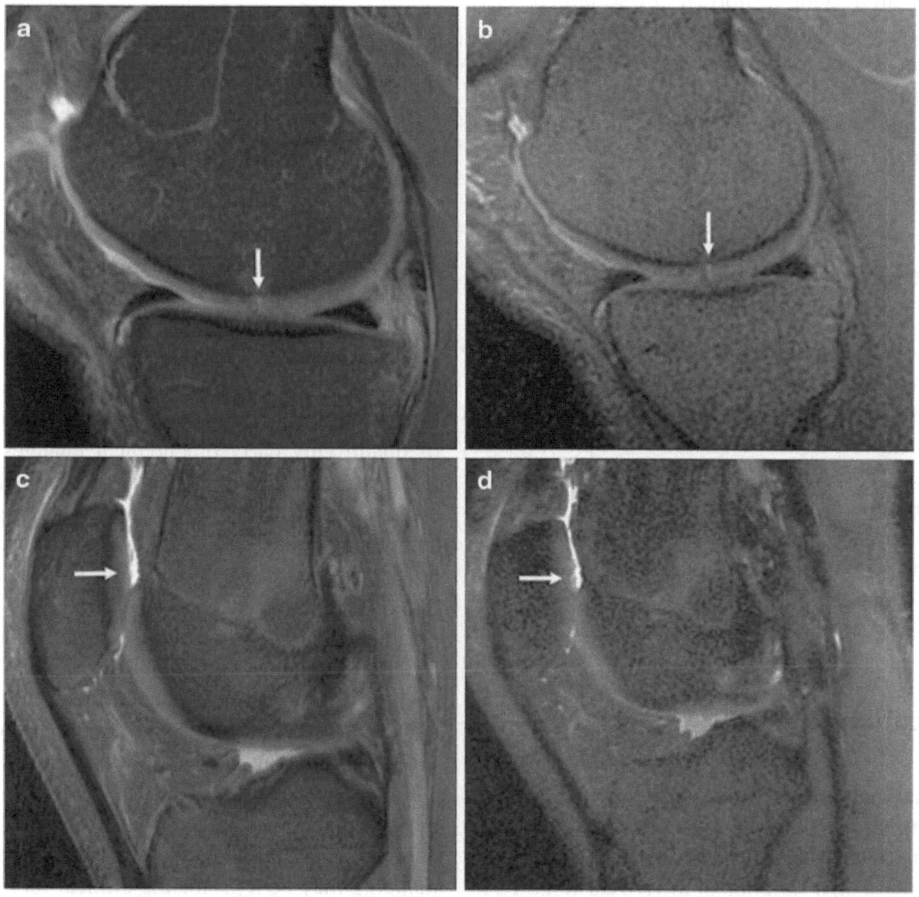

Fig. 6.16 Sagittal 2D (4,200/51 ms) (**a**, **c**) and 3D (2,500/38 ms) (**b**, **d**) FSE sequences of the knee. Focal cartilage lesion at the medial femoral condyle and the patella. The cartilage fissures are well depicted on (**b**, **d**) but not as well visualized on (**a**, **c**) due to reduced slice thickness. Also note that contrast between cartilage and bone is limited in (**b**, **d**) and bone marrow appears noisy

MR Arthrography

Direct MR arthrography with use of T1-weighted pulse sequences following intraarticular injection of gadolinium chelates has been shown to represent a reliable imaging technique for the detection of surface lesions of articular cartilage with sensitivity and specificity ranging from 85% to 100% [56, 57]. The injected fluid produces high contrast between joint space, cartilage, and subchondral bone, and at the same time distends the joint and thus, improves the separation of corresponding joint surfaces, such as the chondral surfaces of the femur and the acetabulum at the hip joint. Given its invasive nature, however, this technique is of limited use for OA imaging.

A simple method to produce artificial arthrographic contrast in a T1-like fast spin-echo (FSE) sequence with the use of a driven equilibrium pulse (DRIVE) has recently been described. In contrast to the 3D DEFT sequence mentioned above, this 2D technique provides bright signal intensity of joint fluid with otherwise unchanged signal intensities compared with a normal T1-weighted FSE sequence at high spatial resolution and short scan times [58]. DRIVE can also be used to increase the contrast and/or spatial resolution of IM-weighted FSE images. However, this new technique and its value for cartilage imaging are still under clinical evaluation.

Quantitative Imaging of the Cartilage Matrix

In addition to assessing cartilage pathology as well as thickness and volume, recent studies have shown the potential of MRI parameters to reflect changes in biochemical composition of cartilage with early OA. These techniques include T2 quantification [59], T1rho quantification [14, 60], and delayed Gadolinium-enhanced MRI of cartilage (dGEMRIC) [61, 62]. These techniques allow characterization of the cartilage matrix and, potentially, quality before morphological damage occurs.

T2 Quantification

It was shown that increasing T2 relaxation time was proportional to the distribution of cartilage water and is sensitive to small water content changes [63]. In an early study Dardzinski et al. examined the spatial variation of in vivo cartilage T2 in young asymptomatic adults and found a reproducible pattern of increasing T2 that was proportional to the known spatial variation in cartilage water and was inversely proportional to the distribution of proteoglycans [64]. These authors postulated that the regional T2 differences were secondary to the restricted mobility of cartilage water within an anisotropic solid matrix. Thus measurement of the spatial distribution of the T2 reflecting areas of increased and decreased water content may be used to quantify cartilage degeneration before morphologic changes are appreciated.

In a preliminary study Mosher et al. showed that aging is associated with an asymptomatic increase in T2 of the transitional zone of articular cartilage [65]. The results of this study indicated that the diffuse increase in T2 in senescent cartilage is different in appearance than the focally increased T2 observed in damaged articular cartilage [65]. Dunn et al. analyzed 55 participants who were categorized with radiography as healthy ($n=7$), having mild OA ($n=20$), or severe OA ($n=28$) [59]. They found that healthy participants had mean T2 values of 32.1–35.0 ms, while patients with mild and severe OA had mean T2 values of 34.4–41.0 ms. All cartilage compartments except the lateral tibia showed significant ($P<.05$) increases in T2 relaxation time between healthy and diseased knees. Correlation of T2 values with clinical symptoms and cartilage morphology was found predominantly in medial compartments.

T1rho Quantification

A different parameter that has been proposed to measure cartilage composition is 3D T1rho relaxation mapping. T1rho describes the spin-lattice relaxation in the rotating frame and changes in the extracellular matrix of cartilage, like loss of glycosaminglycans (GAG), may be reflected in measurements of T1rho due to less-restricted motion of water protons. Preliminary results demonstrated the in vivo feasibility of quantifying early biochemical changes in symptomatic OA participants using T1rho-weighted MRI on a 1.5 T clinical scanner [14, 60]. In a study with a limited number of symptomatic participants it was shown that T1rho-weighted MRI provided a noninvasive marker for quantification of early degenerative changes of cartilage in vivo [14]. Li et al. examined ten healthy volunteers, and nine OA patients at 3.0 T and found a significant difference ($P=0.002$) in the average T1rho within patellar and femoral cartilage between controls (45.04 ± 2.59 ms) and OA patients (53.06 ± 4.60 ms) [66]. A significant correlation was found between T1rho and T2 relaxation measurements; however, the difference of T2 measurements was not significant between controls and OA patients. These initial results suggested that T1rho relaxation mapping may be a promising clinical tool for OA detection and treatment monitoring. Stahl et al. [67] analyzed the diagnostic value of T2- and T1rho-measurements in identifying asymptomatic physically active subjects with and without

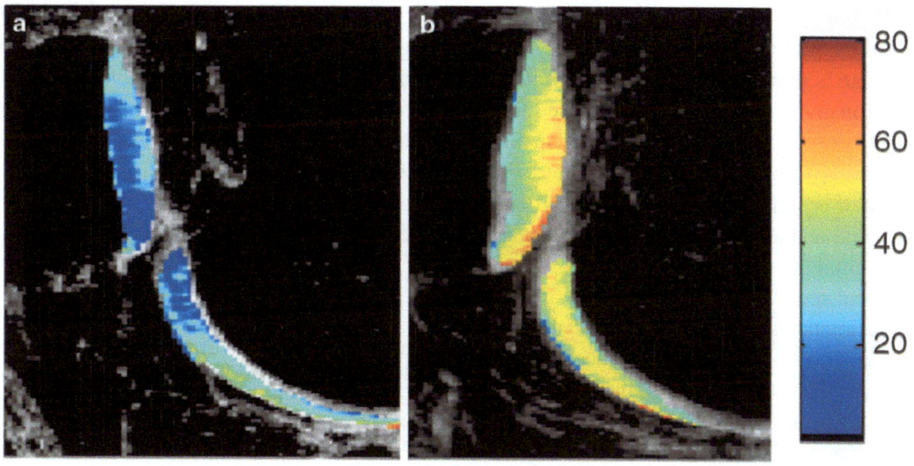

Fig. 6.17 T1rho color map (ms) of the patellofemoral cartilage. Asymptomatic subject without focal cartilage pathology (low T1rho values) (**a**) and asymptomatic subject with early, diffuse cartilage degeneration (high T1rho) and focal cartilage defects (not shown) (**b**) from reference [63]

focal cartilage pathology. These investigators found that subjects with and without focal cartilage pathology had different T1rho and T2 composition of cartilage and concluded that T1rho and T2 may be parameters suited to identify asymptomatic subjects at higher risk for developing cartilage degeneration (Fig. 6.17).

Further studies are currently underway to correlate T1rho measurements with early OA determined from arthroscopy, as a standard of reference, in larger symptomatic populations. The advantage of T1rho and T2 measurements is that these techniques are noninvasive and do not require contrast injection.

dGEMRIC

Cartilage consists of approximately 70% water and the remainder predominantly of type II collagen fibers and GAG. These GAG macromolecules contain negative charges that attract sodium ions (Na^+). One of the most commonly used MRI contrast agents Gd-DTPA^{2-} (Magnevist, Berlex, Wayne, New Jersey) has a negative charge and will therefore not penetrate cartilage in areas of high GAG concentrations. In fact it will be distributed in higher concentrations in areas with lower GAG concentration and thus pathologic cartilage composition. Gd-DTPA^{2-} concentrations in cartilage can be quantified and this technique has been defined as dGEMRIC or delayed Gadolinium-enhanced MRI of cartilage. Initial studies have shown that the dGEMRIC measurement of GAG corresponds to the true GAG concentration as measured with biochemistry and histology [61, 68]. This technique has also been used in a number of clinical studies and variations of this measurement have been shown in patients with OA, trials of autologous chondrocyte implants, and participants with sedentary lifestyle versus those with regular exercise [12, 69–71].

MR Imaging in Relation to Joint Specific Requirements

MRI to assess cartilage currently concentrates mostly on the knee joint, with an increasing number of studies, however, also focusing on the hip joint [72–76]. Given the reduced thickness, MRI is limited in visualizing *wrist* cartilage [77]; however, with new developments in coil design and sequences this has been improved in recent years. With multichannel wrist coils SNR can be greatly improved. One caveat of wrist imaging is positioning; off center imaging is frequently not possible and superman positioning is uncomfortable especially in patients with osteoarthritis or inflammatory arthropathies. Scanners with larger gantry sizes may allow positioning of the wrist and hand at the side of the patient and if patients are small and thin this may also work with standard scanners.

Similar problems are found at the *elbow* given reduced cartilage thickness and difficulty in positioning. While wrist coils are technically advanced, however, development of elbow coils has not received similar attention. It has been suggested to use flex coils or knee coils but flex coils have limitations in SNR and knee coils are challenging with patient positioning. Fortunately clinical indications to evaluate cartilage at the elbow are restricted.

Similarly cartilage imaging of the *shoulder* has a limited clinical role as this non-weight-bearing joint rarely is affected by cartilage pathology and repair is not a standard procedure. However, coil technology at the shoulder is advanced with the availability of 8-channel shoulder coils that allow high SNR and high spatial resolution imaging.

Though the cartilage is thin, imaging of the *ankle* is getting increasing attention giving advances in coil and sequence design. A number of conditions affect the ankle cartilage including osteochondritis dissecans and sport-related injuries; also cartilage repair is performed at the ankle. Dedicated ankle coils are available and alternatively knee coils can be used for high-quality imaging of the ankle.

While morphological sequences are standard for imaging of the cartilage at the joints less experience is available with *quantitative sequences*. Given the clinical relevance and cartilage thickness, the knee was studied most frequently [59, 65, 78–82]. Studies have also focused on the hip but less experience is available and imaging has been limited by the reduced cartilage thickness with pronounced partial volume effects [72, 73, 76, 83]. Segmentation of the femoral and acetabular cartilage layers at the hip is challenging and frequently differentiation of the two cartilage layers is not possible. To better assess the cartilage layers at the acetabulum and femoral head, distraction has been used with weights attached to the leg during imaging, but given the increased pain, this is not recommended as a routine procedure in patients with symptomatic hips. Quantitative imaging of the other joints has received less attention because of limited clinical indications and challenges due to reduced cartilage thickness.

An optimal MRI cartilage protocol would include morphological IM-weighted FSE sequences in a coronal and sagittal orientation as well as quantitative sequences for volumetric and cartilage matrix assessment (SPGR/FLASH sequence as well as T1rho, T2, or dGEMRIC maps). Axial IM-weighted sequences may be included to better assess the patella, depending on clinical or research indications. At the hip oblique axial images are useful in assessing cartilage damage and measuring the alpha angle, which is helpful for assessment of femoroacetabular impingement (FAI) [83]. FAI has a major role in the evolution of accelerated cartilage loss and OA. It should be noted that morphological evaluation of cartilage and labrum at the hip joint without intraarticular contrast is limited.

Conclusion

Standard MR imaging of cartilage relies on morphological 2D IM-weighted FSE sequences that are well suited not only to detect focal cartilage abnormalities but also those of menisci, bone marrow, ligaments, and tendons. 3D gradient-echo (such as DESS) and FSE sequences, which allow thinner sections and reformations in different imaging planes are available; these have an increasing role in morphological imaging. Quantitative imaging of cartilage is achieved with SPGR, and FLASH sequences, which are used to assess cartilage Volume; T2, T1rho, and dGEMRIC techniques are used to analyse cartilage biochemical composition. Dedicated surface coils are required to best visualize joint cartilage, in particular at the knee joint, and multichannel phased-array coils with parallel imaging have been shown to be beneficial in improving image quality and/or shortening acquisition time. Image quality also benefits from increased field strength and 3.0 T MRI is increasingly used for assessing joint cartilage.

Acknowledgments This article was based on a previous publication by the same author in Magnetic Resonance Imaging Clinics of North America (Magn Reson Imaging Clin N Am. 2010 Feb;18(1):95–110) and Radiologic Clinics of North America (Radiol Clin North Am. 2009 Jul;47(4):617–32).

References

1. Kladny B, Gluckert K, Swoboda B, Beyer W, Weseloh G. Comparison of low-field (0.2 Tesla) and high-field (1.5 Tesla) magnetic resonance imaging of the knee joint. Arch Orthop Trauma Surg. 1995;114:281–6.
2. Rand T, Imhof H, Turetschek K, Schneider B, Vögele T, Gäbler C, et al. Comparison of low field (0.2 T) and high field (1.5 T) MR imaging in the differentiation of torned from intact menisci. Eur J Radiol. 1999;30:22–7.
3. Woertler K, Strothmann M, Tombach B, Reimer P. Detection of articular cartilage lesions: experimental evaluation of low- and high-field-strength MR imaging at 0.18 and 1.0 T. J Magn Reson Imaging. 2000;11:678–85.
4. Ahn JM, Kwak SM, Kang HS, Muhle C, Pedowitz RA, Frank LR, et al. Evaluation of patellar cartilage in cadavers with a low-field-strength extremity-only magnet: comparison of MR imaging sequences, with macroscopic findings as the standard. Radiology. 1998;208:57–62.
5. Felson D, Chaisson C, Hill C, Totterman SM, Gale ME, Skinner KM, et al. The association of bone marrow lesions with pain in knee osteoarthritis. Ann Intern Med. 2001;134:541–9.
6. Hunter DJ, Lo GH, Gale D, Grainger AJ, Guermazi A, Conaghan PG. The reliability of a new scoring system for knee osteoarthritis MRI and the validity of bone marrow lesion assessment: BLOKS (Boston Leeds Osteoarthritis Knee Score). Ann Rheum Dis. 2008;67:206–11.
7. Link TM, Steinbach LS, Ghosh S, Ries M, Lu Y, Lane N, et al. Osteoarthritis: MR imaging findings in different stages of disease and correlation with clinical findings. Radiology. 2003;226:373–81.
8. Phan CM, Link TM, Blumenkrantz G, Dunn TC, Ries MD, Steinbach LS, et al. MR imaging findings in the follow-up of patients with different stages of knee osteoarthritis and the correlation with clinical symptoms. Eur Radiol. 2006;16:608–18.
9. Recht M, Kramer J, Marcelis S, Pathria MN, Trudell D, Haghighi P, et al. Abnormalities of articular cartilage in the knee: analysis of available MR technique. Radiology. 1993;187:473–8.
10. Eckstein F, Heudorfer L, Faber SC, Burgkart R, Englmeier KH, Reiser M. Long-term and resegmentation precision of quantitative cartilage MR imaging (qMRI). Osteoarthritis Cartilage. 2002;10:922–8.
11. Peterfy CG, Guermazi A, Zaim S, Tirman PF, Miaux Y, White D, et al. Whole-Organ Magnetic Resonance Imaging Score (WORMS) of the knee in osteoarthritis. Osteoarthritis Cartilage. 2004;12:177–90.

12. Burstein D, Gray M. New MRI techniques for imaging cartilage. J Bone Joint Surg Am. 2003;85-A Suppl 2:70–7.
13. Mosher TJ, Dardzinski BJ. Cartilage MRI T2 relaxation time mapping: overview and applications. Semin Musculoskelet Radiol. 2004;8:355–68.
14. Regatte RR, Akella SV, Wheaton AJ, Lech G, Borthakur A, Kneeland JB, et al. 3D-T1rho-relaxation mapping of articular cartilage: in vivo assessment of early degenerative changes in symptomatic osteoarthritic subjects. Acad Radiol. 2004;11:741–9.
15. Barr C, Bauer JS, Malfair D, Ma B, Henning TD, Steinbach L, et al. MR imaging of the ankle at 3 Tesla and 1.5 Tesla: protocol optimization and application to cartilage, ligament and tendon pathology in cadaver specimens. Eur Radiol. 2007;17:1518–28.
16. Bauer JS, Barr C, Henning TD, Malfair D, Ma CB, Steinbach L, et al. Magnetic resonance imaging of the ankle at 3.0 Tesla and 1.5 Tesla in human cadaver specimens with artificially created lesions of cartilage and ligaments. Invest Radiol. 2008;43:604–11.
17. Bauer JS, Krause SJ, Ross CJ, Krug R, Carballido-Gamio J, Ozhinsky E, et al. Volumetric cartilage measurements of porcine knee at 1.5-T and 3.0-T MR imaging: evaluation of precision and accuracy. Radiology. 2006;241:399–406.
18. Kijowski R, Blankenbaker D, Davis K, Shinki K, Kaplan L, De Smet AA. Comparison of 1.5 T and 3 T magnetic resonance imaging systems for evaluating the articular cartilage of the knee joint. Chicago: RSNA; 2007. VS21-14.
19. Link TM, Sell CA, Masi JN, Phan C, Newitt D, Lu Y, et al. 3.0 vs 1.5 T MRI in the detection of focal cartilage pathology – ROC analysis in an experimental model. Osteoarthritis Cartilage. 2005;14:63–70.
20. Masi JN, Sell CA, Phan C, Han H, Newitt D, Steinbach L, et al. Cartilage MR imaging at 3.0 versus that at 1.5 T: preliminary results in a porcine model. Radiology. 2005;236:140–50.
21. Kijowski R, Blankenbaker DG, Davis KW, Shinki K, Kaplan LD, De Smet AA. Comparison of 1.5- and 3.0-T MR imaging for evaluating the articular cartilage of the knee joint. Radiology. 2009;250:839–48.
22. Wong S, Steinbach L, Zhao J, Stehling C, Ma CB, Link TM. Comparative study of imaging at 3.0 T versus 1.5 T of the knee. Skeletal Radiol. 2009;38:761–9.
23. Eckstein F, Charles HC, Buck RJ, Kraus VB, Remmers AE, Hudelmaier M, et al. Accuracy and precision of quantitative assessment of cartilage morphology by magnetic resonance imaging at 3.0 T. Arthritis Rheum. 2005;52:3132–6.
24. Peterfy CG, Schneider E, Nevitt M. The osteoarthritis initiative: report on the design rationale for the magnetic resonance imaging protocol for the knee. Osteoarthritis Cartilage. 2008;16:1433–41.
25. Kraff O, Theysohn JM, Maderwald S, Saylor C, Ladd SC, Ladd ME, et al. MRI of the knee at 7.0 Tesla. Rofo. 2007;179:1231–5.
26. Krug R, Carballido-Gamio J, Banerjee S, Stahl R, Carvajal L, Xu D, et al. In vivo bone and cartilage MRI using fully-balanced steady-state free-precession at 7 tesla. Magn Reson Med. 2007;58:1294–8.
27. Roemer FW, Guermazi A, Lynch JA, Peterfy CG, Nevitt MC, Webb N, et al. Short tau inversion recovery and proton density-weighted fat suppressed sequences for the evaluation of osteoarthritis of the knee with a 1.0 T dedicated extremity MRI: development of a time-efficient sequence protocol. Eur Radiol. 2005;15:978–87.
28. Yamamura M, Miki H, Nakamura N, Murai M, Yoshikawa H, Sugano N. Open-configuration MRI study of femoro-acetabular impingement. J Orthop Res. 2007;25:1582–8.
29. Hinterwimmer S, von Eisenhart-Rothe R, Siebert M, Welsch F, Vogl T, Graichen H. Patella kinematics and patello-femoral contact areas in patients with genu varum and mild osteoarthritis. Clin Biomech (Bristol, Avon). 2004;19:704–10.
30. Nishii T, Kuroda K, Matsuoka Y, Sahara T, Yoshikawa H. Change in knee cartilage T2 in response to mechanical loading. J Magn Reson Imaging. 2008;28:175–80.
31. Amin S, Guermazi A, Lavalley MP, Niu J, Clancy M, Hunter DJ, et al. Complete anterior cruciate ligament tear and the risk for cartilage loss and progression of symptoms in men and women with knee osteoarthritis. Osteoarthritis Cartilage. 2008;16:897–902.
32. Logan M, Dunstan E, Robinson J, Williams A, Gedroyc W, Freeman M. Tibiofemoral kinematics of the anterior cruciate ligament (ACL)-deficient weightbearing, living knee employing vertical access open "interventional" multiple resonance imaging. Am J Sports Med. 2004;32:720–6.
33. Logan MC, Williams A, Lavelle J, Gedroyc W, Freeman M. Tibiofemoral kinematics following successful anterior cruciate ligament reconstruction using dynamic multiple resonance imaging. Am J Sports Med. 2004;32:984–92.
34. Stehling C, Souza RB, Hellio Le Graverand-Gastineau MP, Wyman BT, Li X, Majumdar S, Link TM. Loading of the knee during 3.0 Tesla MRI is associated with significantly increased medial meniscus extrusion in mild and moderate osteoarthritis. ECR 2010, Scientific Program S212.
35. Lutterbey G, Behrends K, Falkenhausen MV, Wattjes MP, Morakkabati N, Gieseke J, et al. Is the body-coil at 3 Tesla feasible for the MRI evaluation of the painful knee? A comparative study. Eur Radiol. 2007;17:503–8.
36. Bauer JS, Banerjee S, Henning TD, Krug R, Majumdar S, Link TM. Fast high-spatial-resolution MRI of the ankle with parallel imaging using GRAPPA at 3 T. AJR Am J Roentgenol. 2007;189:240–5.
37. Zuo J, Li X, Banerjee S, Han E, Majumdar S. Parallel imaging of knee cartilage at 3 Tesla. J Magn Reson Imaging. 2007;26:1001–9.
38. Naraghi A, White L. MRI evaluation of the postoperative knee: special considerations and pitfalls. Clin Sports Med. 2006;25:703–25.
39. Saadat E, Jobke B, Chu B, Lu Y, Cheng J, Li X, et al. Diagnostic performance of in vivo 3 T Fast Spin Echo MRI for articular cartilage abnormalities in human osteoarthritic knees using histology as standard of reference. Eur Radiol. 2008;18:2292–302.
40. Kawahara Y, Uetani M, Nakahara N, Doiguchi Y, Nishiguchi M, Futagawa S, et al. Fast spin-echo MR of the articular cartilage in the osteoarthrotic knee. Correlation of MR and arthroscopic findings. Acta Radiol. 1998;39:120–5.
41. Link TM, Sell CA, Masi JN, Phan C, Newitt D, Lu Y, et al. 3.0 vs 1.5 T MRI in the detection of focal cartilage pathology – ROC analysis in an experimental model. Osteoarthritis Cartilage. 2006;14:63–70.
42. Potter HG, Linklater JM, Allen AA, Hannafin JA, Haas SB. Magnetic resonance imaging of articular cartilage in the knee. An evaluation with use of fast-spin-echo imaging. J Bone Joint Surg Am. 1998;80:1276–84.
43. Ramnath RR, Magee T, Wasudev N, Murrah R. Accuracy of 3-T MRI using fast spin-echo technique to detect meniscal tears of the knee. AJR Am J Roentgenol. 2006;187:221–5.
44. Bredella MA, Tirman PF, Peterfy CG, Zarlingo M, Feller JF, Bost FW, et al. Accuracy of T2-weighted fast spin-echo MR imaging with fat saturation in detecting cartilage defects in the knee: comparison with arthroscopy in 130 patients. AJR Am J Roentgenol. 1999;172:1073–80.
45. Yoshioka H, Stevens K, Genovese M, Dillingham MF, Lang P. Articular cartilage of knee: normal patterns at MR imaging that mimic disease in healthy subjects and patients with osteoarthritis. Radiology. 2004;231:31–8.
46. Yoshioka H, Stevens K, Hargreaves BA, Steines D, Genovese M, Dillingham MF, et al. Magnetic resonance imaging of articular cartilage of the knee: comparison between fat-suppressed three-dimensional SPGR imaging, fat-suppressed FSE imaging, and fat-suppressed three-dimensional DEFT imaging, and correlation with arthroscopy. J Magn Reson Imaging. 2004;20:857–64.
47. Eckstein F, Burstein D, Link TM. Quantitative MRI of cartilage and bone: degenerative changes in osteoarthritis. NMR Biomed. 2006;19:822–54.
48. Ruehm S, Zanetti M, Romero J, Hodler J. MRI of patellar articular cartilage: evaluation of an optimized gradient echo sequence (3D-DESS). J Magn Reson Imaging. 1998;8:1246–51.

49. Hargreaves BA, Gold GE, Lang PK, Conolly SM, Pauly JM, Bergman G, et al. MR imaging of articular cartilage using driven equilibrium. Magn Reson Med. 1999;42:695–703.
50. Gold GE, Fuller SE, Hargreaves BA, Stevens KJ, Beaulieu CF. Driven equilibrium magnetic resonance imaging of articular cartilage: initial clinical experience. J Magn Reson Imaging. 2005;21:476–81.
51. Hargreaves BA, Gold GE, Beaulieu CF, Vasanawala SS, Nishimura DG, Pauly JM. Comparison of new sequences for high-resolution cartilage imaging. Magn Reson Med. 2003;49:700–9.
52. Kornaat PR, Reeder SB, Koo S, Brittain JH, Yu H, Andriacchi TP, et al. MR imaging of articular cartilage at 1.5 T and 3.0 T: comparison of SPGR and SSFP sequences. Osteoarthritis Cartilage. 2005;13:338–44.
53. Bauer J, Barr C, Steinbach L, Malfair, D, Krug, R, Ma, C, Link, TM. Imaging of the articular cartilage of the ankle at 3.0 and 1.5 Tesla. Eur Radiol Suppl. 2006;16(S1):238.
54. Ristow O, Steinbach L, Sabo G, Krug R, Huber M, Rauscher I, et al. Isotropic 3D fast spin-echo imaging versus standard 2D imaging at 3.0 T of the knee-image quality and diagnostic performance. Eur Radiol. 2009;19:1263–72.
55. Stevens KJ, Busse RF, Han E, Brau AC, Beatty PJ, Beaulieu CF, et al. Ankle: isotropic MR imaging with 3D-FSE-cube – initial experience in healthy volunteers. Radiology. 2008;249:1026–33.
56. Gagliardi JA, Chung EM, Chandnani VP, Kesling KL, Christensen KP, Null RN, et al. Detection and staging of chondromalacia patellae: relative efficacies of conventional MR imaging, MR arthrography, and CT arthrography. AJR Am J Roentgenol. 1994;163:629–36.
57. Kramer J, Recht MP, Imhof H, Stiglbauer R, Engel A. Postcontrast MR arthrography in assessment of cartilage lesions. J Comput Assist Tomogr. 1994;18:218–24.
58. Woertler K, Rummeny EJ, Settles M. A fast high-resolution multislice T1-weighted turbo spin-echo (TSE) sequence with a DRIVen equilibrium (DRIVE) pulse for native arthrographic contrast. AJR Am J Roentgenol. 2005;185:1468–70.
59. Dunn TC, Lu Y, Jin H, Ries MD, Majumdar S. T2 relaxation time of cartilage at MR imaging: comparison with severity of knee osteoarthritis. Radiology. 2004;232:592–8.
60. Regatte RR, Akella SV, Borthakur A, Kneeland JB, Reddy R. In vivo proton MR three-dimensional T1rho mapping of human articular cartilage: initial experience. Radiology. 2003;229:269–74.
61. Bashir A, Gray ML, Hartke J, Burstein D. Nondestructive imaging of human cartilage glycosaminoglycan concentration by MRI. Magn Reson Med. 1999;41:857–65.
62. Burstein D, Bashir A, Gray ML. MRI techniques in early stages of cartilage disease. Invest Radiol. 2000;35:622–38.
63. Liess C, Lusse S, Karger N, Heller M, Gluer CC. Detection of changes in cartilage water content using MRI T2-mapping in vivo. Osteoarthritis Cartilage. 2002;10:907–13.
64. Dardzinski BJ, Mosher TJ, Li S, Van Slyke MA, Smith MB. Spatial variation of T2 in human articular cartilage. Radiology. 1997;205:546–50.
65. Mosher TJ, Dardzinski BJ, Smith MB. Human articular cartilage: influence of aging and early symptomatic degeneration on the spatial variation of T2 – preliminary findings at 3 T. Radiology. 2000;214:259–66.
66. Li X, Han ET, Ma CB, Link TM, Newitt DC, Majumdar S. In vivo 3 T spiral imaging based multi-slice T(1rho) mapping of knee cartilage in osteoarthritis. Magn Reson Med. 2005;54:929–36.
67. Stahl R, Luke A, Li X, Carballido-Gamio J, Ma CB, Majumdar S, et al. T1rho, T(2) and focal knee cartilage abnormalities in physically active and sedentary healthy subjects versus early OA patients-a 3.0-Tesla MRI study. Eur Radiol. 2009;19:132–43.
68. Trattnig S, Mlynarik V, Breitenseher M, Huber M, Zembsch A, Rand T, et al. MRI visualization of proteoglycan depletion in articular cartilage via intravenous administration of Gd-DTPA. Magn Reson Imaging. 1999;17:577–83.
69. Gillis A, Bashir A, McKeon B, Scheller A, Gray ML, Burstein D. Magnetic resonance imaging of relative glycosaminoglycan distribution in patients with autologous chondrocyte transplants. Invest Radiol. 2001;36:743–8.
70. Williams A, Gillis A, McKenzie C, Po B, Sharma L, Micheli L, et al. Glycosaminoglycan distribution in cartilage as determined by delayed gadolinium-enhanced MRI of cartilage (dGEMRIC): potential clinical applications. AJR Am J Roentgenol. 2004;182:167–72.
71. Williams A, Sharma L, McKenzie CA, Prasad PV, Burstein D. Delayed gadolinium-enhanced magnetic resonance imaging of cartilage in knee osteoarthritis: findings at different radiographic stages of disease and relationship to malalignment. Arthritis Rheum. 2005;52:3528–35.
72. Carballido-Gamio J, Link TM, Li X, Han ET, Krug R, Ries MD, et al. Feasibility and reproducibility of relaxometry, morphometric, and geometrical measurements of the hip joint with magnetic resonance imaging at 3 T. J Magn Reson Imaging. 2008;28:227–35.
73. Cheng Y, Wang S, Yamazaki T, Zhao J, Nakajima Y, Tamura S. Hip cartilage thickness measurement accuracy improvement. Comput Med Imaging Graph. 2007;31:643–55.
74. Kim YJ, Bixby S, Mamisch TC, Clohisy JC, Carlisle JC. Imaging structural abnormalities in the hip joint: instability and impingement as a cause of osteoarthritis. Semin Musculoskelet Radiol. 2008;12:334–45.
75. Taljanovic MS, Graham AR, Benjamin JB, Gmitro AF, Krupinski EA, Schwartz SA, et al. Bone marrow edema pattern in advanced hip osteoarthritis: quantitative assessment with magnetic resonance imaging and correlation with clinical examination, radiographic findings, and histopathology. Skeletal Radiol. 2008;37:423–31.
76. Tiderius CJ, Jessel R, Kim YJ, Burstein D. Hip dGEMRIC in asymptomatic volunteers and patients with early osteoarthritis: the influence of timing after contrast injection. Magn Reson Med. 2007;57:803–5.
77. Eckstein F, Siedek V, Glaser C, Al-Ali D, Englmeier KH, Reiser M, et al. Correlation and sex differences between ankle and knee cartilage morphology determined by quantitative magnetic resonance imaging. Ann Rheum Dis. 2004;63:1490–5.
78. Blumenkrantz G, Stahl R, Carballido-Gamio J, Link T, Majumdar S. Longitudinal changes in the heterogeneity of cartilage T2 in osteoarthritis subjects. In: Proceedings of 14th Annual Scientific Meeting of ISMRM. Berlin, Germany; 2007.
79. Li X, Benjamin Ma C, Link TM, Castillo DD, Blumenkrantz G, Lozano J, et al. Benjamin Ma C, Link TM, et al. In vivoT(1rho) and T(2) mapping of articular cartilage in osteoarthritis of the knee using 3 T MRI. Osteoarthritis Cartilage. 2007;15:789–97.
80. Li X, Han ET, Busse RF, Majumdar S. In vivo T(1rho) mapping in cartilage using 3D magnetization-prepared angle-modulated partitioned k-space spoiled gradient echo snapshots (3D MAPSS). Magn Reson Med. 2008;59:298–307.
81. Mosher TJ, Liu Y, Yang QX, Yao J, Smith R, Dardzinski BJ, et al. Age dependency of cartilage magnetic resonance imaging T2 relaxation times in asymptomatic women. Arthritis Rheum. 2004;50:2820–8.
82. Regatte RR, Akella SV, Lonner JH, Kneeland JB, Reddy R. T1rho relaxation mapping in human osteoarthritis (OA) cartilage: comparison of T1rho with T2. J Magn Reson Imaging. 2006;23:547–53.
83. Pfirrmann CW, Mengiardi B, Dora C, Kalberer F, Zanetti M, Hodler J. Cam and pincer femoroacetabular impingement: characteristic MR arthrographic findings in 50 patients. Radiology. 2006;240:778–85.

Chapter 7
MRI of Cartilage: Pathological Findings

Thomas M. Link

Keywords MRI • Cartilage • Pathologies • Associated findings • Osteoarthritis • Osteochondritis dissecans • Trauma • Osteochondral defects

The most important clinical indications for magnetic resonance imaging (MRI) are assessment of cartilage in osteoarthritis (OA), chronic or acute osteochondral injury including sports injuries, osteochondritis dissecans, chondromalacia patellae, and inflammatory arthropathies (in particular before invasive therapy). In addition dedicated cartilage imaging is required after invasive cartilage repair procedures or conservative therapies, including pharmacological therapies, to monitor treatment effect. MR studies are required to tailor therapies and in the future new quantitative techniques may have significance in indicating treatment as well as monitoring therapy similar to bone mineral density currently used in the setting of osteoporosis.

Most of these indications focus on imaging of the knee, which has the thickest cartilage and is most accessible to MR imaging. As outlined previously in Chap. 6, cartilage imaging of the hip is more challenging because of the limited thickness of the hip cartilage with a mean thickness of around 1.5–2 mm. The same applies for imaging of the ankle and elbow with the cartilage at the hand being even thinner. In general indications for cartilage imaging at the shoulder and wrist are limited given the non-weight-bearing function of these joints. Rarely trauma-induced cartilage injury requires direct visualization of cartilage defects or fragments. At the elbow and ankle visualization of the cartilage is more important as osteochondritis dissecans and cartilage injury are not infrequently found at these sites. Hip cartilage imaging is getting increasing interest because of femoroacetabular impingement and its role in the evolution of osteoarthritis. Cam-type femoroacetabular impingement typically leads to injury of the anterosuperior cartilage of the femoral head and the labrum.

Osteoarthritis

One of the most significant health problems in our aging society is degenerative joint disease. Interestingly, the risk for disability attributable to knee OA is as great as that attributable to cardiovascular disease and greater than that caused by any other medical condition in elderly persons [1]. Knee OA is already the leading cause of functional disability, and its prevalence is projected to double by the year 2020, caused in part by increases in obesity and longevity [2].

Radiographs have been used for many years as a standard technique to diagnose and grade OA; the Kellgren–Lawrence (KL) scale is a standard, well-established classification system to score OA and has been used in multiple studies over the last decades [3]. We have learned, however, that early findings of joint degeneration are missed on radiographs and that MRI provides a substantially better evaluation of joint disease by including information on tissues not visualized with radiographs including cartilage, menisci, ligaments, and bone marrow [4]. Figure 7.1 shows a relatively normal appearing lateral radiograph of the knee, however, extensive, near full thickness cartilage loss at the patella and trochlea as well as a focal area of delamination at the posterior aspect of the lateral femoral condyle. Expected pathologies associated with OA, however, do not only encompass cartilage loss, but also abnormalities of the menisci, the bone marrow, the ligaments as well as pathologies in the soft tissues around the joint with joint effusion, synovitis, and popliteal cysts being the major findings.

T.M. Link (✉)
Department of Radiology and Biomedical Imaging,
University of California at San Francisco, 400 Parnassus Avenue,
A-367, San Francisco, CA 94131, USA
e-mail: thomas.link@radiology.ucsf.edu; tmlink@radiology.ucsf.edu

T.M. Link (ed.), *Cartilage Imaging: Significance, Techniques, and New Developments*,
DOI 10.1007/978-1-4419-8438-8_7, © Springer Science+Business Media, LLC 2011

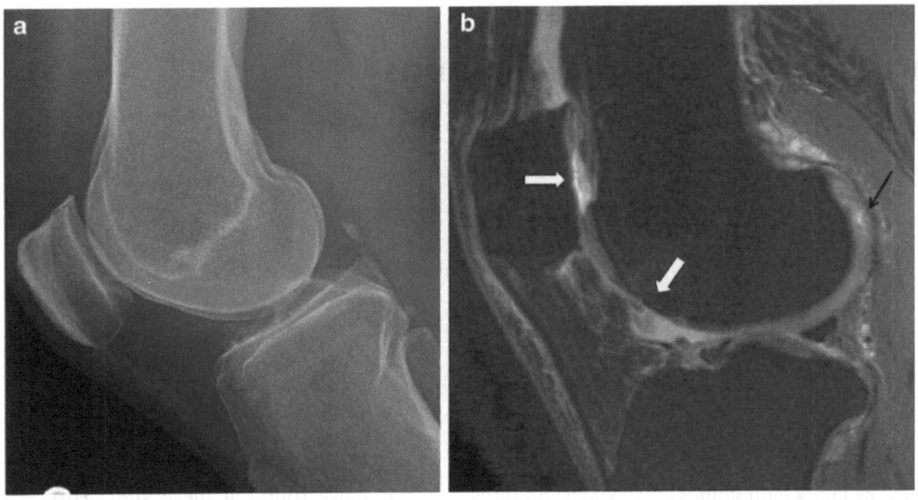

Fig. 7.1 (**a**, **b**). Radiograph and sagittal magnetic resonance imaging (MRI) of a patient with osteoarthritis (OA) show a relatively normal appearing lateral radiograph of the knee with small patellar osteophytes, however, extensive, near full thickness cartilage loss at the patella and trochlea (*white arrows*) as well as a focal area of partial thickness delamination (*black arrow*) at the posterior aspect of the lateral femoral condyle

Please note, that the extent of these abnormalities is not well associated with *clinical findings* of pain and limited function. According to the American College of Rheumatology guidelines osteoarthritis (OA) of the knee is defined and classified based on clinical, radiographic, and laboratory findings [5]. Chronic or recurrent pain in the knee is of central importance in the disease process of OA. A number of studies were performed correlating presence and degree of joint pain with findings on conventional radiographs and magnetic resonance imaging (MRI). Using Kellgren–Lawrence grades to quantify osteoarthritis on conventional radiographs and correlating these with the degree of pain (using the established Western Ontario and McMasters Universities (WOMAC) osteoarthritis index), however, did not show significant correlations [4, 6, 7]. Studies have investigated associations between the different MR abnormalities and pain [4, 8–12]. One of the early studies correlating MR findings and WOMAC pain scores in 50 subjects with varying degree of osteoarthritis [4] could not demonstrate significant results for semiquantitatively assessed cartilage, bone marrow, ligamentous, and meniscal abnormalities. Interestingly this study, however, showed increased WOMAC pain scores at early stages of cartilage loss, while more advanced cartilage loss was associated with lower WOMAC scores. Zhai et al. [13] also found non-full-thickness, early focal cartilage lesions of the femur and the patella in younger subjects (average age 45 years) to be associated with pain. Kornaat et al. [10, 11] could not demonstrate significant correlations between pain and semiquantitatively assessed MRI findings in 368 subjects with varying degrees of symptomatic osteoarthritis of the knee. Two other studies, on the other hand, found correlations between bone marrow edema pattern and knee pain [8, 9]. Felson et al. studied subjects with osteoarthritis or high risk for osteoarthritis over a period of 15 months and found the development of pain to be associated with an increase in the size of bone marrow edema–like lesions. In summary bone marrow edema pattern and early cartilage lesions may be associated to some extent with clinical symptoms of pain.

Typical MR findings associated with OA do not only include cartilage abnormalities but also meniscal, ligamentous, and bone marrow lesions. The following five paragraphs provide an overview of the MR findings related to OA.

Cartilage Abnormalities

Table 7.1 shows the presence and severity of cartilage lesions in relation to radiographic KL scores of OA. This table clearly indicates that with increasing OA cartilage lesions are more numerous and more severe. Different patterns of cartilage loss are identified and loss can be focal or diffuse. The standard classification system of cartilage lesions [14] differentiates four different grades according to their signal and their depths and is analogous

Table 7.1 Presence and severity of cartilage lesions assessed on FSE and SPGR sequences in relation to radiographic Kellgren–Lawrence (KL) scores of osteoarthritis (OA) ($n = 50$ patients). Cartilage score: 0 = no cartilage defect, 1 = signal inhomogeneity in the cartilage, 2 = cartilage defect less than 50%, 3 = cartilage defect more than 50%, 4 = full thickness lesion) (Modified from Phan et al. [4])

		KL-1 ($n = 10$)	KL-2 ($n = 11$)	KL-3 ($n = 13$)	KL-4 ($n = 16$)	All ($n = 50$)
No defects	0	20% (2/10)	36% (4/11)	8% (1/13)	0	14% (7/50)
Lesions	1	10% (1/10)	0	0	0	2% (1/50)
	2	20% (2/10)	18% (2/11)	8% (1/13)	0	10% (5/50)
	3	40% (4/10)	28% (3/11)	31% (4/13)	19% (3/16)	28% (14/50)
	4	10% (1/10)	18% (2/11)	55% (7/13)	81% (13/16)	46% (23/50)
Average score		2.1	1.9	3.2	3.8	
Standard deviation		±1.4	±1.6	±1.2	±0.4	

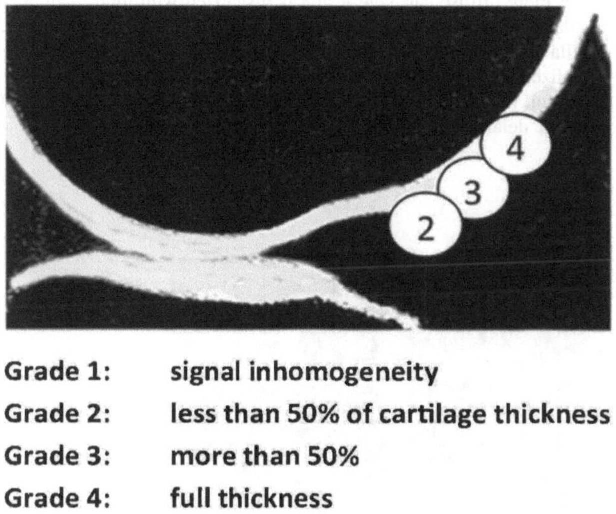

Fig. 7.2 The standard classification system of cartilage lesions differentiates four different grades according to their signal and their depths and is analogous to the arthroscopic classification system defined by Noyes et al.: grade 1 is defined as signal abnormalities within the cartilage (arthroscopically corresponding to softening of the cartilage), grade 2 as a focal cartilage lesion less than 50% of the diameter of the cartilage, grade 3 as a lesion of more than 50% of the cartilage diameter and grade 4 as a full thickness cartilage lesion

to the arthroscopic classification system defined by Noyes et al. [15]: grade 1 is defined as signal abnormalities within the cartilage (arthroscopically corresponding to softening of the cartilage), grade 2 as a focal cartilage lesion less than 50 % of the diameter of the cartilage, grade 3 as a lesion of more than 50% of the cartilage diameter and grade 4 as a full thickness cartilage lesion (Fig. 7.2). Figure 7.3 illustrates the different grades in patients with varying degrees of OA. Given differences in signal characteristics between different sequences identification of grade 1 lesions is not very reproducible and histological correlation of grade 1 lesions with cartilage proteoglycan loss is very limited [16]. While the above-mentioned scoring system is used for cartilage lesions in general other classification systems have been developed which also evaluate the size of the cartilage defects and were specifically developed for OA such as the WORMS and BLOKS but these will be described in Chap. 8 of this book.

MRI usually performs well in detecting full thickness cartilage lesions, however, it is limited in detecting superficial and partial thickness lesions. Saadat et al. [16] analyzed the performance of a fat-saturated intermediate-weighted (iw) fast spin echo sequence obtained at 3T in detecting cartilage lesions using histology as a standard of reference. All patients underwent MRI before undergoing total knee replacement and the histological sections of the resected specimens (safranin [Saf]-O [specific for proteoglycans], hematoxylin and eosin [H&E] for histological analysis) were rigorously matched with the preoperative MRI. In addition to the standard classification system described above these investigators also studied surface fraying and more severe fibrillation. Figure 7.4 shows representative images from this study. In diagnosing lesions affecting cartilage thickness and surface fraying and fibrillation accuracy was in the order of 70–73% with the highest sensitivities for cartilage thickness lesions and highest specificities for surface fraying and fibrillation. Substantially better performance was found for high-grade (3 and 4) lesions while limitations were found for low-grade lesions and in differentiating grade 2 and 3 lesions.

Interestingly, however, analyzing MR signal abnormalities of the cartilage performance was very limited in relation to histological findings with a sensitivity of 36%, a specificity of 62%, and an accuracy of 45%. This means that signal abnormalities visualized in the cartilage are in less than 50% associated with histological degeneration; however, if the signal is normal histological findings are also in the normal range in 62%. Figure 7.5 shows an

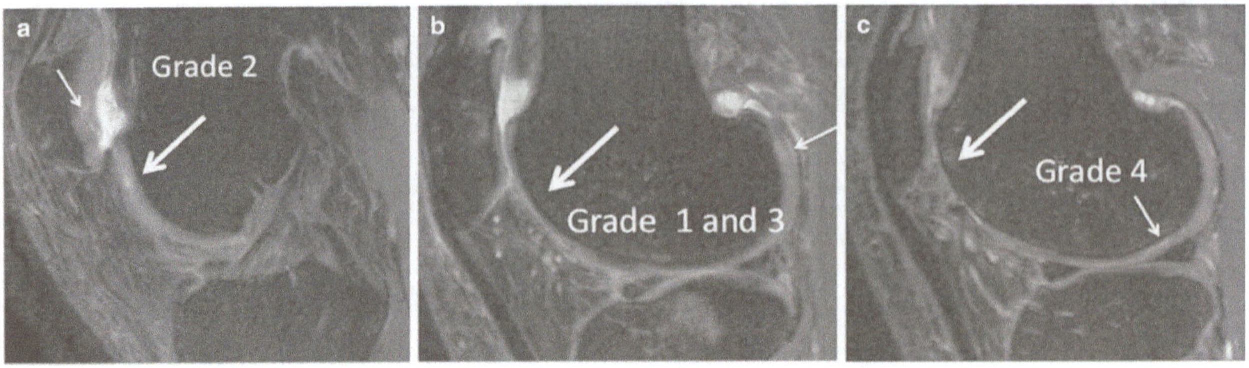

Fig. 7.3 (**a–c**). Sagittal fat-saturated intermediate-weighted (iw) FSE sequences showing different grades of cartilage lesions at the trochlea in patients with varying degrees of osteoarthritis (OA). In (**a**) a subtle focal lesion is shown at the trochlea (*arrow*), which is superficial and only affects less than 50% of the cartilage diameter. In addition partial thickness cartilage delamination at the patella (*small arrow*). In (**b**) a larger more diffuse cartilage lesion is visualized with more than 50% cartilage loss (*arrow*). Also note more than 50% cartilage loss at the patella and bone marrow edema pattern at the tibia. A grade 1 lesion is visualized at the posterior aspect of the femoral condyle (*small arrow*). In (**c**) full thickness cartilage loss is shown at the trochlea (*arrow*) and cartilage delamination at the femoral condyle (*small arrow*)

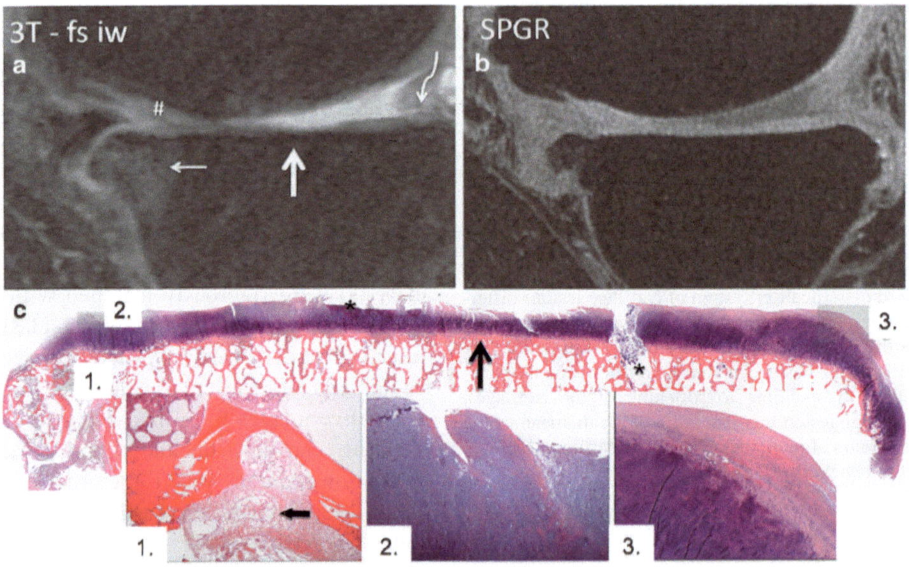

Fig. 7.4 (**a–c**). Sagittal fat-saturated intermediate-weighted (iw) FSE (**a**) and SPGR (**b**) sequences obtained at 3T with histology as a standard of reference (H&E stain) (**c**). In (**a**) indistinct cartilage is shown at the central tibia corresponding to an area of cartilage fraying on histology (**c**) (*arrow*). Bone marrow edema pattern at the anterior aspect of the tibia (*small arrow* in **a**) corresponds to an area of fibrovascular ingrowth (1). Fraying and degeneration of the anterior tibial cartilage is shown in (2) corresponding to an area of bright, indistinct cartilage in the intermediate-weighted (iw) FSE sequence (# in **a**). At the posterior aspect of the tibia (*curved arrow*) signal abnormality of the cartilage is visualized (**a**), which corresponds to an area of fibrocartilage and pannus overgrowth (3) (From Saadat et al. [16])

example were signal abnormalities in the MRI actually corresponded to histological abnormalities (synovial tissue overgrowth).

In general studies using arthroscopy as a standard of reference have found higher sensitivities and specificities compared to the above-mentioned histological study. Clearly, however, arthroscopy has limitations in particular in differentiating grade 2 and 3 lesions, and there is also inter-observer variability. In a study by Yoshioka et al. [17], iw FSE sequences were found to have a sensitivity of 100%

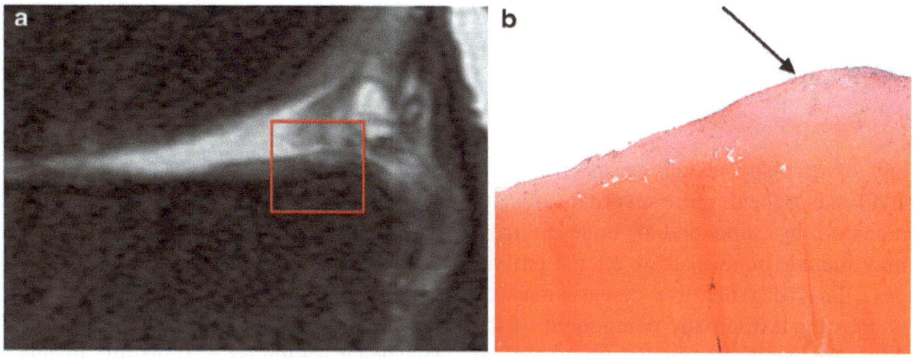

Fig. 7.5 (**a**, **b**). Sagittal fat-saturated intermediate-weighted (fs iw) FSE (**a**) of the medial joint compartment and corresponding tibial histological section (safranin [Saf]-O) (**b**) in a 54-year-old female patient. Cartilage thickening/swelling at the posterior aspect of the tibia with high signal intensity region (*highlighted area* in **a**). The corresponding Saf-O staining (**b**) shows an area of cartilage thickening due to synovial overgrowth (pannus tissue) with proteoglycan loss (From Saadat et al. [16].)

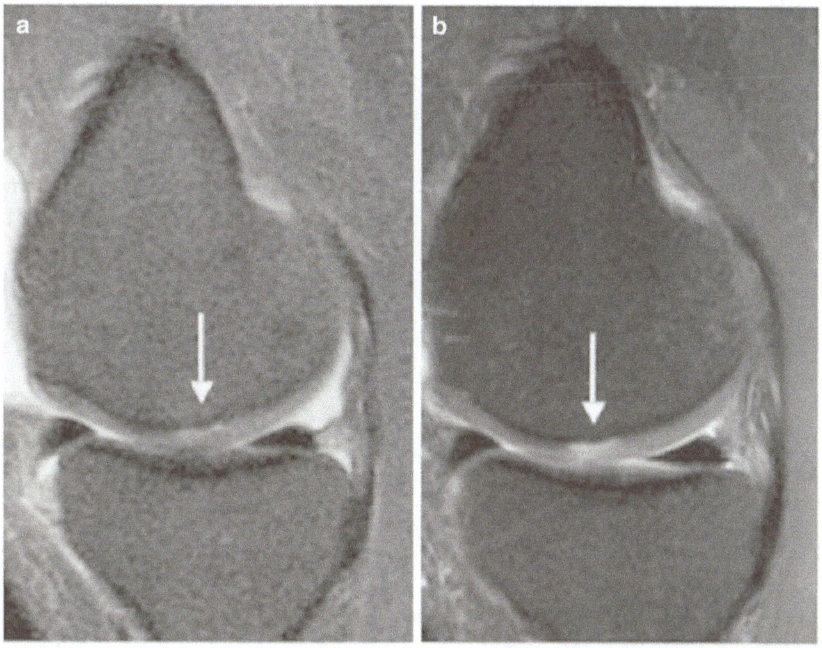

Fig. 7.6 (**a**, **b**). A 36-year-old male patient with a clinical history of left knee pain and suspected osteochondritis dissecans. At 1.5 T (**a**; sagittal fat-saturated intermediate-weighted [fs iw] FSE sequence, TR 3,200 ms, TE 46 ms) an area of high signal is shown along the subchondral bone underneath the cartilage suggesting delamination (*arrow*) without a focal cartilage defect. The 3.0 T study (**b**; TR 4,300 ms, TE 51 ms) clearly shows a full thickness cartilage defect along with delamination (*arrow*). Findings were confirmed by arthroscopy after both imaging studies were obtained (From Wong et al. [47])

and specificity of 68%. Potter et al. [18] found 87% sensitivity and 92% specificity for the ability of FSE in detection of lesions. Kijowski et al. compared 1.5 and 3.0 T imaging using arthroscopy as a standard of reference and found respective sensitivity, specificity, and accuracy of MR imaging for detecting cartilage lesions of 69.3%, 78.0%, and 74.5% at 1.5 T and 70.5%, 85.9%, and 80.1% at 3.0 T. Wong et al. had similar results and found that diagnosis of cartilage abnormalities was improved at 3.0 T with higher sensitivity (75.7% vs 70.6%) and accuracy (88.2% vs 86.4%) (Fig. 7.6).

It should be noted that diagnostic performance in correctly grading the lesions in MR images yields significantly lower results, for example, Wong et al. found a correct grading of cartilage lesions only in 51.3% of the cases at 3.0 T versus 42.9% of the cases at 1.5 T.

The morphology of cartilage lesions in osteoarthritis varies and may be diffuse or focal; more severe lesions are frequently accompanied by subchondral bone marrow changes, which may include bone marrow edema pattern and cystic changes. Early degenerative disease may be more focal also suggesting a traumatic component of the disease process. Most frequently the medial femoro-tibial joint compartment is affected as varus osteoarthritis is most frequent. In valgus osteoarthritis the lateral compartment is affected. Not infrequently severe degenerative changes are found at the patello-femoral joint compartment, which is a non-weight-bearing compartment. The latter distribution is found in patellar tracking disorders and this may also be associated with high-impact activities such as running, which particularly affect this joint (Fig. 7.7). Also it should be noted that calcium pyrophosphate deposition disease (CPPD) is a disease, which typically affects the femoro-patellar joint and can be associated with severe cartilage loss (Fig. 7.8) and degeneration. Cartilage MR signal in CPPD may vary, however, is mostly low, and diagnosis is challenging. In a previous human cadaver study with histological validation Abreu et al. [19] found that radiographs were superior in diagnosing calcium deposits compared to MRI and MRI was insensitive to the presence of CPPD deposits in the knee, even when such deposits are widespread. Also they demonstrated that the sensitivity of MRI was significantly better in detecting CPPD deposits in the hyaline cartilage of the femoral condyles when compared with other knee internal structures, even when such structures contained a higher amount of calcification.

Another finding not infrequently associated with cartilage degeneration is delamination. In delamination a separation of the articular cartilage from the underlying subchondral bone at the tidemark is found, or delamination may occur if a layer of cartilage is separated from underlying cartilage. These findings have been reported at the knee in athletes and younger physically active subjects [20, 21] but with improving MR techniques are also frequently found in cartilage degeneration. The delamination line runs parallel to the joint surface, but the overlying articular cartilage remains initially intact as shown in Fig. 7.9. In particular if the cartilage layer gets unstable maceration may occur resulting in accelerated OA.

Delamination has been reported as a typical finding in cam-type femoroacetabular impingement and may be found in up to 52% of these patients [22, 23]. However, sensitivity

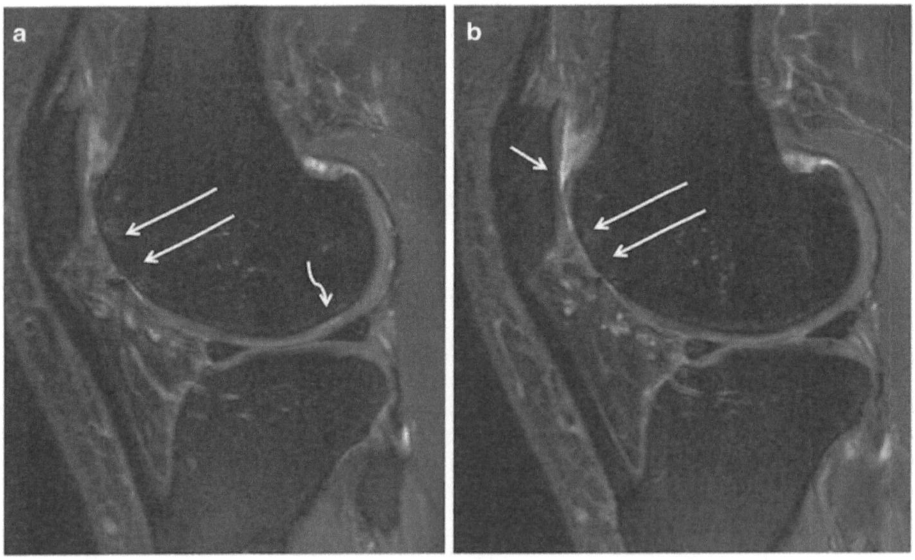

Fig. 7.7 (**a**, **b**). Sagittal fat-saturated intermediate-weighted (fs iw) FSE sequences of a middle-aged woman with a history of being an avid runner and a patellar tracking disorder. Severe up to full thickness cartilage loss at the trochlea (*large arrows*) and more than 50% cartilage loss at the patella (*small arrow*). In addition cartilage inhomogeneity, swelling, and an area of delamination (*curved arrow* in **a**) at the femoral condyle

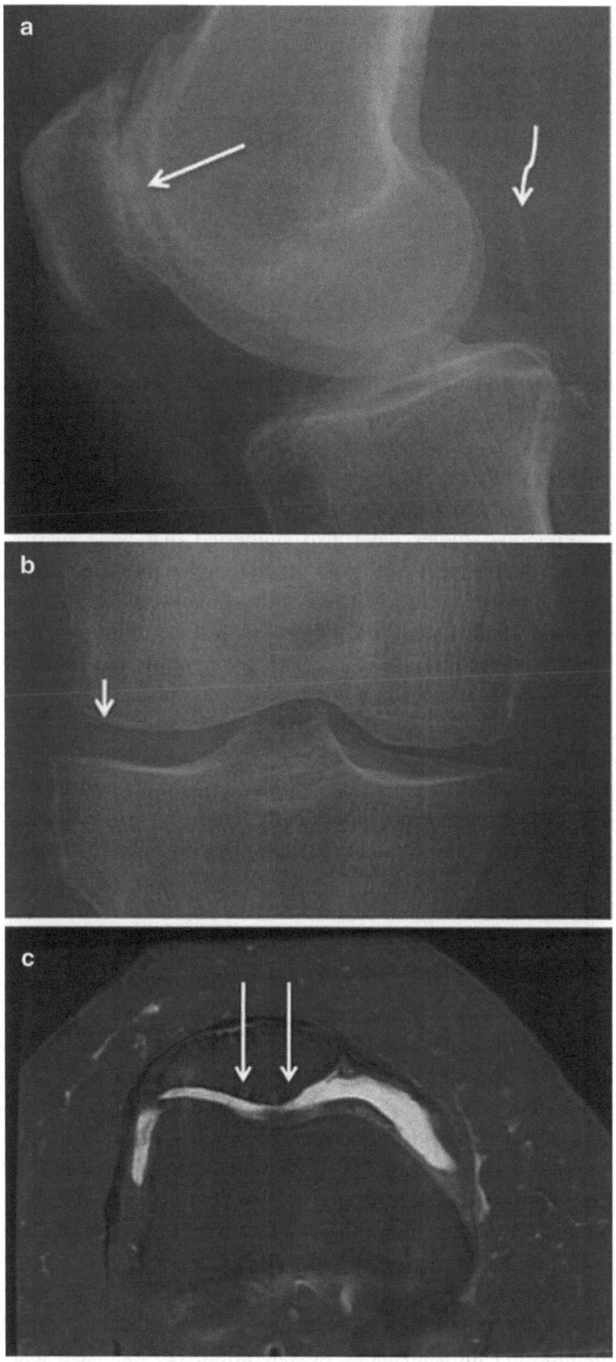

Fig. 7.8 (**a**–**c**). Anteroposterior (**a**) and lateral (**b**) radiographs as well as axial fat-saturated intermediate-weighted (fs iw) FSE sequence (**c**) in a patient with calcium pyrophosphate deposition disease (CPPD), which typically affects the femoro-patellar joint and can be associated with severe cartilage loss (*large arrows* in **a** and **c**). In addition meniscal calcifications (*small arrow* in **b**) and calcifications in the gastrocenemius muscles (*curved arrow* in **a**) are shown

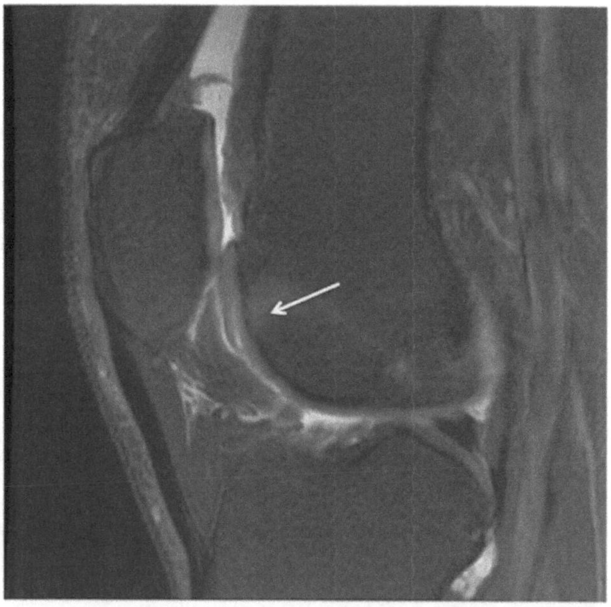

Fig. 7.9 Sagittal fat-saturated intermediate-weighted (fs iw) FSE sequence showing cartilage delamination, which is frequently associated with cartilage degeneration. The delamination line runs parallel to the joint surface (*arrow*), but the overlying articular cartilage may initially appear intact. Also note subtle bone marrow edema pattern in the trochlear region and mild joint effusion in the supra-patellar recess

even with MR arthrography is low: Pfirrmann et al. used MR arthrography of the hip to study acetabular cartilage delamination in 23 patients with surgically confirmed cartilage delamination. At MR, a diagnosis of fluid signal intensity under the cartilage delamination had a sensitivity of 22–30% but a high specificity of 95%. A MR hypointense line in the acetabular cartilage demonstrated on sagittal three-dimensional (3D) double-echo steady-state images with water excitation had a better diagnostic performance with a sensitivity of 70% but a specificity of 5–62%. Hypointense areas in the acetabular cartilage were quite specific (90%) on both coronal intermediate-weighted fat-saturated (iw fs) images but the sensitivity varied between 54% and 70%.

Quantitative imaging of cartilage is of major significance in OA, but will be described separately in Chaps. 10–14. Both volumetric measurements and molecular MR imaging techniques focusing on the cartilage matrix have been used to study early and more advanced stages of OA.

Table 7.2 Prevalence of bone marrow edema pattern (edema) in relation to radiographic evidence of osteoarthritis (OA) (Kellgren–Lawrence [KL] scores) (Modified from Phan et al. [4]). Maximum diameter of bone marrow edema pattern was measured on fluid-sensitive coronal and sagittal FSE sequences. Total number of patients was 50

	KL-1 (*n* = 10)	KL-2 (*n* = 11)	KL-3 (*n* = 13)	KL-4 (*n* = 16)	All (*n* = 50)
No edema	70% (7/10)	64% (7/11)	23% (3/13)	19% (3/16)	40% (20/50)
Edema, all	30% (3/10)	36% (4/11)	77% (10/13)	81% (13/16)	60% (30/50)
– Mild (<1 cm)	20% (2/10)	9% (1/11)	23% (3/13)	25% (4/16)	20% (10/50)
– Moderate (1–2 cm)	10% (1/10)	9% (1/11)	31% (4/13)	44% (7/16)	26% (13/50)
– Severe (>2 cm)		18% (2/11)	23% (3/13)	12% (2/16)	14% (7/50)

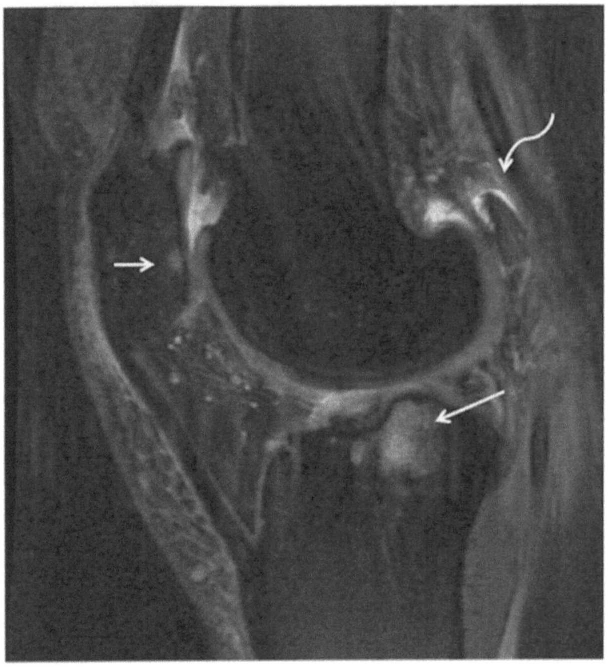

Fig. 7.10 Extensive bone marrow edema pattern at the tibia (*large arrow*) demonstrated in a sagittal fat-saturated intermediate-weighted (fs iw) FSE sequence with overlying cartilage loss. In addition small amount of bone marrow edema pattern at the patella with cartilage loss (*small arrow*). Inhomogeneity of the trochlear cartilage and loose body in the posterior-superior aspect of the joint capsule (*curved arrow*)

Bone Marrow Edema Pattern and Other Bone Marrow Lesions

Bone marrow edema pattern is a typical finding associated with cartilage defects in degenerative disease. Link et al. [4] found bone marrow edema pattern in 79% of patients with moderate and severe OA as defined by radiographic findings (Table 7.2, Fig. 7.10) but only in 33% of patients with mild OA. Previous studies analyzing resected tissue in patients undergoing total knee arthroplasty found mostly normal tissue underlying MRI findings of bone marrow edema pattern, but also abnormalities such as fibrovascular ingrowth, bone marrow fibrosis and necrosis, bone remodeling, bone marrow bleeding, and cystic changes [16, 24]. Similar findings were published by Taljanovic et al. for hip osteoarthritis, but these authors also found that microfractures in different stages of healing were associated with bone marrow edema pattern [25].

Previous studies have also suggested that bone marrow edema may be related to pain yet findings in the literature are contradictory and inconclusive at this time [4, 8, 10, 26]. One of these studies analyzed subjects with osteoarthritis or high risk for osteoarthritis over a period of 15 months and found the development of pain to be associated with an increase in the size of bone marrow edema–like lesions. Also insufficiency fractures and avascular necrosis present with bone marrow edema pattern. In particular in older, female patients insufficiency fractures are not infrequently found and lead to accelerated OA (see Section on Nonspecific Osteochondral Lesions).

Meniscal Degeneration

Meniscal degeneration is similar to cartilage abnormalities a frequent finding encountered with OA. As previously demonstrated meniscal lesions are found in a very high percentage of patients with moderate and severe OA (96.6%) with mostly severe abnormalities including displaced tears and maceration [4]. Interestingly prevalence of meniscal lesions in mild OA is still high (85.7%) yet abnormalities mostly are mild and include intrasubstance degeneration [4].

Different classification systems have been used to grade meniscal abnormalities. Standard abnormalities described include (1) intrasubstance degeneration, (2) meniscal tears that extend to the meniscal surface and do not change the shape of the meniscus, these include horizontal, oblique, and vertical tears, (3) complex tears with deformity of the meniscus, and (4) complete maceration/destruction of the meniscus. In addition meniscal extrusion is frequently present as the meniscal tissue is degenerating. Extrusion is mostly found at the medial compartment (meniscal body) and defined as 3 mm or more measured from the tibial border. Figure 7.11 shows different grades of meniscal degeneration and tears.

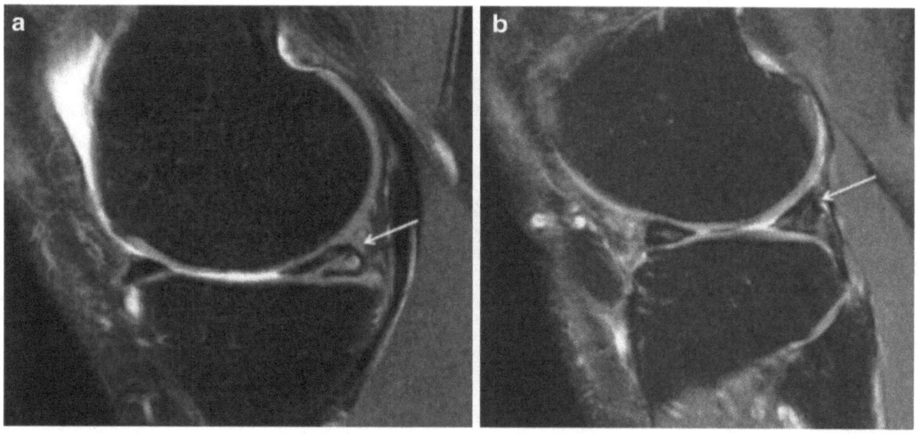

Fig. 7.11 (**a**, **b**). Different grades of meniscal degeneration and tears visualized in sagittal fat-saturated intermediate-weighted (fs iw) FSE sequences. In (**a**) an oblique tear with intrasubstance degeneration of the posterior horn of the medial meniscus is shown (*arrow*). In (**b**) intrasubstance degeneration is demonstrated of the posterior and anterior horn of the lateral meniscus; in addition there is a degenerative swelling of the posterior horn with an intrasubstance tear (*arrow*)

Meniscal abnormalities may also be graded according to the WORMS [27] or BLOKS [28] classification systems. Using WORMS six compartments are defined based on sagittal and coronal fast spin echo sequences and in each of these are graded according to five levels: 0 = intact; 1 = minor radial tear or parrot-beak tear; 2 = nondisplaced tear or prior surgical repair; 3 = displaced tear or partial resection; 4 = complete maceration/destruction or complete resection. Using BLOKS meniscal signal, extrusion and tears are separately classified.

Ligamentous Abnormalities

Osteoarthritis is frequently associated with ligamentous abnormalities; according to a previous study [4] ACL tears are found in 48% of patients with moderate and severe OA and collateral ligament abnormalities in approximately 20%. In addition ACL tears are more commonly associated with symptomatic knee OA and interestingly fewer than half of patients with ACL rupture recall a knee injury, suggesting that this risk factor for knee OA is underrecognized [29]. It is also generally accepted that the presence of ACL tears is associated with more rapid cartilage loss; in particular, cartilage lesions located in the central region of the medial compartment show more rapid progression of cartilage loss than cartilage lesions in the anterior and posterior portions of the medial compartment [30]. Different types of ACL degeneration are differentiated including full thickness tears, partial tears, and mucoid degeneration. Figure 7.12 shows examples of different types of ACL abnormalities associated with osteoarthritis.

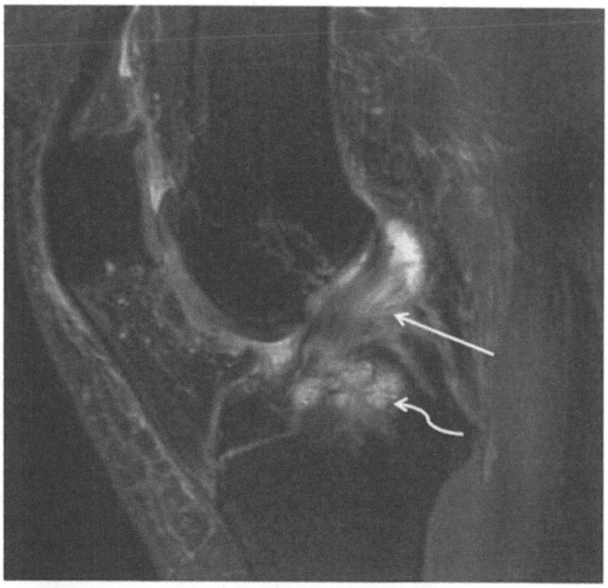

Fig. 7.12 ACL abnormality associated with osteoarthritis (OA) shown in a sagittal fat-saturated intermediate-weighted (fs iw) FSE sequence. The ACL is thickened and abnormally high in signal consistent with mucoid degeneration (*arrow*); in addition bone marrow abnormalities at the tibia including edema pattern and cystic changes (*curved arrow*)

Joint Effusion and Synovitis

Joint effusion and synovitis are typical findings associated with OA and it is generally accepted that these findings play an important role in symptomatic OA. Moderate and severe OA are associated in more than 90% with joint effusion and even in mild OA joint effusion is present in approximately

50% of patients [4]. While cartilage loss shows inconsistent association with joint pain previous studies found that joint effusion and synovitis were associated with clinical symptoms of OA including joint pain [10, 31] and may be an important parameter in monitoring treatment of OA. Interestingly while cartilage loss occurs in over 50% of knees with joint effusion and synovitis, these findings appear not to be associated with progression of cartilage loss in either tibiofemoral or patello-femoral compartment [31].

Inflammatory Arthropathies

Inflammatory arthropathies include rheumatoid arthritis and the seronegative spondylarthropathies ankylosing spondylitis, reactive arthritis, and psoriasis arthritis. MRI is helpful in assessing the degree of inflammatory changes of the joints and in monitoring therapy by directly visualizing synovitis, joint effusion, pannus tissue, and joint erosion. However, given that frequently small joints are affected the role of evaluating cartilage as a MRI biomarker in these inflammatory arthropathies, contrary to osteoarthritis, is limited.

The most frequent inflammatory arthropathy is *rheumatoid arthritis*, which typically affects the hands (radiocarpal, intercarpal, and metacarpophalangeal joints) and the feet (metatarsophalangeal joints). The central joints such as the knee and hip joints are less frequently affected by rheumatoid arthritis.

Standard 2D FSE sequences are not well suited for cartilage imaging of small joints as minimum slice thickness and in plane spatial resolution are limited. Previously 3D gradient-echo techniques were found to be best suited for the detection and grading of hyaline cartilage and subchondral bone lesions in rheumatoid arthritis [32]. Currently 3D FSE sequences may offer a viable alternative to cartilage imaging of small joints. In addition contrast administration is generally recommended to best visualize synovial proliferation and disease activity.

Figure 7.13 shows fat-saturated T2-weighted and contrast-enhanced T1-weighted MR images of the knee in a patient

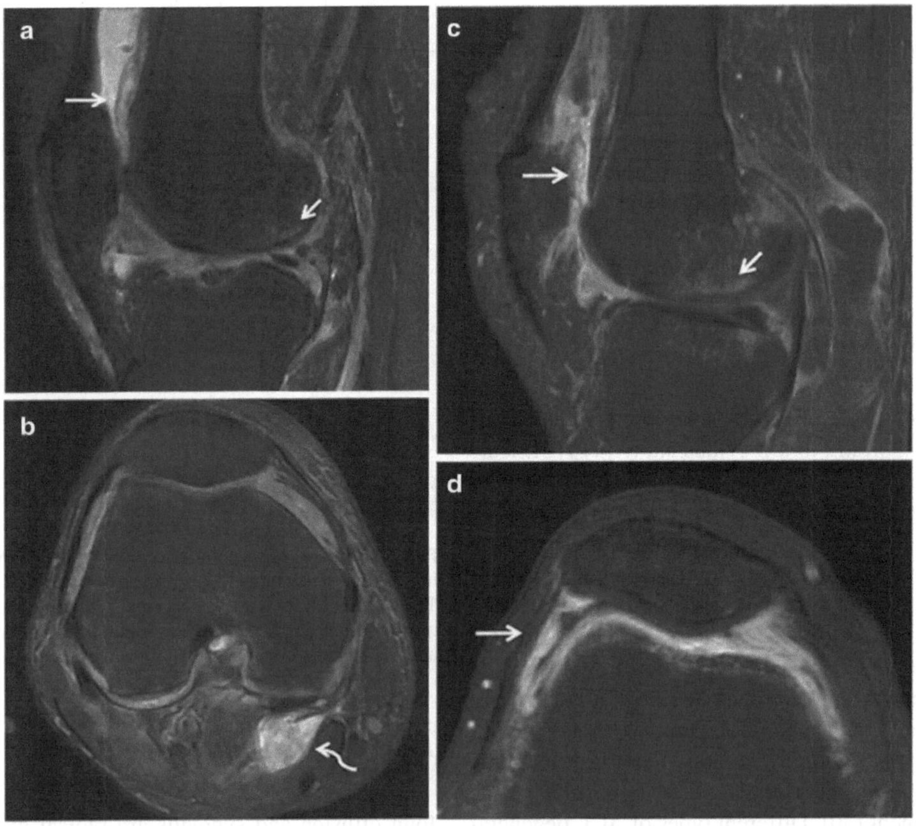

Fig. 7.13 (**a–d**). Fat-saturated intermediate-weighted (fs iw) (**a, b**) and contrast-enhanced T1-weighted (**c, d**) magnetic resonance (MR) images in a sagittal (**a–c**) and axial (**b–d**) orientation of the knee in a patient with active rheumatoid arthritis and synovitis. Thickened synovial pannus tissue (*arrows* in **a, c**) covers the hyaline cartilage and bone, which eventually erodes these tissues. Pannus tissue shows avid contrast enhancement (*arrows* **c, d**). Subtle reactive bone marrow edema pattern (*small arrows*) in the lateral femoral condyle. Joint effusion in the supra-patellar recess and popliteal cyst with pannus tissue (*curved arrow*)

with active rheumatoid arthritis. The pannus tissue covers the hyaline cartilage and erodes it. Cartilage protects the subchondral bone, which explains why the marginal bony regions of the joints, which are not covered by cartilage are eroded first. The slow erosion of the cartilage leads to concentric joint space narrowing and finally to focal erosions of the subchondral bone accompanied by bone marrow edema pattern. The bone marrow edema pattern is an important MRI finding predicting progression of rheumatoid arthritis [33]. While erosions and cartilage destruction are a frequent MR finding in adult rheumatoid arthritis, cartilage lesions are not so frequently visualized in juvenile idiopathic arthritis [34].

The typical MR imaging findings related to rheumatoid arthritis were published by the Outcome Measures in Rheumatology (OMERACT) MR Imaging Group and the so-called the RA-MRI scoring system (RAMRIS) was developed to better quantify and monitor joint inflammation [35, 36]. RAMRIS incorporates measures of joint inflammation and damage including bone erosion, edema pattern, and synovitis. The RAMRIS has demonstrated good reliability for bone erosion and synovitis at the wrists and metacarpophalangeal joints subject to reader training, with slightly lower levels of reader agreement for bone marrow edema pattern.

Quantitative, volumetric assessment of cartilage at the hands and feet required for assessment and monitoring of rheumatoid arthritis is challenging. In a previous study [37] the accuracy and reproducibility of a noninvasive technique for quantifying the volume of articular cartilage in the metacarpophalangeal joints of the hand by use of three-dimensional fat-suppressed gradient-echo sequence was studied in cadaver specimens. Accuracy errors for quantifying cartilage volume were –1.8% (95% confidence interval, –3.5% to –0.7%) for metacarpal cartilage and 9.1% (4.3–14.7%) for proximal phalangeal cartilage. Reproducibility errors were 5.2% (95% confidence interval, 2.9–7.6%) and 9.9% (5.4–15.1%), respectively. The authors concluded that fat-suppressed gradient-echo imaging provided sufficient contrast and spatial resolution to allow accurate and reproducible quantification of articular cartilage volume in the metacarpophalangeal joints of the hand. Thus, this technique may be useful for monitoring cartilage loss in patients with arthritis yet the technique and the postprocessing to determine cartilage volume in small joints are challenging.

A previous study calculated cartilage volume at the knee in patients with rheumatoid arthritis [38]; reproducibility of cartilage volume measurements and cartilage loss in 1 year was determined. Imaging was performed at 1.0 T using a three-dimensional spoiled gradient-echo sequence with fat-suppression. Manual image segmentation was performed once or twice on the lateral tibial, medial tibial, patellar, and femoral compartment by either one or two segmenters. Coefficients of variation for repeated volume measurement of total cartilage were 2.2% (same segmenter, same scan), 5.2% (different segmenter, same scan), 4.9% (same segmenter, different scan, same session), and 4.4% (same segmenter, different scan, different session). Over the 12 month duration of the study there was neither significant change in total cartilage volume nor were there significant changes in volume in any individual compartment. These investigators concluded that the volume measurement technique is reproducible, but any net change in cartilage volume over 1 year is very small. This study shows that even in inflammatory arthropathies cartilage loss is mild over time and comparable to this found in osteoarthritis.

Data concerning T1rho and T2 relaxation time measurements to study the cartilage matrix in inflammatory arthropathies is limited. *T2 relaxation time measurements* were used to study the weight-bearing cartilage of the distal femur in healthy children and in children with idiopathic juvenile arthritis [39]. An increased average T2 relaxation time in children with idiopathic juvenile arthritis was found, which suggests that T2 relaxation time maps may reflect cartilage microstructure differences that occur in idiopathic juvenile arthritis [39]. T2 relaxation time mapping may allow for early detection of cartilage changes and provide an objective, quantitative method of monitoring disease progression, with the long-term potential to guide therapy.

While cartilage imaging may play a similar role in psoriasis arthritis compared to rheumatoid arthritis, it is of minor significance in other inflammatory arthropathies such as ankylosing spondylitis and reactive arthritis. Ankylosing spondylitis mostly affects the spine and sacroiliac joints, however, it may also affect the hip joints and lead to cartilage with erosions, joint space narrowing, and eventually severe secondary degenerative disease.

Osteochondritis Dissecans

Osteochondritis dissecans is a disease of adolescents and young adults and is seen with increased frequency which is in part due to earlier and increasingly competitive sports participation. Despite much speculation, the cause of both juvenile and adult osteochondritis dissecans remains unclear, but early recognition is essential. Several causes have been postulated responsible for the development of osteochondritis dissecans, which include inflammation, genetics, ischemia, and repetitive trauma. It has been suggested that repetitive trauma may induce a stress reaction resulting in a stress fracture within the underlying subchondral bone. If repetitive loading persists and exceeds the ability of the subchondral bone to heal, necrosis of the fragment may occur and lead to fragment dissection, separation, and nonunion.

Whereas adult osteochondritis dissecans lesions have a greater propensity to instability, juvenile osteochondritis dissecans lesions are typically stable, and those with an intact articular surface have a potential to heal with nonoperative treatment through cessation of repetitive impact loading [40]. Although the exact prevalence of osteochondritis dissecans is unknown, reports of between 15 and 29 per 100,000 have been made and gender differences have also been highlighted, with a preponderance among male patients in a ratio of 5:3 [40]. Osteochondritis dissecans is found typically at the knee, ankle, and elbow in typical locations. These include the mesial aspect of the medial femoral condyle at the knee, the medial talar dome, and the capitellum humeri at the elbow. An arthroscopic grading system was developed [41] which differentiates four grades: a Grade 1 lesion shows intact cartilage, which, however, is partially soft and ballottable, grade 2 lesions demonstrate early separation with cartilage defects, grade 3 lesions are partially detached, and grade 4 lesions show craters with loose bodies. Figure 7.14 shows an osteochondral body at the capitellum humeri, which is completely detached and can be removed with a surgical instrument.

MR imaging is essential in characterizing osteochondritis dissecans, planning treatment, predicting prognosis after nonoperative management, and monitoring the success of surgical treatment. MRI in particular has a central role in the early diagnosis of osteochondritis dissecans. It can accurately assess bone marrow abnormalities, the status of the overlying cartilage, the lesion size, to some extent the stability of a lesion and the presence of loose bodies.

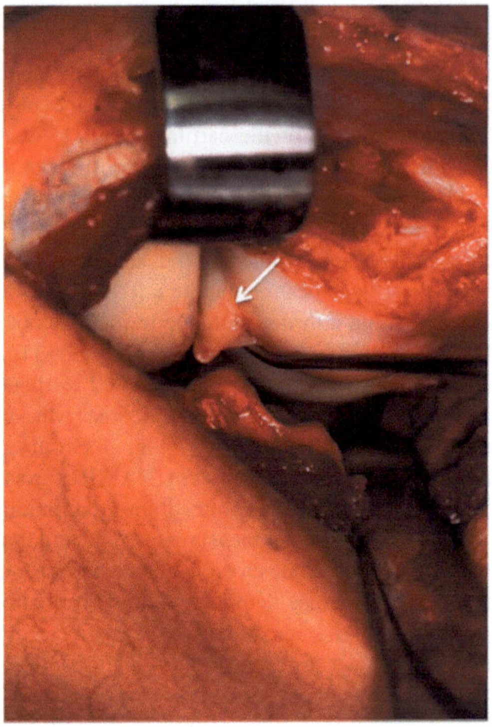

Fig. 7.14 Osteochondritis dissecans of the elbow. Intra-operative image of an osteochondral body at the capitellum humeri is pulled out with a surgical probe (*arrow*)

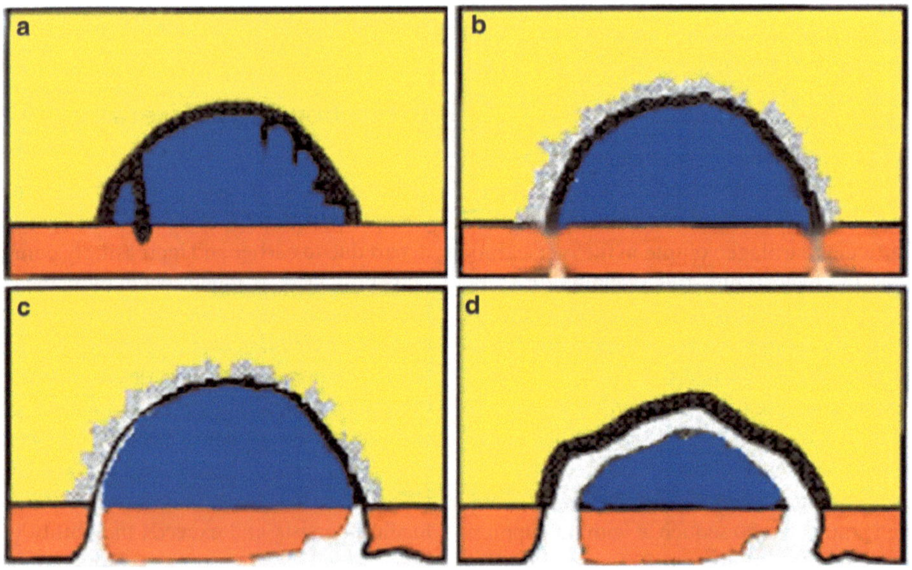

Fig. 7.15 (**a–d**). Osteochondritis dissecans classification described by Bohndorf [43] differentiates three grades. In *grade 1* (**a**) a convex subchondral bone marrow abnormality with central necrosis is found with intact overlying cartilage. In grade 2 (**b**) cartilage abnormalities are shown with swelling or thinning, focal areas of degeneration and eventually focal cartilage defects. In grade 3 (**c, d**) the osseous fragment is dissected from the surrounding healthy bone. Initially the osteochondral element is partially (**c**) and eventually completely detached from the bone (**d**)

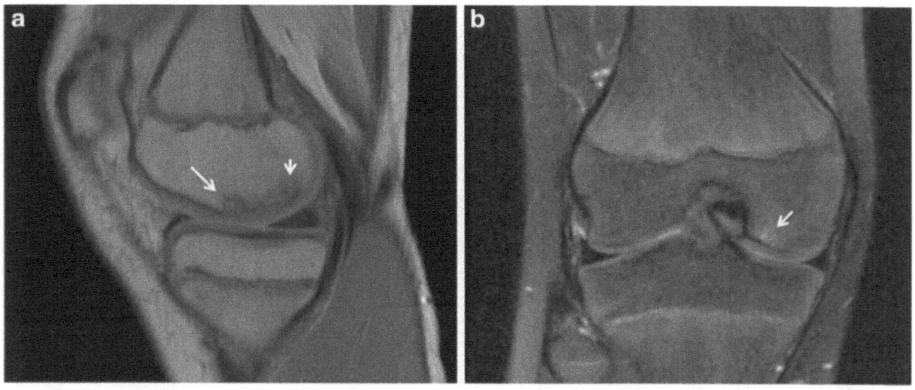

Fig. 7.16 (**a**, **b**). Sagittal proton-density (**a**) and coronal fat-saturated intermediate-weighted (fs iw) (**b**) FSE sequence of a *grade 1 osteochondritis dissecans lesion* at the right knee. Bony lesion in a subchondral region at the mesial aspect of the medial femoral condyle (*arrows*), the overlying cartilage is intact

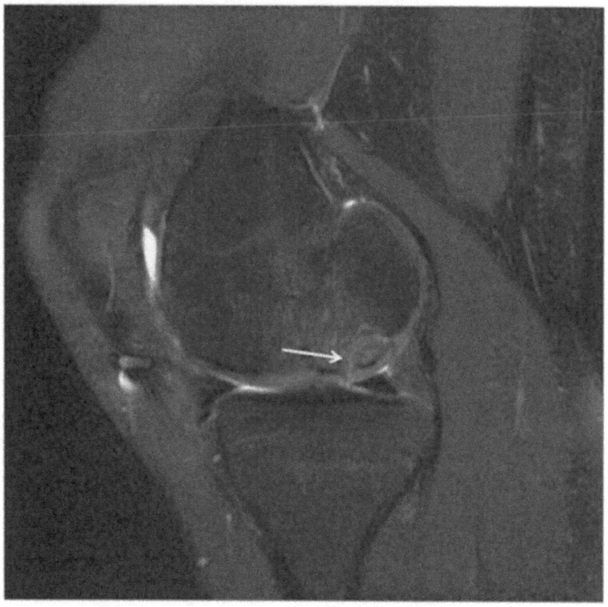

Fig. 7.17 Sagittal fat-saturated intermediate-weighted (fs iw) FSE sequence of the knee showing a *grade 3 osteochondritis dissecans* lesion [43] at the medial femoral condyle with focal cartilage defect and partial dissection of the bone from the surrounding healthy bone in the anterior aspect (*arrow*). In addition there is substantial bone marrow edema pattern in this region, most pronounced of the partially dissected lesion

To visualize osteochondritis dissecans standard 2D T1-weighted and intermediate-weighted sequences with fat saturation have been used. Fluid-sensitive and high-resolution sequences best allow to assess partial dissection and to evaluate whether the overlying cartilage layer is intact; a previous study suggested that 3D FSE sequences could be useful to better assess the cartilage layer given its reduced slice thickness [42].

Different MRI grading systems have been published including those by Bohndorf and Hughston et al. [43, 44]. Hughston et al. described five MR stages for juvenile osteochondritis dissecans: stage 1: small signal changes without clear margins of a fragment; stage 2: osteochondral fragment with clear margins but without fluid between fragment and underlying bone; stage 3: fluid is visible partially between fragment and underlying bone; stage 4: fluid is completely surrounding the fragment, but the fragment is still in situ; stage 5: fragment is completely detached and displaced (loose body). Bohndorf's MRI classification differentiates three stages (Fig. 7.15). In *stage* 1 a demarcated crescentic subchondral osseous region with central necrosis is found and the cartilage coverage is macroscopically intact. Figure 7.16 illustrates this finding and shows a patient with a bony lesion in a subchondral region at the medial femoral condyle, the overlying cartilage is intact. This lesion is T2 bright and T1 low with a relatively wide zone of transition and has a convex border to the subchondral bone. These lesions typically show contrast enhancement after Gadolinium application. In *stage* 2 cartilage abnormalities are evident, there may be swelling or thinning of the cartilage with focal areas of degeneration and eventually focal cartilage defects. Eventually a zone of separation forms between surrounding healthy and substituting necrotic bone. The dissection in this border zone is first visualized on the articular side. Figure 7.17 shows a stage 2 lesion with a focal cartilage defect and partial dissection of the bone from the surrounding healthy bone in the anterior aspect. There is also swelling of the cartilage in the posterior region. The osseous lesion is T2 bright and there is mild surrounding bone marrow edema pattern. In *stage* 3 the osseous fragment is detached from the surrounding healthy bone and eventually will become unstable and a loose body will develop. Figures 7.18 and 7.19 show stage 3 osteochondral lesions, which are completely separated from the surrounding bone.

To date there is limited information on the use of quantitative or molecular imaging techniques in the early diagnosis, therapeutic management, and prognostic evaluation of osteochondritis dissecans lesions.

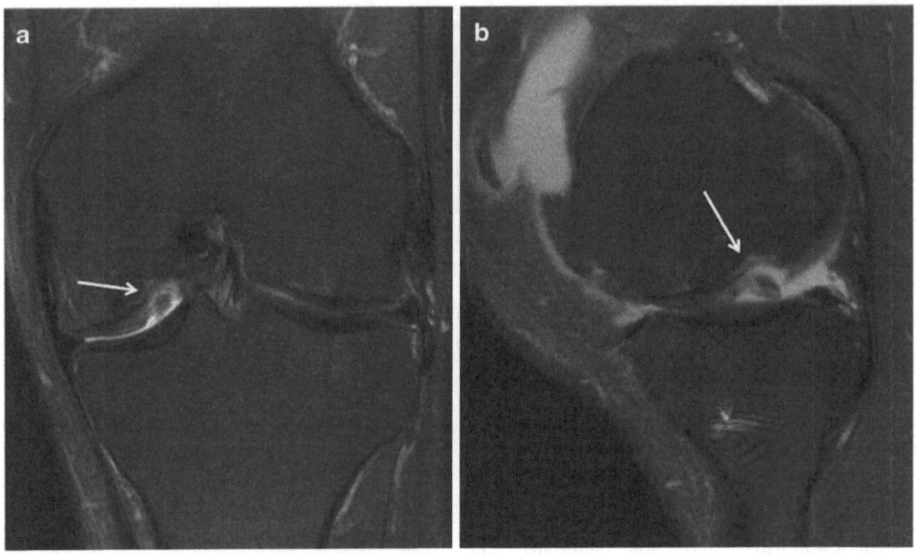

Fig. 7.18 Coronal (**a**) and sagittal (**b**) fat-saturated intermediate-weighted (fs iw) FSE sequence of the knee demonstrating a *grade 3 osteochondritis dissecans* lesion [43] at the mesial aspect of the medial femoral condyle, which is completely separated from the surrounding bone (*arrows*) and is completely surrounded by fluid. Large joint effusion but no significant bone marrow edema pattern

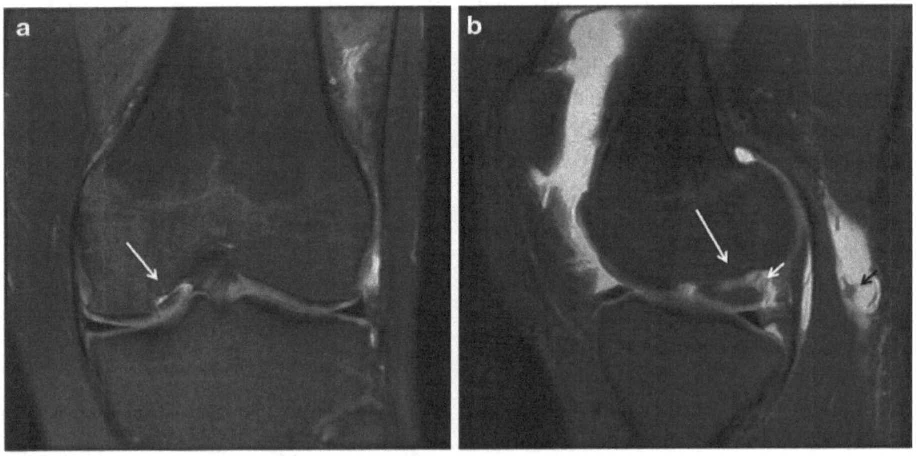

Fig. 7.19 Coronal (**a**) and sagittal (**b**) fat-saturated intermediate-weighted (fs iw) FSE sequence of the knee demonstrating a large *grade 3 osteochondritis dissecans* lesion [43] at the mesial aspect of the medial femoral condyle (*large arrows*). This lesion is also completely separated from the surrounding bone, has a large bony component, and is responsible for a large joint effusion with a popliteal cyst. Adjacent to the dissected lesion on the sagittal image and in the popliteal cyst (*small arrows*) are small cartilage elements

Traumatic Cartilage Injury

Detecting acute osteochondral injuries, which frequently accompany ligament tears, may modify patient treatment and ultimately may prevent secondary osteoarthritis [45]. Osteochondral injuries may also be due to chronic overuse with mild clinical symptoms. Osteochondral injuries are most frequently found at the lower extremities, the knee but also ankle and hip joint are frequent sites. Throwing athletes and gymnasts suffer osteochondral injuries at the elbow and shoulder. Osteochondral injuries are rarely found in the small joints of the hands and feet. When they do occur in these locations, they are generally the result of unique injuries, or are the result of mechanical abnormalities of joint movement or stress distribution [45]. Interestingly within one joint there are also areas that are more prone to injury; this includes for example the capitellum humeri at the elbow and the talar dome at the ankle joint. Osteochondral and chondral injuries are mostly prevalent in physically very active individuals, particularly in younger, skeletally immature athletes.

Previously osteochondral injuries were difficult to diagnose as spatial resolution and image quality of MRI were limited and osteochondral fractures in particular at the joints with thin cartilage (e.g. hip and ankle joint) were difficult to visualize. High-resolution fluid-sensitive sequences are best suited to visualize osteochondral injuries as they provide high contrast between cartilage and surrounding joint fluid as well as direct visualization of bone marrow abnormalities. Standard 2D intermediate-weighted FSE sequences are restricted to higher slice thicknesses (2–4 mm) which limit evaluation of smaller defects or fragments; fluid-sensitive 3D-gradient-echo and FSE sequences may help to overcome these limitations. Three tesla imaging will also improve visualization and grading of cartilage defects and fragments [46, 47]. Given that traumatized joints frequently have a large amount of joint effusion dedicated MR arthrography is usually not required.

MR findings of osteochondral injury range from cartilage contusion to delamination and osteochondral fragments. The imaging appearance of chondral/osteochondral injury differs, based on the severity and acuity of the trauma, and the reparative response of the tissue as described by Mosher et al. [48]: A single episode of high-impact trauma may result in a chondral or osteochondral fracture. In certain locations, with appropriate mechanisms of injury, the forces applied to the bone/cartilage unit result in a debonding or delamination of the cartilage from the underlying bone. Acute trauma may alter the biomechanical properties of the bone/cartilage complex, leading to progressive focal loss of articular cartilage and degenerative change in the subchondral bone. In the absence of an acute traumatic insult, chronic repetitive microtrauma may produce focal microfracture, necrosis, and healing response of subchondral bone, with localized degenerative changes in the overlying cartilage.

Several classifications have been used to grade cartilage lesions yet one of the most complex approaches has been published by Bohndorf [49]. This classification (Fig. 7.20) differentiates five grades and includes also underlying bony injury.

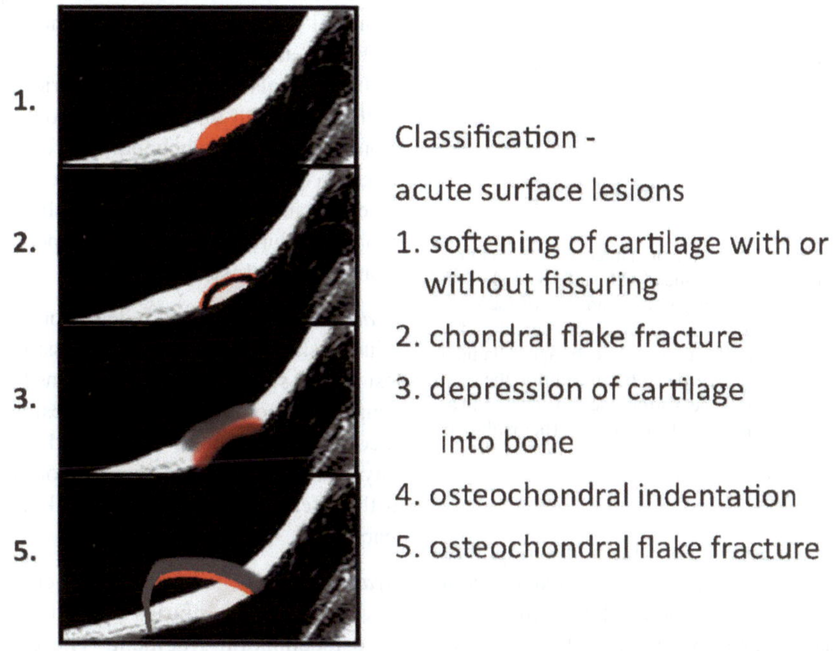

Fig. 7.20 Bohndorf's classification for traumatic cartilage and osteochondral lesions [49] differentiates five grades. Grade 1 represents cartilage softening, grade 2 a cartilage flake fracture, grade 3 a depression of cartilage into bone, and grade 5 an osteochondral flake fracture (see detailed definitions in the text)

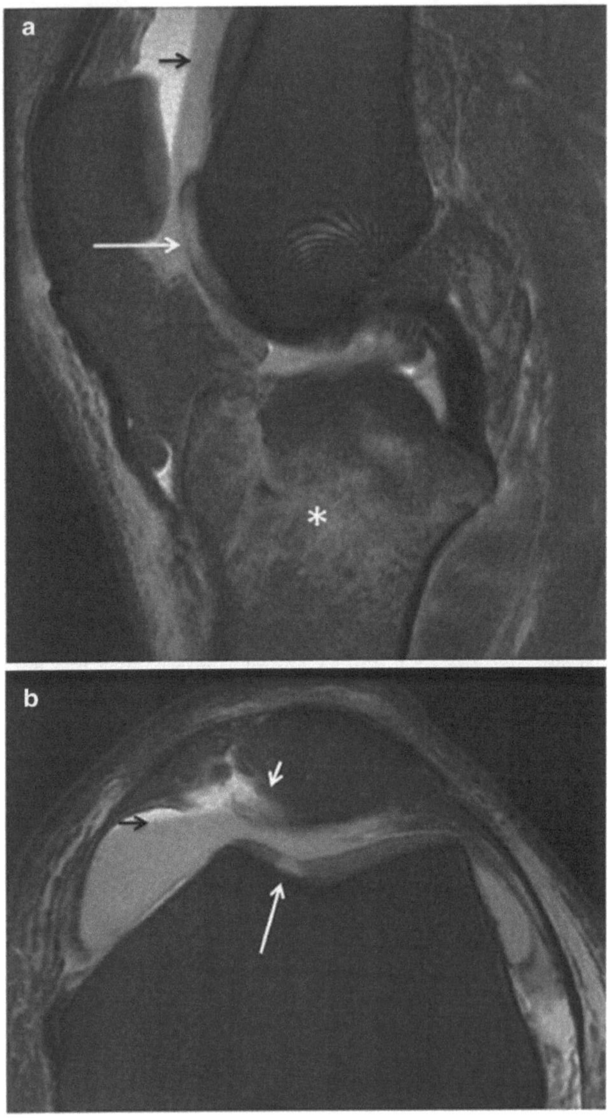

Fig. 7.21 Sagittal (**a**) and axial (**b**) fat-saturated intermediate-weighted (fs iw) FSE sequence of the knee in a patient who suffered a ski accident. The magnetic resonance (MR) images show an area of increased cartilage signal at the trochlea (*large white arrows*) corresponding to a focal cartilage contusion/softening. Posttraumatic cartilage delamination at the medial patella (*small white arrow* in **b**). In addition there is a proximal tibia fracture with extensive bone marrow edema pattern (* in **a**). Fluid–fluid levels indicate joint effusion with hemorrhage (hemarthrosis) (*small black arrow*)

Grade 1: Softening of cartilage with or without fissuring/fibrillation. These lesions demonstrate focal increased signal compared to the surrounding cartilage or focal fissuring of the cartilage in the traumatized area. Arthroscopically this would correspond to an area of softening [49] and may show surface fibrillations. Figures 7.21 and 7.22 show grade 1 lesions. Figure 7.21 shows an area of increased cartilage signal at the trochlea in a patient who suffered a ski accident with a tibial plateau fracture.

Grade 2: Chondral flap or overt chondral fracture ("flake"). Figures 7.22 and 7.23 show chondral flake fractures. In Fig. 7.22 the cartilage is completely separated from the bone and is a loose body within the joint. In Fig. 7.23, there is posttraumatic cartilage delamination after dislocation of the patella. Please note that in these lesions the bone is not affected and no bony fracture or bruise is visualized. These cartilage fragments may be reattached or removed, otherwise they will form loose bodies which may grow given that cartilage is nourished through the synovial fluid. Secondary synovial osteochondromatosis may be the consequence [50]. Figure 7.24 shows a MR image of the knee in a patient with a posttraumatic chondral body, which is shaped like a pebble stone.

Grade 3: Depression of cartilage into bone (condensing of cartilage and immediate subchondral bone). The typical mechanism of these injuries is that of an ACL tear, where "kissing" contusions are observed at the lateral femoral condyle and the posterior aspect of the lateral tibia. There is cartilage contusion, which results in apparent thinning of the cartilage diameter and injury to the subchondral bone and tidemark. In addition to cartilage thinning fraying may be observed. These findings are typical at the lateral femoral condyle, while at the tibia a shear injury is observed. Figure 7.25 shows an example of a focal osteochondral injury of the lateral femoral condyle in a patient with ACL tear.

It should also be noted that injuries of the articular surface of the knee with intact cartilage may progress after several months to chronic subchondral defects or chondrolysis, even when no chondral abnormality is seen arthroscopically at the time of trauma [51]. Figure 7.26 shows a small focal osteochondral injury at the posterior aspect of the femoral head 3 months after a bike injury.

Grade 4: Osteochondral indentation. Grade 4 osteochondral injuries show a focal bony impression–type fracture. These lesions are similar to grade 3 lesions but have a more prominent bony component. These lesions are also typically accompanied by bone bruises and there is thinning and/or fraying of the cartilage. These lesions are also typically seen at the lateral compartment of the knee after complete ACL tears.

Grade 5: Osteochondral flake fracture (partially or totally detached). These injuries lead to avulsion/detachment of an osteochondral fragment. These lesions are typically found at the ankle as shown in Fig. 7.27. Osteochondral fractures of the talar dome should be ruled out in all ankle

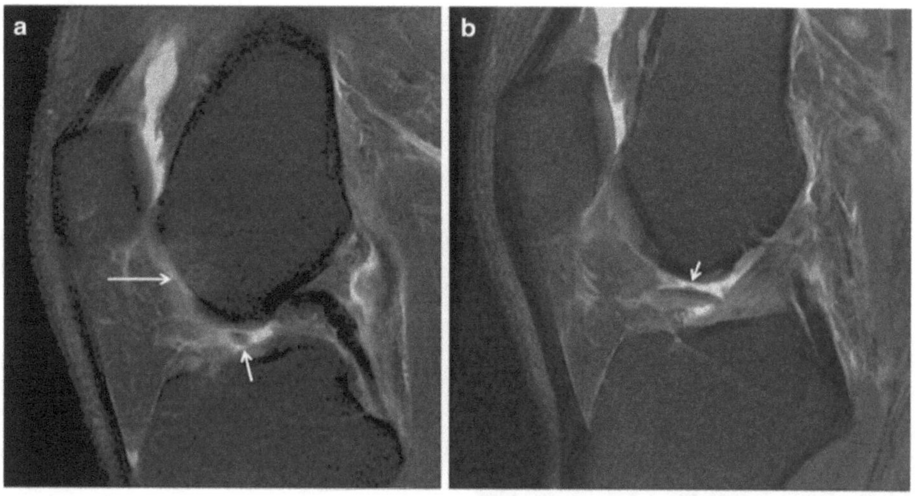

Fig. 7.22 Sagittal fat-saturated intermediate-weighted (fs iw) FSE sequence showing large chondral flake fracture. The donor side is demonstrated in (**a**) at the trochlea (*large arrow*) with underlying subchondral bone marrow edema pattern. The full size of the cartilage fragment is best identified in (**b**) (*small arrow*) but partially also in (**a**) (*small arrow*)

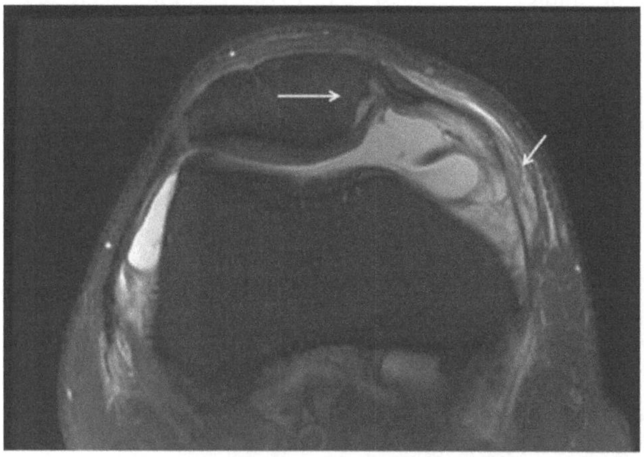

Fig. 7.23 Axial fat-saturated intermediate-weighted (fs iw) FSE sequence of the knee demonstrating posttraumatic cartilage delamination (*large white arrow*) after transient dislocation of the patella. In addition a high-grade partial tear of the patello-femoral ligament (*small arrow*) is shown

sprains since the reported incidence in acute sprains is about 2–6% [52]. These lesions are usually found in a medial location and typically associated with tears of the anterior talofibular and/or calcaneofibular ligaments. If not treated they may result in accelerated osteoarthritis of the ankle joint. It should be noted that these injuries are frequently also well seen with conventional radiographs, as they have a bony component.

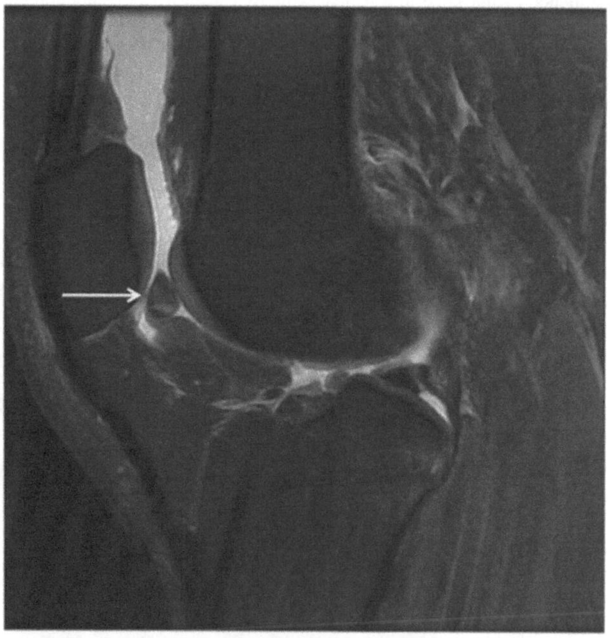

Fig. 7.24 Sagittal fat-saturated intermediate-weighted (fs iw) FSE sequence of the knee in a patient with a posttraumatic chondral body (*arrow*), which is shaped like a pebble stone, indicating remote trauma. In addition a large joint effusion is shown in the supra-patellar recess

Given the acute nature of osteochondral injuries and the frequently required arthroscopic surgery, quantitative assessment of these lesions has limited significance in the early phase to plan therapy. However, quantitative/molecular imaging is used to study cartilage repair after osteochondral injury [53–55] and research studies have demonstrated the potential of quantitative imaging to diagnose cartilage injury not visualized with standard MRI techniques [56–58]. Bolbos et al. showed significantly increased T1rho values in cartilage overlying bone bruises when compared with surrounding cartilage at the lateral tibia, but no difference was found in the lateral femoral condyle [57]. These findings indicate that biochemical abnormalities of hyaline cartilage are already present following initial ACL injuries over the lateral tibia and that these may be due to shear stress during the injury. Interestingly while T1rho values were increased in this location focal morphological MR abnormalities were frequently not found. In addition to quantitative changes of the hyaline cartilage at the tibia T1rho abnormalities were also found in the posterior horn of the lateral meniscus after ACL injury [56]. Significantly higher T1rho values were found at the posterior horn compared with the anterior horn of patients' meniscus ($P = 0.005$). A significant correlation ($P = 0.007$) was found between T1rho values of the posterior horn of the lateral meniscus and T1rho values of the posterior subcompartment of the lateral tibial cartilage in patients. The authors concluded that T1rho mapping techniques provide tools to quantitatively evaluate meniscus and cartilage matrix in patients with ACL injuries.

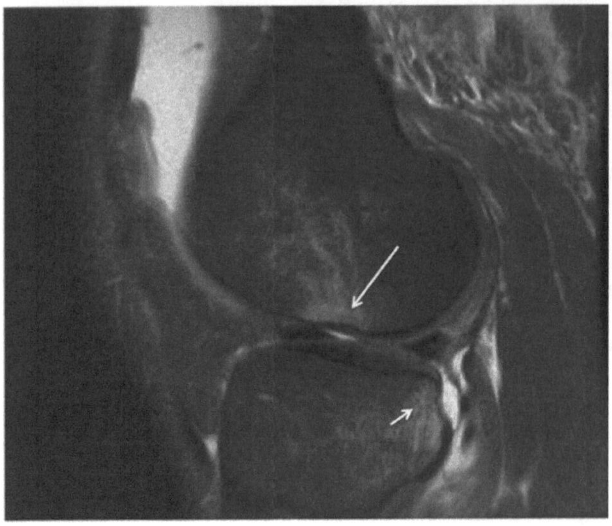

Fig. 7.25 Sagittal fat-saturated intermediate-weighted (fs iw) FSE sequence of the knee in a patient with ACL tear. Focal osteochondral injury at the lateral femoral condyle (*arrow*) with focal bony impression, cartilage contusion, bone marrow edema pattern, and subtle fracture lines. In addition bone marrow edema pattern at the lateral, posterior tibia (*arrow*) and large joint effusion in the supra-patellar recess

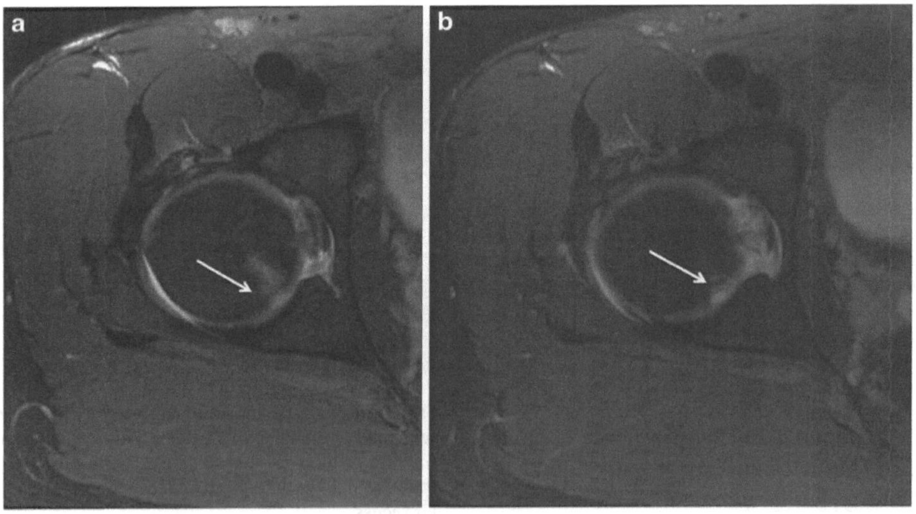

Fig. 7.26 Axial fat-saturated intermediate-weighted (fs iw) FSE sequence of the right hip joint shows a small focal osteochondral injury at the posterior, medial aspect of the femoral head 3 months after a bike injury. In (**a**) both the small cartilage defect and the accompanying bone marrow edema pattern (*arrow*) are shown, while in (**b**) the cartilage defect is better shown but without bone marrow edema pattern

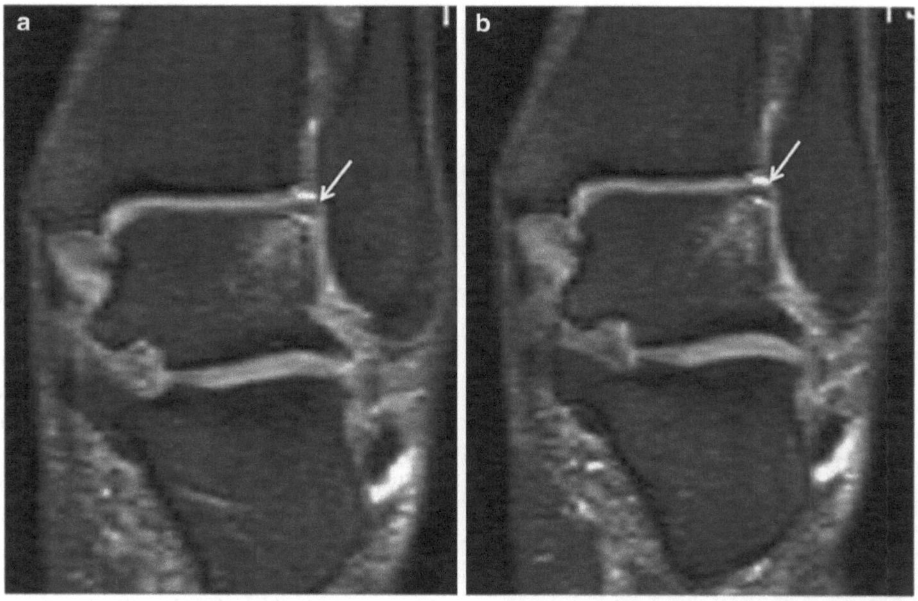

Fig. 7.27 Coronal dual-echo steady-state (DESS) sequence of the left ankle joint demonstrating a partially detached osteochondral flake fracture (*arrow* in **a** and **b**) at the lateral talar dome. Accompanying bone marrow edema pattern in the talus

Nonspecific Osteochondral Lesions

Osteochondral lesions are a common finding in particular at the knee, which are frequently of uncertain significance and not necessarily related to patients' symptoms. Most frequently these lesions are related to a previous injury or focal cartilage degeneration, they may also be related to insufficiency fractures or reflect incomplete or early osteochondritis dissecans. The long-term prognosis of these lesions is not fully understood and only a small number of studies have investigated the evolution of these lesions. Faber et al. investigated 23 patients with acute anterior cruciate ligament injuries, normal radiographs, and occult osteochondral lesions revealed by magnetic resonance imaging 6 years after initial injury and anterior cruciate ligament hamstring autograft reconstruction [59]. A significant number of patients had evidence of cartilage thinning adjacent to the site of the initial osteochondral lesion. Marrow signal changes persisted in 15 (65%) of the patients. Their results suggested that the initial injury resulted in irreversible changes in the knee. Injuries associated with persistent marrow signal indicate ongoing bone remodeling and alteration in the load-bearing properties of subchondral bone, which in turn allow for changes in the overlying cartilage. An additional study investigated isolated osteochondral defects at the femoral condyles in 15 knees that were not treated surgically [60]. In 33% of the cases osteochondral lesions were observed after a significant trauma including soccer and football injuries. The average period of follow-up was 109 months, the range being 54–282 months. Six patients (seven knees) were under the age of 18 at the onset of symptoms. Of these, MRI of six knees showed either no abnormality or a healed lesion. If the onset was after skeletal maturity, six of the eight knees showed features of osteoarthritis on the MRI scan. The results of this study suggest that osteochondral lesions in children and adolescents may heal while in adults they will progress to joint degeneration and eventually to osteoarthritis.

These lesions are most frequently found at the lower extremity, in particular at the knee and the talus. Figure 7.28 shows an example of an osteochondral lesion at the trochlea in a 35-year-old male runner with irregularity and signal abnormality of the cartilage with bone marrow edema pattern of the underlying cartilage. In fluid-sensitive, intermediate-weighted FSE sequences abnormal cartilage is typically bright and appears inhomogeneous. Even without definite evidence of a cartilage defect subchondral bone marrow edema pattern is a sign of significant damage of the overlying cartilage, which leads to bone remodeling.

In younger subjects and athletes diagnosis of an osteochondral lesion may lead to interventions, most frequently arthroscopic and aimed at repairing the cartilage surface. These interventions include microfracture, drilling procedures, mosaicplasty, or autologous chondrocyte implantation.

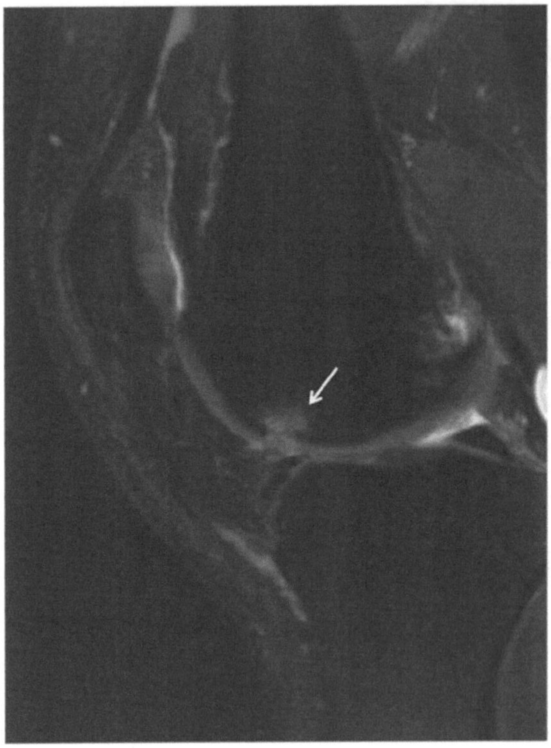

Fig. 7.28 Sagittal fat-saturated intermediate-weighted (fs iw) FSE sequence of the knee demonstrating a nonspecific osteochondral lesion at the trochlea in a 35 year-old male runner with irregularity and signal abnormality of the cartilage and underlying bone marrow edema pattern (*arrow*)

Osteonecroses and Insufficiency Fractures

While osteochondritis dissecans typically affects male adolescents and adults, insufficiency fractures, previously termed spontaneous necrosis of the knee (SONK), are typically found in middle-aged and older individuals. These osteochondral lesions at the femoral condyles of the knee were originally termed Ahlbaeck's disease in 1968 [61], and subsequently the disease was termed SONK. The disease characterized by sudden onset of pain and lucency at the medial femoral condyle was thought to be similar to avascular necrosis of the femoral head. Currently, however, this disease entity is thought to originate from insufficiency fractures [62–65], which lead to osteochondral abnormalities, pain, and accelerated osteoarthritis. Using histo-pathological analyses obtained from patients undergoing surgery for spontaneous osteonecrosis of the knee Yamamoto et al. found that the primary event leading to spontaneous osteonecrosis of the knee is a subchondral insufficiency fracture and that the localized osteonecrosis seen in association with this disease is the result of a fracture [64]. Similar findings were obtained at the hip and a number of focal, subchondral abnormalities of the femoral head are now also attributed to insufficiency fractures and not to avascular necrosis of the femoral head [65, 66].

SONK/insufficiency fractures are typically found in older patients, above the age of 50, are commonly associated with osteoporosis, and are more frequent in women than in men. They may also be found after arthroscopic surgery, in particular

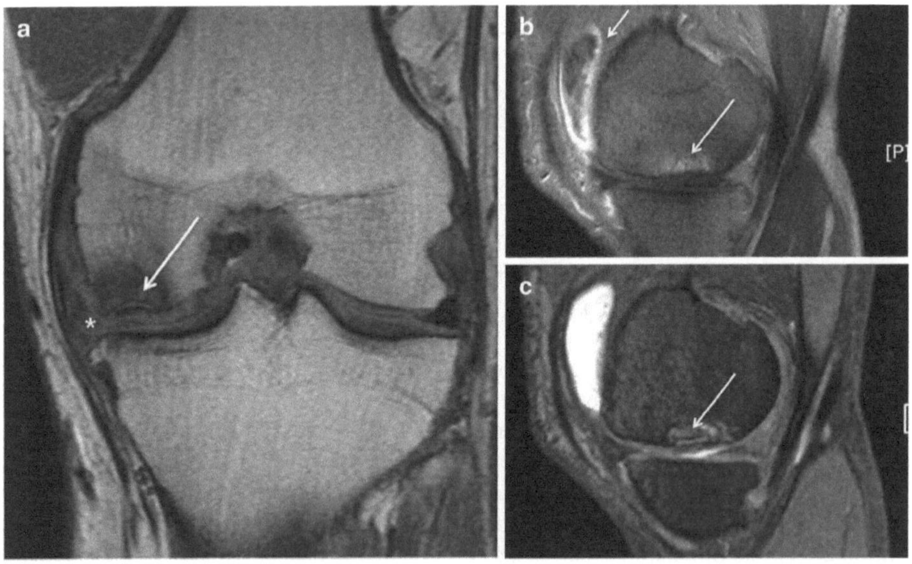

Fig. 7.29 Coronal T1-weighted FSE sequence (**a**), sagittal contrast-enhanced fat-saturated (fs) T1-weighted FSE sequence (**b**) and dual-echo steady-state (DESS) sequence (**c**) of the knee in a patient with an insufficiency fracture (previously SONK) at the medial femoral condyle (*large arrows*). The fracture line and flattening of the femoral condyle are well shown. Maceration of the medial meniscus (*). In addition there is a large supra-patellar joint effusion with synovitis (contrast enhancement with *small arrow* in **b**)

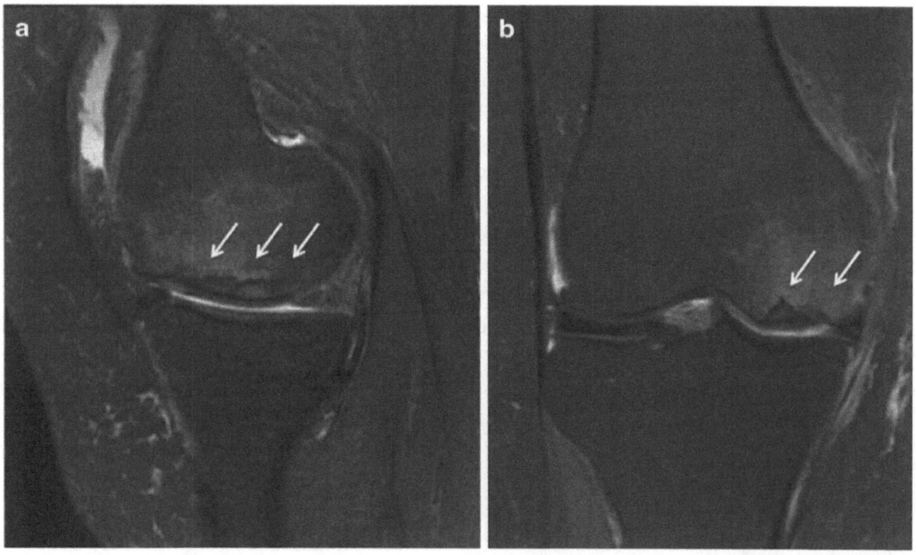

Fig. 7.30 Sagittal (**a**) and coronal (**b**) fat-saturated intermediate-weighted (fs iw) FSE sequences of the right knee in a patient with an insufficiency fracture at the medial femoral condyle (*arrows*). The fracture line is well shown and there is adjacent bone marrow edema pattern

after meniscal resection due to altered biomechanical loading of the knee.

Standard *MR imaging sequences* are used to visualize these osteochondral lesions; the fracture line may be best assessed with T1-weighted or fat-saturated intermediate-weighted (fluid-sensitive) fast spin echo sequences and the overlying cartilage is best analyzed using fat-saturated intermediate-weighted fast spin echo sequences. Coronal and sagittal orientations will best characterize the lesion and overlying cartilage.

MRI findings include bone marrow edema pattern, a linear signal abnormality in the subchondral region, overlying cartilage irregularities, contour abnormalities of the bone, and synovitis with joint effusion. The patients tend to develop accelerated osteoarthritis, which eventually requires total joint replacement. Figures 7.29 and 7.30 show MR images of patients with insufficiency fractures.

Assessment of cartilage overlying these lesions using quantitative MRI techniques has not yet been performed but may potentially help to better characterize damage of the cartilage due to deformity with altered biomechanical loading and alteration of the viability of the subchondral bone.

Femoroacetabular Impingement

Femoroacetabular impingement may be due to abnormalities at the femoral head–neck junction (cam-type impingement) or due to abnormalities of the bony acetabulum (pincer-type impingement) [67]. Both disease entities lead to cartilage damage and accelerated osteoarthritis. *Cam-type impingement* is typically found in younger to middle-aged, male patients and is characterized by a bump at the head–neck junction, which is congenital or related to acquired abnormalities such as slipped capital femoral epiphysis. This leads to abutment of the femoral head–neck junction against the acetabular rim [68]. The abnormality results in cartilage injury at the anterior and lateral, superior aspects of the hip joint, with delamination and focal defects. In addition to the hyaline cartilage the labrum is damaged with tears, deformity, and reactive hypertrophy. *Pincer-type impingement* is associated with protrusio acetabuli or an abnormally deep acetabulum and is typically found in middle-aged or older women. In pincer-type impingement acetabular overcoverage limits the range of motion and leads to a conflict between the acetabulum and the femur [69]. Cartilage loss is typically found at the inferior, medial, and posterior aspects of the joint. Pincer and cam-type impingement require different surgical management and differentiation of these entities is therefore important.

To best assess deformities, cartilage and labral injury sagittal and oblique axial sequences (Fig. 7.31) have been shown to be most useful. Oblique axial sequences can also be used to calculate the so-called alpha angles, which help in making the diagnosis of cam-type impingement. Proton-density- or T1-weighted as well as fat-saturated intermediate-weighted fast spin echo sequences have been applied and it has been shown that MR arthrography improves visualization of the cartilage and labrum [70]. In addition 3D gradient-echo sequences (such as dual-echo steady-state [DESS] sequences) have been used to improve visualization of labrum and cartilage [71]. It should be noted, however, that due to the limited thickness of the cartilage even with 3T MRI and optimized sequences evaluation of the cartilage at the hip is challenging and not infrequently the interface between acetabular and femoral head cartilage is not well shown. The cartilage thickness at the acetabulum and femoral head varies from 1 to 3 mm with the thickest diameter in the anterior, anterolateral, and superior regions [72].

Morphological findings associated with cam-type impingement include (1) cartilage lesions at the superior and anterosuperior aspect of the femoral head and acetabulum, (2) tears and degeneration of the labrum in the superior and anterosuperior region and (3) bony abnormalities at the head–neck junction and nonspherical shape of the femoral head with enlarged alpha angles. Compared to pincer-type impingements mean alpha angles were significantly larger in cam-type impingement in the anterior (68° vs 54°, respectively; $P < 0.005$) and anterosuperior (81° vs 66°, respectively; $P < 0.018$) region [23]. The triad of these findings is present in 88% of patients with cam-type femoroacetabular impingement [73]. Additional less-frequent findings include paralabral cysts, presence of an os acetabuli, synovial herniation pits, and bone marrow edema pattern at the anterosuperior aspect of the femoral head. Figure 7.32 shows images of a patient with severe femoroacetabular impingement.

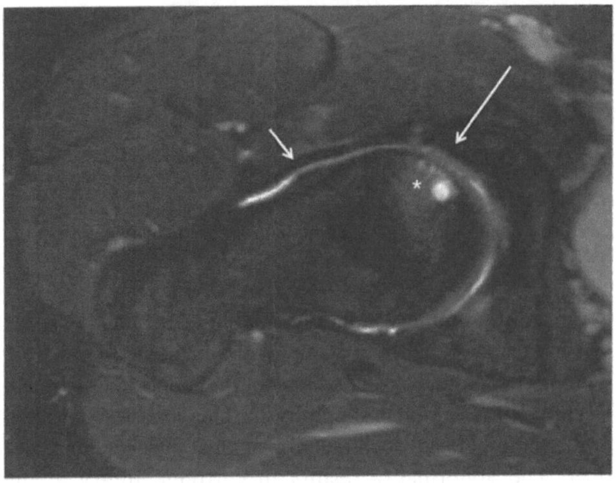

Fig. 7.31 Fluid-sensitive, fat-saturated (fs) oblique axial FSE sequence (magnetic resonance [MR] arthrogram) of the right hip in a patient with femoroacetabular impingement. The typical findings include a bump at the head–neck junction (*small arrow*) and cartilage thinning and irregularity at the anterior, supero-lateral aspect of the hip joint (*large arrow*). In addition there are subchondral cysts (*) and bone marrow edema pattern at the anterior aspect of the femoral head

In pincer-type impingement (1) cartilage lesions are found to be significantly larger in the posteroinferior position than in cam-type impingment, (2) labral tears and degeneration are located in the posterior and posteroinferior positions, and (3) the acetabulum is significantly deeper (mean depth, 4.8 mm vs mean depth in cam-type impingement, 0.7 mm) [23].

In general a cut-off of 55° is used to differentiate normal and abnormal alpha angles based on a study by Notzli et al. who found an average alpha angle of 74° in patients with cam-type impingement and of 42° in control subjects using MR images [74].

Quantitative assessment of the hip cartilage matrix has been performed to better characterize biochemical changes in femoroacetabular impingement using delayed gadolinium-enhanced magnetic resonance imaging (dGEMRIC) and T2* mapping [75–79]. Jessel et al. [79] studied 37 hips in 30 patients with femoroacetabular impingement and found significant correlations between dGEMRIC index, pain ($P < 0.05$), and alpha angle ($P < 0.05$). They concluded that the correlation of dGEMRIC with alpha angle suggests that hips with more femoral deformity show signs of early OA.

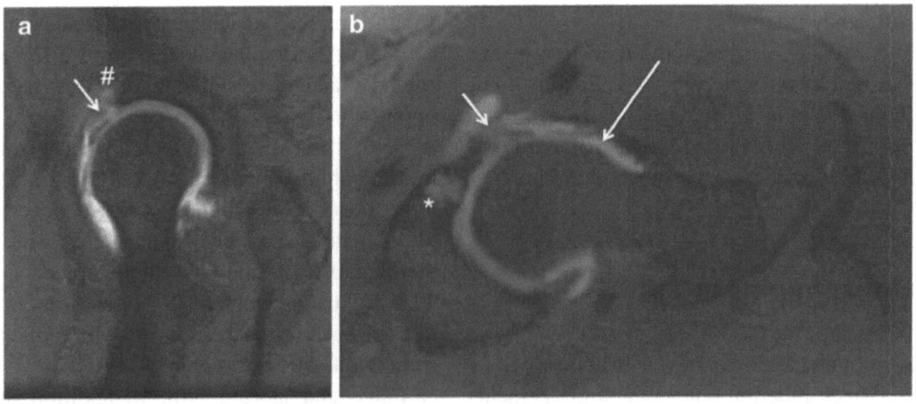

Fig. 7.32 Fluid-sensitive, fat-saturated (fs) sagittal (**a**) and oblique axial (**b**) FSE sequences (magnetic resonance [MR] arthrogram) of the left hip in a patient with severe femoroacetabular impingement. Bump at the head–neck junction (*large arrow*), severe anterior-superior labral tear (*small arrow*), subchondral cysts at the acetabulum (*) and paralabral cysts (#)

Bittersohl et al. [78] studied ten asymptomatic young-adult volunteers and 26 symptomatic femoroacetabular impingement with dGEMRIC. In their study both cam- and pincer-type femoroacetabular impingement revealed remarkably lower T1 mean values in comparison to asymptomatic volunteers in all regions of interest. Distribution of the T1 dGEMRIC values was in accordance with the specific femoroacetabular impingement damage pattern. In cam types, there was a significant drop ($P < 0.05$) of T1 in the anterior to superior location. In pincer types, there was a generalized circumferential decrease noted. In an additional study reproducibility for dGEMRIC was studied and found to be high using intra-class correlation (ICC) measurements (ICC range, 0.667–0.915). Intra- and Inter-observer analyses also demonstrated a high agreement for T1(Gd) assessment (0.973 and 0.932) [75].

Summary and Conclusion

Recent new therapeutic modalities, such as cartilage repair and surgery for femoroacetabular impingement, have made cartilage MR imaging an exciting field of clinical interest and research. Cartilage pathology is found in a large number of disease entities and abnormalities, which include osteoarthritis, inflammatory arthropathies, osteochondritis dissecans, trauma, and femoroacetabular impingement. As these entities have different therapies it is important to understand their epidemiology and characteristical MR morphology. In addition it is critical to optimize imaging for these individual entities and to be familiar with new molecular imaging techniques, which is in addition to morphologic visualization allow quantification of the biochemical cartilage composition.

References

1. Guccione AA, Felson DT, Anderson JJ, Anthony JM, Zhang Y, Wilson PW, et al. The effects of specific medical conditions on the functional limitations of elders in the Framingham Study. Am J Public Health. 1994;84:351–8.
2. From the Centers for Disease Control and Prevention. Arthritis prevalence and activity limitations – United States, 1990. JAMA. 1994;272:346–7.
3. Kellgren J, Lawrence J. Radiological assessment of osteoarthritis. Ann Rheum Dis. 1957;16:494–501.
4. Link TM, Steinbach LS, Ghosh S, Ries M, Lu Y, Lane N, et al. Osteoarthritis: MR imaging findings in different stages of disease and correlation with clinical findings. Radiology. 2003;226:373–81.
5. Altman R, Asch E, Bloch D, Bole G, Borenstein D, Brandt K, et al. Development of criteria for the classification and reporting of osteoarthritis. Classification of osteoarthritis of the knee. Diagnostic and Therapeutic Criteria Committee of the American Rheumatism Association. Arthritis Rheum. 1986;29:1039–49.
6. Barker K, Lamb SE, Toye F, Jackson S, Barrington S. Association between radiographic joint space narrowing, function, pain and muscle power in severe osteoarthritis of the knee. Clin Rehabil. 2004;18:793–800.
7. Phan CM, Link TM, Blumenkrantz G, Dunn TC, Ries MD, Steinbach LS, Majumdar S. MR imaging findings in the follow-up of patients with different stages of knee osteoarthritis and the correlation with clinical symptoms. Eur Radiol. 2006;16:608–18.
8. Felson D, Chaisson C, Hill C, Totterman S, Gale M, Skinner K, et al. The association of bone marrow lesions with pain in knee osteoarthritis. Ann Intern Med. 2001;134:541–9.
9. Felson DT, Niu J, Guermazi A, Roemer F, Aliabadi P, Clancy M, et al. Correlation of the development of knee pain with enlarging bone marrow lesions on magnetic resonance imaging. Arthritis Rheum. 2007;56:2986–92.
10. Kornaat PR, Bloem JL, Ceulemans RY, Riyazi N, Rosendaal FR, Nelissen RG, et al. Osteoarthritis of the knee: association between clinical features and MR imaging findings. Radiology. 2006;239:811–7.
11. Kornaat PR, Kloppenburg M, Sharma R, Botha-Scheepers SA, Le Graverand MP, Coene LN, et al. Bone marrow edema-like lesions change in volume in the majority of patients with osteoarthritis; associations with clinical features. Eur Radiol. 2007;17:3073–8.
12. Phan CM, Link TM, Blumenkrantz G, Dunn TC, Ries MD, Steinbach LS, et al. MR imaging findings in the follow-up of patients with different stages of knee osteoarthritis and the correlation with clinical symptoms. Eur Radiol. 2006;16:608–18.
13. Zhai G, Cicuttini F, Ding C, Scott F, Garnero P, Jones G. Correlates of knee pain in younger subjects. Clin Rheumatol. 2007;26:75–80.
14. Recht M, Kramer J, Marcelis S, Pathria M, Trudell D, Haghigi P, et al. Abnormalities of articular cartilage in the knee: analysis of available MR techniques. Radiology. 1993;187:473–8.
15. Noyes FR, Stabler CL. A system for grading articular cartilage lesions at arthroscopy. Am J Sports Med. 1989;17:505–13.
16. Saadat E, Jobke B, Chu B, Lu Y, Cheng J, Li X, et al. Diagnostic performance of in vivo 3T Fast Spin Echo MRI for articular cartilage abnormalities in human osteoarthritic knees using histology as standard of reference. Eur Radiol. 2008;18:2292–302.
17. Yoshioka H, Stevens K, Hargreaves BA, Steines D, Genovese M, Dillingham MF, et al. Magnetic resonance imaging of articular cartilage of the knee: comparison between fat-suppressed three-dimensional SPGR imaging, fat-suppressed FSE imaging, and fat-suppressed three-dimensional DEFT imaging, and correlation with arthroscopy. J Magn Reson Imaging. 2004;20:857–64.
18. Potter HG, Linklater JM, Allen AA, Hannafin JA, Haas SB. Magnetic resonance imaging of articular cartilage in the knee. An evaluation with use of fast-spin-echo imaging. J Bone Joint Surg Am. 1998;80:1276–84.
19. Abreu M, Johnson K, Chung CB, De Lima Jr JE, Trudell D, Terkeltaub R, et al. Calcification in calcium pyrophosphate dihydrate (CPPD) crystalline deposits in the knee: anatomic, radiographic, MR imaging, and histologic study in cadavers. Skeletal Radiol. 2004;33:392–8.

20. Kendell SD, Helms CA, Rampton JW, Garrett WE, Higgins LD. MRI appearance of chondral delamination injuries of the knee. AJR Am J Roentgenol. 2005;184:1486–9.
21. Levy AS, Lohnes J, Sculley S, LeCroy M, Garrett W. Chondral delamination of the knee in soccer players. Am J Sports Med. 1996;24:634–9.
22. Anderson LA, Peters CL, Park BB, Stoddard GJ, Erickson JA, Crim JR. Acetabular cartilage delamination in femoroacetabular impingement. Risk factors and magnetic resonance imaging diagnosis. J Bone Joint Surg Am. 2009;91:305–13.
23. Pfirrmann CW, Duc SR, Zanetti M, Dora C, Hodler J. MR arthrography of acetabular cartilage delamination in femoroacetabular cam impingement. Radiology. 2008;249:236–41.
24. Zanetti M, Bruder E, Romero J, Hodler J. Bone marrow edema pattern in osteoarthritic knees: correlation between MR imaging and histologic findings. Radiology. 2000;215: 835–40.
25. Taljanovic MS, Graham AR, Benjamin JB, Gmitro AF, Krupinski EA, Schwartz SA, et al. Bone marrow edema pattern in advanced hip osteoarthritis: quantitative assessment with magnetic resonance imaging and correlation with clinical examination, radiographic findings, and histopathology. Skeletal Radiol. 2008;37:423–31.
26. Felson DT, Niu J, Clancy M, Sack B, Aliabadi P, Zhang Y. Effect of recreational physical activities on the development of knee osteoarthritis in older adults of different weights: the Framingham Study. Arthritis Rheum. 2007;57:6–12.
27. Peterfy CG, Guermazi A, Zaim S, Tirman PF, Miaux Y, White D, et al. Whole-Organ Magnetic Resonance Imaging Score (WORMS) of the knee in osteoarthritis. Osteoarthritis Cartilage. 2004;12:177–90.
28. Hunter DJ, Lo GH, Gale D, Grainger AJ, Guermazi A, Conaghan PG. The reliability of a new scoring system for knee osteoarthritis MRI and the validity of bone marrow lesion assessment: BLOKS (Boston Leeds Osteoarthritis Knee Score). Ann Rheum Dis. 2008;67:206–11.
29. Hill CL, Seo GS, Gale D, Totterman S, Gale ME, Felson DT. Cruciate ligament integrity in osteoarthritis of the knee. Arthritis Rheum. 2005;52:794–9.
30. Biswal S, Hastie T, Andriacchi TP, Bergman GA, Dillingham MF, Lang P. Risk factors for progressive cartilage loss in the knee: a longitudinal magnetic resonance imaging study in forty-three patients. Arthritis Rheum. 2002;46:2884–92.
31. Hill CL, Hunter DJ, Niu J, Clancy M, Guermazi A, Genant H, et al. Synovitis detected on magnetic resonance imaging and its relation to pain and cartilage loss in knee osteoarthritis. Ann Rheum Dis. 2007;66:1599–603.
32. Uhl M, Allmann KH, Ihling C, Hauer MP, Conca W, Langer M. Cartilage destruction in small joints by rheumatoid arthritis: assessment of fat-suppressed three-dimensional gradient-echo MR pulse sequences in vitro. Skeletal Radiol. 1998;27:677–82.
33. Hetland ML, Ejbjerg B, Horslev-Petersen K, Jacobsen S, Vestergaard A, Jurik AG, et al. MRI bone oedema is the strongest predictor of subsequent radiographic progression in early rheumatoid arthritis. Results from a 2-year randomised controlled trial (CIMESTRA). Ann Rheum Dis. 2009;68:384–90.
34. Gylys-Morin VM, Graham TB, Blebea JS, Dardzinski BJ, Laor T, Johnson ND, et al. Knee in early juvenile rheumatoid arthritis: MR imaging findings. Radiology. 2001;220:696–706.
35. McQueen F, Lassere M, Edmonds J, Conaghan P, Peterfy C, Bird P, et al. OMERACT Rheumatoid Arthritis Magnetic Resonance Imaging Studies. Summary of OMERACT 6 MR Imaging Module. J Rheumatol. 2003;30:1387–92.
36. Peterfy C, Edmonds J, Lassere M, Conaghan P, Ostergaard M, McQueen F, et al. OMERACT Rheumatoid Arthritis MRI Studies Module. J Rheumatol. 2003;30:1364–5.
37. Peterfy CG, van Dijke CF, Lu Y, Nguyen A, Connick TJ, Kneeland JB, et al. Quantification of the volume of articular cartilage in the metacarpophalangeal joints of the hand: accuracy and precision of three-dimensional MR imaging. AJR Am J Roentgenol. 1995;165:371–5.
38. Gandy SJ, Brett AD, Dieppe PA, Keen MC, Maciewicz RA, Taylor CJ, et al. Measurement of cartilage volumes in rheumatoid arthritis using MRI. Br J Radiol. 2005;78:39–45.
39. Kight AC, Dardzinski BJ, Laor T, Graham TB. Magnetic resonance imaging evaluation of the effects of juvenile rheumatoid arthritis on distal femoral weight-bearing cartilage. Arthritis Rheum. 2004;50:901–5.
40. Kocher MS, Tucker R, Ganley TJ, Flynn JM. Management of osteochondritis dissecans of the knee: current concepts review. Am J Sports Med. 2006;34:1181–91.
41. Guhl JF. Arthroscopic treatment of osteochondritis dissecans. Clin Orthop Relat Res. 1982;167:65–74.
42. Ristow O, Steinbach L, Sabo G, Krug R, Huber M, Rauscher I, et al. Isotropic 3D fast spin-echo imaging versus standard 2D imaging at 3.0 T of the knee-image quality and diagnostic performance. Eur Radiol. 2009;19:1263–72.
43. Bohndorf K. Osteochondritis (osteochondrosis) dissecans: a review and new MRI classification. Eur Radiol. 1998;8:103–12.
44. Hefti F, Beguiristain J, Krauspe R, Moller-Madsen B, Riccio V, Tschauner C, et al. Osteochondritis dissecans: a multicenter study of the European Pediatric Orthopedic Society. J Pediatr Orthop B. 1999;8:231–45.
45. Sanders RK, Crim JR. Osteochondral injuries. Semin Ultrasound CT MR. 2001;22:352–70.
46. Kijowski R, Blankenbaker DG, Davis KW, Shinki K, Kaplan LD, De Smet AA. Comparison of 1.5- and 3.0-T MR imaging for evaluating the articular cartilage of the knee joint. Radiology. 2009;250(3):839–48.
47. Wong S, Steinbach L, Zhao J, Stehling C, Ma CB, Link TM. Comparative study of imaging at 3.0 T versus 1.5 T of the knee. Skeletal Radiol. 2009;38:761–9.
48. Mosher TJ. MRI of osteochondral injuries of the knee and ankle in the athlete. Clin Sports Med. 2006;25:843–66.
49. Bohndorf K. Imaging of acute injuries of the articular surfaces (chondral, osteochondral and subchondral fractures). Skeletal Radiol. 1999;28:545–60.
50. Murphey MD, Vidal JA, Fanburg-Smith JC, Gajewski DA. Imaging of synovial chondromatosis with radiologic-pathologic correlation. Radiographics. 2007;27:1465–88.
51. Vellet AD, Marks PH, Fowler PJ, Munro TG. Occult posttraumatic osteochondral lesions of the knee: prevalence, classification, and short-term sequelae evaluated with MR imaging. Radiology. 1991;178:271–6.

52. Shea MP, Manoli 2nd A. Osteochondral lesions of the talar dome. Foot Ankle. 1993;14:48–55.
53. Trattnig S, Burstein D, Szomolanyi P, Pinker K, Welsch GH, Mamisch TC. T1(Gd) gives comparable information as Delta T1 relaxation rate in dGEMRIC evaluation of cartilage repair tissue. Invest Radiol. 2009;44:598–602.
54. Welsch GH, Mamisch TC, Marlovits S, Glaser C, Friedrich K, Hennig FF, et al. Quantitative T2 mapping during follow-up after matrix-associated autologous chondrocyte transplantation (MACT): full-thickness and zonal evaluation to visualize the maturation of cartilage repair tissue. J Orthop Res. 2009;27:957–63.
55. Welsch GH, Mamisch TC, Quirbach S, Zak L, Marlovits S, Trattnig S. Evaluation and comparison of cartilage repair tissue of the patella and medial femoral condyle by using morphological MRI and biochemical zonal T2 mapping. Eur Radiol. 2009;19:1253–62.
56. Bolbos RI, Link TM, Ma CB, Majumdar S, Li X. T1rho relaxation time of the meniscus and its relationship with T1rho of adjacent cartilage in knees with acute ACL injuries at 3 T. Osteoarthritis Cartilage. 2009;17:12–8.
57. Bolbos RI, Ma CB, Link TM, Majumdar S, Li X. In vivo T1rho quantitative assessment of knee cartilage after anterior cruciate ligament injury using 3 Tesla magnetic resonance imaging. Invest Radiol. 2008;43:782–8.
58. Li X, Ma BC, Bolbos RI, Stahl R, Lozano J, Zuo J, et al. Quantitative assessment of bone marrow edema-like lesion and overlying cartilage in knees with osteoarthritis and anterior cruciate ligament tear using MR imaging and spectroscopic imaging at 3 Tesla. J Magn Reson Imaging. 2008;28:453–61.
59. Faber KJ, Dill JR, Amendola A, Thain L, Spouge A, Fowler PJ. Occult osteochondral lesions after anterior cruciate ligament rupture. Six-year magnetic resonance imaging follow-up study. Am J Sports Med. 1999;27:489–94.
60. Prakash D, Learmonth D. Natural progression of osteo-chondral defect in the femoral condyle. Knee. 2002;9:7–10.
61. Ahlback S, Bauer GC, Bohne WH. Spontaneous osteonecrosis of the knee. Arthritis Rheum. 1968;11:705–33.
62. Kidwai AS, Hemphill SD, Griffiths HJ. Radiologic case study. spontaneous osteonecrosis of the knee reclassified as insufficiency fracture. Orthopedics. 2005;28:236, 333–6.
63. Ramnath RR, Kattapuram SV. MR appearance of SONK-like subchondral abnormalities in the adult knee: SONK redefined. Skeletal Radiol. 2004;33:575–81.
64. Yamamoto T, Bullough PG. Spontaneous osteonecrosis of the knee: the result of subchondral insufficiency fracture. J Bone Joint Surg Am. 2000;82:858–66.
65. Yamamoto T, Bullough PG. Subchondral insufficiency fracture of the femoral head and medial femoral condyle. Skeletal Radiol. 2000;29:40–4.
66. Yamamoto T, Schneider R, Bullough PG. Subchondral insufficiency fracture of the femoral head: histopathologic correlation with MRI. Skeletal Radiol. 2001;30:247–54.
67. Pfirrmann CW, Mengiardi B, Dora C, Kalberer F, Zanetti M, Hodler J. Cam and pincer femoroacetabular impingement: characteristic MR arthrographic findings in 50 patients. Radiology. 2006;240:778–85.
68. Ito K, Minka 2nd MA, Leunig M, Werlen S, Ganz R. Femoroacetabular impingement and the cam-effect. A MRI-based quantitative anatomical study of the femoral head-neck offset. J Bone Joint Surg Br. 2001;83:171–6.
69. Ganz R, Parvizi J, Beck M, Leunig M, Notzli H, Siebenrock KA. Femoroacetabular impingement: a cause for osteoarthritis of the hip. Clin Orthop Relat Res. 2003;417:112–20.
70. Vanhoenacker FM, Peeters J, Camerlinck M, Myncke J. MR arthrography of the hip joint: a practical approach. JBR BTR. 2009;92:31–4.
71. Knuesel PR, Pfirrmann CW, Noetzli HP, Dora C, Zanetti M, Hodler J, et al. MR arthrography of the hip: diagnostic performance of a dedicated water-excitation 3D double-echo steady-state sequence to detect cartilage lesions. AJR Am J Roentgenol. 2004;183:1729–35.
72. Kurrat HJ, Oberlander W. The thickness of the cartilage in the hip joint. J Anat. 1978;126:145–55.
73. Kassarjian A, Yoon LS, Belzile E, Connolly SA, Millis MB, Palmer WE. Triad of MR arthrographic findings in patients with cam-type femoroacetabular impingement. Radiology. 2005;236:588–92.
74. Notzli HP, Wyss TF, Stoecklin CH, Schmid MR, Treiber K, Hodler J. The contour of the femoral head-neck junction as a predictor for the risk of anterior impingement. J Bone Joint Surg Br. 2002;84:556–60.
75. Bittersohl B, Hosalkar HS, Haamberg T, Kim YJ, Werlen S, Siebenrock KA, et al. Reproducibility of dGEMRIC in assessment of hip joint cartilage: a prospective study. J Magn Reson Imaging. 2009;30:224–8.
76. Bittersohl B, Hosalkar HS, Hughes T, Kim YJ, Werlen S, Siebenrock KA, et al. Feasibility of T2* mapping for the evaluation of hip joint cartilage at 1.5T using a three-dimensional (3D), gradient-echo (GRE) sequence: a prospective study. Magn Reson Med. 2009;62:896–901.
77. Bittersohl B, Hosalkar HS, Kim YJ, Werlen S, Siebenrock KA, Mamisch TC. Delayed gadolinium-enhanced magnetic resonance imaging (dGEMRIC) of hip joint cartilage in femoroacetabular impingement (FAI): are pre- and postcontrast imaging both necessary? Magn Reson Med. 2009;62:1362–7.
78. Bittersohl B, Steppacher S, Haamberg T, Kim YJ, Werlen S, Beck M, et al. Cartilage damage in femoroacetabular impingement (FAI): preliminary results on comparison of standard diagnostic vs delayed gadolinium-enhanced magnetic resonance imaging of cartilage (dGEMRIC). Osteoarthritis Cartilage. 2009;17:1297–306.
79. Jessel RH, Zilkens C, Tiderius C, Dudda M, Mamisch TC, Kim YJ. Assessment of osteoarthritis in hips with femoroacetabular impingement using delayed gadolinium enhanced MRI of cartilage. J Magn Reson Imaging. 2009;30:1110–5.

Chapter 8
Scoring Systems to Semiquantitatively Grade Cartilage Pathology with MRI

Christoph Stehling

Keywords Scoring Systems • Cartilage • KOSS • UCSF score • MRI • WORMS • BLOKS • Noyes and Stabler score • Recht score

A number of semiquantitative scoring methods for grading cartilage loss on MRI have been developed. Most of these scoring strategies derive from arthroscopy, and grade primarily the depth of focal cartilage loss over a five-point scale. However, newer scores have been developed, which aim at grading osteoarthritis and provide a more complex analysis of cartilage. These include the Whole-Organ MRI score (WORMS) and the Boston–Leeds Osteoarthritis Knee score (BLOKS), in addition to cartilage these scores also grade other tissues involved in osteoarthritis such as bone marrow, menisci, and ligaments.

Arthroscopic Articular Cartilage Rating Scores

Outerbridge Score

Outerbridge published a scoring system about macroscopic changes of chondromalacia of the patella in 1961 [1]. Changes can be classified into four grades: in grade 1 there are softening and swelling of the cartilage; in grade 2 there are fragmentation and fissuring in an area half an inch or less in diameter, grade 3 is the same as grade 2 but an area more than half an inch in diameter is involved, in grade 4 there is full-thickness erosion of cartilage down to bone.

Noyes and Stabler Score

In comparison to the Outerbridge Score Noyes and Stabler established a more detailed scoring system in 1989. Their system was based on four variables: integrity of the cartilage surface, extent (depth) of involvement, location of the lesion, and diameter of the lesion [2].

In their classification system they separated the description of the surface appearance from the depth of involvement. They distinguished three surface grades: articular cartilage surface intact (grade 1), articular cartilage surface damaged, open lesion (grade 2), and bone exposed (grade 3). Each grade is divided into subtypes, A or B, depending upon the depth of involvement.

A type 1A designation corresponds to a moderate degree of softening of the cartilage, and type 1B results in severe softening of the cartilage. Type 2A lesion is characterized by disruption of the cartilage surface less than one-half thickness, and type 2B is greater than one-half thickness. Type 3B indicates any surface with exposed bone but remains with normal bony contour, and type 3B indicates cavitation or erosion of bone surface.

The size of the lesion was ranked by one of five categories from less than 10 mm to more than 25 mm. The anatomic location was recorded and was divided into femur, tibia, and patella. The femoral articular surface was divided into the trochlea and anterior, middle, and posterior thirds of the femoral condyles. The tibial condyles were also divided into an anterior, middle, and posterior part. The patella was categorized in proximal one-third, middle one-third, and distal one-third and according to facet involvement in medial and lateral.

Modified Arthroscopic Cartilage Scores for MRI

Recht Scores

Recht et al. described two cartilage lesion MRI classifications [3, 4]. The first one according to a modification of the arthroscopic scoring scheme proposed by Outerbridge [1] in 1993 and a second classification system based on Noyes and Stabler's grading system (2) in 1996. Both classification systems are still in use in the literature [5–8].

C. Stehling (✉)
Department of Clinical Radiology, University of Muenster,
Albert-Schweitzer-Strasse 33, Muenster 48149, Germany
e-mail: cstehling@uni-muenster.de

T.M. Link (ed.), *Cartilage Imaging: Significance, Techniques, and New Developments*,
DOI 10.1007/978-1-4419-8438-8_8, © Springer Science+Business Media, LLC 2011

The modified Outerbridge Score [3] is a five-point scale: grade 0, normal cartilage; grade 1, cartilage softening and/or swelling; grade 2, mild surface fibrillation and/or less than 50% loss of cartilage thickness; grade 3, severe surface fibrillation and/or loss of more than 50% of cartilage thickness but without exposure of subchondral bone; and grade 4, complete loss of cartilage with subchondral bone exposure (Fig. 8.1). The score has been used in recent publications because of its simplicity [5, 6, 8].

For the modified Noyes classification [4] Recht used the first three variables (integrity of the articular surface, extent (depth) of involvement, location of the lesion), and the diameter of the lesion was not evaluated. The score is used in current manuscripts [7, 9]. Cartilage surface was graded as intact (grade 0), damaged but present (grade 2), or absent with subchondral bone exposed (grade 3). Articular cartilage with an intact surface is further subdivided into normal articular cartilage (grade 0) and softened articular cartilage, characterized morphologically by cartilage swelling and/or signal abnormality (grade 1). Grade 2 lesions were subdivided into grades 2A and 2B, on the basis of the extent of the lesion. Lesions that involved less than half the thickness of the articular cartilage were classified as 2A; lesions that involve more than half but less than the entire thickness of the cartilage were classified as 2B. Grade 3 included any lesion with exposed bone; 3A indicated an intact bone surface with a normal bone contour, and 3B indicated cavitation or erosion of the bone surface. On the MR images, 3B lesions were considered present if there was abnormal subchondral bone marrow signal intensity or if there was an osteophyte present in a region of full cartilage thickness loss.

The patella and femoral trochlea were each subdivided into four regions: proximal medial, proximal lateral, distal medial, and distal lateral.

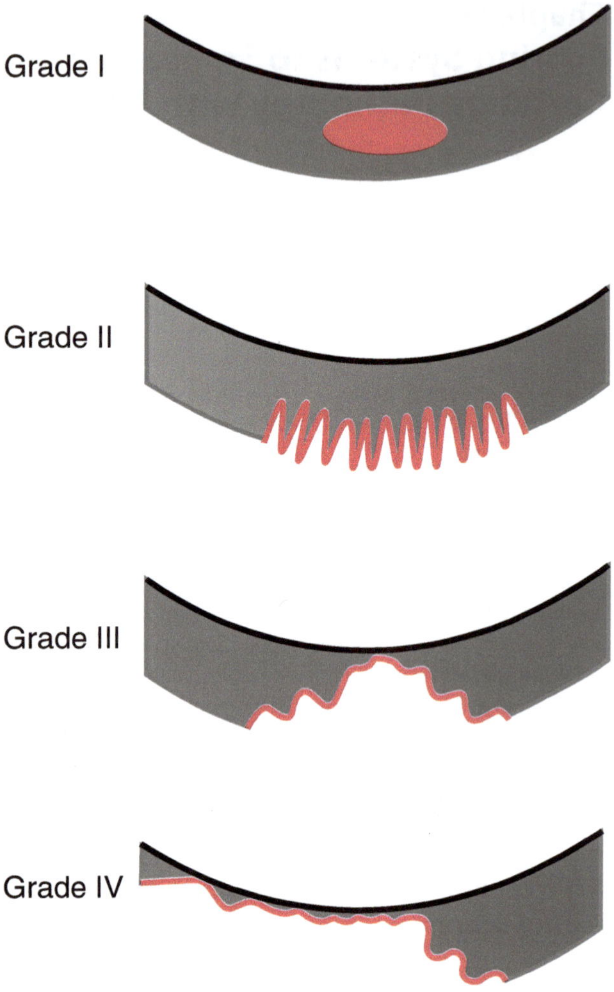

Fig. 8.1 The modified Outerbridge Score (Recht Score 1) is a five-point scale: normal cartilage, *grade 1* cartilage softening and/or swelling, *grade 2* mild surface fibrillation and/or less than 50% loss of cartilage thickness, *grade 3* severe surface fibrillation and/or loss of more than 50% of cartilage thickness but without exposure of subchondral bone, and *grade 4* complete loss of cartilage with subchondral bone exposure

ICRS Score

The International Cartilage Repair Society (ICRS) has set up an arthroscopic grading system, the ICRS Hyaline Cartilage Lesion Classification System, published 2003 by Brittberg [10]. The ICRS classification system focuses on the lesion depth (graded from 0 to 4). Cartilage defects can be ranked: grade 0: (normal) healthy cartilage; grade 1a,b: the cartilage has a soft spot or blisters; grade 2: minor tears visible in the cartilage (less than 50% of cartilage layer); grade 3a–d: lesions have deep crevices (more than 50% of cartilage layer); grade 4a,b: the cartilage tear exposes the underlying (subchronal) bone.

The ICRS Score has also been transferred to MR imaging by Brittberg et al. [10]. ICRS-1a lesions have fibrillation and/or slight softening with intact cartilage surface and it is difficult to differentiate these lesions from normal (ICRS-0) cartilage using MRI. ICRS-1b lesions (superficial lacerations and fissures) are deeper, and they are more easily detectable with MRI. The spatial resolution of MRI is usually adequate to determine whether a cartilage defect involves >50% of the cartilage thickness (ICRS 3) or <50% of the cartilage thickness (ICRS 2).

The deepest layers of articular cartilage usually appear dark on MR images, similar to the appearance of the subchondral bone plate. Therefore, it has been assumed unlikely that MRI will be able to differentiate among ICRS-3a lesions (which do not extend into the calcified cartilage layer), ICRS-3b lesions (which extend down to the calcified layer), and ICRS-3c lesions (which extend down to but not through the subchondral bone plate). Blistering (ICRS-3d lesions) may be detected as a bulge and swelling on the cartilage surface.

ICRS-4 cartilage lesions, which extend into the subchondral bone, are often detected by the presence of a subchondral cyst beneath them. Even if the direct communication between the cartilage defect and the cyst cannot be identified on the images, direct communication should be strongly suspected. Similarly, except in the setting of acute trauma when a bone bruise may be present, if there is a focal edema–like signal in the marrow beneath a cartilage lesion, it may indicate that the lesion extends to, or into, the subchondral bone plate (suggesting a classification of ICRS 3 or ICRS 4). As with the arthroscopic grading of lesions, the grading of the depth of a lesion found with MRI should be recorded as the greatest depth observed within the lesion.

Semiquantitative Whole Organ Scores

WORMS Score

Peterfy and colleagues published the Whole-Organ Magnetic Resonance Imaging Score (WORMS) in 2004 [11]. Many epidemiologic studies and clinical trials have used WORMS to assess several OA features of the knee [5, 12–18].

It can be used to capture different patterns of regional cartilage loss and provides more information about the extent of the surface involvement. The WORMS method takes into account a variety of features that are currently believed to be relevant to the functional integrity of the knee and potentially involved in the pathophysiology of OA.

WORMS is used to semiquantitatively evaluate MR images of the knee with 14 independent articular features: cartilage signal and morphology, subarticular bone marrow abnormality, subarticular cysts, subarticular bone attrition, marginal osteophytes, medial and lateral meniscal integrity, anterior and posterior cruciate ligament (PCL) integrity, medial and lateral collateral ligament (LCL) integrity, synovitis, loose bodies, and periarticular cysts/bursae.

Five of the features examined are related to the articular surfaces.

These features are evaluated in 15 different regions subdivided by anatomical landmarks in the fully extended knee (Fig. 8.2). The patella is divided into the lateral facet (LP) and medial facet (MP). The patellar ridge is considered part of the MP. The subchondral component of each patellar region includes the full thickness of the bone to the opposite cortex. The femoral articular surface is divided into medial (MF) and lateral (LF) condyles, with the trochlear groove considered part of MF. The boundary between MF and LF is defined by a plane aligned with the lateral wall of the femoral notch. MF and LF are each divided into three regions: (1) anterior (a): extending from the anterior-superior osteochondral junction to the anterior margin of the anterior horn of the meniscus; (2) central (c): extending from the anterior margin of the anterior horn of the meniscus to the posterior capsular attachment of the posterior horn of the meniscus; and (3) posterior (p): extending from the posterior capsular attachment of the posterior horn of the meniscus to the posterior-superior osteochondral junction. The subchondral component of each femoral region extends perpendicularly from the articular surface to the level of an imaginary line connecting the anterior and posterior osteochondral junctions. The medial tibial plateau (MT) and lateral tibial plateau (LT) are each divided into three equal regions: anterior (a), central (c) and posterior (p). Based on these subdivisions, the patellofemoral joint (PFJ) comprises regions MP, LP, MFa (medial femur anterior), and LFa (lateral femur anterior); the medial femorotibial joint (MFTJ) comprises regions MFc, MFp, MTa, MTc, and MTp; and the lateral femorotibial joint (LFTJ) comprises regions LFc, LFp, LTa, LTc, and LTp. The nonarticulating portion of the tibial plateau beneath the tibial spines is designated region 'S' (subspinous). The subchondral component of each tibial region extends 2 cm beneath the articular surface.

Cartilage signal and morphology are scored in each of the 14 articular-surface regions (excluding region S) using an eight-point scale (Fig. 8.3): 0 = normal thickness and signal; 1 = normal thickness but abnormal signal on fluid sensitive sequences; 2.0 = partial-thickness focal defect <1 cm in greatest width; 2.5 = full-thickness focal defect <1 cm in greatest width; 3 = multiple areas of partial-thickness (grade 2.0) defects intermixed with areas of normal thickness, or a grade 2.0 defect wider than 1 cm but <75% of the region; 4 = diffuse (≥75% of the region) partial-thickness loss; 5 = multiple areas of full-thickness loss (grade 2.5) or a grade 2.5 lesion wider than 1 cm but <75% of the region; 6 = diffuse (≥75% of the region) full-thickness loss.

The WORMS Score does not only grade the depth of focal cartilage loss but also expands the scale to eight points in order to capture different patterns of regional cartilage loss and more information about extent of surface involvement. Each point on the scale is one integer, except for grade 2.5. This point interval is smaller than the others are because the difference in cartilage loss between a small focal partial-thickness defect (2.0) and a small focal full-thickness defect (2.5) is proportionately smaller than the difference between the other intervals. The adjustment, accordingly, improves linearity of the scale. WORMS also incorporates changes in cartilage signal on T2-weighted images, which have been shown to represent areas of chondromalacia that may precede focal tissue loss. Intraclass correlation coefficients (ICC) were determined for each feature as a measure of interobserver agreement and an early study found good performance (cartilage = 0.99) [11].

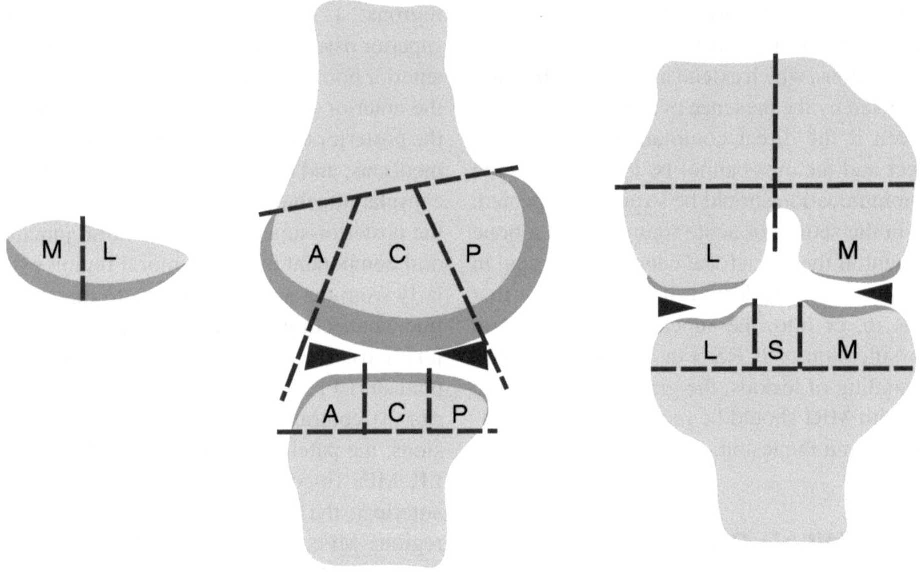

Fig. 8.2 Regional subdivision of the articular surfaces. The patella (*left image*) is divided into medial (M) and lateral (L) regions, with the ridge considered part of the M region. The femur and tibia are also divided into M and L regions (*right image*), with the trochlear groove of the femur considered part of the M region. Region S represents the portion of the tibia beneath the tibial spines. The femoral and tibial surfaces are further subdivided into anterior (a), central (c), and posterior (p) regions (*middle image*). Region A of the femur corresponds to the patellofemoral articulation; region C the weight bearing surface, and region P the posterior convexity that articulates only in extreme flexion. Region C of the tibial surface corresponds to the uncovered portion between the anterior and posterior horns of the meniscus centrally and the portion covered by the body of the meniscus peripherally

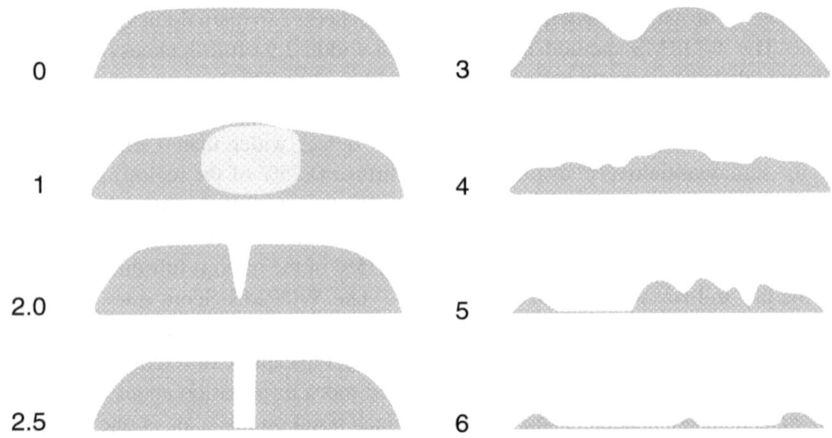

Fig. 8.3 Eight-point scale for scoring articular cartilage signal and morphology. Each region of the knee surface is scored independently

Because of the very time-consuming analysis of the 15 subregions some authors modified the score to grade cartilage lesions in patients where only a relatively small number of lesions is expected, such as the incidence cohort of the Osteoarthritis Initiative [5, 16–18]. In these studies the number of anatomical compartments was reduced from 15 to 6, respectively seven compartments, and included the patella, trochlea, medial and lateral femur, and medial and lateral tibia [5, 16–18].

Alterations in meniscal morphology are also assessed with the WORMS, separately in six regions (medial and lateral: anterior, body, posterior) [11]. The different regions are graded separately from 0 to 4 based on both the sagittal and coronal images: 0 = intact; 1 = minor radial tear or parrot-beak tear; 2 = nondisplaced tear or prior surgical repair; 3 = displaced tear or partial resection; 4 = complete maceration/destruction or complete resection.

A cumulative grade for each meniscus is determined: 0 = all 0; 1 = at least one 1, but no >1; 2 = 2 in only one region; 3 = 2 in more than one region; 4 = 3 in one or more regions; 5 = 4 in only one region; 6 = 4 in more than one region. Peterfy et al. pointed out that an algorithm was needed in order to adjust for nonlinearity among the regional grades, which could lead to inconsistencies if the grades were simply summarized. The meniscus scoring system offers a high inter-reader agreement with ICC values of 0.87 [11].

The score does not include intrasubstance degeneration and does not classify tear morphology well such as longitudinal, horizontal, vertical, and radial tears as limitations and it does not include extrusion, meniscal root, and meniscal shape abnormalities (like discoid meniscus). Recent publications have included intrasubstance degeneration and meniscal extrusion in the evaluation of the meniscus [5, 16].

Subarticular bone marrow abnormality was defined as poorly marginated areas of increased signal intensity in the normally fatty epiphyseal marrow on fat-suppressed T2-weighted FSE images. Subarticular cysts were identified as foci of markedly increased signal in the subarticular bone with sharply defined, rounded margins and no evidence of internal marrow tissue or trabecular bone. Both features were graded in each of the 14 articular-surface regions as well as the region of the tibia beneath the tibial spines (S) from 0 to 3 based on the extent of regional involvement. Synovial thickening and joint effusion were not distinguished from each other, but graded collectively from 0 to 3 in terms of the estimated maximal distention of the synovial cavity. The anterior cruciate ligament (ACL) and posterior cruciate ligament (PCL) were independently scored as intact (0) or torn (1) using the sagittal T2 FSE images. The medial collateral ligament (MCL) and lateral collateral ligament (LCL) were independently scored as intact (0) or torn (1) using the coronal images. A combined ligament score was calculated by adding the sum of the ACL and PCL scores to half the sum of the MCL and LCL scores. Flattening or depression of the articular surfaces was termed bone attrition and graded from 0 to 3 based on the subjective degree of deviation from the normal contour. Osteophytes along 14 different margins of the knee, the anterior (a), central weight-bearing (c), and posterior (p) margins of the femoral condyles and tibial plateaus, and the medial (M) and lateral (L) margins of the patella were graded from 0 to 7 [11].

KOSS Score

The KOSS Score was introduced by Kornaat et al. in 2005 [19] and is comparable to the WORMS Score. Cartilage status and other abnormalities are scored individually for each subregion, and each score is differentiated by the size of the lesion. KOSS uses a different subregion division than WORMS and differentiates the patellar crest (crista patellae), the medial patellar facet and lateral patellar facet, the medial trochlear articular facet and lateral trochlear articular facet, the medial femoral condyle and lateral femoral condyle (excluding the trochlear groove), and the medial tibial plateau and lateral tibial plateau.

Cartilaginous defects are graded as diffuse, or focal defects, or osteochondral defects. The depth of diffuse and focal cartilage loss is qualitatively graded in relation to the height of the adjacent intact cartilage or the expected, normal cartilage contour. The depth of a cartilaginous defect is graded as: grade 0 = absent (no abnormality in signal intensity or morphology); grade 1 = less than 50% reduction of cartilage thickness; grade 2 = 50% or greater reduction of cartilage thickness; grade 3 = full-thickness or near-full-thickness cartilage defect. The depth of the osseous component of the osteochondral defect is scored by estimating the distance between the actual osteochondral defect and the extrapolated subchondral cortex, and is graded as follows: grade 0 = absent; grade 1 = minimal (<2 mm); grade 2 = moderate (2–5 mm); grade 3 = severe (>5 mm). The surface extent (S) of a diffuse, focal, or osteochondral cartilage defect is estimated by its maximal diameter and graded as follows: grade 0 = absent; grade 1 = minimal (<5 mm); grade 2 = moderate (5–10 mm); grade 3 = severe (>10 mm). A cartilaginous defect is described as focal in the case of an abrupt transition (acute angle) between the cartilage defect and the surrounding cartilage, resembling a crater. It is described as diffuse in the case of a smooth and gradual transition zone (obtuse angle) between normal and thinned cartilage. When a focal chondral or osteochondral defect is superimposed on diffuse cartilage loss, both defects are scored.

A meniscal tear is defined as a region of intermediate signal intensity on proton density-weighted images within the meniscus, communicating with its superior or inferior surface or inner margin [20]. Meniscal tears are classified according to their shape as: 1, horizontal; 2, vertical; 3, radial; 4, complex; and 5, bucket-handle [21].

Meniscal subluxation is defined as protrusion, usually of the body of the meniscus, over the edge of the tibial plateau on coronal proton density-weighted images and is graded as follows: grade 0 = absent; grade 1 = minimal (<1/3 width of the meniscus bulging); grade 2 = moderate (1/3–2/3 meniscal width involved); grade 3 = severe (>2/3 meniscal width involved).

Meniscal intrasubstance degeneration is scored on proton density-weighted images as: grade 0 = absent; grade 1 = when a small, central focus of intermediate signal intensity on proton density-weighted images is noticed in the meniscus; grade 2 = when the intrameniscal focus of intermediate signal intensity on proton density-weighted images is surrounded by a broad, hypointense peripheral rim; grade 3 = when only a thin, hypointense peripheral rim outlines the intermediate signal intensity meniscal center.

The interobserver reproducibility of this classification was described as good with an ICC value of 0.77. The inter- and intraobserver reproducibility for individual parameters such as cartilage scoring was 0.64 for intraobserver reproducibility (interobserver reproducibility 0.78) and for meniscal abnormalities 0.70–0.78 (intraobserver reproducibility 0.76–0.78).

The authors also pointed out a major disadvantage of the KOSS Score [19], which is the fact that it is very time consuming. Depending on the amount of focal chondral and osteochondral defects, each MR examination requires approximately 30 min of careful evaluation.

BLOKS Score

The Boston–Leeds Osteoarthritis Knee Score (BLOKS) is a novel expert-based semiquantitative scoring system specifically developed for knee OA described by Hunter et al. in 2008 [22]. It is a descriptive score for each morphological feature including cartilage integrity, attrition, bone marrow lesions and cysts, osteophytes, ligaments, meniscus, and synovitis.

Two methods for scoring cartilage were developed. The rationale for the development of the first system was to provide separate scores for the size (area affected) and extent of full-thickness loss in each of the regional areas of the knee (Cartilage Score 1). This system is more complex as it requires the reader to integrate many focal abnormalities to arrive at one scale. To improve the reproducible selection of anatomic sites for reading purposes the authors also created a scoring system that facilitates scoring of the thickness at selected sites (Cartilage Score 2). These are sites where articular cartilage loss is most frequently observed.

Cartilage Score 1

The knee is divided into eight articular regions for scoring articular cartilage. The patella is divided into two regions, the medial and lateral patella, where medial delineates medial to the crista. The femur is divided into four regions, medial and lateral trochlea and medial and lateral weight-bearing femur (the weight-bearing femur includes the central and posterior femur) (Figs. 8.4 and 8.5). The tibia is divided into medial and lateral regions.

The BLOKS uses a modified WORMS grading. In WORMS, grade 1 does not represent a change in shape but rather a change in signal in cartilage of an otherwise normal shape. Grades 2 and 3 represent similar types of abnormality of the cartilage, focal defects without overall thinning. Therefore, to create a consistent and logical scale for evaluation of cartilage morphologic change and a fair comparison with radiographic changes in joint space narrowing, the investigators collapsed the WORMS cartilage score to a 0–4 scale, where the original WORMS Score of 0 and 1 are collapsed to 0, the original scores of 2 and 3 are collapsed to 1, and the original scores of 4, 5, and 6 are considered 2 and 3, respectively. In the new scale (Fig. 8.6) grade 0 is defined as no cartilage loss; grade 1 as <10% loss of the region of the cartilage surface area; grade 2 as 10–75% loss of the region of the cartilage surface area and grade 3 as >75% loss of the region of the cartilage surface area.

The score at all five plates in both the medial and lateral TF joint is summarized to give a score with a possible range from 0 to 20. Cartilage loss is defined as a change in the summary score at subsequent follow-up.

Cartilage Score 2

This particular score is for site-specific cartilage loss and it is recommended as an alternative grading scheme that contains less detail but is more easily administered. This particular grade focuses on cartilage at 11 specific sites including: three parts of the patella, medial, lateral patella, and the crista; four sites on the medial and lateral weight-bearing tibia and femur each. For cartilage score 2 the size of any cartilage loss at specified points is graded as follows: grade 0, no cartilage loss; grade 1, partial loss; grade 2, complete loss [22].

The meniscus scoring system contains two parts, extrusion and morphology. Extrusion is scored in four areas: medial meniscus – medial extrusion (coronal image) and anterior extrusion (sagittal image); lateral meniscus – lateral extrusion (coronal image) and anterior extrusion (sagittal image). The delineation of extrusion is graded using a four-point score for the amount of extrusion in millimeters: 0, <2 mm; 1, 2–2.9 mm; 2, 3–4.9 mm; 3, >5 mm.

The morphology of the medial and lateral meniscus is scored for the anterior and posterior horn as well as the body. The anterior and posterior horn regions are scored using the sagittal sequences and body is scored using the coronal sequences. The following morphologic features are scored: (1) signal changes yes/no (not extending through meniscal surface, i.e., not a tear); (2) tear yes/no (defined as high signal extending to an articular surface); (3) vertical tear yes/no (includes radial and longitudinal tears) – must extend to both the femoral and tibial surfaces; (4) horizontal tear yes/no; (5) complex tear yes/no (as defined by high signal that extends to two surfaces and ≥3 points); (6) root tear yes/no (posterior horn); (7) Macerated yes/no (loss of overall normal morphological appearance of the meniscus and with an associated increased diffuse signal in the meniscal tissue); and (8) meniscal cyst: yes/no.

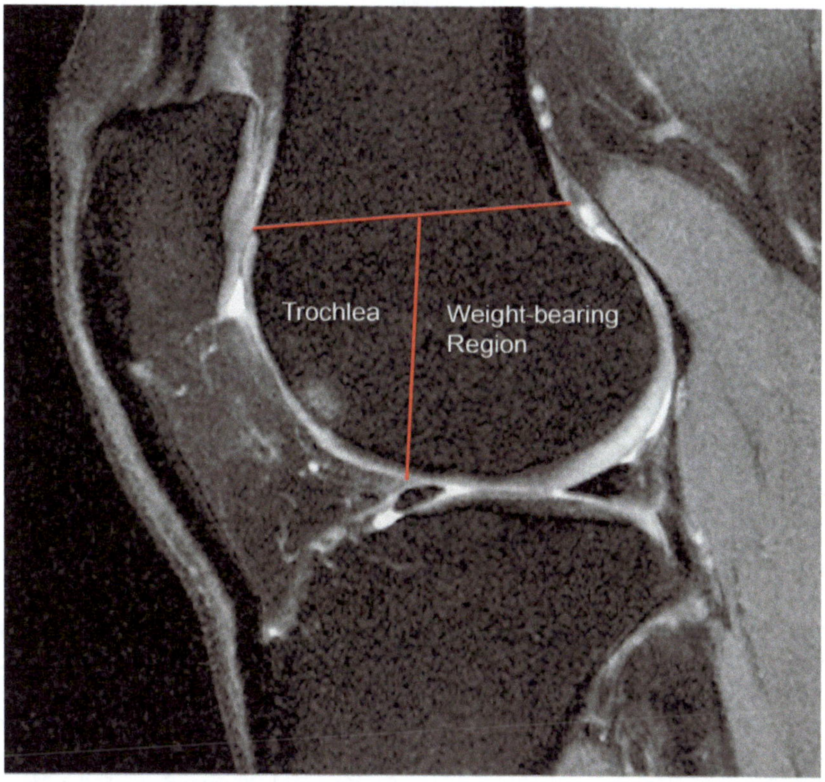

Fig. 8.4 Anatomical delineation of femur into trochlea and weight-bearing regions on sagittal projection in BLOKS score

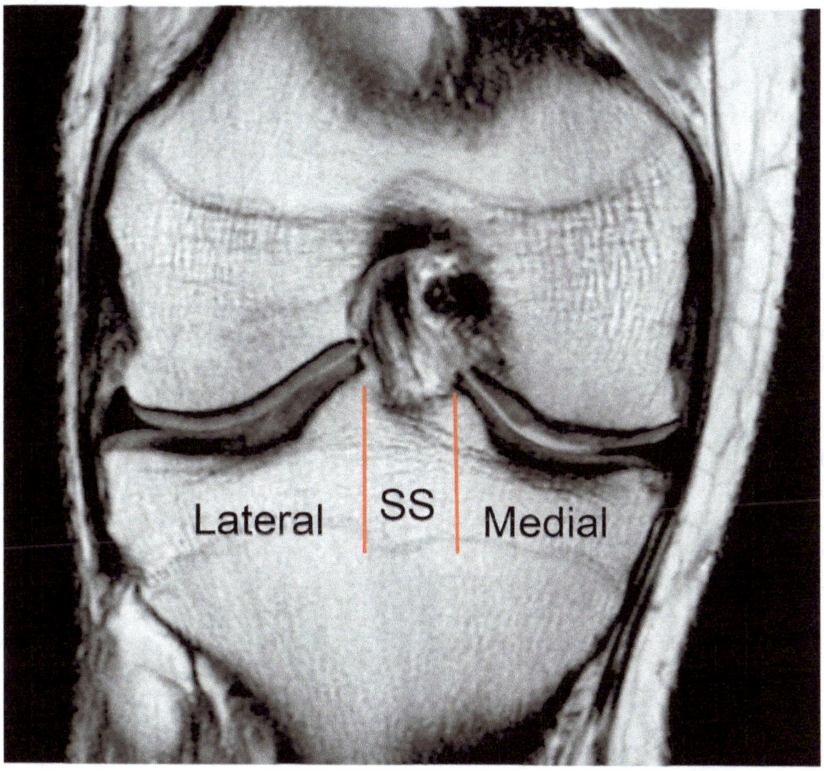

Fig. 8.5 Anatomical delineation of tibia on a coronal projection into medial, subspinous (SS) and lateral regions in BLOKS score

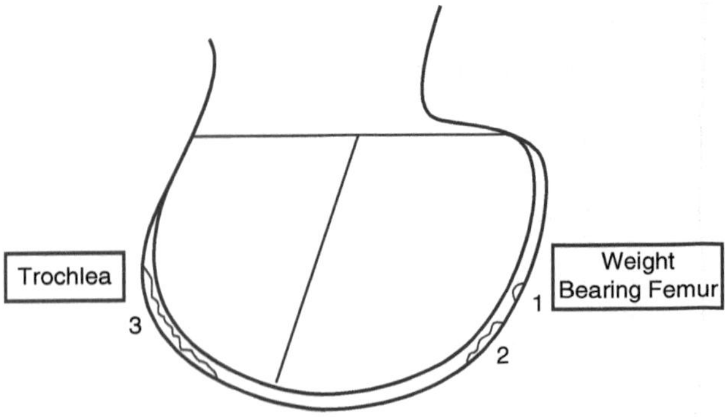

Fig. 8.6 Grade for size of any cartilage loss as a percentage of surface area as related to the size of each individual region in BLOKS score 1. Grade 0 is defined as no cartilage loss; grade 1 as <10% loss of the region of the cartilage surface area; grade 2 as 10–75% loss of the region of the cartilage surface area; and grade 3 as >75% loss of the region of the cartilage surface area

Hunter et al. explored the validity of assessment of different pathologies using the BLOKS instrument and found that it demonstrated reasonable reliability and validity [22]. The inter-reader reliability ranged from 0.51 for meniscal extrusion up to 0.79 for meniscal tears. The reliability for cartilage morphology was 0.72.

UCSF Score

In extension to the WORMS and Recht Score, Link and Stahl developed a UCSF quantitative score in 2008 specifically tailored to evaluate early focal cartilage lesions, as a more sensitive technique to longitudinally monitor cartilage lesions and determine progression of disease [12, 23]. Pathologic findings at the knee joint cartilage and bone marrow are analyzed using a modified WORMS Score. The 15 previously described compartments are merged to a total of seven compartments: the medial and lateral tibia, trochlea, medial and lateral femur, as well as medial and lateral patella. To quantify better the subtle cartilage lesions found in subjects not sufficiently assessed with the WORMS, extent of cartilage inhomogeneity (WORMS = 1) and extent of cartilage defects (WORMS ≥ 2) are calculated. In lesions with a WORMS of 1 the inhomogeneity of the signal intensity is quantified by multiplying its largest diameter by the number of slices that visualizes it (slice thickness in millimeters, including section gap). The extent of lesions with visible cartilage defects (WORMS Score ≥ 2) is approximated by the following equation:

$$\text{Lesion volume} = \text{largest diameter (mm)} \times \text{number of sections} \times \text{section thickness including gap (mm)} \times \text{depth factor} \times \text{shape factor}.$$

To determine the depth factor of the lesion the surrounding normal cartilage was divided into three layers with equal thickness. If the maximum lesion depth did not exceed the thickness of the superficial layer it was assigned as 1/3. It became 2/3 or 3/3 if the maximal lesion depth comprised also the medium or the lowest layer, respectively. The shape factor was 1 if more than 50% of the lesion had the largest depth (assessed in the section with the largest diameter), otherwise a shape factor of 0.5 was assigned. The authors also developed a score to quantify the volume of bone marrow lesions. Figure 8.7a–c shows how cartilage and bone marrow lesions were quantified.

Summary

A number of semiquantitative scoring methods for grading cartilage loss on MRI have been developed. Outerbridge published a scoring system about macroscopic changes of chondromalacia of the patella in 1961. In comparison to the Outerbridge Score Noyes and Stabler established a more detailed scoring system in 1989. Their system was based on four variables: integrity of the cartilage surface, extent (depth) of involvement, location of the lesion, and diameter of the lesion.

Recht et al. described two cartilage lesion MRI classifications. The first one according to a modification of the arthroscopic scoring scheme proposed by Outerbridge in 1993 and a second classification system based on Noyes and Stabler's grading system in 1996.

The International Cartilage Repair Society (ICRS) has set up an arthroscopic grading system, the ICRS Hyaline Cartilage Lesion Classification System, published 2003 by Brittberg.

Peterfy and colleagues published the whole-organ magnetic resonance imaging score (WORMS) in 2004. WORMS is used to semiquantitatively evaluate MR images of the knee with 14 independent articular features: cartilage signal and morphology, subarticular bone marrow abnormality, subarticular cysts, subarticular bone attrition, marginal osteophytes, medial and lateral meniscal integrity, anterior and posterior cruciate ligament integrity, medial and lateral collateral ligament integrity, synovitis, loose bodies, and periarticular cysts/bursae.

The KOSS Score was introduced by Kornaat et al. in 2005 and is comparable to the WORMS Score. Cartilage status and other abnormalities are scored individually for each subregion, and each score is differentiated by the size of the lesion.

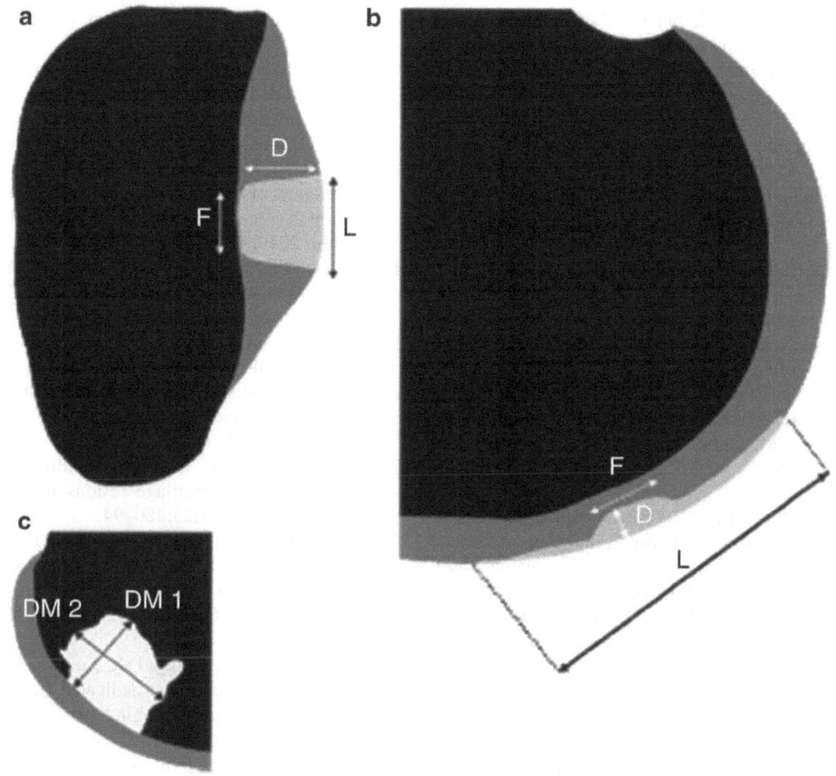

Fig. 8.7 Schematic drawing illustrating how cartilage lesions and bone marrow edema pattern (BMEP) are quantified on iw FSE sequences using the UCSF score (from reference [12]). (**a**) Full-thickness cartilage lesion with a depth factor of 3/3 or 1. Maximum depth across the diameter of more than 50% of the entire lesion, defined as a shape factor of 1 (*D* maximum depth, *F* diameter of deepest part of the lesion, *L* maximum diameter of entire lesion). (**b**) More than 50% partial thickness lesion at the posterior part of the femoral condyle indicating a depth factor of 2/3 or 0.66. Maximum depth across the diameter of less than 50% of the entire lesion, defined as a shape factor of 0.5 (*D* maximum depth, *F* diameter of deepest aspect of the lesion, *L* maximum diameter of entire lesion). (**c**) Subchondral BMEP at the anterior lateral femur condyle. Drawing illustrates the two largest diameters (DM 1 and DM 2)

The Boston–Leeds Osteoarthritis Knee Score (BLOKS) is a novel expert-based semiquantitative scoring system specifically developed for knee OA described by Hunter et al. in 2008. It is a descriptive score for each morphological feature including cartilage integrity, attrition, bone marrow lesions and cysts, osteophytes, ligaments, meniscus, and synovitis.

In extension to the WORMS and Recht Score Link and Stahl developed a UCSF quantitative score in 2008 specifically tailored to evaluate early focal cartilage lesions, as a more sensitive technique to longitudinally monitor cartilage lesions and determine progression of disease. Pathologic findings at the knee joint cartilage and bone marrow are analyzed using a modified WORMS Score.

References

1. Outerbridge RE. The etiology of chondromalacia patellae. J Bone Joint Surg Br. 1961;43-B:752–7.
2. Noyes FR, Stabler CL. A system for grading articular cartilage lesions at arthroscopy. Am J Sports Med. 1989;17:505–13.
3. Recht MP, Kramer J, Marcelis S, Pathria MN, Trudell D, Haghighi P, et al. Abnormalities of articular cartilage in the knee: analysis of available MR techniques. Radiology. 1993;187:473–8.
4. Recht MP, Piraino DW, Paletta GA, Schils JP, Belhobek GH. Accuracy of fat-suppressed three-dimensional spoiled gradient-echo FLASH MR imaging in the detection of patellofemoral articular cartilage abnormalities. Radiology. 1996;198:209–12.
5. Stehling C, Lane NE, Nevitt MC, Lynch J, McCulloch CE, Link TM. Subjects with higher physical activity levels have more severe focal knee lesions diagnosed with 3 T MRI: analysis of a non-symptomatic cohort of the osteoarthritis initiative. Osteoarthritis Cartilage. 2010;18(6):776–86.
6. Wong S, Steinbach L, Zhao J, Stehling C, Ma CB, Link TM. Comparative study of imaging at 3.0 T versus 1.5 T of the knee. Skeletal Radiol. 2009;38(8):761–9.
7. Kijowski R, Blankenbaker DG, Davis KW, Shinki K, Kaplan LD, De Smet AA. Comparison of 1.5- and 3.0-T MR imaging for evaluating the articular cartilage of the knee joint. Radiology. 2009;250:839–48.
8. Phan CM, Link TM, Blumenkrantz G, Dunn TC, Ries MD, Steinbach LS, et al. MR imaging findings in the follow-up of patients with different stages of knee osteoarthritis and the correlation with clinical symptoms. Eur Radiol. 2006;16:608–18.

9. Bauer JS, Barr C, Henning TD, Malfair D, Ma CB, Steinbach L, et al. Magnetic resonance imaging of the ankle at 3.0 Tesla and 1.5 Tesla in human cadaver specimens with artificially created lesions of cartilage and ligaments. Invest Radiol. 2008;43:604–11.
10. Brittberg M, Winalski CS. Evaluation of cartilage injuries and repair. J Bone Joint Surg Am. 2003;85-A Suppl 2:58–69.
11. Peterfy CG, Guermazi A, Zaim S, Tirman PF, Miaux Y, White D, et al. Whole-Organ Magnetic Resonance Imaging Score (WORMS) of the knee in osteoarthritis. Osteoarthritis Cartilage. 2004;12:177–90.
12. Stahl R, Luke A, Ma CB, Krug R, Steinbach L, Majumdar S, et al. Prevalence of pathologic findings in asymptomatic knees of marathon runners before and after a competition in comparison with physically active subjects – a 3.0 T magnetic resonance imaging study. Skeletal Radiol. 2008;37:627–38.
13. Hunter DJ, Conaghan PG, Peterfy CG, Bloch D, Guermazi A, Woodworth T, et al. Responsiveness, effect size, and smallest detectable difference of Magnetic Resonance Imaging in knee osteoarthritis. Osteoarthritis Cartilage. 2006;14(Suppl A): A112–15.
14. Conaghan PG, Tennant A, Peterfy CG, Woodworth T, Stevens R, Guermazi A, et al. Examining a whole-organ magnetic resonance imaging scoring system for osteoarthritis of the knee using Rasch analysis. Osteoarthritis Cartilage. 2006;14(Suppl A):A116–21.
15. Roemer FW, Zhang Y, Niu J, Lynch JA, Crema MD, Marra MD, et al. Tibiofemoral joint osteoarthritis: risk factors for MR-depicted fast cartilage loss over a 30-month period in the multicenter osteoarthritis study. Radiology. 2009;252:772–80.
16. Stehling C, Liebl H, Krug R, Lane NE, Nevitt MC, Lynch J, et al. Patellar cartilage: T2 values and morphologic abnormalities at 3.0-T MR imaging in relation to physical activity in asymptomatic subjects from the osteoarthritis initiative. Radiology. 2010;254: 509–20.
17. Stahl R, Luke A, Li X, Carballido-Gamio J, Ma CB, Majumdar S, et al. T1rho, T2 and focal knee cartilage abnormalities in physically active and sedentary healthy subjects versus early OA patients – a 3.0-Tesla MRI study. Eur Radiol. 2009;19:132–43.
18. Zhao J, Li X, Bolbos RI, Link TM, Majumdar S. Longitudinal assessment of bone marrow edema-like lesions and cartilage degeneration in osteoarthritis using 3 T MR T1rho quantification. Skeletal Radiol. 2010;39:523–31.
19. Kornaat PR, Ceulemans RY, Kroon HM, Kroon HM, Riyazi N, Kloppenburg M, et al. MRI assessment of knee osteoarthritis: Knee Osteoarthritis Scoring System (KOSS)–inter-observer and intra-observer reproducibility of a compartment-based scoring system. Skeletal Radiol. 2005;34:95–102.
20. Stoller DW, Martin C, Crues 3rd JV, Kaplan L, Mink JH. Meniscal tears: pathologic correlation with MR imaging. Radiology. 1987;163:731–5.
21. Lewandrowski KU, Muller J, Schollmeier G. Concomitant meniscal and articular cartilage lesions in the femorotibial joint. Am J Sports Med. 1997;25:486–94.
22. Hunter DJ, Lo GH, Gale D, Grainger AJ, Guermazi A, Conaghan PG. The reliability of a new scoring system for knee osteoarthritis MRI and the validity of bone marrow lesion assessment: BLOKS (Boston Leeds Osteoarthritis Knee Score). Ann Rheum Dis. 2008;67:206–11.
23. Stahl R, Krug R, Kelley DA, Zuo J, Ma CB, Majumdar S, et al. Assessment of cartilage-dedicated sequences at ultra-high-field MRI: comparison of imaging performance and diagnostic confidence between 3.0 and 7.0 T with respect to osteoarthritis-induced changes at the knee joint. Skeletal Radiol. 2009;38:771–83.

Chapter 9
Atlas: Cartilage Abnormalities and Scores

Hans Liebl and Thomas M. Link

Keywords Atlas • Typical MRI findings • Noyes and Stabler MRI classification • WORMS • Recht score • Grades • Cartilage abnormalities

The following chapter illustrates cartilage abnormalities and provides semiquantitative scores for these lesions. The focus of this chapter is on the most frequently used Recht (modified Noyes and Stabler) score [1, 2] and Whole-Organ-MRI-Score (WORMS) [3]. These scores have been used in a number of previous studies and have been found helpful in assessing the grade of cartilage lesions, in particular in degenerative joint disease, and in monitoring cartilage abnormalities [4–7]. The individual scores were explained in detail in the previous chapter.

The standard modified Noyes and Stabler MRI classification [1, 2] differentiates four grades: a grade 1 cartilage lesion is defined as a focal signal abnormality of the cartilage with or without swelling; a grade 2a lesion is a focal defect involving less than half of the cartilage thickness; a grade 2b lesion affects more than 50% of the cartilage layer; and a grade 3 lesion is defined as involving the entire cartilage layer and exposing the bone. Grade 3A lesions have a normal bony surface, and 3B lesions include an erosion of the bony surface (Figs. 9.1–9.23).

The whole-organ magnetic resonance imaging score (WORMS) [3] assesses both depth and size of the cartilage lesions using an eight-point scale: grade 1 lesions have a normal thickness but abnormal signal on fluid sensitive sequences; grade 2.0 lesions are partial-thickness focal defects, which are smaller than 1 cm in the greatest width; grade 2.5 are full-thickness focal defects smaller than 1 cm in greatest width; grade 3 lesions are defined as multiple areas of partial-thickness (grade 2.0) defects intermixed with areas of normal thickness, or a Grade 2.0 defect wider than 1 cm but affecting <75% of the region; grade 4 lesions are diffuse partial-thickness lesions affecting more than 75% of the region; grade 5 lesions show multiple areas of full-thickness cartilage loss (grade 2.5) or a grade 2.5 lesion wider than 1 cm but <75% of the region; and finally, grade 6 lesions demonstrate full-thickness cartilage loss in more than 75% of the region (Figs. 9.1–9.23).

Alterations in meniscal morphology are also assessed with the WORMS. The different meniscal regions are graded separately from 0 to 4 based on both sagittal and coronal images: grade 1 is defined as a minor radial tear or parrot-beak tear; grade 2 as a nondisplaced tear or prior surgical repair; grade 3 as a displaced tear or partial resection; and finally, grade 4 as complete maceration/destruction or complete resection of the meniscus. Intrasubstance degeneration is not assessed in the WORMS, but since it is of substantial importance to report early meniscal degeneration we included it in this chapter (Figs. 9.24–9.32).

In summary in this chapter we show examples of different grades of cartilage abnormalities with different defined scores, which will help investigators to better apply the different cartilage lesion classification scores. We focused on the most frequently applied and in our opinion most versatile and easiest to use scores that are currently available.

T.M. Link (✉)
Department of Radiology and Biomedical Imaging, University of California at San Francisco, 400 Parnassus Avenue, A-367, San Francisco, CA 94131, USA
e-mail: Thomas.Link@radiology.ucsf.edu; tmlink@radiology.ucsf.edu

T.M. Link (ed.), *Cartilage Imaging: Significance, Techniques, and New Developments*,
DOI 10.1007/978-1-4419-8438-8_9, © Springer Science+Business Media, LLC 2011

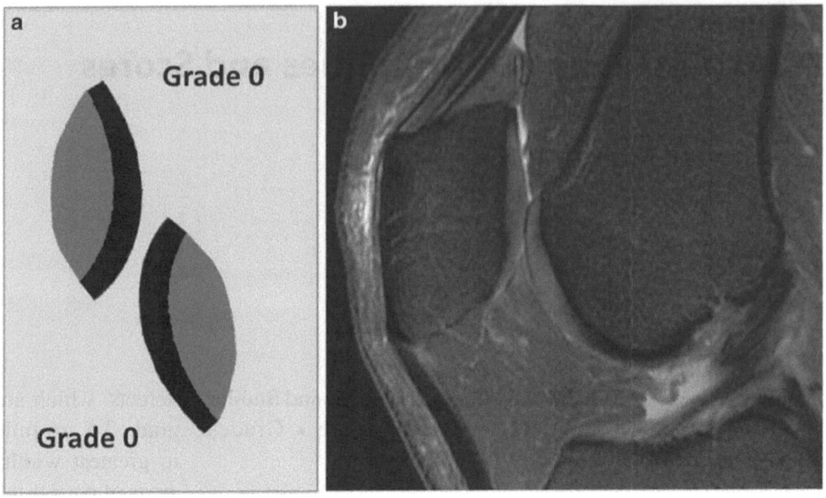

Fig. 9.1 *Whole-Organ-MRI-Score (WORMS) grade 0 cartilage.* Graph of normal knee cartilage (**a**) and sagittal fat saturated intermediate weighted fast spin echo sequence of the knee (**b**) showing healthy cartilage at the patella and trochlea. Both signal and thickness of the cartilage are normal

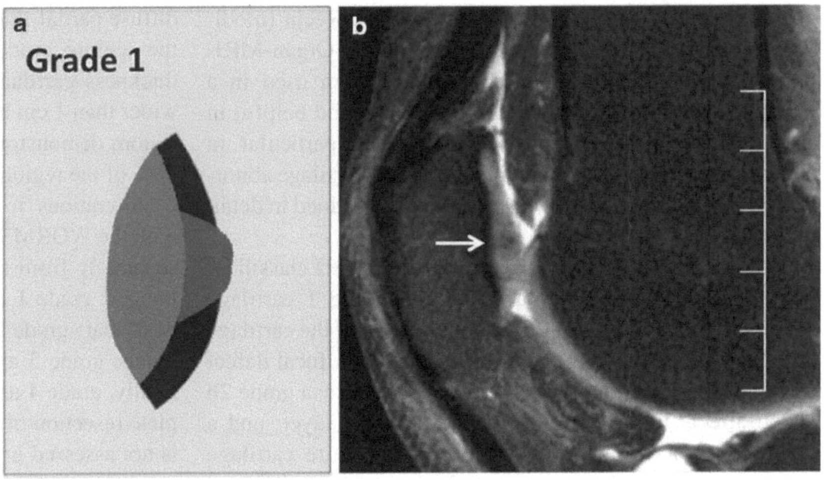

Fig. 9.2 *Whole-Organ-MRI-Score (WORMS) grade 1 lesion.* Graph of grade 1 knee cartilage lesion (**a**) and sagittal fat saturated intermediate weighted fast spin echo sequence of the knee (**b**) showing a cartilage WORMS grade 1 lesion at the patella characterized by signal abnormality and mild swelling (*arrow*). This lesion would be classified as a grade 1 lesion according to the modified Noyes and Stabler MRI score

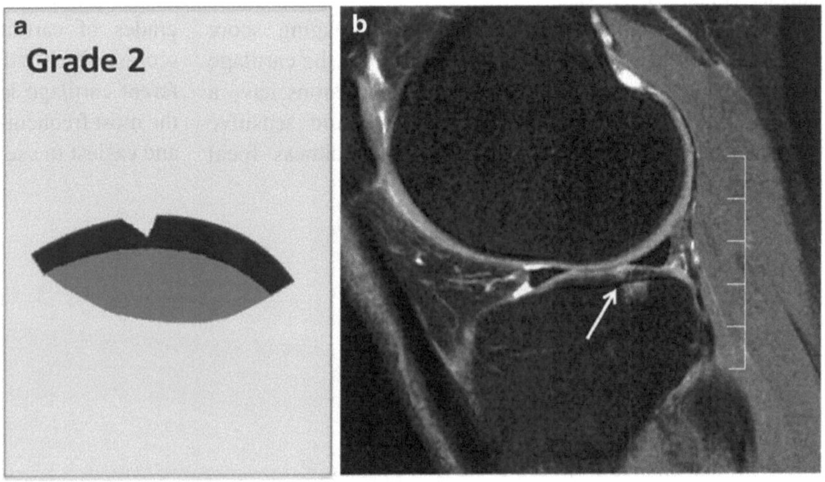

Fig. 9.3 *Whole-Organ-MRI-Score (WORMS) grade 2 lesion.* Graph of grade 2 knee cartilage lesion (**a**) and sagittal fat saturated intermediate weighted fast spin echo sequence of the knee (**b**) showing a cartilage WORMS grade 2 lesion at the posterior aspect of the lateral tibia. The focal lesion measures less than 1 cm and is less than full thickness (*arrow*). This lesion would be classified as a grade 2b lesion according to the modified Noyes and Stabler MRI score as it affects more than 50% of the cartilage layer. In addition, there is adjacent bone marrow edema pattern

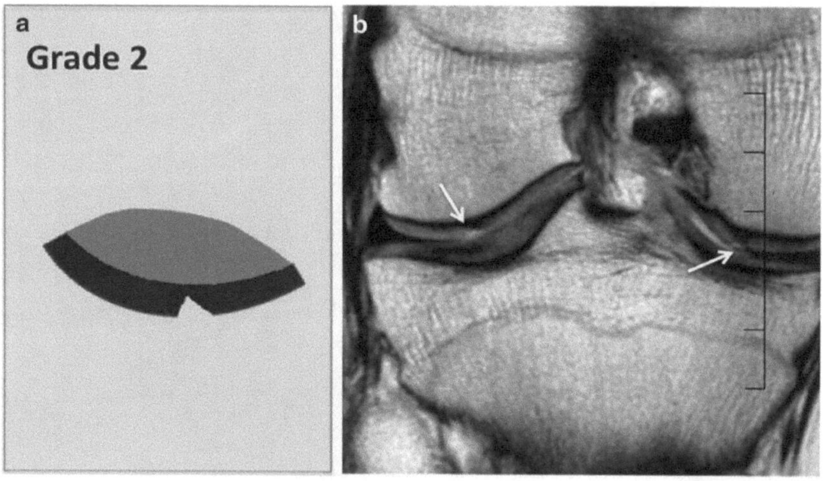

Fig. 9.4 *Whole-Organ-MRI-Score (WORMS) grade 2 lesion*. Graph of grade 2 knee cartilage lesion (**a**) and coronal proton density weighted fast spin echo sequence of the knee (**b**) showing two cartilage WORMS grade 2 lesions at the medial and lateral femoral condyles. The focal lesions measure less than 1 cm and are less than full thickness (*arrows*). The lateral lesion would be classified as a grade 2b lesion according to the modified Noyes and Stabler MRI score as it affects more than 50% of the cartilage layer and the medial lesion (medial aspect of the medial femoral condyle) would be graded as a 2a lesion as it affects less than 50% of the cartilage thickness

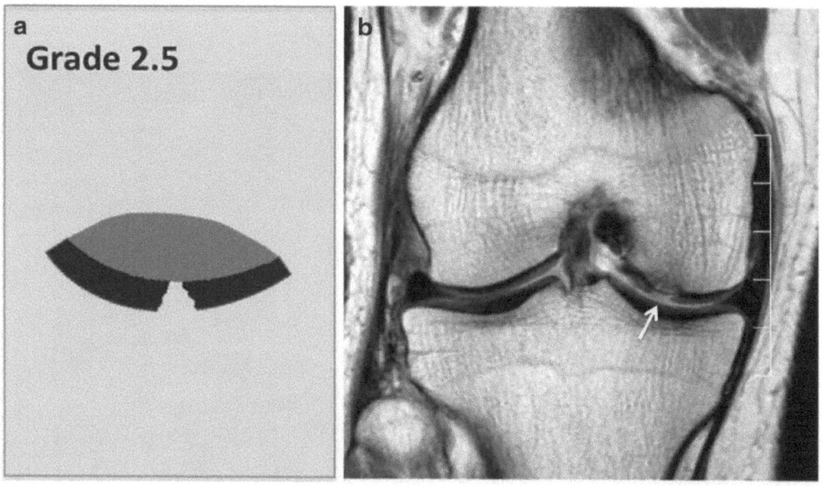

Fig. 9.5 *Whole-Organ-MRI-Score (WORMS) grade 2.5 lesion*. Graph of grade 2.5 knee cartilage lesion (**a**) and coronal proton density weighted fast spin echo sequence of the knee (**b**) showing a cartilage WORMS grade 2.5 lesion at the medial femoral condyle. The focal lesion measures less than 1 cm and extends to the subchondral bone (full thickness) (*arrow*). The lesion would be classified as a grade 3 lesion according to the modified Noyes and Stabler MRI score as it affects the entire cartilage layer and extends to the subchondral bone. Additional subchondral bone changes are consistent with a 3b lesion

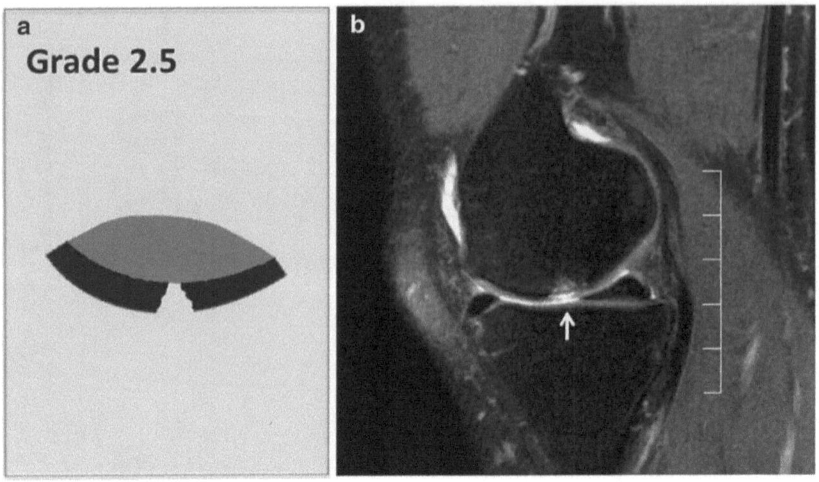

Fig. 9.6 *Whole-Organ-MRI-Score (WORMS) grade 2.5 lesion.* Graph of grade 2.5 knee cartilage lesion (**a**) and sagittal fat saturated intermediate weighted fast spin echo sequence of the knee (**b**) showing a cartilage WORMS grade 2.5 lesion at the central weight-bearing portion of the medial femoral condyle. The focal lesion measures less than 1 cm and is a full-thickness lesion (*arrow*). This lesion would be classified as a grade 3b lesion according to the modified Noyes and Stabler MRI score as it affects the entire cartilage layer and is associated with subchondral cystic changes and bone marrow edema pattern

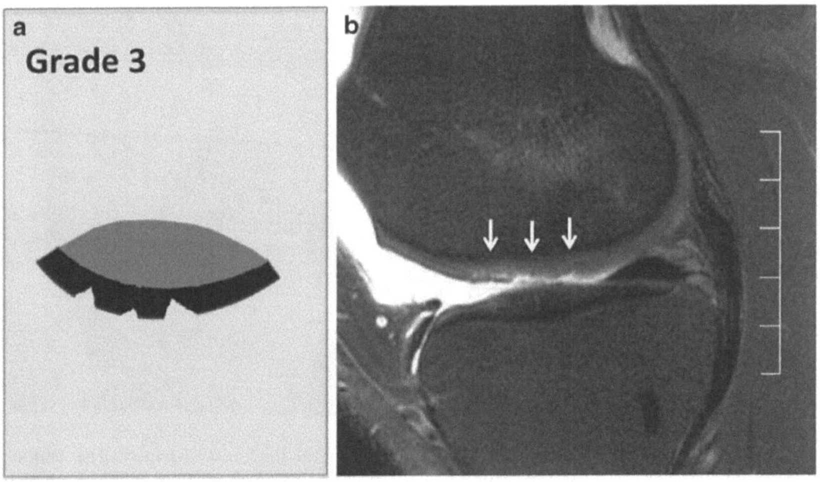

Fig. 9.7 *Whole-Organ-MRI-Score (WORMS) grade 3 lesion.* Graph of grade 3 knee cartilage lesion (**a**) and sagittal fat saturated intermediate weighted fast spin echo sequence of the knee (**b**) showing a cartilage WORMS grade 3 lesion at the central weight-bearing portion of the medial femoral condyle. The focal lesion measures more than 1 cm but affects less than 75% of the central portion of the medial femoral condyle; it is also a partial-thickness lesion (*arrows*). This lesion would be classified as a grade 2a lesion according to the modified Noyes and Stabler MRI score as it affects less than 50% of the cartilage layer

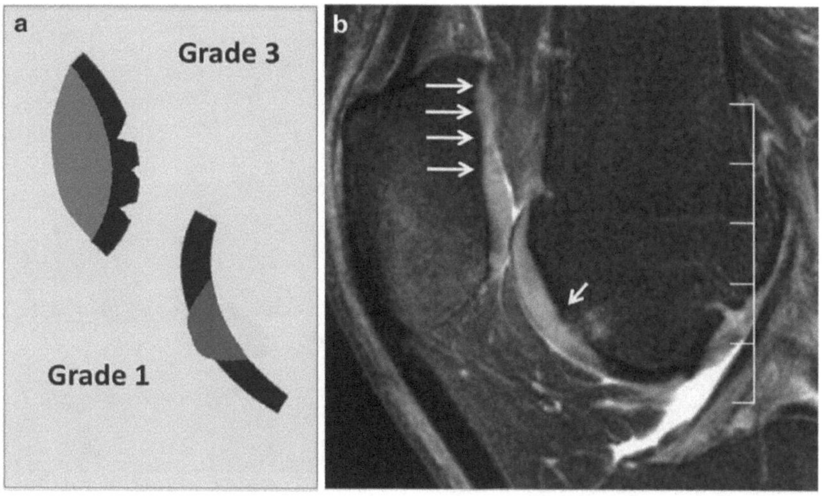

Fig. 9.8 *Whole-Organ-MRI-Score (WORMS) grade 3 and 1 lesion.* Graph of grade 3 and 1 knee cartilage lesions (**a**) and sagittal fat saturated intermediate weighted fast spin echo sequence of the knee (**b**) showing a cartilage WORMS grade 3 lesion at the patella and a grade 1 lesion at the trochlea. The lesion at the patella measures more than 1 cm but affects less than 75% of the central portion of the patella joint surface; it is also a partial-thickness lesion (*arrows*). In addition, there is cartilage signal abnormality at the trochlea (*small arrow*) consistent with a grade 1 lesion. The underlying bone marrow edema pattern at the trochlea in this region suggests significant cartilage matrix abnormality

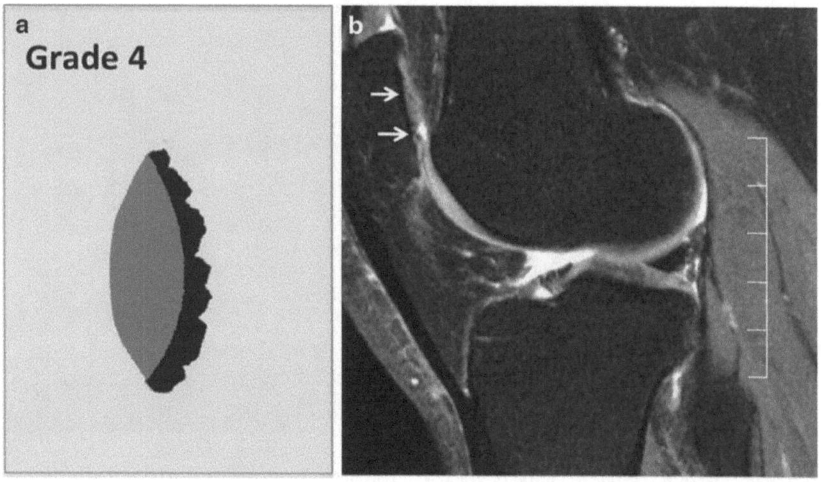

Fig. 9.9 *Whole-Organ-MRI-Score (WORMS) grade 4.* Graph of grade 4 knee cartilage lesion (**a**) and sagittal fat saturated intermediate weighted fast spin echo sequence of the knee (**b**) showing a cartilage WORMS grade 4 lesion at the patella. The lesion affects more than 75% of the patella joint surface and is partial thickness (*arrows*). This lesion would be classified as a grade 2b lesion according to the modified Noyes and Stabler MRI score as it affects more than 50% of the cartilage layer. In addition, there are signal inhomogeneities and swelling in the central portion of the lateral tibial cartilage

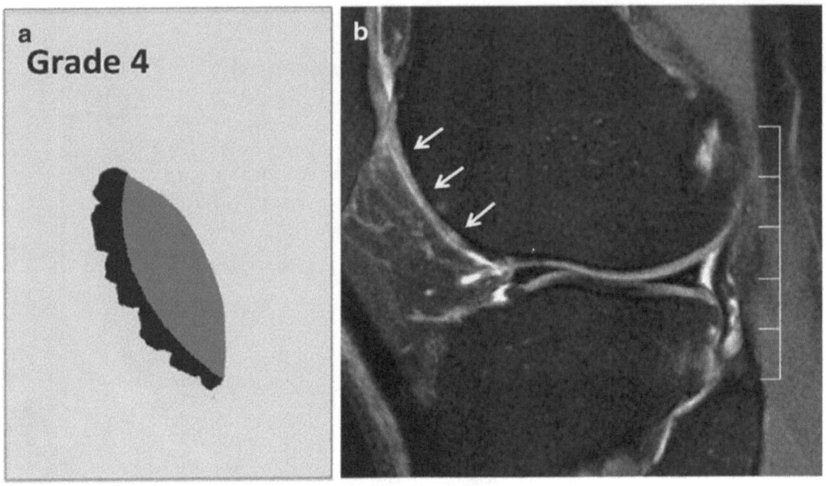

Fig. 9.10 *Whole-Organ-MRI-Score (WORMS) grade 4*. Graph of grade 4 knee cartilage lesion (**a**) and sagittal fat saturated intermediate weighted fast spin echo sequence of the knee (**b**) showing a cartilage WORMS grade 4 lesion at the trochlea. The lesion affects more than 75% of the trochlea joint surface and is partial thickness (*arrows*). This lesion would be classified as a grade 2a lesion according to the modified Noyes and Stabler MRI score as it affects less than 50% of the cartilage layer. In addition, there is subtle bone marrow edema pattern at the trochlea

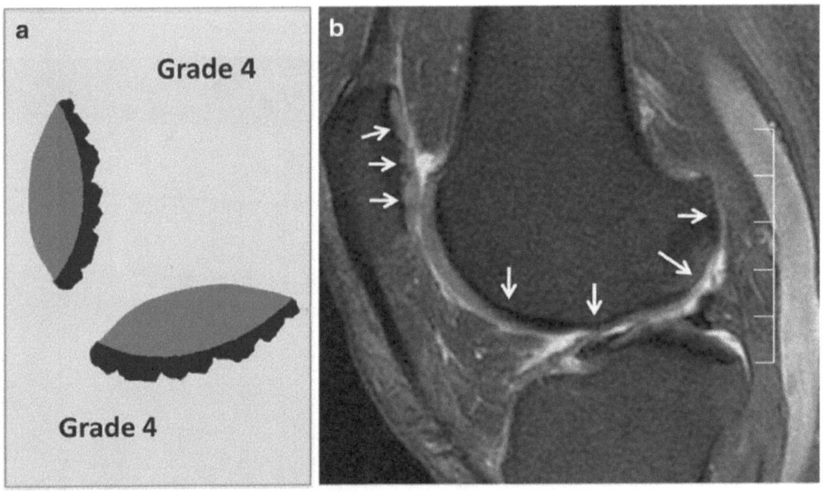

Fig. 9.11 *Whole-Organ-MRI-Score (WORMS) grade 4*. Graph of grade 4 knee cartilage lesions (**a**) and sagittal fat saturated intermediate weighted fast spin echo sequence of the knee (**b**) showing cartilage WORMS grade 4 lesions at the patella, the central, and posterior portion of the lateral femoral condyle. The lesions affect more than 75% of the joint surfaces and are partial thickness (*arrows*). This lesion at the patella would be classified as a grade 2a lesion according to the modified Noyes and Stabler MRI score as it affects less than 50% of the cartilage layer. The lesions at the central and posterior portion of the lateral femoral condyle would be classified as grade 2b lesions as they affect more than 50% of the cartilage layer

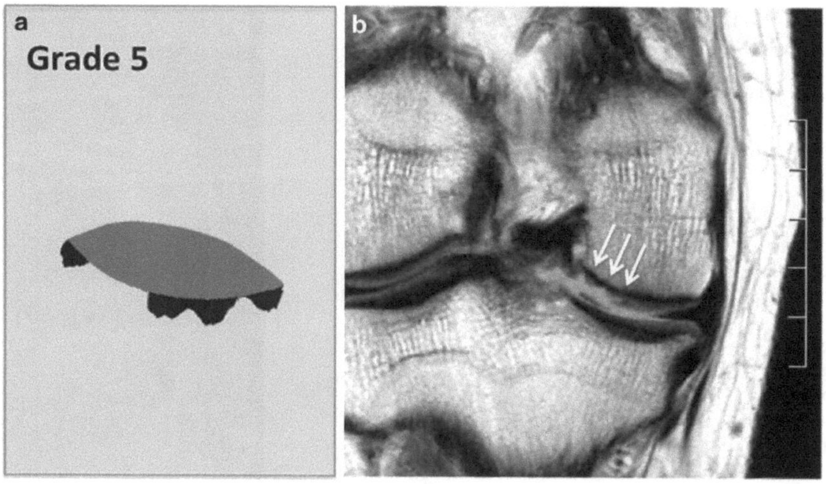

Fig. 9.12 *Whole-Organ-MRI-Score (WORMS) grade 5.* Graph of grade 5 knee cartilage lesion (**a**) and coronal proton density weighted fast spin echo sequence of the knee (**b**) showing a cartilage WORMS grade 5 lesion at the medial femoral condyle. The focal lesion measures more than 1 cm and extends to the subchondral bone (full thickness) (*arrows*). The lesion would be classified as a grade 3a lesion according to the modified Noyes and Stabler MRI score as it affects the entire cartilage layer and does not demonstrate subchondral bone changes

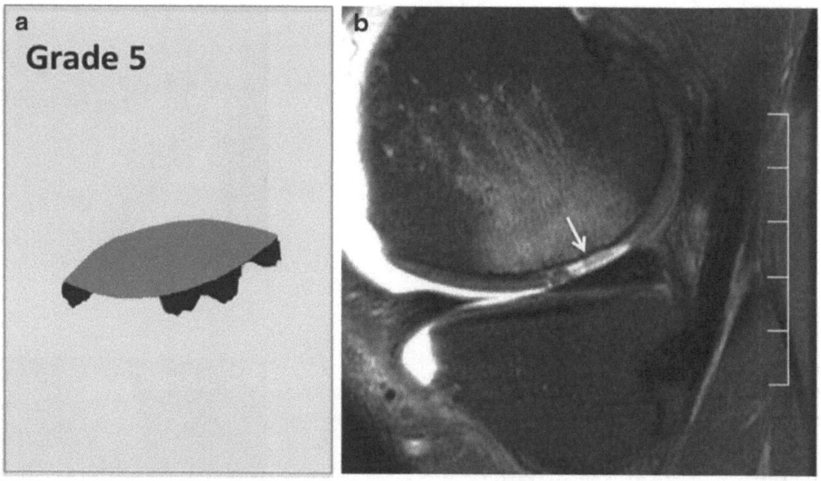

Fig. 9.13 *Whole-Organ-MRI-Score (WORMS) grade 5.* Graph of grade 5 knee cartilage lesion (**a**) and sagittal fat saturated intermediate weighted fast spin echo sequence of the knee (**b**) showing a cartilage WORMS grade 5 lesion at the posterior weight-bearing portion of the medial femoral condyle. The full-thickness lesion measures more than 1 cm (*arrows*) but affects less than 75% of the central portion of the medial femoral condyle. This lesion would be classified as a grade 3b lesion according to the modified Noyes and Stabler MRI score as it affects the entire cartilage layer and is associated with subchondral bone marrow edema pattern

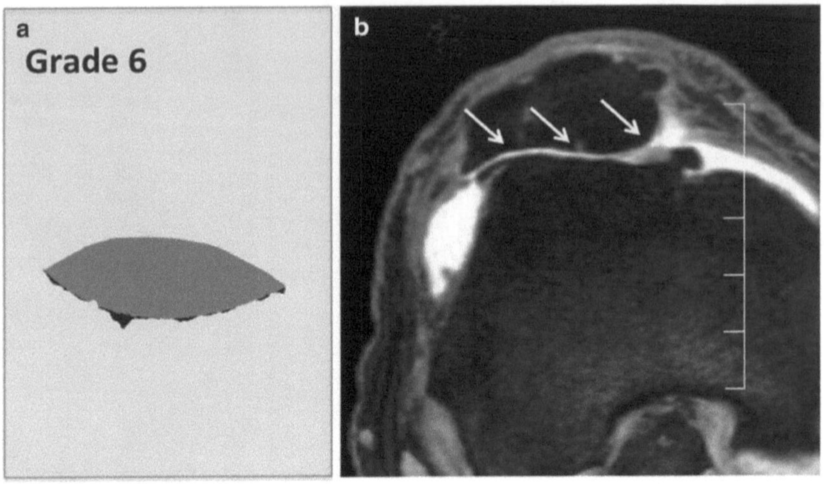

Fig. 9.14 *Whole-Organ-MRI-Score (WORMS) grade 6*. Graph of grade 6 knee cartilage lesion (**a**) and axial reconstruction of a fat saturated dual echo steady state (DESS) sequence of the knee (**b**) showing a cartilage WORMS grade 6 lesion at the patella (*arrows*) and trochlea. The patella full-thickness lesion affects the entire patellar joint surface, and the trochlea lesion affects more than 75% of the joint surface. The lesions would be classified as grade 3 lesions according to the modified Noyes and Stabler MRI score; grade 3b at the patella given subchondral cystic change

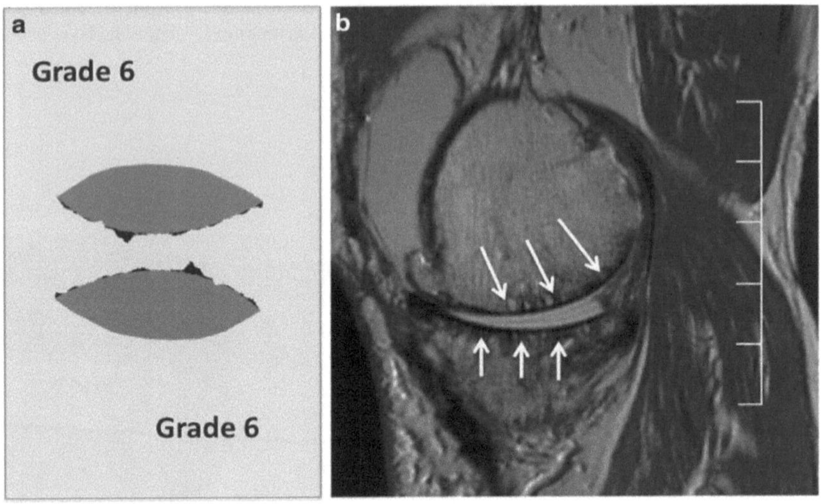

Fig. 9.15 *Whole-Organ-MRI-Score (WORMS) grade 6*. Graph of grade 6 knee cartilage lesions (**a**) and sagittal proton density fast spin echo sequence of the knee (**b**) showing cartilage WORMS grade 6 lesions at the medial femoral condyle and tibia (*arrows*). The full-thickness lesions affect more than 75% of the joint surfaces. Also note subchondral bone marrow edema pattern and cystic changes. In addition, large osteophytes are demonstrated

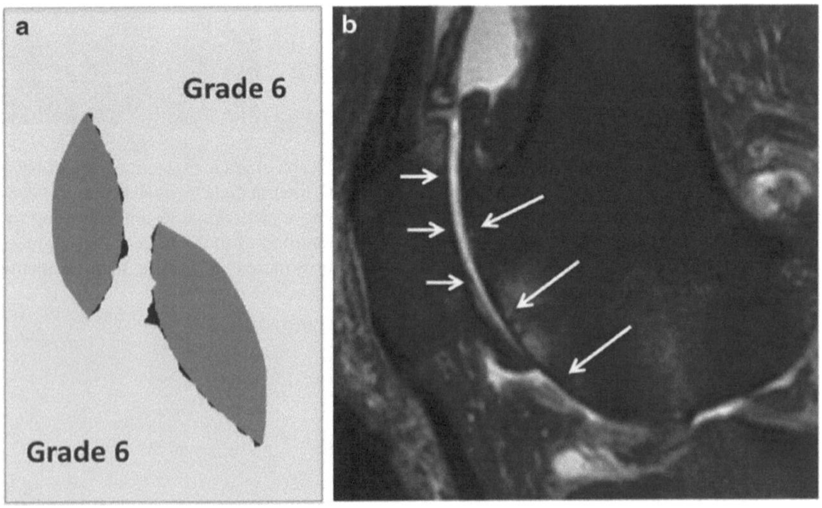

Fig. 9.16 *Whole-Organ-MRI-Score (WORMS) grade 6*. Graph of grade 6 knee cartilage lesions (**a**) and sagittal fat saturated intermediate weighted fast spin echo sequence of the knee (**b**) showing cartilage WORMS grade 6 lesions at the trochlea and patella (*arrows*). The full-thickness lesions affect more than 75% of the joint surfaces. The lesions would be classified as grade 3b lesions according to the modified Noyes and Stabler MRI score as they affect the entire cartilage layer and are associated with subchondral bone marrow edema pattern and cystic changes (trochlea). In addition, large osteophytes are demonstrated

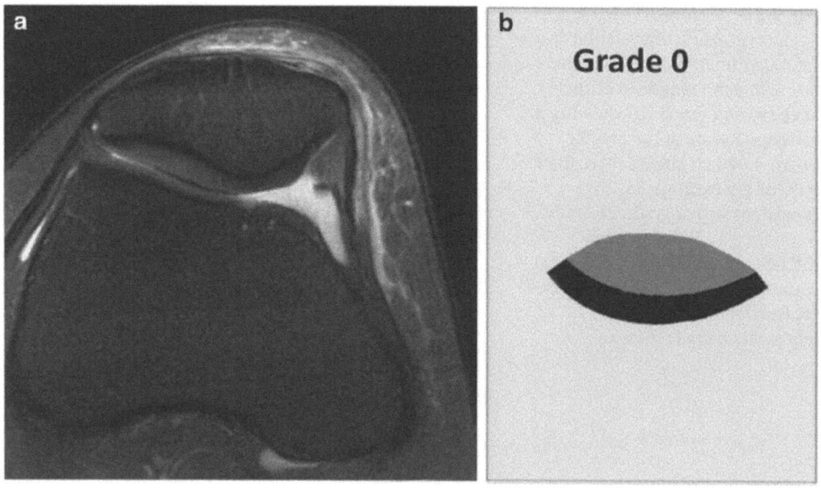

Fig. 9.17 *Modified Noyes and Stabler grade 0.* Axial fat saturated intermediate weighted fast spin echo sequence of the knee (**a**) and graph (**b**) showing healthy cartilage at the patella and trochlea. Both signal and thickness of the cartilage are normal

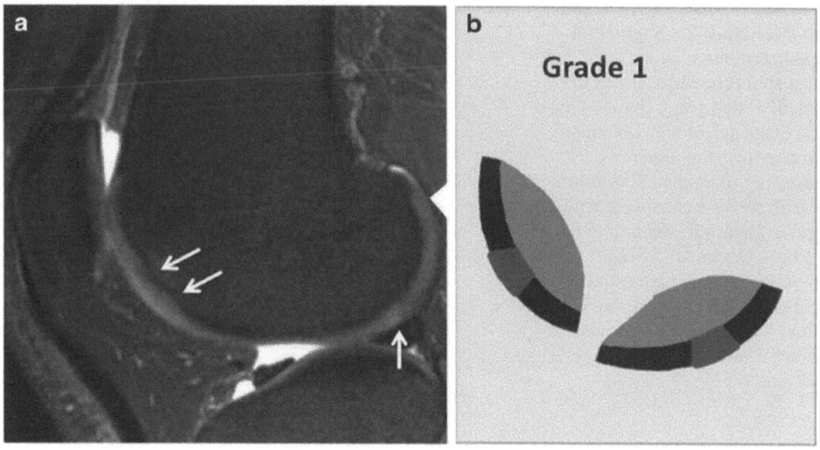

Fig. 9.18 *Modified Noyes and Stabler grade 1.* Sagittal fat saturated intermediate weighted fast spin echo sequence of the knee (**a**) and graph (**b**) showing cartilage signal inhomogeneity and swelling at the trochlea and at the posterior weight-bearing portion of the lateral femoral condyle (*arrows*) consistent with grade 1 lesions. According to Whole-Organ-MRI-Score (WORMS), these lesions would be classified as grade 1

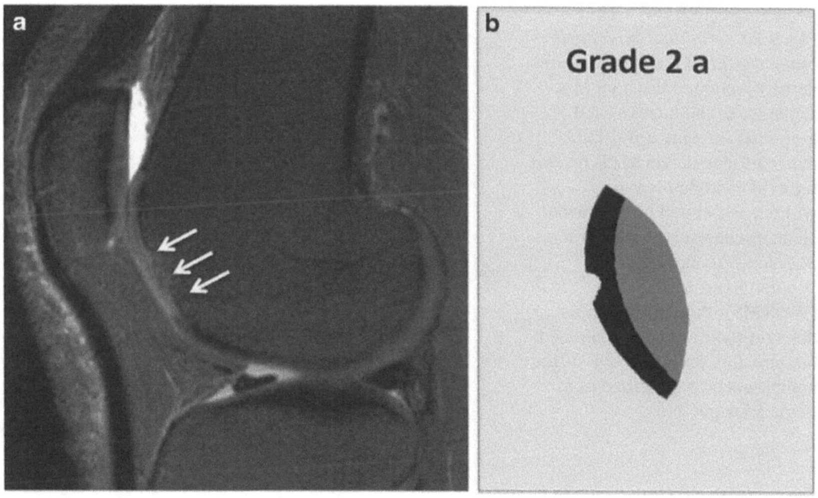

Fig. 9.19 *Modified Noyes and Stabler grade 2a.* Sagittal fat saturated intermediate weighted fast spin echo sequence of the knee (**a**) and graph (**b**) showing a cartilage defect at the trochlea (*arrows*), which affects less than 50% of the cartilage layer consistent with a grade 2a lesion. This lesion would be classified as grade 3 according to Whole-Organ-MRI-Score (WORMS) showing a partial-thickness cartilage defect greater than 1 cm in width but affecting less than 75% of the compartment

Fig. 9.20 *Modified Noyes and Stabler grade 2b.* Sagittal fat saturated intermediate weighted fast spin echo sequence of the knee (**a**) and graph (**b**) showing a cartilage fissure at the patella (*arrow*), which affects more than 50% of the cartilage layer consistent with a grade 2b lesion. According to Whole-Organ-MRI-Score (WORMS), this focal partial-thickness cartilage defect measuring less than 1 cm represents a grade 2 lesion

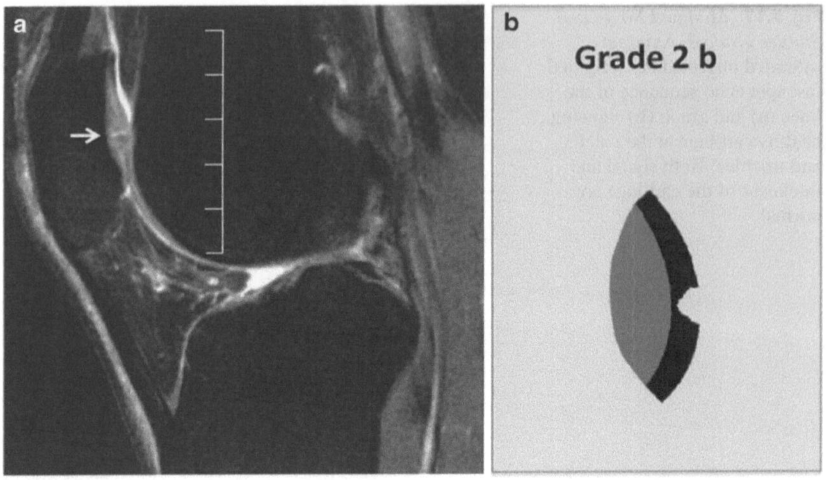

Fig. 9.21 *Modified Noyes and Stabler grade 2b.* Sagittal fat saturated intermediate weighted fast spin echo sequence of the knee (**a**) and graph (**b**) showing a cartilage defect with delamination at the patella (*arrow*) affecting more than 50% of the cartilage layer consistent with a grade 2b lesion. According to Whole-Organ-MRI-Score (WORMS), this partial-thickness cartilage defect measuring more than 1 cm in width represents a grade 3 lesion

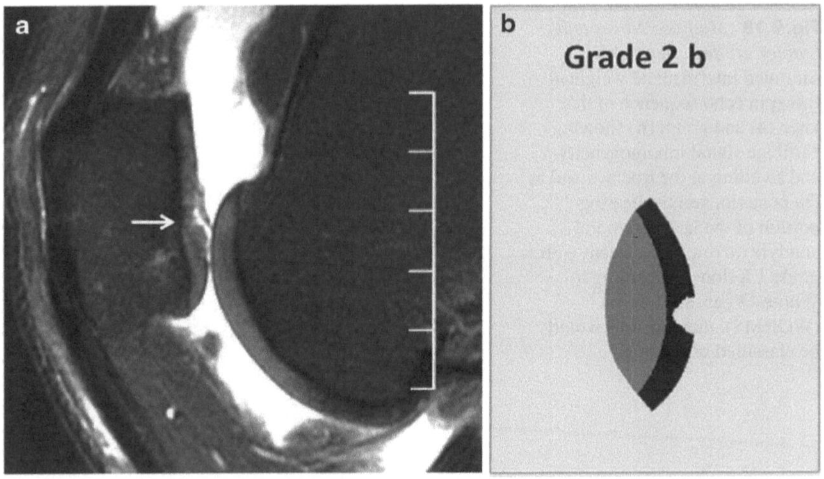

Fig. 9.22 *Modified Noyes and Stabler grade 3a.* Coronal proton density weighted fast spin echo sequence of the knee (**a**) and graph (**b**) showing a full-thickness cartilage defect at the medial femoral condyle (*arrows*) without associated bone marrow changes consistent with a grade 3a lesion. According to Whole-Organ-MRI-Score (WORMS), this full-thickness defect measuring more than 1 cm but affecting less than 75% of the compartment is classified as a grade 5 lesion

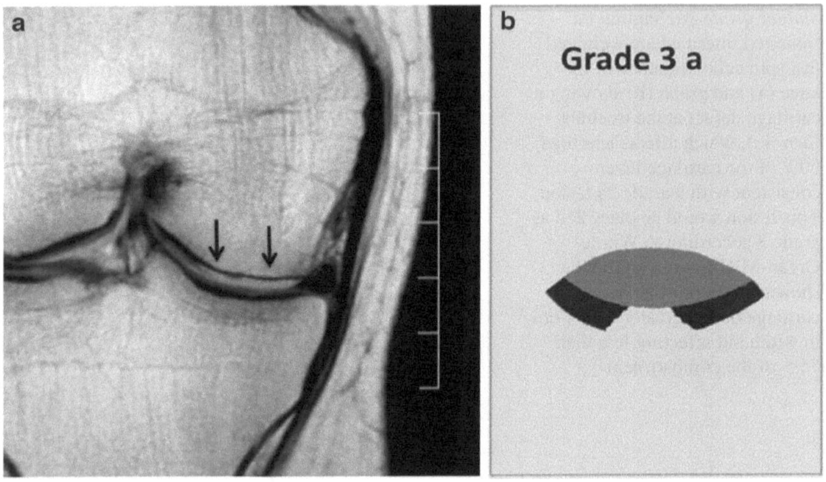

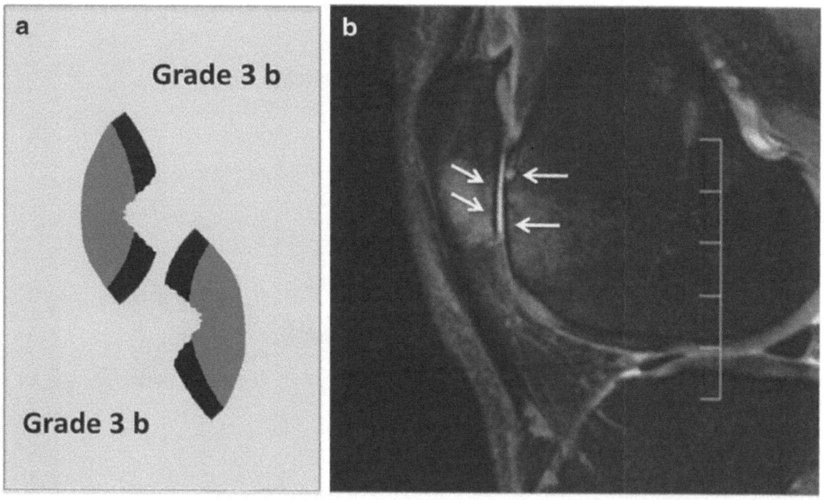

Fig. 9.23 *Modified Noyes and Stabler grade 3b*. Sagittal fat saturated intermediate weighted fast spin echo sequence of the knee (**a**) and graph (**b**) showing a full-thickness cartilage defect at the patella and trochlea (*arrows*) with associated bone marrow changes consistent with a grade 3b lesion. Small subchondral cyst at the trochlea and large osteophyte at the superior patellar joint surface. Both patella and trochlea show full-thickness cartilage defects with more than 75% of the compartments affected representing grade 6 lesions according to Whole-Organ-MRI-Score (WORMS)

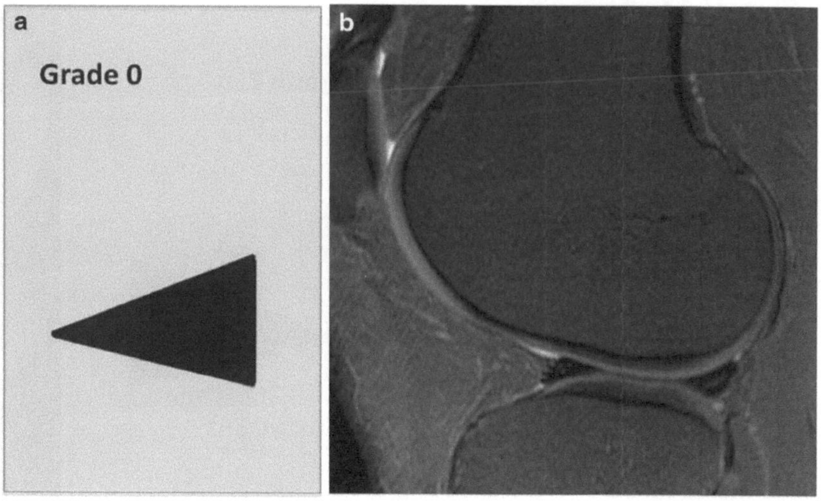

Fig. 9.24 *Normal meniscus, Whole-Organ-MRI-Score (WORMS) grade 0*. Graph (**a**) and sagittal fat saturated intermediate weighted fast spin echo sequence of the knee (**b**) showing normal anterior and posterior horn of the lateral meniscus with no tears and normal shape. Subtle focal increase in signal at the posterior horn suggests vessels in the *red zone*

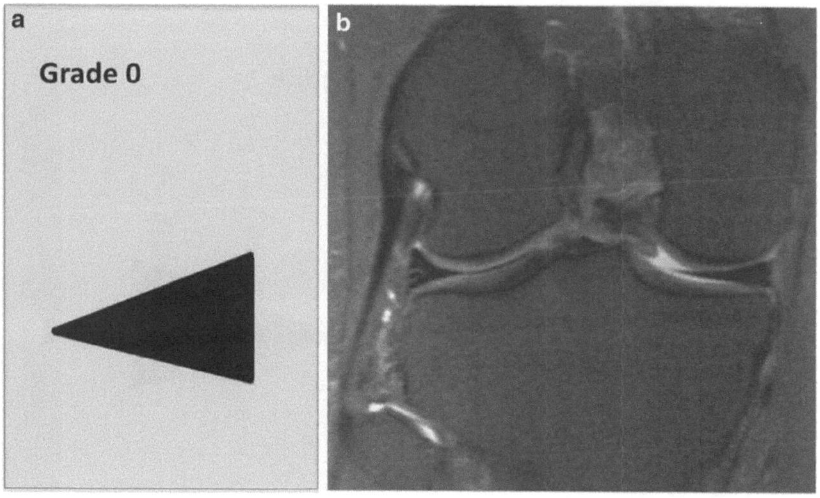

Fig. 9.25 *Normal meniscus, Whole-Organ-MRI-Score (WORMS) grade 0*. Graph (**a**) and coronal fat saturated intermediate weighted fast spin echo sequence of the knee (**b**) showing normal meniscal bodies with no tears and normal shape. Linear focal increases in signal at the lateral meniscus body are consistent with vessels in the *red zone*

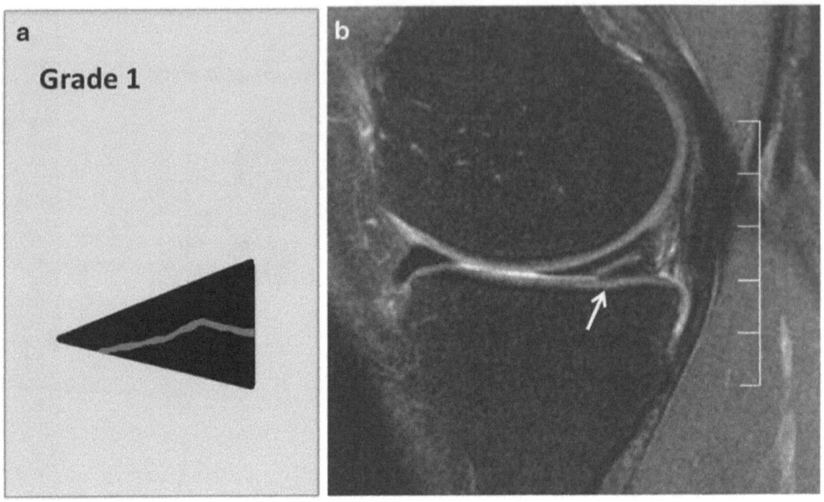

Fig. 9.26 Normal meniscus, *Whole-Organ-MRI-Score (WORMS) grade 1*. Graph (**a**) and sagittal fat saturated intermediate weighted fast spin echo sequence of the knee (**b**) showing a longitudinal/oblique, nondisplaced tear of the posterior horn of the medial meniscus that was classified as a grade 1 tear (*arrow*), according to a previously published, modified WORMS classification [6, 7]

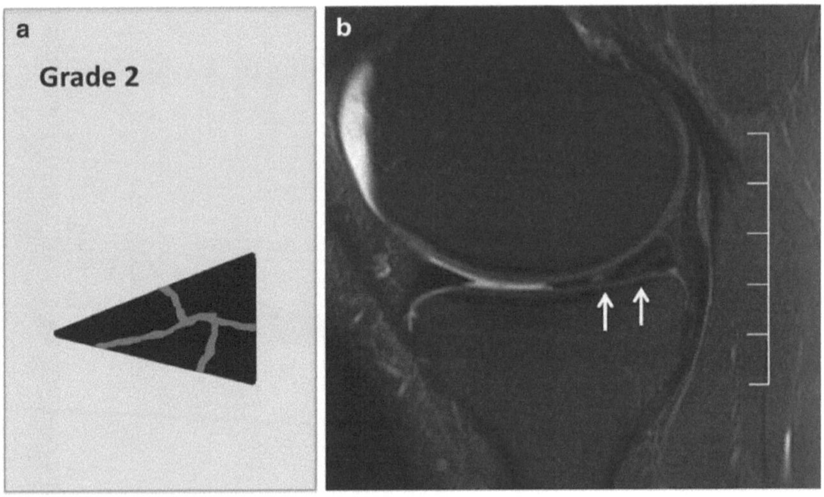

Fig. 9.27 *Meniscus with complex tear without deformity, Whole-Organ-MRI-Score (WORMS) grade 2*. Graph (**a**) and sagittal fat saturated intermediate weighted fast spin echo sequence of the knee (**b**) showing a complex, nondisplaced tear of the posterior horn of the medial meniscus that was classified as a grade 2 tear (*arrows*)

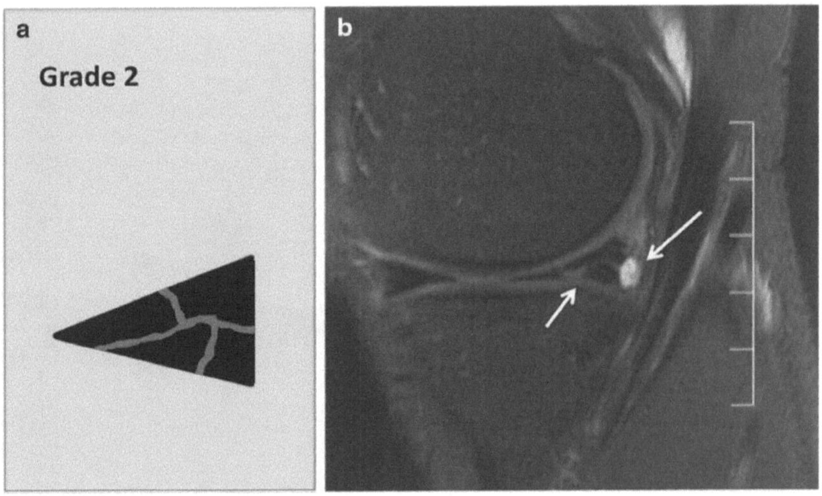

Fig. 9.28 *Meniscus with complex tear without deformity, Whole-Organ-MRI-Score (WORMS) grade 2*. Graph (**a**) and sagittal fat saturated intermediate weighted fast spin echo sequence of the knee (**b**) showing a complex, nondisplaced tear of the posterior horn of the medial meniscus that was classified as a grade 2 tear (*short arrow*). In addition, a parameniscal cyst is demonstrated posterior to the meniscus in direct contact with the meniscal tear (*long arrow*)

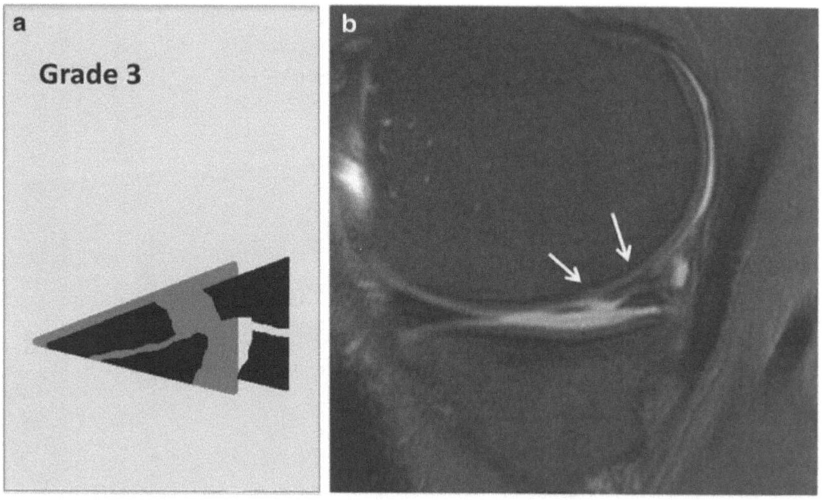

Fig. 9.29 *Meniscus with complex tear and deformity, Whole-Organ-MRI-Score (WORMS) grade 3*. Graph (**a**) and sagittal fat saturated intermediate weighted fast spin echo sequence of the knee (**b**) showing a complex tear of the posterior horn of the medial meniscus with deformity that was classified as a grade 3 tear (*arrows*)

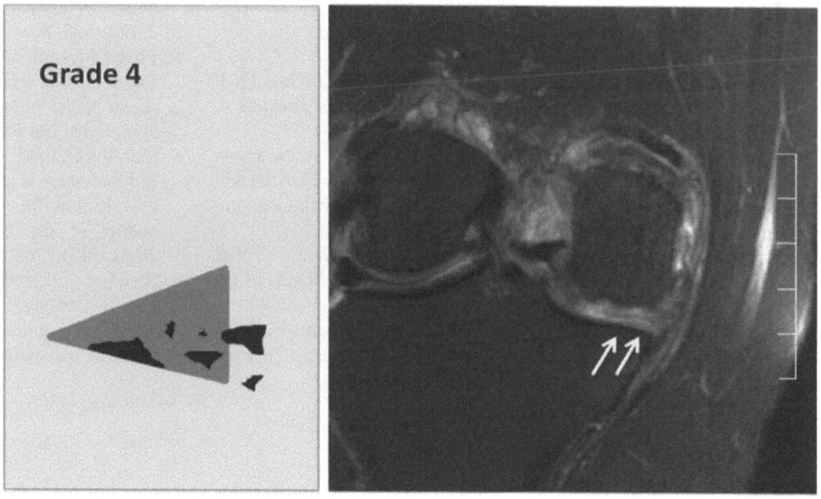

Fig. 9.30 *Meniscus with severe tear and maceration, Whole-Organ-MRI-Score (WORMS) grade 4*. Graph (**a**) and coronal fat saturated intermediate weighted fast spin echo sequence of the knee (**b**) showing maceration of the body of the medial meniscus, which is nearly completely destroyed (*arrows*). There is also extensive cartilage destruction at the medial femoral condyle and cartilage thinning at the tibia

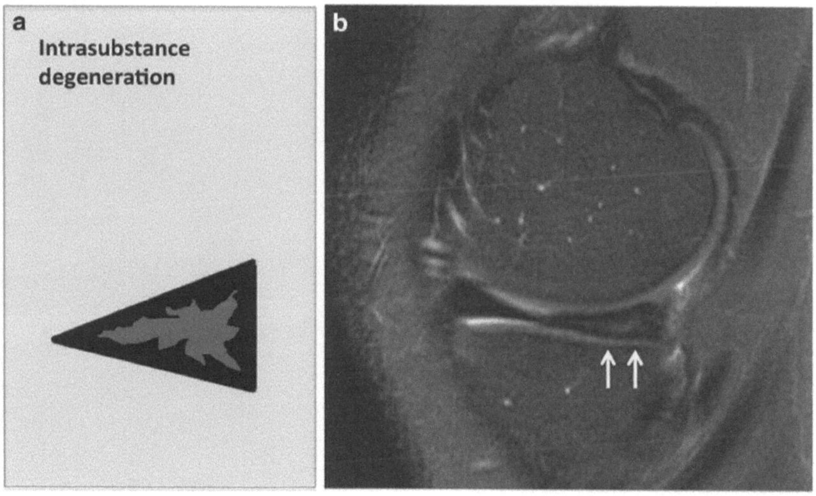

Fig. 9.31 *Meniscus with intrasubstance degeneration*. Graph (**a**) and sagittal fat saturated intermediate weighted fast spin echo sequence of the knee (**b**) showing increased signal of the posterior horn of the medial meniscus (*arrows*) without a tear extending to the meniscal surface consistent with intrasubstance degeneration. Intrasubstance degeneration was not listed in the Whole-Organ-MRI-Score (WORMS) classification, but was part of recently published modified WORMS classification [6, 7]

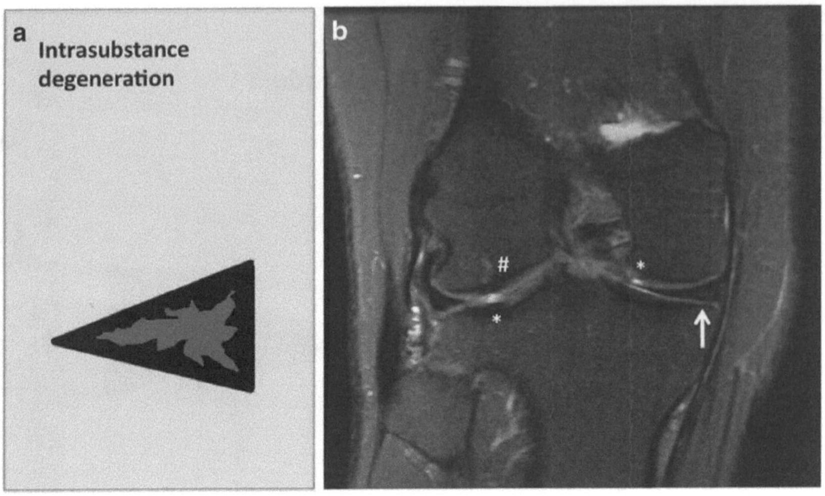

Fig. 9.32 *Meniscus with intrasubstance degeneration.* Graph (**a**) and coronal fat saturated intermediate weighted fast spin echo sequence of the knee (**b**) showing increased signal of the body of the medial meniscus (*arrow*) without a tear extending the meniscal surface consistent with intrasubstance degeneration. In addition, subtle cartilage defects are noted at the medial femoral condyle (mesial aspect) and the lateral tibia (*) as well as signal abnormality at the lateral femoral condyle with underlying bone marrow edema pattern (#)

References

1. Recht M, Kramer J, Marcelis S, Pathria M, Trudell D, Haghigi P, et al. Abnormalities of articular cartilage in the knee: analysis of available MR techniques. Radiology. 1993;187:473–8.
2. Recht M, Piraino D, Paletta G, Schils J, Belhobek G. Accuracy of fat-suppressed three-dimensional spoiled gradient-echo FLASH MR Imaging in the detection of patellofemoral articular cartilage abnormalities. Radiology. 1996;198:209–12.
3. Peterfy CG, Guermazi A, Zaim S, Tirman PF, Miaux Y, White D, et al. Whole-Organ Magnetic Resonance Imaging Score (WORMS) of the knee in osteoarthritis. Osteoarthritis Cartilage. 2004;12(3):177–90.
4. Link TM, Steinbach LS, Ghosh S, Ries M, Lu Y, Lane N, et al. Osteoarthritis: MR imaging findings in different stages of disease and correlation with clinical findings. Radiology. 2003; 226(2):373–81.
5. Phan CM, Link TM, Blumenkrantz G, Dunn TC, Ries MD, Steinbach LS, et al. MR imaging findings in the follow-up of patients with different stages of knee osteoarthritis and the correlation with clinical symptoms. Eur Radiol. 2006;16:608–18.
6. Stehling C, Lane NE, Nevitt MC, Lynch J, McCulloch CE, Link TM. Subjects with higher physical activity levels have more severe focal knee lesions diagnosed with 3T MRI: analysis of a non-symptomatic cohort of the osteoarthritis initiative. Osteoarthritis Cartilage. 2010;18(6):776–86.
7. Stehling C, Liebl H, Krug R, Lane NE, Nevitt MC, Lynch J, et al. Patellar cartilage: T2 values and morphologic abnormalities at 3.0-T MR imaging in relation to physical activity in asymptomatic subjects from the osteoarthritis initiative. Radiology. 2010;254(2):509–20.

Chapter 10
Cartilage Segmentation

Julio Carballido-Gamio and Thomas M. Link

Keywords Cartilage morphology • Cartilage segmentation • Pulse sequence • Radiography • Cross-sectional studies • Cartilage volume • Radiography

Magnetic Resonance Imaging for Quantitative Cartilage Morphology

Magnetic Resonance Imaging (MRI) offers unique opportunities for direct visualization and quantification of cartilage morphology. MRI enables three-dimensional (3D) acquisitions with contiguous slices, an essential feature for 3D quantification, resulting in improved accuracy and precision of morphological metrics. MRI has unique tomographic capabilities, excellent soft tissue contrast, high signal to noise ratio (SNR), and high-spatial resolution making it the imaging modality of choice to quantify cartilage morphology in vivo. However, the anatomic location of articular cartilage, small size, special geometry, and short transverse relaxation time (T_2) represent also a challenge for MRI.

Pulse Sequence Requirements

A pulse sequence suitable for cartilage imaging has to comply at least with the following requirements. It has to have high SNR, high contrast to noise ratio (CNR), high-spatial resolution, should be fast, and should minimize image distortions. Compliance with these requirements translates into easier cartilage segmentations that also require less user interaction, yielding more accurate and precise measurements. Unfortunately, there is interdependency among these MRI parameters, so improvement of one factor results in detrimental of another.

High SNR means that the cartilage signal should be considerably higher than that of the background noise. High CNR is needed so cartilage is easily distinguished from other tissues. High SNR together with high CNR facilitate the delineation of cartilage boundaries during segmentation. Usage of high field magnets (≥1.0 T) as well as dedicated knee coils or surface coils for the special case of hip cartilage are essential to acquire images with high SNR and CNR. Further increase in SNR and CNR is accomplished by eliminating fat signal from surrounding bone structures. This is usually accomplished with frequency-selective spectral fat suppression by a prepulse or with frequency-selective water excitation techniques, increasing the cartilage intensity dynamic range. Elimination of the fat signal also helps to minimize image distortions due to the different magnetic susceptibilities of fat and cartilage, as well as to minimize the chemical shift artifact.

The average cartilage thickness in healthy human knees is in the order of 1.3–2.5 mm, and in a recent 3.0 T study of the hip, a mean composite value of 3.1 mm was reported for healthy human subjects that included both the acetabular and proximal femoral cartilage [1]. A pulse sequence designed for cartilage quantification must therefore have high-spatial resolution. This requirement is even more important when dealing with cartilage of osteoarthritis (OA) patients, so thin sections can be reliably segmented and quantified. In fact, some studies have demonstrated that is more important to have high-spatial resolution at the expense of lower SNR to improve the detection of cartilage lesions [2, 3]. The usage of high field magnets and dedicated coils also contribute to fulfill this requirement. In-plane spatial resolutions of ≤0.3 mm and slice thickness of 1.5 and 1 mm are common for knee cartilage acquisitions at 1.5 and 3.0 T, respectively. In-plane spatial resolution of 0.312 mm × 0.312 mm and slice thickness of 1.5 mm were recently reported in a feasibility and reproducibility study of hip cartilage at 3.0 T [1].

Involuntary as well as voluntary patient motion during and between acquisitions is common in MRI. Even small motion can result in substantial data contamination because

J. Carballido-Gamio (✉)
Grupo Tecnológico Santa Fe, S.A. de C.V., Mexico City, Mexico
and
Department of Radiology and Biomedical Imaging,
University of California at San Francisco, 400 Parnassus Avenue, A-367, San Francisco, CA 94131, USA
e-mail: JCarballido@gtsf.com.mx

T.M. Link (ed.), *Cartilage Imaging: Significance, Techniques, and New Developments*,
DOI 10.1007/978-1-4419-8438-8_10, © Springer Science+Business Media, LLC 2011

of the small cartilage dimensions and complex geometry. Although proper patient immobilization certainly reduces patient motion, pulse sequences that are fast are desirable. This requirement has recently received more attention due to intense research in the field of parallel imaging, which is a special acquisition technique that takes into account the sensitivity of receiver coils to reduce imaging acquisition times [4]. Since cartilage T_2 relaxation time is short, pulse sequences with short echo time (TE) are also needed to acquire signal soon after proton excitation.

Current and Emerging Pulse Sequences for Cartilage Morphology

Fast low angle shot (FLASH), also known as spoiled gradient recalled acquisition at steady state (SPGR), is a T_1-weighted spoiled gradient echo sequence that fulfills most of the above mentioned requirements, and since it is widely available in clinical scanners, it has become the pulse sequence of choice for most research groups in the field of MRI and OA. Fat suppression or water excitation is commonly performed with this sequence to avoid signal from fat, so bone displays background signal, while cartilage and joint fluid show bright and low signal, respectively. Figure 10.1a, b shows sagittal and axial fat-suppressed SPGR images of the knee joint, respectively.

Imaging of hip cartilage morphology using water excitation SPGR was also recently reported at 3.0 T displaying similar tissue contrast as for the knee [1]. Figure 10.2 shows a sagittal acquisition of the hip joint at 3.0 T.

The relatively long acquisition times, but especially the low tissue contrast between cartilage and fluid, led to the proposal of alternative pulse sequences for cartilage morphology such as DEFT (driven equilibrium Fourier transform). DEFT enhances signal from fluid rather than attenuating that of the cartilage and provides contrast dependent on the ratio of the longitudinal and transverse relaxation times of a given tissue. DESS-WE (double echo-steady state with water excitation) provides high fluid-to-cartilage contrast such as DEFT and has been suggested to provide higher SNR efficiency than SPGR [5]. This imaging technique was selected for the Osteoarthritis Initiative (OAI), a multicenter, longitudinal, prospective observational study of knee OA designed to develop a public domain research resource to facilitate the scientific evaluation of biomarkers for OA as potential surrogate endpoints for disease onset and progression. Figure 10.3 shows a sagittal DESS-WE image and a coronal FLASH-WE image of the knee joint from the OAI.

Iterative decomposition of water and fat with echo asymmetry and least squares estimation, better known as IDEAL, has been combined with bSSFP (balanced steady-state free precession) yielding a pulse sequence relatively insensitive to field variations, showing superior SNR, fast acquisition times, and contrast similar to DEFT, thus becoming a strong candidate for quantitative morphological imaging of cartilage.

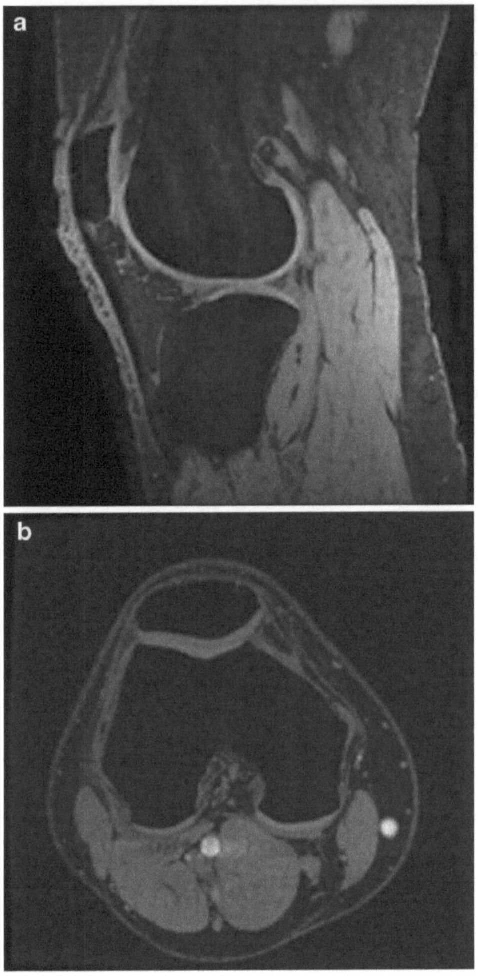

Fig. 10.1 Sagittal (**a**) and axial (**b**) fat-suppressed SPGR images of the knee joint at 3.0 T with in-plane spatial resolution of 0.312 mm × 0.312 mm and slice thickness of 1.0 mm

Cartilage Quantification

The emphasis given in the previous section with respect to the pulse sequence requirements for cartilage imaging will become more apparent in this and the following section. In the field of quantitative MRI, having an image of good quality that unambiguously displays the tissues and/or pathology in question is only the first step. Quantitative information has to be extracted from the images accurately and precisely.

Cartilage morphology using MRI is quantified with different metrics, the most common being its thickness and volume, since cartilage thinning and loss are common pathophysiological elements of OA. However, before any morphological measurement can be performed, cartilage must be isolated from the rest of the image, a process called image segmentation.

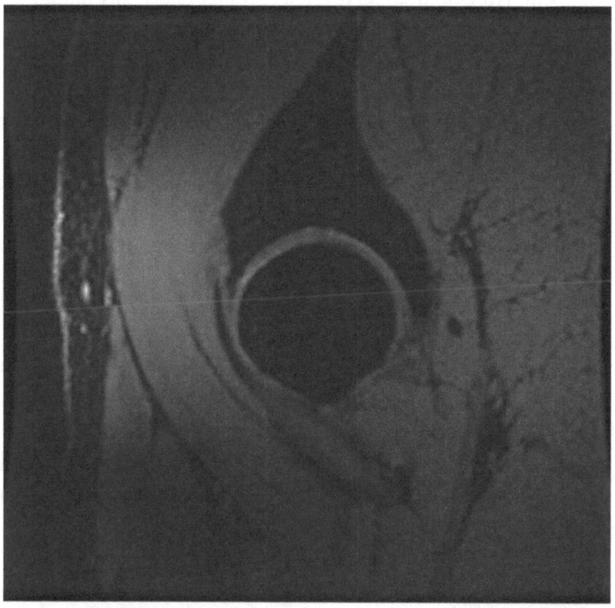

Fig. 10.2 Sagittal water excitation of the hip joint at 3.0 T with in-plane spatial resolution of 0.312 mm × 0.312 mm and slice thickness of 1.5 mm

Cartilage Segmentation

Cartilage segmentation, and consequently morphological quantification, is usually performed using FLASH/SPGR images. Although these images are in general of high SNR and CNR, cartilage segmentation is not easy. Sections such as the patello-femoral articulation, tibio-femoral articulation, as well as the posterior part of the femoral condyles represent a challenge even to the trained human eye. This challenge increases when segmentation involves cartilage of OA patients, since there are signal changes, cartilage surface fibrillation, tissue thinning, appearance of repair tissue, and osteophytes.

Cartilage segmentation is most of the times performed manually by delineating its boundaries. This is consequently a time consuming process. An MRI scan of the knee with slice thickness of 1 mm usually involves the segmentation of about 60 slices for the femoral compartment only. Together, tibial, femoral, and patellar cartilage segmentation could take up to several hours to complete. Up to date, there is no fully automatic cartilage segmentation technique published in the scientific literature that works well for patients with knee OA. However, scientific literature is vast with respect to semiautomatic cartilage segmentation techniques. The main goals of these techniques have been to reduce user interaction while preserving accuracy and precision. It is important to note that whenever a new segmentation technique is developed, its accuracy as well as precision must be measured. These evaluations should be done matching in vivo conditions as close as possible because some image artifacts are only present when the actual tissue is placed in the magnetic field. This is the main reason why amputated and cadaveric joints present unique opportunities to validate new techniques, since cartilage volume or thickness can be measured after scrapping, using direct or indirect methods such as stereophotogrammetry and water displacement techniques.

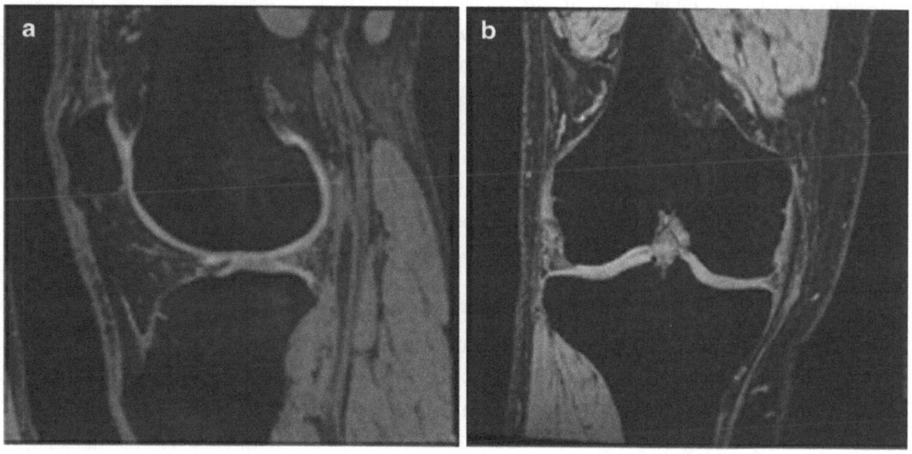

Fig. 10.3 MR images of the knee joint at 3.0 T for cartilage morphological quantification in the OAI. (**a**) DESS-WE in the sagittal orientation with in-plane spatial resolution of 0.365 mm × 0.365 mm and slice thickness of 0.7 mm. (**b**) FLASH-WE in the coronal orientation with in-plane spatial resolution of 0.312 mm × 0.312 mm and slice thickness of 1.5 mm

Most of the current knee cartilage semiautomatic segmentation techniques operate on a slice-by-slice basis relying on edge information. Some of them, prior to cartilage segmentation, also perform image enhancement techniques such as anisotropic diffusion [6] or median filtering to smooth pixel intensities inside regions but not across regions or eliminate texture, respectively. It is also common to use the segmentation of a given slice as the initialization of the contiguous one.

Stammberger and colleagues [7] implemented a quadratic B-spline snake. A B-spline of order k is a continuous and smooth parametric curve that depends only on a number of control points $\bar{v}_1,\ldots,\bar{v}_N \in R2$ and is defined as:

$$\bar{x}(u) = \sum_{i=1}^{N} \bar{v}_i B_i(u) \tag{10.1}$$

where $B_i(u)$ are the polynomial basis functions, u is the curve parameter, and $\bar{x}(u) = (x(u), y(u))^T$ is a point in the 2D image. Three energy terms guide the deformation of the B-spline to fit the cartilage boundaries. An internal energy term controls the rigidity of the contour; an external energy term attracts the contour to the cartilage edges; and a coupling force enforces smooth changes from one slice to another. A scale-space approach was also implemented, going from a coarse to a fine scale. In another 2D segmentation approach, Lynch and colleagues [8] developed a hybrid segmentation method combining expert knowledge with directionally oriented Canny filters, cost functions, and cubic splines, reporting better reproducibility than conventionally used region-growing techniques as well as less user interaction.

Three-dimensional approaches for cartilage segmentation have also been explored. Grau and colleagues [9] proposed an improvement to the watershed transform. The idea behind the watershed transform is that any gray-level image can be considered as a topographic surface. Flooding this surface from its minima, and preventing the merging of water coming from different sources, partitions the image into catchment basins and watershed lines. By using markers, sensitivity to noise and over-segmentation are reduced. The watershed transform is usually applied to the gradient image, however, in the work of Grau and colleagues [9] the watershed was extended to examining difference in class probability of neighboring pixels, further alleviating some of the drawbacks of the watershed transform in medical images: over-segmentation, sensitivity to noise, and poor detection of thin and low SNR structures. Another 3D segmentation approach was proposed by Pakin and colleagues [10] based on a region-growing technique. Regions were labeled as cartilage or noncartilage using a voting procedure depending on local two-class clustering and making use of prior knowledge about cartilage regions.

A more sophisticated segmentation approach was proposed by Warfield and colleagues: adaptive, template moderated, spatially varying statistical classification [11]. The algorithm is a form of spatially varying statistical classification. An explicit template is used to moderate the segmentation obtained by statistical classification. A user performs interactive registration of a knee template to a test scan, and the technique then iterates between a classification step and a template registration step yielding an adaptive, template moderated, spatially varying statistical classification.

Currently, there is no consensus with respect to which orientation is best for knee cartilage segmentation: sagittal, coronal, or axial. Since sagittal acquisitions display both, the femoro-tibial and patello-femoral articulations, they have become the most commonly used for knee OA. However, it has also been suggested that coronal images are better for segmenting cartilage of the femoro-tibial articulation because partial volume effects are minimized in that region [12]. It is also well known that axial acquisitions are optimal for patellar cartilage analysis. Figure 10.4 shows a representative segmentation of knee cartilage segmentation on a sagittal fat-suppressed SPGR image.

In terms of hip cartilage, most of the above segmentation approaches should yield similar performance as for the knee cartilage after some adjustments, since FLASH/SPGR magnetic resonance images of hip cartilage display similar tissue contrast (Fig. 10.2). Carballido-Gamio and colleagues [1] used a segmentation approach based on edge detection and Bezier splines in combination with image enhancement techniques such as anisotropic diffusion filtering, median filtering, and power law transformations. The main difficulty with hip cartilage is, however, the distinction between femoral and acetabular cartilage, which is the main reason why hip cartilage has been segmented as a composite entity [1, 13]. In terms of image orientation, initial work at 1.5 T was done in coronal images using a leg traction device during image acquisition to evaluate femoral and acetabular cartilage individually [14, 15].

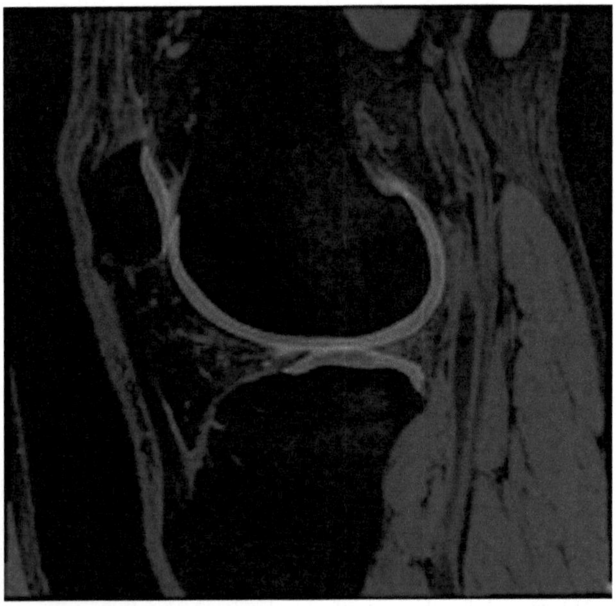

Fig. 10.4 Patellar, femoral, and tibial cartilage segmentation of the knee joint on a fat-suppressed SPGR image

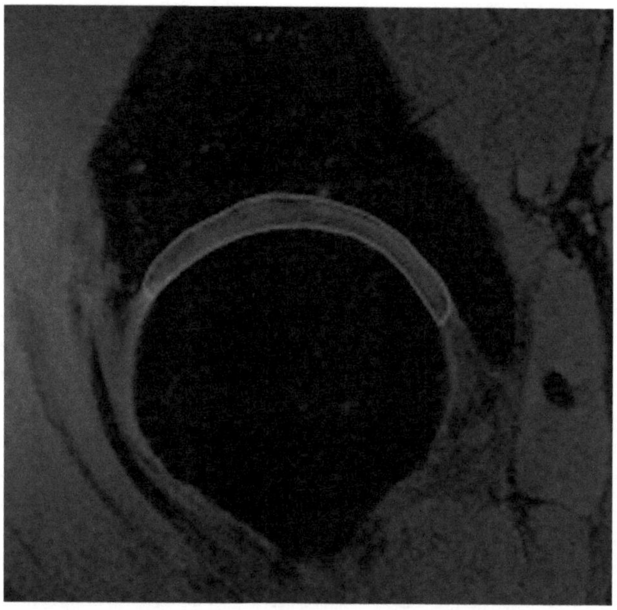

Fig. 10.5 Femoral and acetabular cartilage segmentation are segmented as a single unit on a sagittal water excitation SPGR image

However, later Nishii and colleagues [16] demonstrated that cartilage imaging of the hip joint in the sagittal plane allowed detailed assessment of early cartilage abnormalities. Figure 10.5 shows a representative hip cartilage segmentation on a sagittal water excitation SPGR image, where femoral and acetabular cartilage are segmented as a single unit.

A recent increasing interest in local analysis of cartilage morphological properties has resulted in the development of image processing methods that further subdivide commonly used compartments (medial femoral, lateral femoral, medial tibia plateau, lateral tibia plateau, and patella) into smaller units. In the work of Wirth and Eckstein [17], the tibial plateau was divided into a central area of the total subchondral bone area and anterior, posterior, internal, and external subregions surrounding it. In the weight-bearing femoral condyles, central, internal, and external subregions were determined. Similar weight-bearing regions were previously reported in the scientific literature [18, 19]. In the work of Stahl and colleagues [19], femoral weight-bearing regions were defined based on the local angles of the intersection of inner normal vectors of the bone–cartilage interface with the long axis of the shaft of the femur. Sections with absolute angles of $\leq 30°$ were considered weight bearing, while the rest of cartilage was labeled as nonweight bearing. Going one step farther, Carballido-Gamio and colleagues developed a technique based on the registration of bone shapes that allows point-to-point or regional comparisons of cartilage morphological and relaxation time properties at different time points for intrasubject (longitudinal) or intersubject studies (cross-sectional) [20, 21].

Cartilage Volume

Cartilage volume (units of volume) is perhaps the easiest to compute morphological measure of cartilage. The most straightforward approach consists in summing the number of voxels representing cartilage and then scaling by the corresponding spatial resolution. However, cartilage volume scales with bone size, so it has been suggested that cartilage volume normalized by the total subchondral bone area (units of mm) should also be reported. This normalized metric has shown to perform better than cartilage volume in differentiating subjects with and without OA [22, 23]. Some authors have also reported the cartilage volume normalized by the epicondylar distance (units of area) [24].

Due to the SNR and high-spatial resolution trade-off in MRI mentioned at the beginning of this chapter, researchers havc preferred improving the in-plane spatial resolution at the expense of thicker slices yielding anisotropic voxels. This represents a limitation when true 3D morphological analysis is required, where isotropic voxels are preferred. Although not equivalent to acquiring images with isotropic voxels, interpolation techniques can be applied to improve the spatial resolution in the slice direction of cartilage acquisitions. The interpolation can be either based on gray-level values or shape. The disadvantage of gray-level interpolation is that since no fully automatic cartilage segmentation techniques are available, the number of slices to be segmented interactively increases dramatically. This is the main reason why shape-based interpolation was proposed by Stammberger and colleagues [25] to obtain cartilage representations with isotropic voxels. Although initially proposed for 3D cartilage thickness calculations, shape-based interpolation to obtain isotropic voxels can also be performed prior to cartilage volume calculations [1, 20]. Shape-based interpolation also reduces the discrepancies between morphological measures obtained from acquisitions with different orientations: sagittal, coronal, and axial. Figure 10.6 shows a 3D representation of knee cartilage plates after shape-based interpolation, where commonly used cartilage compartments have been color encoded.

Clinical Utility of MRI Cartilage Volume

In this section, we will discuss important aspects related to MRI cartilage volume and its potential to be considered as an imaging-based biomarker of knee OA. We will review the concepts of accuracy and precision, including cartilage studies addressing them. We will highlight the superiority of MRI with respect to radiography for morphological quantification of cartilage. Longitudinal and cross-sectional knee OA studies showing the utility of MRI cartilage volume, as well as its potential ability to predict clinical outcome, will also be discussed.

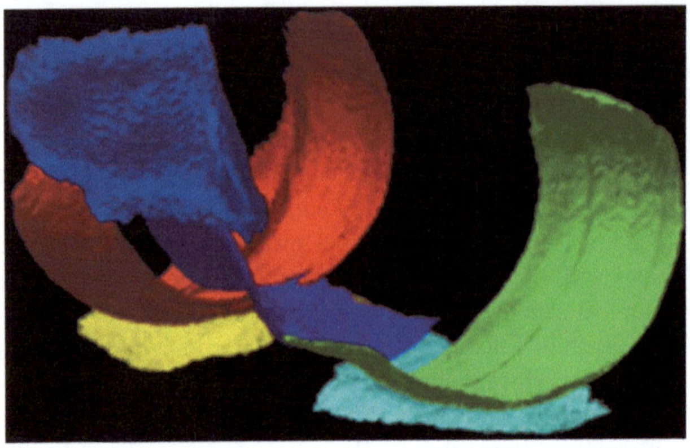

Fig. 10.6 Knee cartilage plates after shape-based interpolation. Commonly used cartilage compartments are color encoded: patella = *blue*; medial femoral compartment = *green*; trochlea = *purple*; lateral femoral compartment = *red*; medial tibial plateau = *cyan*; lateral tibial plateau = *yellow*

MRI Cartilage Volume: Accuracy and Precision

For any given imaging-based parameter to be considered of clinical utility, it should lie directly on the disease pathway and should be measurable with accuracy and precision. Accuracy refers to the degree to which the measurement, e.g., cartilage volume, corresponds to the true value. Precision refers to the ability of reproducing measurements under conditions in which the measured parameter remains constant, and it is usually expressed as a coefficient of variation (CV%), which is the ratio of the standard deviation to the mean of the measurements. However, Glüer et al. [26] proposed reporting the square root of the mean of the variances or the square root of the mean of the squared CV% to give more weight to large precision errors, thus avoiding underestimation of the true precision error in the population. These values can also be expressed in percentages.

Accuracy of knee cartilage volume assessed with MRI has been demonstrated showing correlation values of up to 0.98 with cartilage volume measurements from surgical and postmortem specimens [27–31]. In terms of the precision of magnetic resonance cartilage volume, studies have also demonstrated good coefficients of variation for intraobserver as well as for interobserver variability for healthy subjects and patients with knee OA (~3%) [12]. A multicentre clinical trial of the precision of 3.0 T quantitative MRI of cartilage morphology yielded similar values [32]. For a comprehensive review of precision studies of MRI knee cartilage volume, please refer to the work of Eckstein and colleagues [12]. A recent study of Carballido-Gamio et al. [1] reported a reproducibility of 3.5% for hip cartilage volume (femoral and acetabular as a single unit) also at 3.0 T.

MRI Cartilage Volume and Radiography

The advantage of using MRI compared to radiography for assessing cartilage morphological changes, e.g., volume, has been established. Cicuttini and colleagues [33] examined the relationship between MRI tibial cartilage volume and radiographic grade of OA, which was given by osteophytes and semiquantitative grade of joint space narrowing (JSN). They studied 252 patients with different stages of OA and reported that the inverse relationship between cartilage volume and the grade of JSN was linear. In fact, this inverse relationship was stronger than that between osteophytes and cartilage volume, and when values were adjusted for age, gender, BMI, and bone size, it became even stronger. Jones et al. [34] supported these findings demonstrating that before the first changes of radiographic JSN could be detected, 11–13% of cartilage volume was lost. No association of cartilage volume change with osteophytes was found. Further evidence of the larger sensitivity of cartilage volume than radiographic JSN as a measure of cartilage loss was given by Raynauld et al. [35], reporting significant loss in cartilage volume documented at 6-month intervals for a period of 2 years in patients with OA, despite no correlation seen between cartilage volume loss and radiographic changes.

Longitudinal Studies

Sensitivity to change has been demonstrated even in people without established knee OA [36]. Three studies have reported longitudinal cartilage volume changes for healthy individuals showing that cartilage volume decreases with aging [36–38]. The mean annual reduction in tibial cartilage volume in healthy males ($n = 28$; mean age 51.9 years) was found to be 2.8% (95% CI, 0.2–5.5%) [38]. The average annual decrease in total tibial cartilage volume in healthy postmenopausal females was similar at 2.4% [36]. Ding et al. [39] demonstrated a significant association between age and loss of cartilage volume by approximately 1.5–4.2% per annum in individuals between ages of 26 and 61 years, with females showing a higher rate of loss than males. However, Beattie and colleagues [40] suggested that despite the age-related declines, it is still plausible that those values lied within what may be considered a normal or healthy range.

As the work of Raynauld and colleagues [35], other studies have demonstrated the capability of MRI cartilage volume to detect longitudinal cartilage loss in OA. Cicuttini and colleagues [41] did not observe significant changes in cartilage volume in 166 healthy volunteers aged 21–79 years over a period of approximately 2 years, but significant cartilage loss (–4.1% per annum) was observed in a group of patients who had undergone partial meniscectomy [42]. An elegant meta-analysis of Eckstein and colleagues [41] showed that in OA patients the combined annual loss of cartilage volume was −136 μl (−4.1%) in the patella, −90 μl (−5.6%) in the medial tibia, and −107 μl (−6.0%) in the lateral tibia. Results varied between studies, showing an annual rate of change ranging from −0.3 to −7.4% in the medial tibia, indicating the heterogeneity of the disease. The heterogeneity of knee OA has also been demonstrated with studies such as that of Gandy and colleagues [43], who reported no loss of MRI cartilage volume over 3 years in patients with knee OA (n = 11). However, in a recent work on a subset of 150 subjects from the Progression subcohort of the OAI, Hunter and colleagues [44] studied cartilage morphological changes (absolute and percentage) from baseline at 1 year, as well as the standardized response mean (SRM), i.e., mean change divided by the standard deviation change. The studied morphological parameters were cartilage volume, normalized cartilage volume to bone surface interface area, and percentage denuded area (total cartilage bone interface area denuded of cartilage). The SRMs for cartilage volume of various locations were central medial tibia −0.096, central medial femur −0.394, and patella −0.198. The SRMs for normalized cartilage volume of the various locations were central medial tibia −0.044, central medial femur −0.338, and patella −0.193. Participants had in general denuded area at baseline in the central medial femur (62%) and central medial tibia (60%). These results indicate small-annualized rates of change, but they also show the greatest consisted change in the central medial femur.

In a cartilage defects study, Cicuttini et al. [45] reported that in subjects with cartilage defects, the annual loss of medial tibial cartilage was 2.5% compared with an annual loss of 1.3% in those with no defects, independent of other known risk factors for OA.

MRI Cartilage Volume: Symptoms and Clinical Outcome

The association between cartilage volume loss with pain and function scores has also been investigated and results have been diverse. Using a sagittal fat-saturated gradient echo T_2-weighted sequence, Hunter et al. [46] studied 133 postmenopausal women and reported significant negative association of patellar cartilage volume with the WOMAC score. However, Phan et al. [47] found no association between longitudinal cartilage loss and change in symptoms given by the WOMAC score in 40 subjects. Similarly, Wluka and colleagues [48] reported no significant associations with the WOMAC score at baseline and subsequent cartilage loss in patients with symptomatic early knee OA (n = 132). In contrast to these results, Cicuttini and colleagues [49], in a study of patellar cartilage changes in 110 patients over a period of almost 2 years, reported that subjects with higher pain scores at baseline showed higher loss than those with lower scores. Similar trend was found for those with higher BMI.

MRI cartilage volume has also shown to be a valid indicator of particular clinical outcomes such as change of symptoms and the likelihood of progression to knee replacement surgery. In an Australian study, the rate of change in cartilage volume between baseline and follow-up at 24 months was found to be significantly associated with knee replacement at 48 months. For every 1% increase in the rate of cartilage loss, a 20% increase risk of undergoing total knee arthroplasty (TKA) was detected. Individuals who were in the top tertile of the rate of cartilage loss were shown to have a sevenfold increased risk of progressing to a TKA compared with those in the lowest tertile [50].

Cross-sectional Studies

In other cross-sectional studies such as that of the Framingham cohort, Hunter et al. [23] reported that cartilage volume divided by the bone interface area yielded the best discrimination between patients with radiographic OA of the femorotibial joint and nonradiographic OA participants. Burgkart et al. [30] compared cartilage volume between eight OA patients prior to TKA with a group of 28 healthy subjects and reported a difference of approximately 1,300 μl in the medial tibia in patients with varus OA and differences of approximately 1,800 μl in the lateral tibia in patients with valgus or bicompartmental OA.

T-scores, an indicator of the difference between patients and young healthy subjects, and Z-scores, an indicator of the difference between patients and age-matched healthy subjects, have been also proposed in cross-sectional studies of cartilage morphology [22]. However, a recent publication of Beattie and colleagues [40] reported a pilot study in healthy individuals to estimate reference values of medial minimum joint space width (mJSW) using radiography and medial tibial cartilage morphology using peripheral MRI at 1.0 T. They studied 119 participants (73 female and 43 male; 38.2 ± 13.2 years), and their results suggest that there may be no need to differentiate a T-score and a Z-score in OA diagnosis because cartilage thickness and JSW remain constant throughout life in the absence of OA.

Cicuttini and colleagues [45], in a prospective study, investigated the association of cartilage defects with loss of knee cartilage in healthy, middle-aged adults (n = 86; 53.8 ± 8.8 years) cross-sectionally and longitudinally based on MRI at baseline and 2-year follow-up. Subjects with cartilage defects had a 25% reduction in medial tibial cartilage volume, 15%

reduction in lateral tibial cartilage volume, and 19% reduction in total femoral cartilage volume relative to those with no cartilage defects in cross-sectional analyses. The authors concluded that the presence of asymptomatic, nonfull-thickness medial tibio-femoral cartilage defects might identify healthy individuals most likely to lose knee cartilage in the absence of radiographic knee OA. On a different study, knee cartilage defects were also associated with decreased cartilage volume on a cross-sectional sample of 372 subjects [51].

Cartilage Volume and Its Relationship with Other Tissues

Magnetic resonance studies have also evaluated the relationship between cartilage changes and other tissues in the knee joint. Lindsey et al. [52] and Blumenkrantz et al. [53] studied the association of knee cartilage morphology and trabecular bone, reporting that cartilage loss on one side of the knee joint is related to trabecular bone loss on the opposite side of the knee joint. Cartilage degeneration and its association with changes in subchondral bone architecture and with changes in the trabecular bone proximal to the joint line have also been observed [53, 54].

Wluka et al. [55] studied 271 asymptomatic subjects having no history of knee injury, knee pain, or clinical knee OA. Magnetic resonance images at baseline and 2 years later were acquired to assess the relationship between the presence of bone marrow lesions (BMLs) at baseline and change in tibial cartilage volume over 2 years. Fourteen percent of the participants ($n = 37$) had BMLs, and results indicated a trend for increased annual tibial cartilage volume loss where very large BMLs were present. In another longitudinal study of Hunter et al. [56], an association between enlargement of bone marrow lesions with cartilage loss in OA was also observed. Raynauld et al. [57] demonstrated that size changes in bone edema over 24 months were strongly and independently associated with medial cartilage volume loss.

The possible influence of knee angle on the rate of medial tibial cartilage volume loss in knee OA was demonstrated by Teichtahl and colleagues [58]. They studied 78 adults with symptomatic knee OA and obtained radiographs at baseline and 2 years later to determine change in knee alignment on a continuous scale. Magnetic resonance images for tibial cartilage volume quantification were obtained at 2 and 4.5 years after baseline to determine annual percentage change. Results demonstrated that for every 1° change toward genu valgum, there was an associated 0.44% reduction in the rate of annual medial tibial cartilage volume loss; and that for every 1° change toward genu varum, there was an associated 0.44% increase in the rate of annual medial tibial cartilage volume loss. There were no effects of knee angle on the rate of loss of the lateral tibia cartilage volume. Sharma et al. [59] also observed that varus malalignment predicted medial tibial cartilage volume and thickness loss, and tibial and femoral denuded bone increase.

The relationship between meniscal damage and extrusion with knee cartilage loss in knee OA was investigated by Sharma et al. [59] on 251 knees of 153 subjects. After fully adjusting for other factors (age, sex, body mass index, medial/lateral meniscal extrusion, varus/valgus malalignment, and lateral/medial laxity), medial and lateral meniscal damage predicted medial/lateral tibial cartilage volume loss, and medial/lateral tibial and medial/lateral weight-bearing femoral denuded bone increase. No significant associations were found between cartilage volume and meniscal extrusion after adjustment of other parameters. On the other hand, Ding and colleagues [60], in a 2-year longitudinal study of a largely nonosteoarthritic cohort of 294 individuals, observed an association between meniscal extrusion at baseline with greater rate of loss of medial tibio-femoral cartilage volume.

In terms of hip cartilage, no morphological studies involving subjects with OA have yet been reported, either longitudinally or cross-sectionally.

Summary

In this chapter, we have given a brief overview of the most relevant concepts of MRI cartilage segmentation and volume quantification. There are important aspects that we considered worth to remember. In terms of pulse sequences for imaging of cartilage morphology, they should have high SNR, high CNR, high-spatial resolution, need to be fast, and should minimize image distortions. Emerging cartilage segmentation techniques need to be validated simulating in vivo conditions as close as possible. An imaging-based marker, in order to be considered of clinical utility, must be on the disease pathway, and the technique for its quantification must be accurate and precise. Cartilage volume using MRI is a potential imaging-based biomarker for knee OA because it is a pathophysiological element of OA, its quantification is accurate and precise, and different longitudinal and cross-sectional studies have demonstrated its relevance in OA, as well as its relationships with clinical symptoms, clinical outcome, other joint tissues, as well as with cartilage defects. It is also important to remember that besides cartilage volume, and in general, besides cartilage morphology, there are other promising imaging-based biomarkers under investigation for a better understanding of OA, such as MRI relaxation times like T_2 and $T_{1\rho}$.

References

1. Carballido-Gamio J, Link TM, Li X, Han ET, Krug R, Ries MD, et al. Feasibility and reproducibility of relaxometry, morphometric, and geometrical measurements of the hip joint with magnetic resonance imaging at 3T. J Magn Reson Imaging. 2008;28(1):227–35.
2. Link TM, Majumdar S, Daldrup HE, Peterfy C, Uffmann M, Dowling C, et al. High resolution MRI of small joints: impact of spatial resolution on diagnostic performance and SNR. Magn Reson Imaging. 1998;16(2):147–55.
3. Hardya PA, Newmark R, Liu YM, Meier D, Norris S, Piraino DW, et al. The influence of the resolution and contrast on measuring the articular cartilage volume in magnetic resonance images. Magn Reson Imaging. 2000;18(8):965–72.
4. Zuo J, Li X, Banerjee S, Han E, Majumdar S. Parallel imaging of knee cartilage at 3 Tesla. J Magn Reson Imaging. 2007;26(4):1001–9.
5. Gold GE, Hargreaves BA, Reeder SB, Vasanawala SS, Beaulieu CF. Controversies in protocol selection in the imaging of articular cartilage. Semin Musculoskelet Radiol. 2005;9(2):161–72.
6. Perona P, Malik J. Scale-space and edge detection using anisotropic diffusion. IEEE Trans Pattern Anal Mach Intell. 1990;12(17):629–39.
7. Stammberger T, Eckstein F, Michaelis M, Englmeier KH, Reiser M. Interobserver reproducibility of quantitative cartilage measurements: comparison of B-spline snakes and manual segmentation. Magn Reson Imaging. 1999;17(7):1033–42.
8. Lynch JA, Zaim S, Zhao J, Stork A, Peterfy CG, Genant HK. Cartilage segmentation of 3D MRI scans of the osteoarthritic knee combining user knowledge and active contours. Paper presented at: SPIE, Medical Imaging2000; San Diego.
9. Grau V, Mewes AU, Alcaniz M, Kikinis R, Warfield SK. Improved watershed transform for medical image segmentation using prior information. IEEE Trans Med Imaging. 2004;23(4):447–58.
10. Pakin SK, Tamez-Pena JG, Totterman S, Parker KJ. Segmentation, surface extraction, and thickness computation of articular cartilage. Paper presented at: SPIE, Medical Imaging2002; San Diego.
11. Warfield SK, Kaus M, Jolesz FA, Kikinis R. Adaptive, template moderated, spatially varying statistical classification. Med Image Anal. 2000;4(1):43–55.
12. Eckstein F, Burstein D, Link TM. Quantitative MRI of cartilage and bone: degenerative changes in osteoarthritis. NMR Biomed. 2006;19(7):822–54.
13. Naish JH, Xanthopoulos E, Hutchinson CE, Waterton JC, Taylor CJ. MR measurement of articular cartilage thickness distribution in the hip. Osteoarthritis Cartilage. 2006;14(10):967–73.
14. Nishii T, Nakanishi K, Sugano N, Masuhara K, Ohzono K, Ochi T. Articular cartilage evaluation in osteoarthritis of the hip with MR imaging under continuous leg traction. Magn Reson Imaging. 1998;16(8):871–5.
15. Nakanishi K, Tanaka H, Nishii T, Masuhara K, Narumi Y, Nakamura H. MR evaluation of the articular cartilage of the femoral head during traction. Correlation with resected femoral head. Acta Radiol. 1999;40(1):60–3.
16. Nishii T, Sugano N, Tanaka H, Nakanishi K, Ohzono K, Yoshikawa H. Articular cartilage abnormalities in dysplastic hips without joint space narrowing. Clin Orthop Relat Res Feb. 2001;383:183–90.
17. Wirth W, Eckstein F. A technique for regional analysis of femorotibial cartilage thickness based on quantitative magnetic resonance imaging. IEEE Trans Med Imaging. 2008;27(6):737–44.
18. Kauffmann C, Gravel P, Godbout B, Gravel A, Beaudoin G, Raynauld J-P, et al. Computer-aided method for quantification of cartilage thickness and volume changes using MRI: validation study using a synthetic model. IEEE Trans Biomed Eng. 2003;50(8):978–88.
19. Stahl R, Blumenkrantz G, Carballido-Gamio J, Zhao S, Munoz T, Hellio Le Graverand-Gastineau MP, et al. MRI-derived T2 relaxation times and cartilage morphometry of the tibio-femoral joint in subjects with and without osteoarthritis during a 1-year follow-up. Osteoarthritis Cartilage. 2007;15(11):1225–34.
20. Carballido-Gamio J, Bauer JS, Stahl R, Lee KY, Krause S, Link TM, et al. Inter-subject comparison of MRI knee cartilage thickness. Med Image Anal. 2008;12(2):120–35.
21. Carballido-Gamio J, Link TM, Majumdar S. New techniques for cartilage magnetic resonance imaging relaxation time analysis: texture analysis of flattened cartilage and localized intra- and inter-subject comparisons. Magn Reson Med. 2008;59(6):1472–7.
22. Burgkart R, Glaser C, Hinterwimmer S, Hudelmaier M, Englmeier KH, Reiser M, et al. Feasibility of T and Z scores from magnetic resonance imaging data for quantification of cartilage loss in osteoarthritis. Arthritis Rheum. 2003;48(10):2829–35.
23. Hunter DJ, Niu J, Zhang YQ, McLennan C, LaValley M, Tu X, et al. Cartilage volume must be normalized to bone surface area in order to provide satisfactory construct validity: The Framingham Study. Osteoarthritis Cartilage. 2004;12(Suppl B):S2.
24. Bolbos RI, Zuo J, Banerjee S, Link TM, Ma CB, Li X, et al. Relationship between trabecular bone structure and articular cartilage morphology and relaxation times in early OA of the knee joint using parallel MRI at 3 T. Osteoarthritis Cartilage. 2008;16(10):1150–9.
25. Stammberger T, Eckstein F, Englmeier KH, Reiser M. Determination of 3D cartilage thickness data from MR imaging: computational method and reproducibility in the living. Magn Reson Med. 1999;41(3):529–36.
26. Glüer CC, Blake G, Blunt BA, Jergas M, Genant HK. Accurate assessment of precision errors: how to measure the reproducibility of bone densitometry techniques. Osteoporos Int. 1995;5:262–70.
27. Teichtahl AJ, Wluka AE, Davies-Tuck ML, Cicuttini FM. Imaging of knee osteoarthritis. Best Pract Res Clin Rheumatol. 2008;22(6):1061–74.
28. Cicuttini F, Forbes A, Morris K, Darling S, Bailey M, Stuckey S. Gender differences in knee cartilage volume as measured by magnetic resonance imaging. Osteoarthritis Cartilage. 1999;7(3):265–71.
29. Peterfy CG, van Dijke CF, Janzen DL, Glüer CC, Namba R, Majumdar S, et al. Quantification of articular cartilage in the knee with pulsed saturation transfer subtraction and fat-suppressed MR imaging: optimization and validation. Radiology. 1994;192(2):485–91.
30. Burgkart R, Glaser C, Hyhlik-Durr A, Englmeier KH, Reiser M, Eckstein F. Magnetic resonance imaging-based assessment of cartilage loss in severe osteoarthritis: accuracy, precision, and diagnostic value. Arthritis Rheum. 2001;44(9):2072–7.
31. Graichen H, von Eisenhart-Rothe R, Vogl T, Englmeier KH, Eckstein F. Quantitative assessment of cartilage status in osteoarthritis by quantitative magnetic resonance imaging: technical validation for use in analysis of cartilage volume and further morphologic parameters. Arthritis Rheum. 2004;50(3):811–6.
32. Eckstein F, Buck RJ, Burstein D, Charles HC, Crim J, Hudelmaier M, et al. Precision of 3.0 Tesla quantitative magnetic resonance imaging of cartilage morphology in a multicentre clinical trial. Ann Rheum Dis. 2008;67(12):1683–8.
33. Cicuttini FM, Wluka AE, Forbes A, Wolfe R. Comparison of tibial cartilage volume and radiologic grade of the tibiofemoral joint. Arthritis Rheum. 2003;48(3):682–8.
34. Jones G, Ding C, Scott F, Glisson M, Cicuttini F. Early radiographic osteoarthritis is associated with substantial changes in cartilage volume and tibial bone surface area in both males and females. Osteoarthritis Cartilage. 2004;12(2):169–74.
35. Raynauld JP, Martel-Pelletier J, Berthiaume MJ, V F, Beaudoin G, de Guise JA, et al. Quantitative magnetic resonance imaging evaluation of knee osteoarthritis progression over two years and correlation with clinical symptoms and radiologic changes. Arthritis Rheum. 2004;50(2):476–87.
36. Wluka AE, Wolfe R, Davis SR, Stuckey S, Cicuttini FM. Tibial cartilage volume change in healthy postmenopausal women: a longitudinal study. Ann Rheum Dis. 2004;63(4):444–9.

37. Cicuttini FM, Wluka A, Bailey M, O'Sullivan R, Poon C, Yeung S, et al. Factors affecting knee cartilage volume in healthy men. Rheumatology (Oxford). 2003;42(2):258–62.
38. Hanna F, Ebeling PR, Wang Y, O'Sullivan R, Davis S, Wluka AE, et al. Factors influencing longitudinal change in knee cartilage volume measured from magnetic resonance imaging in healthy men. Ann Rheum Dis. 2005;64(7):1038–42.
39. Ding C, Cicuttini F, Blizzard L, Scott F, Jones G. A longitudinal study of the effect of sex and age on rate of change in knee cartilage volume in adults. Rheumatology (Oxford). 2007;46(2):273–9.
40. Beattie KA, Duryea J, O'Neill J, Pui M, Boulos P, Webber CE, et al. Minimum joint space width and tibial cartilage morphology in the knees of healthy individuals: a cross-sectional study. BMC Musculoskelet Disord. 2008;9:119.
41. Eckstein F, Cicuttini F, Raynauld JP, Waterton JC, Peterfy C. Magnetic resonance imaging (MRI) of articular cartilage in knee osteoarthritis (OA): morphological assessment. Osteoarthritis Cartilage. 2006;14(Suppl A):A46–75.
42. Cicuttini FM, Forbes A, Yuanyuan W, Rush G, Stuckey SL. Rate of knee cartilage loss after partial meniscectomy. J Rheumatol. 2002;29(9):1954–6.
43. Gandy SJ, Dieppe PA, Keen MC, Maciewicz RA, Watt I, Waterton JC. No loss of cartilage volume over three years in patients with knee osteoarthritis as assessed by magnetic resonance imaging. Osteoarthritis Cartilage. 2002;10(12):929–37.
44. Hunter DJ, Niu J, Zhang Y, Totterman S, Tamez J, Dabrowski C, et al. Change in cartilage morphometry: a sample of the progression cohort of the Osteoarthritis Initiative. Ann Rheum Dis. 2009;68(3):349–56.
45. Cicuttini F, Ding C, Wluka A, Davis S, Ebeling PR, Jones G. Association of cartilage defects with loss of knee cartilage in healthy, middle-age adults: a prospective study. Arthritis Rheum. 2005;52(7):2033–9.
46. Hunter DJ, March L, Sambrook PN. The association of cartilage volume with knee pain. Osteoarthritis Cartilage. 2003;11(10):725–9.
47. Phan CM, Link TM, Blumenkrantz G, Dunn TC, Ries MD, Steinbach LS, et al. MR imaging findings in the follow-up of patients with different stages of knee osteoarthritis and the correlation with clinical symptoms. Eur Radiol. 2006;16(3):608–18.
48. Wluka AE, Wolfe R, Stuckey S, Cicuttini FM. How does tibial cartilage volume relate to symptoms in subjects with knee osteoarthritis? Ann Rheum Dis. 2004;63(3):264–8.
49. Cicuttini F, Wluka A, Wang Y, Stuckey S. The determinants of change in patella cartilage volume in osteoarthritic knees. J Rheumatol. 2002;29(12):2615–9.
50. Cicuttini FM, Jones G, Forbes A, Wluka AE. Rate of cartilage loss at two years predicts subsequent total knee arthroplasty: a prospective study. Ann Rheum Dis. 2004;63(9):1124–7.
51. Ding C, Garnero P, Cicuttini F, Scott F, Cooley H, Jones G. Knee cartilage defects: association with early radiographic osteoarthritis, decreased cartilage volume, increased joint surface area and type II collagen breakdown. Osteoarthritis Cartilage. 2005;13(3):198–205.
52. Lindsey CT, Narasimhan A, Adolfo JM, Jin H, Steinbach LS, Link T, et al. Magnetic resonance evaluation of the interrelationship between articular cartilage and trabecular bone of the osteoarthritic knee(1). Osteoarthritis Cartilage. 2004;12(2):86–96.
53. Blumenkrantz G, Lindsey CT, Dunn TC, Jin H, Ries MD, Link TM, et al. A pilot, two-year longitudinal study of the interrelationship between trabecular bone and articular cartilage in the osteoarthritic knee. Osteoarthritis Cartilage. 2004;12(12):997–1005.
54. Bobinac D, Spanjol J, Zoricic S, Maric I. Changes in articular cartilage and subchondral bone histomorphometry in osteoarthritic knee joints in humans. Bone. 2003;32(3):284–90.
55. Wluka AE, Wang Y, Davies-Tuck M, English DR, Giles GG, Cicuttini FM. Bone marrow lesions predict progression of cartilage defects and loss of cartilage volume in healthy middle-aged adults without knee pain over 2 yrs. Rheumatology (Oxford). 2008;47(9):1392–6.
56. Hunter DJ, Zhang Y, Niu J, Goggins J, Amin S, LaValley MP, et al. Increase in bone marrow lesions associated with cartilage loss: a longitudinal magnetic resonance imaging study of knee osteoarthritis. Arthritis Rheum. 2006;54(5):1529–35.
57. Raynauld JP, Martel-Pelletier J, Berthiaume MJ, Abram F, Choquette D, Haraoui B, et al. Correlation between bone lesion changes and cartilage volume loss in patients with osteoarthritis of the knee as assessed by quantitative magnetic resonance imaging over a 24-month period. Ann Rheum Dis. 2008;67(5):683–8.
58. Teichtahl AJ, Davies-Tuck ML, Wluka AE, Jones G, Cicuttini FM. Change in knee angle influences the rate of medial tibial cartilage volume loss in knee osteoarthritis. Osteoarthritis Cartilage. 2009;17(1):8–11.
59. Sharma L, Eckstein F, Song J, Guermazi A, Prasad P, Kapoor D, et al. Relationship of meniscal damage, meniscal extrusion, malalignment, and joint laxity to subsequent cartilage loss in osteoarthritic knees. Arthritis Rheum. 2008;58(6):1716–26.
60. Ding C, Martel-Pelletier J, Pelletier JP, Abram F, Raynauld JP, Cicuttini F, et al. Knee meniscal extrusion in a largely non-osteoarthritic cohort: association with greater loss of cartilage volume. Arthritis Res Ther. 2007;9(2):R21.

Chapter 11
Quantitative MR Imaging of Cartilage Morphology in Osteoarthritis

Felix Eckstein, Martin Hudelmaier, and Wolfgang Wirth

Keywords Osteoarthritis • MR imaging • Cartilage • Knee • Progression • Morphology • Quantitative

Preamble and Introduction

Osteoarthritis (OA) is a degenerative disease of synovial joints that is associated with symptoms (pain) and functional impairment as well as with structural changes in various articular tissues. The articular cartilage provides the weight-bearing surface of joints and its mechanical properties are unmet by any artificial (man-made) material. These properties ensure optimal load transfer to the subchondral bone and an almost frictionless surface in healthy joints. Cartilage volume consists of 80–90% water, which is undergoing hydrostatic pressurization during load transmission [1]. This hydrostatic pressurization mechanism prevents focal load peaks at the subchondral bone interface, it protects the vulnerable cartilage matrix from damage, and it provides the cartilage with a friction coefficient that is 10 times lower than that of ice on ice. It is for this reason that articular cartilage is integral to appropriate joint function and that its loss is associated with functional impairment. Cartilage also is the tissue that has generated most interest in context of quantitative measurement in OA with MRI.

Throughout this chapter, the term "cartilage morphology" will be used to collectively encompass three-dimensional (3D) quantitative measurement of structural properties of articular cartilage tissue dimensions (Fig. 11.1). These include cartilage thickness, surface areas, volume of joint compartments, cartilage plates, or cartilage plate subregions, but not focal cartilage lesions, as also sometimes referred to as "morphologic" cartilage changes in the literature. Also, this chapter will not cover quantitative MRI techniques on cartilage composition, such as dGEMRIC, T2, T1rho, and others, and it will be focused on cartilage in the human knee, as this is where most of the work has been performed to date. Morphological measurements of cartilage structure fully exploit the 3D nature of MRI data sets; their strength is that they are potentially less observer-dependent and more objective than scoring methods, and that relatively small changes in cartilage thickness and volume over time (that occur relatively homogeneously over larger areas) may be detected, which are not apparent to the naked eye. This is important, as the progression of structural changes in OA has generally been shown to be slow, both when being evaluated by radiography [2–4] and MRI [4–8]. A recent study found that quantitative measures of cartilage morphology [9] were more powerful in revealing relationships between local risk factors (meniscal damage and malalignment) and knee cartilage loss than a semiquantitative approach using ordinal data (WORMS) [10]. The disadvantage of quantitative measurement, however, is that it requires specialized software and is more time intensive, because tissue boundaries need to be tracked (i.e., segmented) throughout large series of slices using trained technical personnel. Also, quantitative measurements are less sensitive to the occurrences of small focal changes within larger structures (i.e., cartilage lesions), which may be readily picked up by an expert reader, particularly if the location within the larger structure is variable from joint to joint. A recent study showed, for instance, that MRI-based semiquantitative scoring of cartilage status was able to differentiate between knees with and without early (i.e., Kellgren–Lawrence grade [KLG] 2) radiographic OA in a community-based cohort, whereas quantitative measures of cartilage morphology displayed no or little difference between healthy and KLG2 knees [11]. It therefore depends on the particular context and research question whether semiquantitative or quantitative cartilage assessment are better suited as outcome measures for a particular study, or whether both are needed to

F. Eckstein (✉)
Institute of Anatomy & Musculoskeletal Research, Paracelsus Medical University, Strubergasse 21, Salzburg 5020, Austria
and
Chondrometrics GmbH, Ainring, Germany
e-mail: felix.eckstein@pmu.ac.at

T.M. Link (ed.), *Cartilage Imaging: Significance, Techniques, and New Developments*,
DOI 10.1007/978-1-4419-8438-8_11, © Springer Science+Business Media, LLC 2011

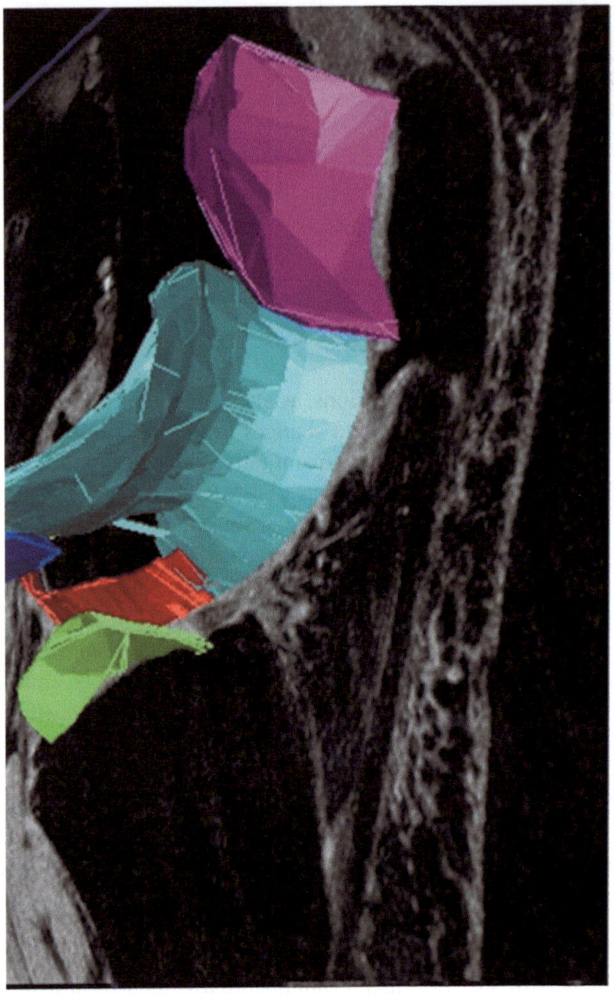

Fig. 11.1 3D reconstruction of the knee cartilages after segmentation: cartilage of the medial tibia (MT) is depicted *dark blue*, that of the lateral tibia (LT) *green*, that of the medial weight-bearing femoral condyles (cMF) *yellow*, that of the lateral weight-bearing femoral condyles (cLF) *red*, that of the patella (P) *magenta*, and that of the femoral trochlea (TrF) *turquoise* (also see Table 11.1 and Fig. 11.3). Segmentation was performed based on a 3D-DESS knee imaging data set from the Osteoarthritis Initiative (OAI), a public–private partnership funded by the National Institutes of Health and conducted by the OAI Study Investigators. For anatomical (region of interest) labels, also see Fig. 11.2

obtain a comprehensive picture. Generally, quantitative measures are more powerful where small changes occur homogeneously throughout larger structures or at highly predictable locations, whereas semiquantitative scoring is more powerful when local changes (in tissue dimensions or signal intensity) occur at unpredictable locations and involve only smaller parts of this structure. Ideally, therefore, both approaches should be used in complimentary rather than competing fashion in studies assessing either the status or the progression of OA.

Table 11.1 Anatomical (region of interest), morphological (metrics) and statistical labels commonly used in cartilage morphology publications on the knee

Abbreviation	Explanation	Unit
Anatomical (region of interest) labels		
Total cartilage plates		
P	Patella	
MT	Medial tibia	
LT	Lateral tibia	
F	Femur	
TrF	Femoral trochlea	
MF	Medial femoral condyle	
cMF	Weight-bearing portion of MF	
pMF	Posterior portion of MF	
LF	Lateral femoral condyle	
cLF	Weight-bearing portion of LF	
pLF	Posterior portion of LF	
MFTC	Aggregate values for MT and cMF (MT + cMF)	
LFTC	Aggregate values for LT and cLF (LT ± cLF)	
Subregions (to be combined with above total plate labels, i.e., cMT or ccMF)		
c	Central	
e	External	
i	Internal	
a	Anterior	
p	Posterior	
Morphological (metrics) label		
VC	Volume of the cartilage	mm^3/ml
tAB	Total area of subchondral bone	cm^2
AC	Area of cartilage surface	cm^2
cAB	Area of tAB covered by AC	cm^2
dAB%	Percent of tAB denuded (not covered by AC)	%
VCtAB	Volume of the cartilage divided by tAB	mm
ThCtAB	Thickness of the cartilage over the entire tAB	mm
ThCcAB	Thickness of cartilage over cAB	mm
dAB%	Percent of tAB denuded (not covered by AC)	%
VCtAB	Volume of the cartilage divided by tAB	mm
ThCtAB	Thickness of the cartilage over the entire tAB	mm
ThCcAB	Thickness of cartilage over cAB	mm
Statistical labels		
Me	Mean (i.e., thickness)	
Max	Maximum (i.e., thickness)	
Mav	Maximal averaged, e.g., mean of the top 1% values	
Min	Minimum (i.e., thickness)	
Miv	Minimum averaged, e.g., mean of the lowest 1% values	
SD	Standard deviation (i.e., thickness)	
CV%	Coefficient of variation (i.e., thickness)	
c(Me, Mav)	Thickness measured from cartilage surface (AC) to bone interface (tAB)	
b(Me, Mav)	Thickness measured from bone interface (tAB) to cartilage surface (AC)	
a(Me, Mav)	Average of the two above (b, c)	

For anatomical (region of interest) labels, also see Figs. 11.1 and 11.2

Cartilage Morphology Outcomes and Regions of Interest in the Knee

Cartilage morphology outcomes commonly include: the size of the total area of subchondral bone (tAB), the area of the cartilage surface (AC), the denuded (dAB) and cartilage-covered (cAB) area of subchondral bone, the cartilage thickness over the tAB (ThCtAB) or over the cAB (ThCcAB), the cartilage volume (VC), the cartilage volume normalized to the tAB (VCtAB), the cartilage signal intensity [12–14], and others (Table 11.1). A consensus-based nomenclature for the above-mentioned structural (i.e., morphological metric labels) or compositional features as well as definition for regions of interest in the knee (i.e., anatomical labels, see Table 11.1 and Fig. 11.2) and has been proposed by a group of experts [15]. The above nomenclature will be used throughout this review, and important abbreviations for morphology metrics and anatomical regions of interests including recent extensions (i.e., statistical labels and subregional labels, i.e., [16]) are summarized in Table 11.1.

To obtain the above quantitative morphological measures of cartilage, the relevant cartilage plates of a joint need to be segmented by a trained user with the choice of several input devices, such as a computer mouse, a graphical tablet, or a touch-sensitive screen [17], and with or without assistance from (semiautomated) segmentation software [18–26]. Since the relative performance of different segmentation algorithms has been discussed in previous reviews [7], this point will not be covered in depth in this chapter. Using the above tools, an operator needs to accurately trace both the bone–cartilage interface (i.e., the subchondral bone surface), and the surface of the cartilage, respectively (AC). The tracing of the subchondral bone surface should ideally include the tAB, including dABs, but it should exclude osteophyte surfaces. As there are various sources of artifacts on MRI, and because signal intensity and contrast may vary substantially between baseline and follow-up acquisitions (for an example, see Fig. 11.3), there is consensus that expert quality control is important for an accurate analysis, with the time required for segmentation or the correction of computer-generated segmentation taking several hours per joint. After all slices of interest have been segmented, image analysis software can be used to compute the three-dimensional morphological features listed in Table 11.1.

In terms of anatomical regions of interest (Table 11.1), MT is used for the medial tibia, LT for the lateral tibia, MF for medial femoral condyle, LF for the lateral femoral condyle, cMF/cLF for the central (weight-bearing) portions of the medial/lateral femoral condyle, and pMF/pLF for the posterior aspects of the medial/lateral femoral condyle (Table 11.1; Fig. 11.2). Since the weight-bearing and posterior aspects of the femoral condyles are continuous and lack a definite anatomical border, different definitions for these ROIs have been proposed: Glaser et al. [27] used the projection of the posterior intercondylar bone bridge as a cut-off between the weight-bearing and posterior zone of MF and LF, respectively, whereas later studies [28] introduced a 60%

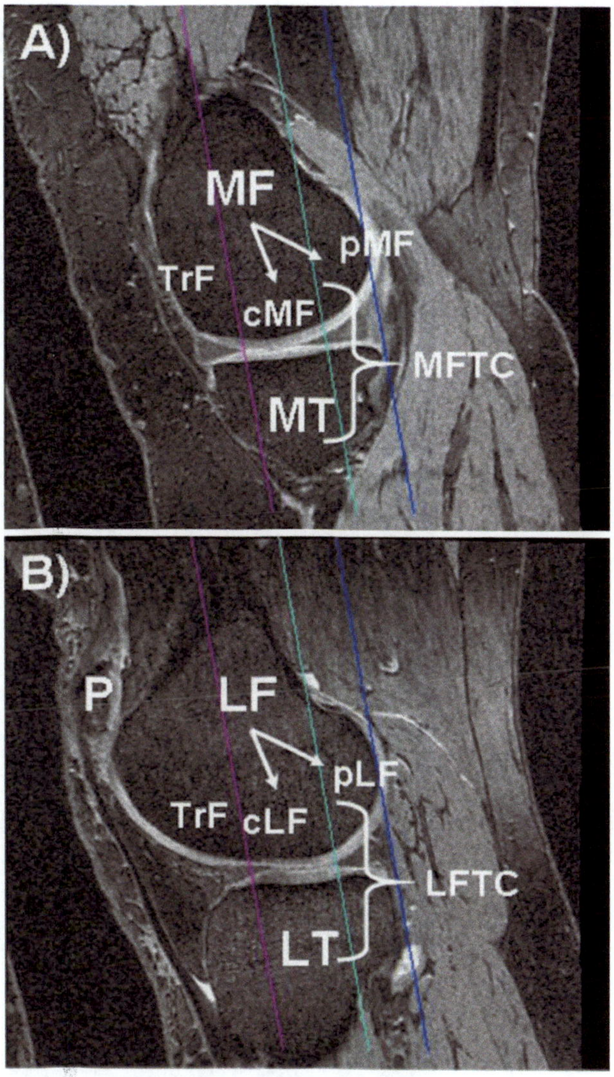

Fig. 11.2 Sagittal 3D DESS MR images showing anatomical regions of interest commonly analyzed: (**a**) medial femorotibial compartment, (**b**) lateral femorotibial compartment; *P* patella, *TrF* femoral trochlear, *MT* medial tibia, *MF* medial femoral condyle, *cMF* weight-bearing part of the medial femoral condyle, *pMF* posterior part of the medial femoral condyle, *MFTC* cMF+MT, *LT* lateral tibia, *LF* lateral femoral condyle, *cLF* weight-bearing part of the lateral femoral condyle, *pMF* posterior part of the lateral femoral condyle, *LFTC* cLF+LT; the magenta line shows the projection of the trochlear notch, the blue line the posterior end of the medial and lateral femoral condyle, and the turquoise line the 60% criterion (of the distance between the trochlear notch and the posterior ends of the condyles) used to separate cMF from pMF, and cLF from pLF, respectively. Images are from the Osteoarthritis Initiative (OAI), a public–private partnership funded by the National Institutes of Health and conducted by the OAI Study Investigators. For anatomical (region of interest) labels, also see Fig. 11.1

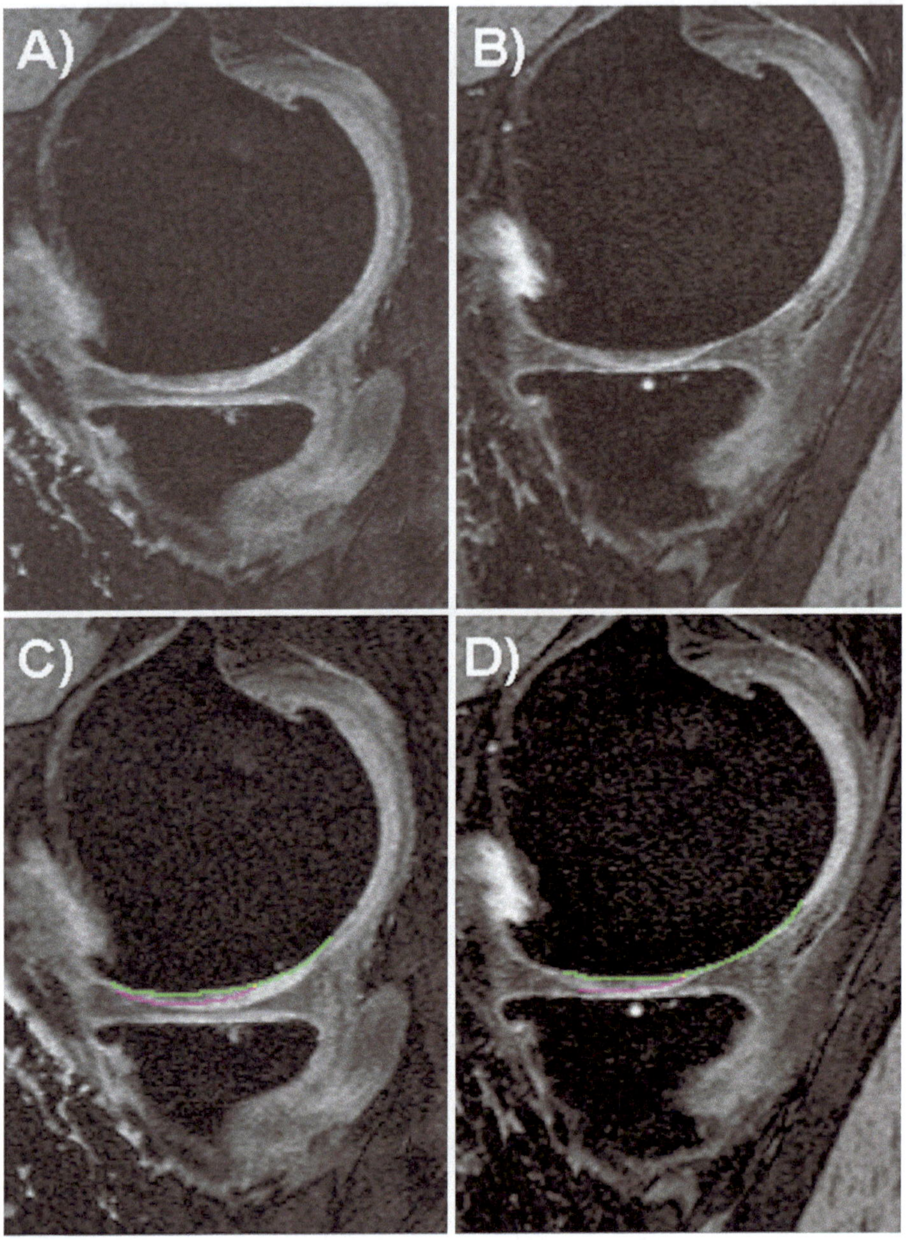

Fig. 11.3 Sagittal 3D DESS MR images acquired at baseline (**a, c**) and at 12-months follow-up (**b, d**). Images (**a**) and (**c**) are without and images (**b**) and (**d**) are with segmentation. The green lines show the outline of the total area of subchondral bone (tAB) in the cMF, and the magenta line shows the outline of the area of the cartilage surface (AC) in the cMF. At the transition of the weight-bearing to the posterior femoral condyle the fluid in image (**a**) could be potentially mistaken for thick cartilage. Images are from the Osteoarthritis Initiative (OAI), a public–private partnership funded by the National Institutes of Health and conducted by the OAI Study Investigators

distance criterion between the trochlear notch and the most posterior aspects of both femoral condyles as a cut-off between both regions (Fig. 11.2). In a direct face-to-face comparison, Hudelmaier et al. [29] reported the tAB of the 60% ROI to be approximately 20% greater and less variable (between subjects) than that based on the bone bridge, with cartilage morphology metrics being generally more reproducible in the 60% ROI. However, thickness measures did not differ significantly between both ROIs, and the longitudinal rate of change and standardized response mean (SRM = mean change/SD of change, as a measure of sensitivity to change) over 2 years were similar for various cartilage morphology metrics in both ROIs. Using sagittal images, both 60% [28] (Fig. 11.2) and 75% [30, 31] cut-offs have been used, the 60% cut-off assigning 36 (±1.8%) of the tAB of MF to the weight-bearing (cMF) and 64% to the posterior portion (pMF), whereas the 75% cut-off assigns 47% (±2.0%) of the tAB to cMF and 53% to pMF, respectively [31]. The mean change and SRM were, however, similar for both ROIs [31]. The (weight-bearing) medial femorotibial compartment (MT+cMF) is commonly addressed as MFTC, and the lateral compartment (LT+cLF) as LFTC (Fig. 11.2). In terms of anatomical labels for the femoropatellar compartment [15], P designates the patella, and TrF the femoral trochlear (=facies articularis patellaris; Fig. 11.2).

Quantitative measures of surface curvature and joint incongruity have also been determined from MR images [32] and were observed to discriminate between subjects with various radiographic OA grades cross-sectionally at 0.2 T [33, 34]. Curvature estimates at different scales (at 0.2 T) were also reported to be associated with the magnitude of cartilage loss longitudinally [35] and cartilage homogeneity (quantified by measuring entropy from the distribution of signal intensities in tibial cartilage from 0.2 T gradient echo images) was reported to discriminate between subjects without and with early radiographic OA [14]. This measure was proposed to be particularly sensitive in peripheral regions, where the cartilage is covered by the meniscus [36]. These results are surprising, because other MRI techniques that have been validated for targeting specific macromolecules of the cartilage, such as collagen, proteoglycans, or water (T2 mapping, T1rho, dGEMRIC, and others) have often been unsuccessful in discriminating between healthy knees and knees with early OA, and they have generally not been able to discriminate between different radiographic OA stages, in particular between early (pre-radiographic) OA and radiographic OA [4, 6, 37].

Relative Performance and Interrelationship of Cartilage Morphology Measures

Most investigations dealing quantitatively with cartilage morphology in OA have focused on the cartilage volume (VC), but this outcome measure has a number of pitfalls: The ability to discriminate between OA and healthy subjects is limited, because cartilage volume is largely determined by bone size, which increases the inter-subject variability and thus limits the ability to discriminate between people with and without cartilage loss [38]. This has led to misinterpretations in the literature, where it has been suggested that a high VC may be protective of OA, because men show higher VCs then women, and women are more susceptible to knee OA than men. However, men have mainly larger joint surfaces than women (and hence also larger VC) [39] even after adjustment for body height and weight [40] and VC can thus not be adequately compared between sexes. In longitudinal studies, the subchondral bone area has been shown to increase with aging, both in healthy reference subjects and in OA patients [41–43]. Such effects may mask a reduction in cartilage thickness in OA when measuring VC, because of the simultaneous expansion of the bone and cartilage layer. Therefore, alternative outcomes have been used, such as the VC normalized to the subchondral bone area (VCtAB), or the cartilage thickness over the entire subchondral bone area (ThCtAB) [38, 44].

In a recent study, Hudelmaier et al. [29] examined the relationship of the above parameters and their test–retest precision (at 3 T) in a set of 33 subjects, both without and with signs of radiographic osteoarthritis (reproducibility study). Further, they compared these parameters at baseline and at 2-year follow-up in 28 subjects with advanced radiographic osteoarthritis (sensitivity study). They found that the AC was larger than the tAB in all cartilage plates. In MT and LT, the cartilage volume divided by the total bone area (VCtAB) was very similar to the mean cartilage thickness over the total bone area (ThCtAB.aMe), whereas in cMF and cLF the VCtAB was somewhat greater than the ThCtAB.aMe. Different implementations of measuring the cartilage thickness (e.g., minimal distance from bone to cartilage, or minimal distance from cartilage to bone, or the average of both) produced very similar values in all cartilage plates. The maximal thickness over the total bone area (ThCtAB.Max) was found to be almost twice as high as the mean thickness (ThCtAB.Me) in the femorotibial plates. Reproducibility errors for cartilage volume divided by the tAB (VCtAB) were similar to those for the cartilage thickness over the total bone area (ThCtAB) and tended to be smaller than those for cartilage volume (VC). The reproducibility errors were also very similar for different implementations of the thickness measurements (see above). The maximal thickness over the total bone area (ThCtAB.Max) and the average of the top 1% greatest thickness values (ThCtAB.Mav) displayed larger reproducibility errors than the averaged mean cartilage thickness over the total bone area (ThCtAB.Me) in all cartilage plates, but reproducibility errors for ThCtAB.Mav tended to be smaller than those for ThCtAB.Max. In terms of the rate of (and sensitivity to) change, the cartilage volume divided by the total bone area (VCtAB) and the mean cartilage thickness over the total bone area (ThCtAB.aMe) exhibited higher rates of change and greater SRMs (greater sensitivity) than cartilage volume (VC) in MT, but the difference was only marginal in cMF. The rates of change and SRMs for cartilage thickness over the covered bone area (ThCcAB) tended to be less than for cartilage thickness over the total bone area (ThCtAB) and cartilage volume (VC), independent of the specific implementation, but tended to be greater than those for cartilage surface area (AC) and the cartilage-covered bone area (cAB). ThCtAB.Max and ThCtAB.Mav showed

Table 11.2 Rate of change and sensitivity to change over 2 years in 28 participants with Kellgren–Lawrence grade (KLG) 3, and test–retest reproducibility in 33 participants with KLG0 to KLG3 for various cartilage morphology metrics and regions of interest in the medial femorotibial compartment

	MT				cMF (60%)			
	MC%	SRM	*p*	RMSCV%	MC%	SRM	*p*	RMSCV%
VC	−2.3	−0.44	0.03	2.5	−3.5	−0.32	0.10	2.6
tAB	0.5	0.37	0.06	1.0	−0.1	−0.04	0.84	1.1
AC	−0.9	−0.33	0.09	1.0	−1.7	−0.22	0.26	1.3
cAB	−1.0	−0.29	0.14	1.0	−3.0	−0.36	0.07	1.1
VCtAB	−2.7	−0.59	0.00	1.9	−4.0	−0.33	0.09	2.0
ThCtAB.aMe	−2.6	−0.58	0.01	1.9	−3.6	−0.31	0.12	1.7
ThCtAB.bMe	−2.8	−0.62	0.00	1.9	−3.3	−0.29	0.13	1.9
ThCtAB.cMe	−2.5	−0.56	0.01	2.0	−3.9	−0.33	0.10	1.7
ThCcAB.aMe	−1.4	−0.43	0.03	1.9	−1.5	−0.18	0.34	1.7
ThCcAB.bMe	−1.5	−0.48	0.02	1.9	−1.2	−0.15	0.43	1.9
ThCcAB.cMe	−1.3	−0.42	0.04	2.0	−2.0	−0.23	0.23	1.7
ThCtAB.aMax	−1.4	−0.27	0.17	4.4	0.0	0.00	0.99	2.8
ThCtAB.bMax	−1.7	−0.30	0.12	4.2	0.7	0.10	0.61	3.3
ThCtAB.cMax	−1.1	−0.18	0.35	5.3	−0.5	−0.09	0.65	3.2
ThCtAB.aMav	−1.4	−0.31	0.11	3.8	−0.3	−0.05	0.79	2.5
ThCtAB.bMav	−1.7	−0.35	0.07	3.5	0.0	0.00	0.98	2.8
ThCtAB.cMav	−1.3	−0.25	0.19	4.5	−0.5	−0.09	0.65	2.8

MC% mean change in percent, *SRM* standardized response mean (= mean change/SD of change), *p* level of significance of change using a paired *t*-test without adjustment for multiple comparisons, *RMSCV%* root mean square coefficient of variation of test–retest acquisitions at baseline, with repositioning in between scans. For other abbreviations, please see Table 11.1. Note that values are given for the "long" femoral region of interest, i.e., a 60% distance between the trochlear notch and the posterior end of both femoral condyles

low rates of change and SRMs, in particular in cMF. Table 11.2 lists the percent change, the SRM, the significance level, and the precision error (test–retest) in MT and cMF (60% ROI) for different morphological variables from this study [29]. In summary, the normalized cartilage volume (VCtAB) and the mean cartilage thickness over the entire subchondral bone area (ThCtAB.Me) tended to be more reproducible and more sensitive to change (SRM up to −0.62) than cartilage volume (SRM up to −0.44), cartilage thickness over the cartilaginous area (ThCcAB; SRM up to −0.48), or maximal cartilage thickness (SRM up to −0.35) [29].

Other publications also reported that the sensitivity to change for ThCtAB or VCtAB was greater than for VC [45, 46], whereas others found comparable SRMs for VC, VCtAB, or ThCtAB [47, 48]. A recent paper [45] reported that, when cartilage loss was relatively rapid (due to high mechanical challenge), "horizontal" cartilage loss (increase in denuded area = dAB) made a stronger contribution to the total cartilage loss (= reduction in ThCtAB), whereas when cartilage loss was relatively slow, the "vertical" cartilage loss (reduction ThCcAB) made a stronger contribution. This finding will need to be confirmed, however, in other cohorts and patho-phyiological conditions. Wirth et al. [49] recently explored the rate and sensitivity to change of the minimal cartilage thickness (ThCtAB.Min) and applied the measurement to central subregions of MT, LT, cMF, and cLF, respectively. In 156 participants of the Osteoarthritis Initiative (OAI), they found the 1-year rate of the ThCtAB.Min changes to be greater than those of ThCtAB.Me, but also reported a greater standard deviation, so that ThCtAB.Min turned out to be less sensitive to change than ThCtAB.Me.

A recent paper [50] investigated the mathematical relationship between the above morphologic measurements and explored whether a subset of the above variables fully reflects differences observed in cartilage in cross-sectional and longitudinal studies. The benefits of this reduction in variables are (a) increased statistical power due to less multiple comparison issues, (b) improved understanding of relationships between the morphologic measures of knee cartilage, and (c) greater efficiency in reporting the results in the literature. Buck et al. used cross-sectional [51] and longitudinal (baseline to 2-year follow-up) 3 T MR image data [52] from 152 women (77 healthy and 75 with knee OA) and found that ThCtAB.tAB, and the percentage of denuded area of the subchondral bone (%dAB) explained >90% of the cross-sectional and longitudinal variation observed in the larger set of cartilage morphology measures, both in healthy and in osteoarthritic knees. The authors therefore recommended these three variables as an efficient subset for describing structural status and change in knee cartilage [50].

In the context of cross-sectional studies, several groups have reported reference values of cartilage morphology in healthy volunteers [38, 53, 54], including templates/atlases for comparison of cartilage thickness distribution patterns between healthy reference subjects and OA patients [44, 55] and reference values for the radiographic joint space width (JSW) [56]. Beattie et al. [56] found that measures of JSW did not significantly decrease with increasing decade, but remained fairly constant throughout the lifespan in either sex; the same was observed for cartilage morphometry measures. The authors suggested that there may therefore be no need to differentiate a T- or Z-score in OA diagnosis, because cartilage thickness and JSW remain constant throughout life in the absence of OA.

Recently, several authors have proposed the measurement of certain anatomically defined subregions within cartilage plates to determine the spatial pattern of cartilage loss [16, 57, 58]. Results obtained with these tools will be presented below.

Imaging Protocols for Measurement of Cartilage Morphology and Their Validation

Quantitative work performed on cartilage with MRI between 1994 and 2006 has been summarized previously [6, 7, 59–65] and will not be reiterated in this review. Briefly, for quantifying cartilage morphology, water-excitation (or fat-suppressed) T1-weighted spoiled gradient recalled echo acquisition in the steady state (SPGR) or fast low angle shot (FLASH) at 1.5 or 3 T represent the current gold standard [7, 64, 66]. Double-echo steady-state imaging (DESS) with water excitation has recently gained interest, because of the faster acquisition time and lower slice thickness that can be achieved (Figs. 11.2 and 11.3) [28, 67–69]. SPGR/FLASH sequences are readily available on virtually all MRI scanners and do not require specific hard- or software, whereas the DESS is currently only available from one vendor [28]. Because the DESS acquires two separate images with different echo times simultaneously, this additionally provides potential opportunity to estimate T2, and to obtain morphological and compositional information of the cartilage from a single high-resolution data set [70]. This approach, however, is still undergoing validation.

The previously mentioned Osteoarthritis Initiative (OAI) (http://www.niams.nih.gov/ne/oi/) is a large research endeavor jointly sponsored by the National Institute of Health (NIH), the National Institute of Arthritis and Musculoskeletal and Skin Diseases (NIAMS), and the pharmaceutical industry. This study in a cohort of 4,800 participants is currently focusing on identifying imaging (and other) biomarkers for predicting and monitoring the onset and progression of symptomatic knee OA using 3 T MRI over a 4-year period. The OAI relies on the previously mentioned nearly isotropic sagittal DESS sequence with water excitation in both knees for quantifying cartilage morphology, and on a coronal FLASH sequence with water excitation in one knee of all participants [71]. Sagittal images have the advantage that all cartilage plates of the knee (including the femoropatellar and femorotibial compartment) are visualized, but suffer from partial volume effects in the internal and external subregions (Fig. 11.4) of the knee cartilage plates. Coronal images, in contrast, can delineate the femorotibial joint and axial images visualize the patella with little partial volume effects, but there is currently no consensus, which of the above is the preferred orientation. However, a direct face-to-face comparison of 2-year changes measured in coronal and sagittal (SPGR) images revealed similar rates and patterns of cartilage loss in the femorotibial joint [72].

The technical accuracy (validity) and test–retest precision (reproducibility) of quantitative cartilage measurements at 1.5 T have been summarized in previous reviews [6, 7]. Analyses based on images acquired with a dedicated 1.0 T extremity scanner were found to be consistent with 1.5 T imaging, albeit less precise (reproducible) [73]. Use of peripheral MRI scanners at lower field potentially permits more widespread distribution of this technology, especially when access to high-field MRI is limited. Also, quantitative cartilage measurements at 0.2 T have been proposed [14, 25, 26, 33–35] but have not been validated versus external standards or measurements at higher field strength, and have shown to display substantially larger precision errors than measurements performed at higher field strength. 3 T cartilage imaging has been cross-calibrated with 1.5 T, and lower precision errors than for 1.5 T imaging were reported when acquiring thinner (coronal) slices of 1.0 mm on a 3 T system [74]. Morphometric analysis from DESS images, as acquired at 3 T in the OAI, was found to be consistent with that from FLASH images and to display similar test–retest precision errors as FLASH in the femorotibial joint, both using unpaired [28] and paired reading approaches [68, 69]. In terms of sensitivity to change, a small comparative study in the OAI pilot study [69], and a comparison of two studies performed on the first release of baseline and year 1 follow-up data in the OAI progression subcohort by two groups [46, 48] found similar rates of change, sensitivity to change, and patterns of cartilage loss in the femorotibial joint. Recently, Wirth et al. [31] performed a direct face-to-face comparison between FLASH and DESS over 1 year longitudinally in 80 knees: The study confirmed a high agreement between cartilage thickness measures as determined from FLASH and DESS cross-sectionally [28] and a similar sensitivity to change of coronal FLASH and sagittal DESS. Further, the study revealed a moderate correlation of the longitudinal 1-year changes, indicating that it may be adequate to pool analyses obtained with FLASH and DESS in larger statistical analyses [31]. Also, the authors found that analysis of every second slice (i.e., obtaining information every 1.4 mm) of the sagittal DESS displayed similar SRMs as compared with segmentation of every 0.7 mm slice, both when either using odd or even slice numbers [31]. Due to the

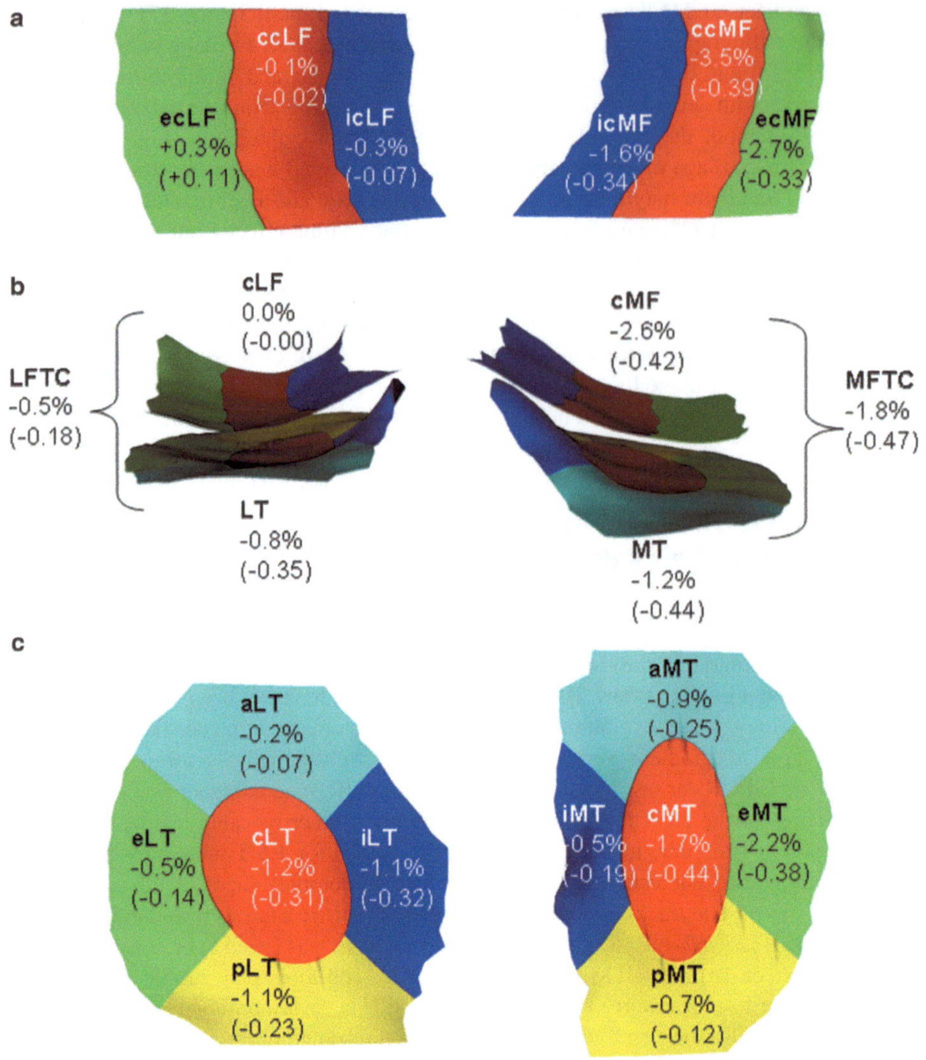

Fig. 11.4 Display of the rates of change (%/annum) and standardized response mean (SRM) in femorotibial cartilage compartments, plates, and subregions. (**a**) View of the weight-bearing part of the medial (cMF) and lateral femoral condyle (cLF) from inferior, (**b**) view of the weight-bearing part of the cMF and cLF and of the medial (MT) and lateral tibia (LT) from posterior and (**c**) view of the MT and LT from superior. For an explanation of the subregion abbreviations, please see Table 11.1. The data represent mean values from three studies: the KLG3 participants of the A 9001140 study ($n=28$) [52] the high risk (BMI > 30; KLG ≥ 2) subcohort from a first release of OAI participants ($n=54$) [46] knees with neutral alignment from the MAK study ($n=74$) [45]

near-isotropic resolution of the sagittal DESS, multiplanar reconstruction (MPR) in the coronal and axial planes is feasible [28, 68, 69]. The rates of (and sensitivity to) change of coronal MPR DESS, however, was similar to that of coronal FLASH and sagittal DESS and did not provide an advantage over the direct analysis of the sagittal DESS [31].

Generally, results from different vendors for cartilage morphometry were shown to be comparable at 1.5 T [75] and at 3 T [76], although one study reported slight offsets between different scanners and protocols from the same vendor [77]. At 3 T, precision errors of cartilage morphometry were observed to be similar for different vendors and scanners in a multicenter trial, and measurements were relatively stable over a 3-month observation period [42]. The stability of geometric measurements over longer periods on phantoms was found to be satisfactory and comparable between several scanners of the same manufacturer over a 3-year period in the OAI [78].

Use of different coils has been evaluated at 3 T: Although the test–retest precision was similar between a phased array and quadrature coil, certain offsets in cartilage morphology outcomes were observed [68]; these prohibit changes of the coil between baseline and follow-up measurements. Cartilage morphometry on images acquired 2 h after intravenous Gd-DTPA injection (for the purpose of simultaneous dGEMRIC imaging) was reported to be highly correlated (r = 0.85–0.95) with that on images obtained before the injection of the contrast agent at baseline [79]. However, a 2-year longitudinal analysis in OA participants reported that the sensitivity to change of post-Gd-DTPA cartilage imaging was substantially less than that from images acquired prior to intravenous Gd-DTPA injection [80].

Rate of Change and Sensitivity to Change in OA

Numerous reports on longitudinal changes of cartilage morphology in subjects with different grades of knee OA have been published [6, 7, 31, 45, 46, 48, 49, 52, 58, 81–88]. These studies have revealed variable results with regard to the rates of cartilage loss and SRM [4, 6, 7]: Two studies reported almost no loss in cartilage volume over a 1-year [88] and 3-year period [81], respectively, whereas other studies reported up to 7% annual cartilage loss in the femorotibial joint [83]. Reasons for this may include variability in imaging and image analysis technology, differences in risk factor profiles between cohorts, differences in study duration, experience and blinding of the readers, and others. A recent study [89] tested the hypothesis that smaller, shorter duration "Proof of Concept" studies may be achievable with 3 T MRI, by selecting populations at high risk of rapid medial femorotibial progression, and using advanced image analysis techniques. Female participants with knee pain, a body mass index (BMI) ≥ 25, radiographic evidence of medial OA, and varus malalignment were monitored over 3 and 6 months, respectively, and anatomically corresponding ROIs were identified on each image by using a three-dimensional statistical shape model of the bone surface. The primary outcome was the change in cartilage thickness in the aspect of cMF that is exposed within the meniscal window during articulation, excluding the peripheral aspects of the femoral surface. Despite these efforts, no change in ThCtAB was detected at the 5% significance level at 3 or 6 months follow-up; the mean change at 3 months from a log-scale ANOVA model was −2.1% [95% confidence interval (CI) (−4.4%, +0.2%)] and the change over 6 months was 0.0% [95% CI (−2.7%, +2.8%)]. Changes in the lateral tibia were significant at 6 month follow-up (−1.5%), but only without correction for multiple comparisons. The authors concluded that the small inconsistent compartment changes and the relatively high variability in cartilage thickness changes seen in the study provided no confidence for a 3- or 6-month study, not even based on a patient population selected for rapid progression [89].

Analyses of the first release of 160 participants of the OAI progression cohort (baseline and year 1 follow-up data) found significant change of up to approximately 2% per annum, with substantially higher rates of progression in the cMF than in the MT, and higher rates in LT than in cLF [46, 48, 49]. However, this pattern of change was not entirely consistent across cohorts when focusing on the SRM rather than on the rate of change [8, 45, 52]. Several studies therefore have taken the approach of additionally reporting the aggregate thickness in the tibia and weight-bearing femur (MFTC or LFTC) [45, 46, 52, 68, 90]. One study suggested that longitudinal changes in VC in the tibia and in the weight-bearing femur are highly correlated [83], and that the measurement of only tibial cartilage is therefore sufficient. However, given that at least some cohorts appear to display larger changes and higher SRMs in the weight-bearing femur than in the tibia [46, 48, 49], this approach has limitations.

Medial and lateral femorotibial cartilage loss as well as patellar cartilage loss was found to be not significantly associated with each other [91]. The ratio of medial versus lateral cartilage loss was reported to be 1.4:1 in knees with neutral biomechanical alignment, consistent with higher mechanical loads being transferred across the medial compartment in neutral knees [45]. In varus knees, the ratio was 3.7:1, and in valgus knees it was 1:6.0, confirming that knee alignment is an important determinant of medial versus lateral cartilage loss [45].

After anterior cruciate ligament rupture, a reduction of cartilage volume and thickness was observed in the femoral trochlea, while an increase was found in the weight-bearing medial femur [92]. The latter observation may be consistent with cartilage swelling or hypertrophy observed as a sign of early OA in various animal models [93–97]. A recent cross-sectional study found significantly thicker cartilage in the medial compartment of participants with medial radiographic KLG2 OA compared with healthy knees [51], and significantly thinner cartilage in some subregions in knees with medial radiographic OA with joint space narrowing (JSN, i.e., KLG3). These findings have suggested that there may be an initial phase of cartilage swelling/hypertrophy in knee OA, particularly at the KLG2 stage where osteophytes form, but where no reduction in JSW is yet observed. This has been supported by recent longitudinal observations by Buck et al. [98], who explored whether the 2-year longitudinal change in cartilage thickness in femorotibial subregions (see below) of knees with radiographic osteoarthritis (ROA) differed from that in healthy knees. Knees from 75 women with definite signs of medial radiographic OA were compared with 77 asymptomatic healthy controls without radiographic OA. A substantial portion of ROA knees were classified as having longitudinal cartilage thinning (28%) or thickening (20%) in at least one medial femorotibial subregion compared with longitudinal changes in healthy knees, and only 5% showed both subregional thinning and thickening at the same time, across (different) medial subregions. Whereas the estimated proportion of KLG3 knees with significant medial cartilage thinning (46%) was substantially greater than that with cartilage thickening (18%), the estimated percentages of KLG2 knees with significant medial thinning (20%) and thickening (23%) were similar. The authors concluded that OA may not be a one-way-road of cartilage loss and that particularly in early radiographic OA, cartilage changes may occur in both directions simultaneously, i.e., cartilage thinning and cartilage thickening. This may provide a reason why relatively small (and variable) rates of change have been observed in OA cohorts, and why short-term trials are challenging [89].

Spatial Patterns of Cartilage Loss in OA/Subregional Analysis

As mentioned above, recent efforts have been focused on measuring anatomically defined subregions within cartilages [16, 57, 58], with the aim of elucidating spatial pattern of cartilage thinning, and to potentially identify (sub)regions with increased rates of (and sensitivity to) cartilage loss in intervention trials.

Cross-sectional Studies

The previously mentioned cross-sectional study by Hellio Le Graverand et al. [51] reported that cartilage "thickening" in KLG2 knees with medial osteophytes (compared with controls) was particularly obvious in the anterior subregion of the MT, in the external and internal subregions of cMF and cLF. Cartilage "thinning" in knees with medial JSN (KLG3) was most evident in the central subregion of the cMF and in the external subregion of the MT, and in the internal subregion of the LT. Although these differences were generally not affected when possible effects of demographic covariates (height and BMI) were considered, it is difficult to exclude confounding by inter-person differences in cross-sectional studies. Therefore, Eckstein et al. [99] performed a within-person, between-knee comparison in 80 participants of the OAI who displayed medial JSN in one knee, but no medial or lateral JSN in the contralateral knee. The strength of this approach is that it rules out confounding from person-specific demographic features, and that it is potentially more sensitive to detecting differences cross-sectionally, given the much smaller magnitude of side differences between knees within the same (healthy) person compared with differences across (healthy) subjects [100]. The authors estimated the magnitude of cartilage thickness reductions to be 190 μm (5.2%) in the medial femorotibial compartment (MFTC) with JSN OARSI grade 1, 630 μm (18%) with OARSI grade 2, and 1,560 μm (44%) with OARSI grade 3 [101, 102]. Side differences were greater in cMF than in MT, and greater in MT than in pMT [99]. Within MT, the greatest differences were observed in the external and central subregions, and within MF the greatest differences were observed in the central subregion of the weight-bearing portion of MF. When evaluating A-P subregions in the MF, the greatest differences between mJSN and contralateral no-mJSN knees were observed in regions located between 30° and 75° at the MF.

Longitudinal Studies

A study by Pelletier et al. [58] reported that the rate of change in cartilage morphology in the central aspects of the femorotibial joint exceeded that in total cartilage plates, but found that the SRM was not improved because of the higher variability of subregional changes [47]. Wirth et al. [49] found the sensitivity to change (SRM) in the central MT to be slightly greater than for the total MT, but this was not the case in the cMF.

Figure 11.4 summarizes the rates of change (%/annum) and the sensitivity to change (SRM) for different subregions from three published studies:

(a) A 2-year multicenter study at 3 T (Pfizer A 9001140). Because healthy reference participants and participants with KLG 2 did not show significant changes in cartilage morphology [52], results are shown for KLG 3 participants only ($n=28$).
(b) The second cohort included is a first release of baseline and year 1 follow-up data from the OAI progression subcohort [49]. Results of a subcohort with a high risk of progression (BMI > 30; KLG ≥ 2) were included ($n=54$).
(c) The third cohort included was from the MAK study [9, 45]. Data from a subcohort of participants with neutral knee alignment were included in the analysis ($n=74$).

As reported previously [8], the central and external part of cMF, and the external and central aspect of MT displayed the relatively greatest change across subregions in the MFTC (Fig. 11.4). With the exception of the external medial femur, these regions consistently displayed greater changes than the total cartilage plate across the studies. In the LFTC, the central, internal, and posterior LT displayed the relatively greatest changes, and no relevant average changes (across studies) were observed in the cLF (Fig. 11.4). Rates of change in the central and internal LT were consistently greater than those for the total cartilage plates. Please note that the patterns for the sensitivity to change (SRM; Fig. 11.4) are similar to those of the rates of change, but not identical. Consistent with other observations [47], the authors found that the sensitivity to change in the subregions was not consistently higher than in the total plates across studies. Only the analysis of the central medial and lateral femorotibial compartments revealed consistently greater SRMs than the analysis of the entire MFTC and LFTC, respectively.

Wirth et al. [103] recently presented a method which extended the previously developed method of subregions in the weight-bearing femorotibial joint [16] to anterior-posteriorly spaced subregions across the entire femoral condyle. This method was applied to participants from the OAI and confirmed that cartilage thinning in the anterior (weight-bearing) region of the MF was greater than that in the posterior aspect of the MF. The authors reported the greatest longitudinal changes (and SRM) to be located at 30–60° (from the trochlear notch [0°] to the posterior/superior end of the MF [150°], with a slight variation between knees with different OARSI JSN grades.

Ordered Value Approach (Subregion Ranking)

Buck et al. [104] analyzed patterns of subregional cartilage change [16] in individual knees and found highly variable patterns. For comparing the rate of change between two groups (i.e., ROA knees with healthy knees, or DMOAD treated knees with control knees) he therefore recommended the use of an ordered values (OV) or ranking system, in which the subregional changes (in MFTC) were assigned to ranked orders in each knee, i.e., the subregion with greatest magnitude of cartilage thinning to OV1, the one with the second greatest magnitude to OV2, and the one with the smallest magnitude of cartilage thinning (or with the greatest magnitude of cartilage thickening) to the highest rank order. When averaging longitudinal changes in cartilage thickness (ThCtAB) across these OVs (which vary in location across subjects), the authors found that the minimal p-value (Wilcoxon) for the differences in 2-year change in medial cartilage thickness in a relatively small number of knees with radiographic OA and JSN (KLG3) versus healthy knees (KLG0) was $p=0.001$, with OV1–OV4 displaying significant differences between both groups. When averaging changes across compartments, plates, or subregions (i.e., the conventional approach), in contrast, only one medial subregion displayed significant differences (in the rate of change) between KLG3 and KLG0 knees ($p=0.037$). Cartilage thickening was significantly greater in knees with radiographic OA (definite osteophytes) without JSN (KLG2) versus KLG0 knees in one medial subregion using the conventional approach ($p=0.02$), but in two OVs using the ordered values approach (minimal $p=0.007$). The authors concluded that the ordered values approach was more sensitive in detecting cartilage thinning in KLG3 and cartilage thickening in KLG2 versus KLG0 knees, respectively. The authors also suggested that this method was particularly useful in the context of comparing a cohort treated with a disease-modifying OA drug versus one treated with a placebo, or in detecting risk factors of OA progression.

Wirth [105] recently extended this approach to include eight medial and eight lateral ($n=16$) subregions. They reported significantly greater cartilage loss in KLG3 than in KLG2 knees, the ordered value approach again displaying much smaller p-values than the conventional approach. This opens new possibilities of including participants with medial and lateral OA (or with varus and valgus malalignment) into a study, without the need of defining cartilage thickness changes in a certain compartment, plate, or subregion as the primary endpoint. The relevant question would then *not* be whether a certain risk factor is associated with or whether a drug can modify cartilage thickness changes in a given location (region), *but* whether the risk factor is associated with or whether the drug can modify the change in cartilage thickness wherever it occurs in an individual knee.

Comparison of MRI with Radiographic Changes in OA

Several studies found only weak correlations between MRI-detected cartilage loss and OA progression in radiography [84, 88, 106]. However, a recent publication reported a higher correlation when the longitudinal reduction in JSW in radiographs was compared with cartilage loss in the central aspect of the MFTC [58]. Whereas some studies found a higher rate and sensitivity to change of cartilage morphology compared with radiography [84, 86, 107], a recent one reported a somewhat greater SRM (−0.62) for fluoroscopy-based Lyon Schuss radiography versus ThCtAB of the MT measured with MRI (−0.59) [52]. However, the authors found the SRM for fixed flexion radiography, a commonly used non-fluoroscopic protocol, which is also used in the OAI [108–112], to be substantially less (SRM = −0.20) in the same study [52]. The authors argued that the relatively high SRM of the minimal JSW measured by Lyon Schuss may be due to the fluoroscopic guidance providing optimal alignment of the anterior and posterior tibial rim, and to radiography being performed under weight-bearing conditions where the cartilage tissue is compressed, while MRI is performed in a supine non-weight-bearing position. Also, it must be kept in mind that radiographic assessment of JSW depends also on meniscal extrusion, and not only on cartilage thickness [113–115] and that meniscus pathology, in particularly subluxation, can therefore cause changes in JSW over time in the absence of cartilage loss. Duryea et al. recently compared the responsiveness (=sensitivity to change) of radiography with that of MRI in the first release of the OAI cohort (150 subjects) over 12 months [116]. The radiographic JSW measurements relied on automated software to delineate the femoral and tibial margins [117, 118]. Measures included the medial compartment minimum JSW and JSW at fixed locations, which were compared to previously published cartilage morphology measures [48]. The SRM value for radiographic JSW measured at the optimal fixed location was −0.32 compared to −0.39 for the most responsive MRI measure. For a subgroup with KLG2 or KLG3 knees, the most responsive SRM values were −0.34 and −0.42, respectively. The authors concluded that new (fixed distance) measures of JSW changes provide a similar sensitivity to change as MRI and compare favorably in view of the cost effectiveness of the two imaging modalities.

Risk Factors of Cartilage Loss Identified by Quantitative Cartilage Morphometry

Great interest is directed at identifying risk factors (predictors) of subsequent cartilage loss, both to understand the pathophysiology of the disease and to be able to identify so-called fast progressors for inclusion in pharmacological intervention studies that attempt to show protection from structural change over relatively short periods (e.g., [89]). This paragraph will focus on studies that have reported correlations between risk factors of progression and *quantitative* measures of cartilage morphology, but not those that have relied on semiquantitative scoring of MRI or quantitative measurement of JSW. The list of (potential) risk factors for cartilage loss is not meant to be complete, but encompasses important examples examined both from cross-sectional and longitudinal studies. Risk factors associated with higher rates of progression were the following.

- *Advanced radiographic OA and low cartilage thickness at baseline.* Opposite to earlier assumptions, recent evidence suggests that advanced radiographic OA (JSN) is one of the strongest predictors of fast progression. There has been evidence that knees with higher KL grades and increased JSN [46, 49, 52, 58] display greater rates of (and sensitivity to) change than those with lower KL grades and without baseline JSN. An analysis of specific radiographic features in a sample from the OAI found that osteophyte status (at baseline) was not associated with medial cartilage loss over 12 months, that knees with medial joint space narrowing showed a trend towards higher rates of change than those without, and that knees with medial femoral subchondral bone sclerosis displayed significantly greater rates of progression than those without [119]. The same study also found that low baseline cartilage thickness was a strong predictor of longitudinal loss in cartilage thickness [119], whereas an earlier study had reported that higher baseline cartilage volume [82] was strongly associated with increased cartilage loss. A within-person, between-knee comparison in painful knees selected from the OAI [30] recently reported that the cartilage loss was greater in knee with radiographic JSN than in contralateral knees without JSN in the same subjects, and that the side differences were greater with higher grades of JSN. Progression was particularly fast in the small subgroup with OARSI JSN grade 3 knees [30].
- *Meniscal extrusion and tears/damage* [58, 85, 86]: Meniscal tears were found to be associated with greater tibial plateau bone area, but not with reduced tibial cartilage volume in a 2-year longitudinal study [120]. However, Sharma et al. [9] reported a significant relationship of cartilage loss with meniscal tears, albeit not with meniscal extrusion. A recent analysis found site-specific relationships between local meniscal tears and subregional cartilage loss, suggesting that a tear in the anterior horn, central part, or posterior horn of the meniscus was associated with increased cartilage loss in adjacent tibial subregions [121]. Crema et al. [122] reported grade 2 and 3 medial meniscus lesions to be associated with greater cartilage loss in the femorotibial compartment, but not grade 1 lesion (=intrasubstance meniscal signal changes) and concluded that the protective function of the meniscus was still preserved in cases of these early lesions. Recent evidence suggests that the meniscus may undergo a phase of hypertrophy in OA [123, 124]. Raynauld et al. [125] observed that selecting a subcohort of participants with meniscal tears/extrusion did not improve the ability to identify treatment effects of a potentially structure-modifying drug, because of the larger standard deviation of the change in the participants with meniscal pathology.
- *Knee malalignment and adduction moment.* A strong relationship was observed between (varus and valgus) malalignment and the ratio of cartilage loss in MFTC versus LFTC [9, 45, 126, 127]. After adjustment for meniscal changes, the study by Sharma et al. [9] found that varus malalignment and medial meniscus damage both predicted medial tibial cartilage volume (and thickness) loss. In contrast, medial–lateral joint laxity, measured with a device applying a fixed varus and valgus load, was not found to have consistent effects and was not a significant predictor of cartilage loss in models fully adjusted for alignment and meniscal damage [9]. Teichtahl et al. [128] showed increases in varus malalignment between baseline and follow-up to be associated with an increase in the rate of MT cartilage loss, whereas there was no significant correlation with the rate of cartilage loss of the LT. The authors concluded that methods to reduce progression of varus alignment may also delay the progression of medial

femorotibial OA. Frontal plane knee valgus malalignment was also correlated with patellar cartilage loss [129]. In a largely non-arthritic cohort, in contrast, no correlation between cartilage loss and malalignment was identified [130]. A recent cross-sectional analysis revealed that a higher peak knee adduction moment was observed in participants with medial compared to those with lateral meniscal tears [131]. Participants with a higher knee adduction moment displayed a larger medial meniscus extrusion and lower medial meniscus height, whereas the inverse relationship was observed for the lateral meniscus. A higher knee adduction moment was also associated with a higher ratio of the medial to lateral tibial subchondral bone area, whereas cartilage thickness and denuded areas in the tibia and femur were not related to the knee adduction moment. Similar results were found for the relationship between knee adduction angular impulse and meniscus, cartilage, and bone morphology [131].

- *High BMI* [46, 49, 58, 84, 86, 91, 132]: This relationship was also suggested to exist in the patella in subjects without OA [133].
- *Bone marrow alterations* [58, 86]: Raynauld et al. [125] reported that although bone marrow lesions and cysts did not increase significantly in size over 24 months in an OA cohort, there was a significant correlation between size change of bone marrow lesions and cysts with the loss of cartilage volume in the medial femorotibial compartment. A relationship between very large bone marrow lesions and lateral tibial cartilage loss was also reported in asymptomatic persons [134, 135].
- *Focal cartilage lesions or defects, as graded by visual scoring* [136, 137] *and denuded areas, as determined quantitatively from MRI* [119, 138, 139]: Cartilage defects at baseline (visual scoring) appeared to be associated with longitudinal measurement of quantitative cartilage loss in the same compartment in OA subjects, although the second of the two above studies [137] only found a significant relationship in the femoropatellar but not in the femorotibial joint. Other studies reported that the presence of cartilage defects predicted knee cartilage loss also in asymptomatic individuals without radiographic knee OA [140, 141]. It was hypothesized that tibial subchondral bone area expansion may lead to the development of knee cartilage defects (which are associated with future cartilage loss) and is predictive of the need for knee joint replacement in subjects with knee OA, independent of radiographic change [142]. Morphometric studies have recently provided evidence that areas of denuded subchondral bone (dABs), as determined by segmentation at baseline, were also relatively strong predictors of subsequent cartilage loss [119]. Hunter et al. [143] reported that in a subsample of knees with no denuded area (at baseline) the SRM for subsequent cartilage volume loss was −0.25, whereas it was −0.30 in the knees with intermediate denuded area, and −1.0 in knees with severe denuded area. Denuded areas were observed to either originate from cartilage loss or from internal osteophytes [139]: In an OA cohort from the OAI, almost half of the men and a third of the women displayed dABs; 61% of the dABs represented internal osteophytes. One of 47 knees with KLG0 displayed any dAB, whereas 29 of the 32 KLG4 knees were affected. There were significant relationships of dAB with increasing KL grades ($p < 0.001$) and with ipsi-compartimental JSN. Internal osteophytes were more frequent laterally (mainly posterior tibia and internal femur), whereas full thickness cartilage loss was more frequent medially (mainly external tibia and femur).
- *Other risk factors*: Some evidence has been provided that smoking may be associated with increased cartilage loss [144, 145], but other factors such as age, sex, pain, function, physical activity levels, synovitis (effusion), sex hormone levels, and serum or urine biomarkers were not consistently found to be associated with cartilage thinning measured quantitatively with MRI and studies have produced partially contradictory results.

Correlation of Cartilage Loss with Clinical Outcome, and Treatment Response in OA

Estimates of tibial cartilage loss over 2 years were suggested to be correlated with those over 4.5 years, albeit the authors did not report the consistency of the longitudinal changes in the second versus the first observation period [146]. More importantly, however, the rate of change in VC over 2 years was significantly associated with total knee arthroplasty (TKA) at year 4 [146]: For every 1% increase in the rate of cartilage loss there was a 20% increased risk of undergoing TKA and participants in the highest tertile of tibial cartilage loss had a 7.1 higher odds of TKA than those in the lowest tertile. In contrast, radiographic scores of OA did not predict TKA in the same study. A more recent study concluded from the same sample that when subchondral bone cysts are present, cartilage loss and risk of knee replacement are higher than if only bone marrow lesions are present, suggesting that cysts identify those most likely to benefit from prevention of disease progression [147]. These are principally important findings as they link cartilage morphology, as a potential surrogate measure of disease progression, to a clinical outcome (i.e., how a patient feels or functions, or how long the knee "survives" [TKA]).

Raynauld et al. [107] recently reported that licofelone (a drug that inhibits both cyclooxygenase and lipoxygenase) significantly reduced cartilage loss over time when averaged over both femorotibial compartment, and that MRI was superior to radiographs in demonstrating a structure-modifying effect in this multicentre trial. Interestingly, the effects were significant only in the lateral, but not in the medial compartment, although the participants had been selected for medial femorotibial radiographic OA and the medial compartment had thus been defined as the primary endpoint. To date, no structure- or disease-modifying drug (SMOAD or DMOAD) has yet been approved by regulatory agencies, neither based on radiographic nor on MRI-based evidence of structure modification in knee cartilage.

Future Directions

Baseline, 12-month and 24-month follow-up radiographic and MRI data have been made publicly available for approximately 4,800 participants of the OAI cohort (http://www.niams.nih.gov/ne/oi/), and clinical data have been released for the 36-month time point. Quantitative data on cartilage morphology at baseline and 12-month follow-up from two groups are publicly available for the first release of 160 OA participants (image data sets 0.B.1 and 1.B.1), and baseline, 12-month, and 24-month follow-up data from the first 107 cases of a core sample of approximately 650 knees, for which central radiographic readings, quantitative measurement of JSW, and cartilage morphometry data are available, will be released in the near future. This and the results of other large epidemiological studies will provide ample opportunity for collaborative research and should allow the research community to make rapid progress in understanding the risk factors involved in quantitative cartilage loss in OA. Most importantly, it will allow one to determine which imaging biomarkers can best predict clinical outcomes, such as real or virtual TKA. This will be an important step in validating novel cartilage imaging biomarkers and approaches as surrogate measures of disease progression, particularly in therapeutic intervention trials. Once the clinical importance of these imaging biomarkers are established, further improvements in imaging hardware, coils, sequences, and image analysis algorithms may foster a more automated analysis of cartilage morphology, composition, and other articular tissues than currently possible. This will be of particular importance once structure- or disease-modifying drugs become available, as this may require monitoring the treatment response in large sets of OA patients. Currently, quantitative MRI of articular cartilage represents a very powerful research tool in experimental, epidemiological, and pharmacological intervention studies. Once structure- or disease-modifying drugs (SMOADs or DMOADs) will become available, quantitative MRI of the cartilage may also play a more important role in clinical decision making and practice.

References

1. Ateshian GA, Lai WM, Zhu WB, Mow VC. An asymptotic solution for the contact of two biphasic cartilage layers. J Biomech. 1994;27(11):1347–60.
2. Le Graverand MP, Mazzuca S, Lassere M, Guermazi A, Pickering E, Brandt K, et al. Assessment of the radioanatomic positioning of the osteoarthritic knee in serial radiographs: comparison of three acquisition techniques. Osteoarthritis Cartilage. 2006;14 Suppl A: 37–43.
3. Cline GA, Meyer JM, Stevens R, Buckland-Wright C, Peterfy C, Beary JF. Comparison of fixed flexion, fluoroscopic semi-flexed and MTP radiographic methods for obtaining the minimum medial joint space width of the knee in longitudinal osteoarthritis trials. Osteoarthritis Cartilage. 2006;14(Suppl A):A32–6. Epub 2006 May 8:A32–6.
4. Guermazi A, Burstein D, Conaghan P, Eckstein F, Hellio Le Graverand-Gastineau MP, Keen H, et al. Imaging in osteoarthritis. Rheum Dis Clin North Am. 2008;34(3):645–87.
5. Hunter DJ, Conaghan PG, Peterfy CG, Bloch D, Guermazi A, Woodworth T, et al. Responsiveness, effect size, and smallest detectable difference of Magnetic Resonance Imaging in knee osteoarthritis. Osteoarthritis Cartilage. 2006;14 Suppl 1:112–15. Epub 2006 May 5:112–5.
6. Eckstein F, Burstein D, Link TM. Quantitative MRI of cartilage and bone: degenerative changes in osteoarthritis. NMR Biomed. 2006;19(7):822–54.
7. Eckstein F, Cicuttini F, Raynauld JP, Waterton JC, Peterfy C. Magnetic resonance imaging (MRI) of articular cartilage in knee osteoarthritis (OA): morphological assessment. Osteoarthritis Cartilage. 2006;14 Suppl 1:46–75.
8. Eckstein F, Guermazi A, Roemer FW. Quantitative MR imaging of cartilage and trabecular bone in osteoarthritis. Radiol Clin North Am. 2009;47(4):655–73.
9. Sharma L, Eckstein F, Song J, Guermazi A, Prasad P, Kapoor D, et al. Relationship of meniscal damage, meniscal extrusion, malalignment, and joint laxity to subsequent cartilage loss in osteoarthritic knees. Arthritis Rheum. 2008;58(6):1716–26.
10. Peterfy CG, Guermazi A, Zaim S, Tieman PF, Miaux Y, White D, et al. Whole-Organ Magnetic Resonance Imaging Score (WORMS) of the knee in osteoarthritis. Osteoarthritis Cartilage. 2004;12(3):177–90.
11. Reichenbach S, Yang M, Eckstein F, Niu J, Hunter DJ, McLennan CE, et al. Does cartilage volume or thickness distinguish knees with and without mild radiographic osteoarthritis? The Framingham Study. Ann Rheum Dis. 2010;69(1):143–9.
12. Hohe J, Faber S, Stammberger T, Reiser M, Englmeier KH, Eckstein F. A technique for 3D in vivo quantification of proton density and magnetization transfer coefficients of knee joint cartilage. Osteoarthritis Cartilage. 2000;8(6):426–33.
13. Hohe J, Faber S, Muehlbauer R, Reiser M, Englmeier KH, Eckstein F. Three-dimensional analysis and visualization of regional MR signal intensity distribution of articular cartilage. Med Eng Phys. 2002; 24(3):219–27.
14. Qazi AA, Folkesson J, Pettersen PC, Karsdal MA, Christiansen C, Dam EB. Separation of healthy and early osteoarthritis by automatic quantification of cartilage homogeneity. Osteoarthritis Cartilage. 2007;15(10):1199–206.
15. Eckstein F, Ateshian G, Burgkart R, Burstein D, Cicuttini F, Dardzinski B, et al. Proposal for a nomenclature for magnetic resonance imaging based measures of articular cartilage in osteoarthritis. Osteoarthritis Cartilage. 2006;14(10):974–83.
16. Wirth W, Eckstein F. A technique for regional analysis of femorotibial cartilage thickness based on quantitative magnetic resonance imaging. IEEE Trans Med Imaging. 2008;27(6):737–44.

17. McWalter EJ, Wirth W, Siebert M, Eisenhart-Roth, Hudelmaier M, Wilson DR. Use of novel interactive input devices for segmentation of articular cartilage from magnetic resonance images. Osteoarthritis Cartilage. 2005;13(1):48–53.
18. Solloway S, Hutchinson CE, Waterton JC, Taylor CJ. The use of active shape models for making thickness measurements of articular cartilage from MR images. Magn Reson Med. 1997;37(6): 943–52.
19. Stammberger T, Eckstein F, Michaelis M, Englmeier KH, Reiser M. Interobserver reproducibility of quantitative cartilage measurements: comparison of B-spline snakes and manual segmentation. Magn Reson Imaging. 1999;17(7):1033–42.
20. Cohen ZA, McCarthy DM, Kwak SD, Legrand P, Fogarasi F, Ciaccio EJ, et al. Knee cartilage topography, thickness, and contact areas from MRI: in-vitro calibration and in-vivo measurements. Osteoarthritis Cartilage. 1999;7(1):95–109.
21. Lynch JA, Zaim S, Zhao J, Stork A, Peterfy CG, Genant HK. Cartilage segmentation of 3D MRI scans of the osteoarthritic knee combining juser knowledge and active contours. Proc SPIE (Int Soc Opt Eng). 2000;3979:925–35.
22. Cashman PM, Kitney RI, Gariba MA, Carter ME. Automated techniques for visualization and mapping of articular cartilage in MR images of the osteoarthritic knee: a base technique for the assessment of microdamage and submicro damage. IEEE Trans Nanobioscience. 2002;1(1):42–51.
23. Kauffmann C, Gravel P, Godbout B, Gravel A, Beaudoin G, Raynauld JP, et al. Computer-aided method for quantification of cartilage thickness and volume changes using MRI: validation study using a synthetic model. IEEE Trans Biomed Eng. 2003; 50(8):978–88.
24. Pathak SD, Ng L, Wyman B, Fogarasi S, Racki S, Oelund JC, et al. Quantitative image analysis: software systems in drug development trials. Drug Discov Today. 2003;8(10):451–8.
25. Folkesson J, Dam E, Olsen OF, Pettersen P, Christiansen C. Automatic segmentation of the articular cartilage in knee MRI using a hierarchical multi-class classification scheme. Med Image Comput Comput Assist. 2005;8(Pt 1):327–34.
26. Folkesson J, Dam EB, Olsen OF, Pettersen PC, Christiansen C. Segmenting articular cartilage automatically using a voxel classification approach. IEEE Trans Med Imaging. 2007;26(1):106–15.
27. Glaser C, Burgkart R, Kutschera A, Englmeier KH, Reiser M, Eckstein F. Femoro-tibial cartilage metrics from coronal MR image data: technique, test-retest reproducibility, and findings in osteoarthritis. Magn Reson Med. 2003;50(6):1229–36.
28. Eckstein F, Hudelmaier M, Wirth W, Kiefer B, Jackson R, Yu J, et al. Double echo steady state magnetic resonance imaging of knee articular cartilage at 3 Tesla: a pilot study for the Osteoarthritis Initiative. Ann Rheum Dis. 2006;65(4):433–41.
29. Hudelmaier M, Wirth W, Wehr B, Kraus V, Wyman BT, Hellio Le Graverand MP, et al. Femorotibial cartilage morphology – reproducibility, of different metrics and femoral regions, and sensitivity to change in disease. Cells Tissues Organs. 2010;192(5):340–50.
30. Eckstein F, Benichou O, Wirth W, Nelson DR, Maschek S, Hudelmaier M, et al. Direct comparison of cartilage loss in painful contra-lateral knees with and without joint space narrowing – data from the Osteoarthritis Initiative (OAI). Arthritis Care Res. 2009;61(9):1218–25.
31. Wirth W, Nevitt M, Hellio Le Graverand MP, Benichou O, Dreher D, Davies RY, et al. Sensitivity to change of cartilage morphometry using coronal FLASH, sagittal DESS, and coronal MPR DESS protocols – comparative data from the osteoarthritis initiative (OAI). Osteoarthritis Cartilage. 2010;18(4):547–54. Epub 2009 Dec 21.
32. Hohe J, Ateshian G, Reiser M, Englmeier KH, Eckstein F. Surface size, curvature analysis, and assessment of knee joint incongruity with MRI in vivo. Magn Reson Med. 2002;47(3):554–61.
33. Dam EB, Folkesson J, Pettersen PC, Christiansen C. Automatic morphometric cartilage quantification in the medial tibial plateau from MRI for osteoarthritis grading. Osteoarthritis Cartilage. 2007;15(7):808–18.
34. Folkesson J, Dam EB, Olsen OF, Christiansen C. Accuracy evaluation of automatic quantification of the articular cartilage surface curvature from MRI. Acad Radiol. 2007;14(10):1221–8.
35. Folkesson J, Dam EB, Olsen OF, Karsdal MA, Pettersen PC, Christiansen C. Automatic quantification of local and global articular cartilage surface curvature: biomarkers for osteoarthritis? Magn Reson Med. 2008;59(6):1340–6.
36. Qazi AA, Dam EB, Nielsen M, Karsdal MA, Pettersen PC, Christiansen C. Osteoarthritic cartilage is more homogeneous than healthy cartilage: identification of a superior region of interest colocalized with a major risk factor for osteoarthritis. Acad Radiol. 2007;14(10):1209–20.
37. Eckstein F, Mosher T, Hunter D. Imaging of knee osteoarthritis: data beyond the beauty. Curr Opin Rheumatol. 2007;19(5): 435–43.
38. Burgkart R, Glaser C, Hinterwimmer S, Hudelmaier M, Englmeier KH, Reiser M, et al. Feasibility of T and Z scores from magnetic resonance imaging data for quantification of cartilage loss in osteoarthritis. Arthritis Rheum. 2003;48(10):2829–35.
39. Faber SC, Eckstein F, Lukasz S, Muhlbauer R, Hohe J, Englmeier KH, et al. Gender differences in knee joint cartilage thickness, volume and articular surface areas: assessment with quantitative three-dimensional MR imaging. Skeletal Radiol. 2001;30(3): 144–50.
40. Otterness IG, Eckstein F. Women have thinner cartilage and smaller joint surfaces than men after adjustment for body height and weight. Osteoarthritis Cartilage. 2007;15(6):666–72.
41. Wang Y, Ding C, Wluka AE, Davis S, Ebeling PR, Jones G, et al. Factors affecting progression of knee cartilage defects in normal subjects over 2 years. Rheumatology (Oxford). 2006;45(1): 79–84.
42. Eckstein F, Buck RJ, Burstein D, Charles HC, Crim J, Hudelmaier M, et al. Precision of 3.0 Tesla quantitative magnetic resonance imaging of cartilage morphology in a multicentre clinical trial. Ann Rheum Dis. 2008;67(12):1683–8.
43. Eckstein F, Hudelmaier M, Cahue S, Marshall M, Sharma L. Medial-to-lateral ratio of tibiofemoral subchondral bone area is adapted to alignment and mechanical load. Calcif Tissue Int. 2009;84(3):186–94.
44. Cohen ZA, Mow VC, Henry JH, Levine WN, Ateshian GA. Templates of the cartilage layers of the patellofemoral joint and their use in the assessment of osteoarthritic cartilage damage. Osteoarthritis Cartilage. 2003;11(8):569–79.
45. Eckstein F, Wirth W, Hudelmaier M, Stein V, Lengfelder V, Cahue S, et al. Patterns of femorotibial cartilage loss in knees with neutral, varus, and valgus alignment. Arthritis Rheum. 2008;59(11): 1563–70.
46. Eckstein F, Maschek S, Wirth W, Wyman B, Nevitt M, Le Graverand MP, et al. One year change of knee cartilage morphology in the first release of participants from the Osteoarthritis Initiative progression subcohort: association with sex, body mass index, symptoms and radiographic osteoarthritis status. Ann Rheum Dis. 2009;68(5):674–9.
47. Raynauld JP, Martel-Pelletier J, Abram F, Dorais M, Haraoui B, Choquette D, et al. Analysis of the precision and sensitivity to change of different approaches to assess cartilage loss by quantitative MRI in a longitudinal multicentre clinical trial in patients with knee osteoarthritis. Arthritis Res Ther. 2008;10(6):R129.
48. Hunter DJ, Niu J, Zhang Y, Totterman S, Tamez J, Dabrowski C, et al. Change in cartilage morphometry: a sample of the progression cohort of the Osteoarthritis Initiative. Ann Rheum Dis. 2009;68(3):349–56.

49. Wirth W, Hellio Le Graverand MP, Wyman BT, Maschek S, Hudelmaier M, Hitzl W, et al. Regional analysis of femorotibial cartilage loss in a subsample from the Osteoarthritis Initiative progression subcohort. Osteoarthritis Cartilage. 2009;17(3):291–7.
50. Buck RJ, Wyman BT, Le Graverand MP, Wirth W, Eckstein F. An efficient subset of morphological measures for articular cartilage in the healthy and diseased human knee. Magn Reson Med. 2010;63(3):680–90.
51. Hellio Le Graverand MP, Buck RJ, Wyman BT, E Vignon, Mazzuca SA, Brandt KD, et al. Subregional femorotibial cartilage morphology in women – comparison between healthy controls and participants with different grades of radiographic knee osteoarthritis. Osteoarthritis Cartilage. 2009;17:1177–85.
52. Hellio Le Graverand MP, Buck RJ, Wyman BT, Vignon E, Mazzuca SA, Brandt KD, et al. Change in regional cartilage morphology and joint space width in osteoarthritis participants versus healthy controls – a multicenter study using 3.0 Tesla MRI and Lyon Schuss radiography. Ann Rheum Dis. 2010;69(1):155–62.
53. Hudelmaier M, Glaser C, Hohe J, Englmeier KH, Reiser M, Putz R, et al. Age-related changes in the morphology and deformational behavior of knee joint cartilage. Arthritis Rheum. 2001;44(11): 2556–61.
54. Eckstein F, Reiser M, Englmeier KH, Putz R. In vivo morphometry and functional analysis of human articular cartilage with quantitative magnetic resonance imaging – from image to data, from data to theory. Anat Embryol (Berl). 2001;203(3):147–73.
55. Tameem HZ, Selva LE, Sinha US. Morphological atlases of knee cartilage: shape indices to analyze cartilage degradation in osteoarthritic and non-osteoarthritic population. Conf Proc IEEE Eng Med Biol Soc. 2007;2007:1310–13.
56. Beattie KA, Duryea J, Pui M, O'Neill J, Boulos P, Webber CE, et al. Minimum joint space width and tibial cartilage morphology in the knees of healthy individuals: a cross-sectional study. BMC Musculoskelet Disord. 2008;9:119.
57. Koo S, Gold GE, Andriacchi TP. Considerations in measuring cartilage thickness using MRI: factors influencing reproducibility and accuracy. Osteoarthritis Cartilage. 2005;13(9):782–9.
58. Pelletier JP, Raynauld JP, Berthiaume MJ, Abram F, Choquette D, Haraoui B, et al. Risk factors associated with the loss of cartilage volume on weight-bearing areas in knee osteoarthritis patients assessed by quantitative magnetic resonance imaging: a longitudinal study. Arthritis Res Ther. 2007;9(4):R74.
59. Gray ML, Eckstein F, Peterfy C, Dahlberg L, Kim YJ, Sorensen AG. Toward imaging biomarkers for osteoarthritis. *Clin Orthop.* 2004 October;(427 Suppl):S175-S181.
60. Mosher TJ, Dardzinski BJ. Cartilage MRI T2 relaxation time mapping: overview and applications. Semin Musculoskelet Radiol. 2004;8(4):355–68.
61. Eckstein F, Hudelmaier M, Putz R. The effects of exercise on human articular cartilage. J Anat. 2006;208(4):491–512.
62. Gold GE, Burstein D, Dardzinski B, Lang P, Boada F, Mosher T. MRI of articular cartilage in OA: novel pulse sequences and compositional/functional markers. Osteoarthritis Cartilage. 2006;14 Suppl 1:76–86. Epub 2006 May 23:76–86.
63. Mosher TJ. Musculoskeletal imaging at 3 T: current techniques and future applications. Magn Reson Imaging Clin N Am. 2006;14(1):63–76.
64. Gold GE, Burstein D, Dardzinski B, Lang P, Boada F, Mosher T. MRI of articular cartilage in OA: novel pulse sequences and compositional/functional markers. Osteoarthritis Cartilage. 2006;14 Suppl 1:76–86. Epub 2006 May 23:76–86.
65. Burstein D. MRI for development of disease-modifying osteoarthritis drugs. NMR Biomed. 2006;19(6):669–80.
66. Peterfy CG, Gold G, Eckstein F, Cicuttini F, Dardzinski B, Stevens R. MRI protocols for whole-organ assessment of the knee in osteoarthritis. Osteoarthritis Cartilage. 2006;14 Suppl 1:95–111.
67. Hardy PA, Recht MP, Piraino D, Thomasson D. Optimization of a dual echo in the steady state (DESS) free-precession sequence for imaging cartilage. J Magn Reson Imaging. 1996;6(2):329–35.
68. Eckstein F, Kunz M, Hudelmaier M, Jackson R, Yu J, Eaton CB, et al. Impact of coil design on the contrast-to-noise ratio, precision, and consistency of quantitative cartilage morphometry at 3 Tesla: a pilot study for the osteoarthritis initiative. Magn Reson Med. 2007;57(2):448–54.
69. Eckstein F, Kunz M, Schutzer M, Hudelmaier M, Jackson RD, Yu J, et al. Two year longitudinal change and test-retest-precision of knee cartilage morphology in a pilot study for the osteoarthritis initiative. Osteoarthritis Cartilage. 2007;15(11):1326–32.
70. Welsch GH, Mamisch TC, Hughes T, Domayer S, Marlovits S, Trattnig S. Advanced morphological and biochemical magnetic resonance imaging of cartilage repair procedures in the knee joint at 3 Tesla. Semin Musculoskelet Radiol. 2008;12(3):196–211.
71. Peterfy CG, Schneider E, Nevitt M. The osteoarthritis initiative: report on the design rationale for the magnetic resonance imaging protocol for the knee. Osteoarthritis Cartilage. 2008;16(12):1433–41.
72. Maschek S, Wirth W, Wyman B, Hellio-Le-Graverand MP, Eckstein F. Differences in quantitative MR imaging of cartilage morphology between sagittal versus coronal acquisitions of the femorotibial joint. Osteoarthritis Cartilage. 2009;17 Suppl 1:S 216 [abstract].
73. Inglis D, Pui M, Ioannidis G, Beattie K, Boulos P, Adachi JD, et al. Accuracy and test-retest precision of quantitative cartilage morphology on a 1.0 T peripheral magnetic resonance imaging system. Osteoarthritis Cartilage. 2007;15(1):110–15.
74. Eckstein F, Charles HC, Buck RJ, Kraus VB, Remmers AE, Hudelmaier M, et al. Accuracy and precision of quantitative assessment of cartilage morphology by magnetic resonance imaging at 3.0 T. Arthritis Rheum. 2005;52(10):3132–6.
75. Morgan SR, Waterton JC, Maciewicz RA, Leadbetter JE, Gandy SJ, Moots RJ, et al. Magnetic resonance imaging measurement of knee cartilage volume in a multicentre study. Rheumatology (Oxford). 2004;43(1):19–21.
76. Kornaat PR, Koo S, Andriacchi TP, Bloem JL, Gold GE. Comparison of quantitative cartilage measurements acquired on two 3.0 T MRI systems from different manufacturers. J Magn Reson Imaging. 2006;23(5):770–3.
77. Hudelmaier M, Horger W, Pfau C, Glaser C, Reiser M, Eckstein F, et al. Cross-calibration of magnetic resonance sequences and scanners for quantifying articular cartilage morphology. Osteoarthritis Cartilage. 2003;11(Suppl A):S72 [abstract].
78. Schneider E, NessAiver M, White D, Purdy D, Martin L, Fanella L, et al. The osteoarthritis initiative (OAI) magnetic resonance imaging quality assurance methods and results. Osteoarthritis Cartilage. 2008;16(9):994–1004.
79. Eckstein F, Buck RJ, Wyman BT, Kotyk JJ, Le Graverand MP, Remmers AE, et al. Quantitative imaging of cartilage morphology at 3.0 Tesla in the presence of gadopentate dimeglumine (Gd-DTPA). Magn Reson Med. 2007;58(2):402–6.
80. Eckstein F, Wyman BT, Buck RJ, Wirth W, Maschek S, Hudelmaier M, et al. Longitudinal quantitative MR imaging of cartilage morphology in the presence of gadopentetate dimeglumine (Gd-DTPA). Magn Reson Med. 2009;61(4):975–80.
81. Gandy SJ, Dieppe PA, Keen MC, Maciewicz RA, Watt I, Waterton JC. No loss of cartilage volume over three years in patients with knee osteoarthritis as assessed by magnetic resonance imaging. Osteoarthritis Cartilage. 2002;10(12):929–37.
82. Wluka AE, Stuckey S, Snaddon J, Cicuttini FM. The determinants of change in tibial cartilage volume in osteoarthritic knees. Arthritis Rheum. 2002;46(8):2065–72.
83. Cicuttini FM, Wluka AE, Wang Y, Stuckey SL. Longitudinal study of changes in tibial and femoral cartilage in knee osteoarthritis. Arthritis Rheum. 2004;50(1):94–7.

84. Raynauld JP, Martel-Pelletier J, Berthiaume MJ, Labonté F, Beaudoin G, de Giuse JA, et al. Quantitative magnetic resonance imaging evaluation of knee osteoarthritis progression over two years and correlation with clinical symptoms and radiologic changes. Arthritis Rheum. 2004;50(2):476–87.
85. Berthiaume MJ, Raynauld JP, Martel-Pelletier J, Labonté F, Beaudoin G, Bloch DA, et al. Meniscal tear and extrusion are strongly associated with progression of symptomatic knee osteoarthritis as assessed by quantitative magnetic resonance imaging. Ann Rheum Dis. 2005;64(4):556–63.
86. Raynauld JP, Martel-Pelletier J, Berthiaume MJ, Beaudoin G, Choquette D, Haraoui B, et al. Long term evaluation of disease progression through the quantitative magnetic resonance imaging of symptomatic knee osteoarthritis patients: correlation with clinical symptoms and radiographic changes. Arthritis Res Ther. 2006;8(1):R21.
87. Wluka AE, Forbes A, Wang Y, Hanna F, Jones G, Cicuttini FM. Knee cartilage loss in symptomatic knee osteoarthritis over 4.5 years. Arthritis Res Ther. 2006;8(4):R90.
88. Bruyere O, Genant H, Kothari M, Zaim S, White D, Peterfy C, et al. Longitudinal study of magnetic resonance imaging and standard X-rays to assess disease progression in osteoarthritis. Osteoarthritis Cartilage. 2007;15(1):98–103.
89. Hunter DJ, Bowes MA, Eaton CB, Holmes AP, Mann H, Khow CK, et al. Can cartilage loss be detected in knee osteoarthritis (OA) patients with 3-6 months' observation using advanced image analysis of 3 T MRI? Osteoarthritis Cartilage. 2010;18(5):677–83. Epub 2010 Feb 26.
90. Raynauld JP, Kauffmann C, Beaudoin G, Berthiaume MJ, de Guise JA, Bloch DA, et al. Reliability of a quantification imaging system using magnetic resonance images to measure cartilage thickness and volume in human normal and osteoarthritic knees. Osteoarthritis Cartilage. 2003;11(5):351–60.
91. Cicuttini F, Wluka A, Wang Y, Stuckey S. The determinants of change in patella cartilage volume in osteoarthritic knees. J Rheumatol. 2002;29(12):2615–19.
92. Frobell RB, Le Graverand MP, Buck R, Roos EM, Roos HP, Tamez-Pena J, et al. The acutely ACL injured knee assessed by MRI: changes in joint fluid, bone marrow lesions, and cartilage during the first year. Osteoarthritis Cartilage. 2009;17(2):161–7.
93. Watson PJ, Carpenter TA, Hall LD, Tyler JA. Cartilage swelling and loss in a spontaneous model of osteoarthritis visualized by magnetic resonance imaging. Osteoarthritis Cartilage. 1996;4(3): 197–207.
94. Calvo E, Palacios I, Delgado E, Ruiz-Cabello J, Hernandez P, Sanchez-Pernaute O, et al. High-resolution MRI detects cartilage swelling at the early stages of experimental osteoarthritis. Osteoarthritis Cartilage. 2001;9(5):463–72.
95. Calvo E, Palacios I, Delgado E, Sanchez-Pernaute O, Largo R, Edigo J, et al. Histopathological correlation of cartilage swelling detected by magnetic resonance imaging in early experimental osteoarthritis. Osteoarthritis Cartilage. 2004;12(11):878–86.
96. Vignon E, Arlot M, Hartmann D, Moyen B, Ville G. Hypertrophic repair of articular cartilage in experimental osteoarthrosis. Ann Rheum Dis. 1983;42(1):82–8.
97. Adams ME, Brandt KD. Hypertrophic repair of canine articular cartilage in osteoarthritis after anterior cruciate ligament transection. J Rheumatol. 1991;18(3):428–35.
98. Buck RJ, Wyman BT, Hellio Le Graverand MP, Hudelmaier M, Wirth W, Eckstein F. Osteoarthritis may not be a one-way-road of cartilage loss – comparison of spatial patterns of cartilage change between osteoarthritic and healthy knees. Osteoarthritis Cartilage. 2010;18(3):329–35.
99. Eckstein F, Wirth W, Hunter DJ, Guermazi A, Kwoh CK, Nelson DR, et al. Magnitude and regional distribution of cartilage loss associated with grades of joint space narrowing in radiographic osteoarthritis – data from the Osteoarthritis Initiative (OAI). Osteoarthritis Cartilage. 2010;18(6):760–8. Epub 2010 Feb 18.
100. Eckstein F, Muller S, Faber SC, Englmeier KH, Reiser M, Putz R. Side differences of knee joint cartilage volume, thickness, and surface area, and correlation with lower limb dominance – an MRI-based study. Osteoarthritis Cartilage. 2002;10(12):914–21.
101. Altman RD, Gold GE. Atlas of individual radiographic features in osteoarthritis, revised. Osteoarthritis Cartilage. 2007;15(Suppl A): 1–56.
102. Altman RD, Hochberg M, Murphy Jr WA, Wolfe F, Lequesne M. Atlas of individual radiographic features in osteoarthritis. Osteoarthritis Cartilage. 1995;3(Suppl A):3–70.
103. Wirth W, Benichou O, Kwoh CK, Guermazi A, Hunter D, Putz R, et al. Spatial patterns of cartilage loss in the medial femoral condyle in osteoarthritic knees: data from the Osteoarthritis Initiative. Magn Reson Med. 2010;63(3):574–81.
104. Buck RJ, Wyman BT, Le Graverand MP, Hudelmaier M, Wirth W, Eckstein F. Does the use of ordered values of subregional change in cartilage thickness improve the detection of disease progression in longitudinal studies of osteoarthritis? Arthritis Rheum. 2009;61(7):917–24.
105. Wirth W, Buck R, Hellio Le Graverand-Gastineau MP, Benichou O, Dreher D, Davies RY, et al. Ordered values of cartilge loss in knee subregions more efficiently differentiate progression at different radiographic stages of OA: data from the OA Initiative. Osteoarthritis Cartilage. 2009;17 Suppl 1:S203 [abstract].
106. Cicuttini F, Hankin J, Jones G, Wluka A. Comparison of conventional standing knee radiographs and magnetic resonance imaging in assessing progression of tibiofemoral joint osteoarthritis. Osteoarthritis Cartilage. 2005;13(8):722–7.
107. Raynauld JP, Martel-Pelletier J, Bias P, Laufer S, Haraoui B, Choquette D, et al. Protective effects of licofelone, a 5-lipoxygenase and cyclooxygenase inhibitor, versus naproxen on cartilage loss in knee osteoarthritis: a first Multi-Centre Clinical Trial using quantitative MRI. Ann Rheum Dis. 2009;68(6):938–47. Epub 2008 Jul 23.
108. Peterfy C, Li J, Zaim S, Duryea J, Lynch J, Miaux Y, et al. Comparison of fixed-flexion positioning with fluoroscopic semi-flexed positioning for quantifying radiographic joint-space width in the knee: test-retest reproducibility. Skeletal Radiol. 2003;32(3):128–32.
109. Botha-Scheepers S, Kloppenburg M, Kroon HM, Hellio Le Graverand MP, Breedveld FC, Ravaud P, et al. Fixed-flexion knee radiography: the sensitivity to detect knee joint space narrowing in osteoarthritis. Osteoarthritis Cartilage. 2007;15(3):350–3.
110. Charles HC, Kraus VB, Ainslie M, Hellio Le Graverand-Gastineau MP. Optimization of the fixed-flexion knee radiograph. Osteoarthritis Cartilage. 2007;15(11):1221–4.
111. Nevitt MC, Peterfy C, Guermazi A, Felson DT, Duryea J, Woodworth T, et al. Longitudinal performance evaluation and validation of fixed-flexion radiography of the knee for detection of joint space loss. Arthritis Rheum. 2007;56(5):1512–20.
112. Le Graverand MP, Vignon EP, Brandt KD, Mazzuca SA, Puperno M, Buck R, et al. Head-to-head comparison of the Lyon Schuss and fixed flexion radiographic techniques. Long-term reproducibility in normal knees and sensitivity to change in osteoarthritic knees. Ann Rheum Dis. 2008;67(11):1562–6.
113. Adams JG, McAlindon T, Dimasi M, Carey J, Eustace S. Contribution of meniscal extrusion and cartilage loss to joint space narrowing in osteoarthritis. Clin Radiol. 1999;54(8):502–6.
114. Gale DR, Chaisson CE, Totterman SM, Schwartz RK, Gale ME, Felson D. Meniscal subluxation: association with osteoarthritis and joint space narrowing. Osteoarthritis Cartilage. 1999;7(6): 526–32.
115. Hunter DJ, Zhang YQ, Tu X, Lavalley M, Niu JB, Amin S, et al. Change in joint space width: hyaline articular cartilage loss or alteration in meniscus? Arthritis Rheum. 2006;54(8):2488–95.

116. Duryea J, Neumann G, Niu J, Totterman S, Tamez J, Dabrowski C, et al. Comparison of radiographic joint space width to MRI cartilage morphometry: analysis of longitudinal data from the Osteoarthritis Initiative (OAI). Arthritis Care Res. 2010;62(7):932–7.
117. Duryea J, Li J, Peterfy CG, Gordon C, Genant HK. Trainable rule-based algorithm for the measurement of joint space width in digital radiographic images of the knee. Med Phys. 2000;27(3):580–91.
118. Neumann G, Hunter D, Nevitt M, Chibnik LB, Kwoh K, Chen H, et al. Location specific radiographic joint space width for osteoarthritis progression. Osteoarthritis Cartilage. 2009;17(6):761–5.
119. Eckstein F, Wirth W, Hudelmaier MI, Maschek S, Hitzl W, Wyman BT, et al. Relationship of compartment-specific structural knee status at baseline with change in cartilage morphology: a prospective observational study using data from the osteoarthritis initiative. Arthritis Res Ther. 2009;11(3):R90.
120. Davies-Tuck ML, Martel-Pelletier J, Wluka AE, Pelletier JP, Ding C, Jones G, et al. Meniscal tear and increased tibial plateau bone area in healthy post-menopausal women. Osteoarthritis Cartilage. 2008;16(2):268–71.
121. Chang A, Eckstein F, Moiso K, Moisio K, Chmiel JS, Almagor O, et al. Subegional effects of meniscal tears and subluxation in knee osteoarthritis. Osteoarthritis Cartilage. 2009;17 Suppl 1:S189 [abstract].
122. Crema MD, Guermazi A, Li L, et al. The association of prevalent medial meniscal pathology with cartilage loss in the medial tibiofemoral compartment over a 2-year period. Osteoarthritis Cartilage. 2010;18(3):336–43.
123. Jung KA, Lee SC, Hwang SH, et al. High frequency of meniscal hypertrophy in persons with advanced varus knee osteoarthritis. Rheumatol Int. 2010;30(10):1325–33.
124. Wirth W, Frobell RB, Souza RB, et al. A three-dimensional quantitative method to measure meniscus shape, position, and signal intensity using MR images: a pilot study and preliminary results in knee osteoarthritis. Magn Reson Med. 2010;63(5):1162–71.
125. Raynauld JP, Martel-Pelletier J, Berthiaume MJ, et al. Correlation between bone lesion changes and cartilage volume loss in patients with osteoarthritis of the knee as assessed by quantitative magnetic resonance imaging over a 24-month period. Ann Rheum Dis. 2008;67(5):683–8.
126. Cicuttini F, Wluka A, Hankin J, Wang Y. Longitudinal study of the relationship between knee angle and tibiofemoral cartilage volume in subjects with knee osteoarthritis. Rheumatology (Oxford). 2004;43(3):321–4.
127. Eisenhart-Rothe R, Graichen H, Hudelmaier M, Vogl T, Sharma L, Eckstein F. Femorotibial and patellar cartilage loss in patients prior to total knee arthroplasty, heterogeneity, and correlation with alignment of the knee. Ann Rheum Dis. 2006;65(1):69–73.
128. Teichtahl AJ, Davies-Tuck ML, Wluka AE, Jones G, Cicuttini FM. Change in knee angle influences the rate of medial tibial cartilage volume loss in knee osteoarthritis. Osteoarthritis Cartilage. 2009;17(1):8–11.
129. Teichtahl AJ, Wluka AE, Cicuttini FM. Frontal plane knee alignment is associated with a longitudinal reduction in patella cartilage volume in people with knee osteoarthritis. Osteoarthritis Cartilage. 2008;16(7):851–4.
130. Zhai G, Ding C, Cicuttini F, Jones G. A longitudinal study of the association between knee alignment and change in cartilage volume and chondral defects in a largely non-osteoarthritic population. J Rheumatol. 2007;34(1):181–6.
131. Vanwanseele B, Eckstein F, Smith RM, et al. The relationship between knee adduction moment and cartilage and meniscus morphology in women with osteoarthritis. Osteoarthritis Cartilage. 2010;18(7):894–901. Epub 2010 Apr 22.
132. Cicuttini FM, Wluka A, Bailey M, et al. Factors affecting knee cartilage volume in healthy men. Rheumatology (Oxford). 2003;42(2):258–62.
133. Teichtahl AJ, Wluka AE, Wang Y, et al. Obesity and adiposity are associated with the rate of patella cartilage volume loss over two years in adults without knee osteoarthritis. Ann Rheum Dis. 2009;68(6):909–13. Epub 2008 Jul 16.
134. Wluka AE, Hanna FS, Davies-Tuck M, et al. Bone Marrow Lesions predict increase in knee cartilage defects and loss of cartilage volume in middle-aged women without knee pain over 2 years. Ann Rheum Dis. 2009;68(6):850–5. Epub 2008 Jul 14.
135. Wluka AE, Wang Y, Davies-Tuck M, English DR, Giles GG, Cicuttini FM. Bone marrow lesions predict progression of cartilage defects and loss of cartilage volume in healthy middle-aged adults without knee pain over 2 yrs. Rheumatology (Oxford). 2008;47(9):1392–6.
136. Ding C, Cicuttini F, Scott F, Boon C, Jones G. Association of prevalent and incident knee cartilage defects with loss of tibial and patellar cartilage: a longitudinal study. Arthritis Rheum. 2005;52(12):3918–27.
137. Wluka AE, Ding C, Jones G, Cicuttini FM. The clinical correlates of articular cartilage defects in symptomatic knee osteoarthritis: a prospective study. Rheumatology (Oxford). 2005;44(10):1311–16.
138. Hunter DJ, Li L, Zhang YQ, et al. Region of interest analysis: by selecting regions with denuded areas can we detect greater amounts of change? Osteoarthritis Cartilage. 2010;18(2):175–83.
139. Frobell RB, Wirth W, Nevitt M, et al. Presence, location, type and size of denuded areas of subchondral bone in the knee as a function of radiographic stage of OA – data from the OA initiative. Osteoarthritis Cartilage. 2010;18(5):668–76. Epub 2010 Feb 6.
140. Cicuttini F, Ding C, Wluka A, Davis S, Ebeling PR, Jones G. Association of cartilage defects with loss of knee cartilage in healthy, middle-age adults: a prospective study. Arthritis Rheum. 2005;52(7):2033–9.
141. Ding C, Martel-Pelletier J, Pelletier JP, et al. Two-year prospective longitudinal study exploring the factors associated with change in femoral cartilage volume in a cohort largely without knee radiographic osteoarthritis. Osteoarthritis Cartilage. 2008;16(4):443–9.
142. Ding C, Cicuttini F, Jones G. Tibial subchondral bone size and knee cartilage defects: relevance to knee osteoarthritis. Osteoarthritis Cartilage. 2007;15(5):479–86.
143. Hunter DJ, Li L, Zhang YQ, et al. Region of interest analysis: by selecting regions with denuded areas can we detect greater amounts of change? Osteoarthritis Cartilage. 2010;18(2):175–83. Epub 2009 Aug 29.
144. Ding C, Cicuttini F, Blizzard L, Jones G. Smoking interacts with family history with regard to change in knee cartilage volume and cartilage defect development. Arthritis Rheum. 2007;56(5):1521–8.
145. Davies-Tuck ML, Wluka AE, Forbes A, et al. Smoking is associated with increased cartilage loss and persistence of bone marrow lesions over 2 years in community-based individuals. Rheumatology (Oxford). 2009;48(10):1227–31.
146. Cicuttini FM, Jones G, Forbes A, Wluka AE. Rate of cartilage loss at two years predicts subsequent total knee arthroplasty: a prospective study. Ann Rheum Dis. 2004;63(9):1124–7.
147. Tanamas SK, Wluka AE, Pelletier JP, et al. The association between subchondral bone cysts and tibial cartilage volume and risk of joint replacement in people with knee osteoarthritis: a longitudinal study. Arthritis Res Ther. 2010;12(2):R58.

Chapter 12
MR T2 Relaxation Time Measurements for Cartilage and Menisci

Thomas Baum, Thomas M. Link, and Bernard J. Dardzinski

Keywords MRI • T2 relaxation time • Image acquisition and processing • Compartments • Segmentation • Image analysis • Clinical applications

Introduction

Magnetic Resonance Imaging (MRI) can be used not only for morphologic but also for quantitative assessment of knee cartilage. Quantitative T1rho and T2 relaxation time measurements and dGEMRIC (delayed Gadolinium enhanced MRI of the cartilage) have emerged as potential cartilage biomarkers to assess early degenerative disease. This chapter focuses on the T2-technique and clinical applications of hyaline cartilage and meniscal T2 relaxation time measurements in particular at the knee.

The chapter is structured into four parts: After a brief background section, image acquisition and processing are outlined. Subsequently, image analysis and clinical applications are presented.

Background

Early stages of knee osteoarthritis (OA) are characterized by degradation of components of the extracellular matrix of the cartilage [1, 2]. The proteoglycan content decreases and the collagen network shows signs of disorganization. The latter induces higher water mobility and consequentially increased water content within the cartilage. These initial cartilage changes are subclinical, i.e., individuals do not have symptoms of OA. T1rho and T2 relaxation times are affected by these pathophysiological processes [3, 4]. Whereas T1rho relaxation time is more sensitive to the proteoglycan content of the cartilage, T2 relaxation time is more sensitive to cartilage hydration and orientation and integrity of the collagen network. Therefore, T1rho and T2 are noninvasive biomarkers for cartilage degeneration. These biomarkers may be used to detect early stages of the disease, quantitatively assess disease severity, sensitively monitor disease progression, and monitor OA therapy. Since they are sensitive to tissue components of cartilage that change before morphologic signs are detectable, they are particularly suited for the early disease stages, which are not accessible with standard morphological MR imaging [5]. In one of the early studies, Dardzinski et al. analyzed T2 measurements in asymptomatic volunteers and found a reproducible pattern of increasing T2 that was proportional to the known spatial variation in cartilage water [6]. Based on these findings, the authors postulated that these regional T2 differences were secondary to the restricted mobility of cartilage water within an anisotropic solid matrix. In a subsequent clinical study, Mosher et al. studied asymptomatic volunteers and individuals with symptoms of patellar chondromalacia using quantitative T2 maps of patellar cartilage and found an asymptomatic increase in T2 with aging as well as an increase in cartilage T2 from the radial zone to the articular surface [7]. Based on these studies and findings, investigators adopted T2 relaxation time measurements to assess cartilage degeneration in clinical studies, which culminated in implementing T2 relaxation time measurements in the NIH sponsored Osteoarthritis Initiative (OAI) multicenter trial.

Image Acquisition and Processing

Imaging Sequences and Field Strength

Quantitative T2 relaxation time measurements in vivo are typically performed at 1.5 and 3.0 T. Pai et al. compared several different sequences used for T2 quantification [8]: spin echo (SE), multiecho SE, fast spin echo (FSE), and spiral

T. Baum (✉)
Department of Radiology and Biomedical Imaging, Musculoskeletal and Quantitative Imaging Research Group, University of California, 185 Berry Street, Suite 350, San Francisco, CA 94107, USA
and
Department of Radiology, Technische Universität München, Ismaninger Str. 22, 81675 Munich, Germany
e-mail: thomas-baum@gmx.de

T.M. Link (ed.), *Cartilage Imaging: Significance, Techniques, and New Developments*, DOI 10.1007/978-1-4419-8438-8_12, © Springer Science+Business Media, LLC 2011

and 3D spoiled gradient recalled (SPGR) acquisition. Sequences ranged in scan time, signal-to-noise ratio (SNR) efficiency, and reproducibility. The investigators found that T2 values obtained with these sequences were partly significantly different; consequently, comparisons of T2 values of different studies always have to take into account the used modalities of image acquisition.

Spin echo sequences have been most commonly used for T2 quantification. Various possibilities for the number and values of the echo times (TE) were reported. To give an example, the Osteoarthritis Initiative (OAI), which had 4,796 study participants, used a multislice multiecho (MSME) spin echo sequence with seven echoes (TE = 10, 20, 30, 40, 50, 60, and 70 ms), repetition time (TR) of 2,700 ms, and total acquisition time of 10.6 min [9].

Compared to single-echo spin echo and single-slice multiecho spin echo sequences, the application of a MSME spin echo sequence considerably reduces the acquisition time. This is important for the feasibility of quantitative T2 relaxation time measurements in clinical practice. However, potential error sources are introduced by using a MSME spin echo sequence [10–12]. A multislice sequence requires slice-selective refocusing pulses. First, off-resonance effects are generated by refocusing pulses for other slices. This introduces magnetization transfer contrast (MTC) into the images, resulting in reduced signal intensity in cartilage and thus possibly in inaccuracy of the T2 measurements. Second, slice selective refocusing pulses do not result in rectangular slice profiles, leading to imperfect refocusing throughout the slice and causing stimulated echo contributions. The occurrence of the stimulated echoes causes overestimation of T2 values in multiecho sequences.

Regarding MTC, Watanabe et al. reported that the average T2 value measured with multislice acquisition was shorter than that measured with single-slice acquisition [11]. However, they found only a relatively small decrease in T2 and observed no obvious interslice variation in T2 values when multislice acquisition was used. They concluded that multislice acquisitions for T2 measurements are clinically applicable. Regarding stimulated echo contributions, studies have suggested that excluding the first echo from the fitting process minimizes error from stimulated echoes in calculated T2 values [10, 12, 13].

T2 quantification based on 3D spoiled gradient recalled (SPGR) can be used alternatively to avoid the above-mentioned error sources due to the use of a MSME spin echo sequence [8]. The sequence consists of a nonselective T2 preparation and a 3D SPGR acquisition during the transient signal evolving towards steady state. A recent study used this sequence and reported an acquisition time of 11 min with parallel imaging [14].

By using parallel imaging, scan time can be reduced. Parallel imaging uses spatial encoding from coil elements of the receiver array. Thus, gradient encoding steps are reduced, enabling accelerated image acquisition. Parallel imaging reduces the scan time at the cost of SNR, but image acquisition using parallel imaging with an acceleration factor of 2 showed good accuracy and reproducibility of T2 values [15].

In addition to T2 quantifications at 1.5 and 3.0 T, Welsch et al. demonstrated the feasibility of T2 measurements at 7.0 T [16]. They compared 12 healthy volunteers and 4 patients after matrix-associated autologous chondrocyte transplantation (MACT). T2 values in healthy cartilage increased significantly from deep to superficial cartilage, whereas cartilage repair tissue showed no significant stratification. The authors concluded that optimized protocols and sophisticated coil technology, together with increased signal at 7.0 T MRI, may lead to advanced biochemical cartilage imaging.

Compared to hyaline cartilage, menisci have shorter T2 relaxation times (5–8 ms). Therefore, T2 relaxation time measurements of the menisci were performed using a SPGR sequence with shorter TEs (e.g., TE = 4.1, 14.5, 25.0, and 45.9 ms and TR = 2,000 ms) [17]. Zarin et al. used similar TEs, but excluded the last TE = 44.8 ms for the T2 map calculations due to the very low SNR for the meniscus (SNR < 5) [14]. An alternative to characterize the meniscus is ultrashort echo time (UTE) imaging, which is currently a growing research field [18, 19].

T2 Relaxation Time Measurements

The actual T2 relaxation time value for each pixel is calculated by fitting the measured signal intensity S at each TE to a mono-exponential decay function:

$$S(\mathrm{TE}_i) = S_0 \cdot \mathrm{e}^{(-\mathrm{TE}_i/\mathrm{T2})},$$

where S_0 is the signal intensity at zero TE.

To solve the equation for T2 and S_0, different fitting methods such as linear least squares, weighted linear least squares, or nonlinear least squares algorithms were used in the past [10, 20]. The chosen fitting method has a considerable impact on the resulting T2 values, thus making the comparison of T2 values of different studies using different fitting methods difficult. Furthermore, the measured signal intensity S is always affected by noise. Especially in low SNR images, S does not decay exponentially with increasing TE, which may induce overestimations of T2. Therefore, it was recently suggested to fit the noise-corrected squared signal intensity to an exponential function or even better fit S to a noise-corrected exponential function. Compared to the above-mentioned traditional fitting methods, the noise-corrected fitting methods showed better accuracy and precision in phantom and in vivo measurements [21].

The last step of image processing is the creation of T2 maps containing the calculated T2 values of each pixel. These maps can be presented color-coded where individual colors correspond to specific T2 values to allow visual assessment of hyaline cartilage or meniscal T2.

Image Analysis

Compartments

Quantitative T2 relaxation time measurements of articular cartilage of the knee are performed in distinct compartments. A nomenclature for these anatomical regions of interest has been established [22]. The nomenclature distinguishes between patella, trochlea, medial femur, lateral femur, medial tibia, and lateral tibia compartment. The patella compartment can be subdivided in a medial, central, and lateral subregion, the lateral/medial femur compartment in a central and posterior subregion, and the trochlea in a medial, central, and lateral subregion (Fig. 12.1). The medial and lateral subregion of the trochlea is often added to the medial, respectively, lateral femur compartment [23–25]. Furthermore, different weight-bearing and nonweight-bearing areas were introduced for the medial/lateral femur/tibia. Therefore, it is important to check the particular compartment definitions of each study to allow an adequate comparison of different studies.

The medial/lateral meniscus is usually divided in anterior, posterior, and body compartment [14, 17, 26]. Based on sagittal images, the meniscal body is defined mesially as the first section where the anterior and posterior parts of the meniscus are connected and peripherally as the last section showing the meniscus without partial volume effects. The posterior border of the posterior horn of the lateral meniscus is defined by the hiatus popliteus. The fascicles are not included in the image analysis.

Segmentation

Cartilage compartments/subregions are segmented based on coronal or sagittal images. Two different techniques are commonly used for cartilage segmentation.

The first is a segmentation superimposition technique. Cartilage is segmented on spoiled gradient recalled (SPGR) echo or double-echo steady-state (DESS) images (Figs. 12.2 and 12.3). Software using edge detection or graph-cuts algorithms was developed to perform the segmentation (semi-) automatically [27–30]. These segmentation techniques were primarily developed for cartilage volume measurements. For T2 quantifications, the obtained segmentations need to be superimposed on T2 maps. Software was developed to adjust for different slice thickness of SPGR/DESS images and T2 maps. T2 maps need to be registered on the SPGR/DESS images due to patient movement between DESS/SPGR and T2 mapping acquisitions [28, 31]. Recent studies have used a VTK CISG Registration Toolkit for image registration [14, 32, 33]. After superimposition on the T2 maps, the segmented compartments/subregions often have to be manually corrected due to accidentally included fluid with elevated T2 values, which is a very time-consuming process. An average time duration of 30 min was reported for T2 quantifications of the three compartments of one meniscus using the segmentation superimposition technique [14, 17]. The segmentation and T2 measurements of the six standard compartments of the articular cartilage (patella, trochlea, medial femur, medial tibia, lateral femur, and lateral tibia) require approximately 5 h using this technique [25]. However, this time effort includes not only T2 quantifications but also articular cartilage volume measurements.

This segmentation procedure is not acceptable for researchers who exclusively evaluate T2 relaxation times in large clinical trials like the Osteoarthritis Initiative (OAI). Therefore, an alternative segmentation technique was developed, which

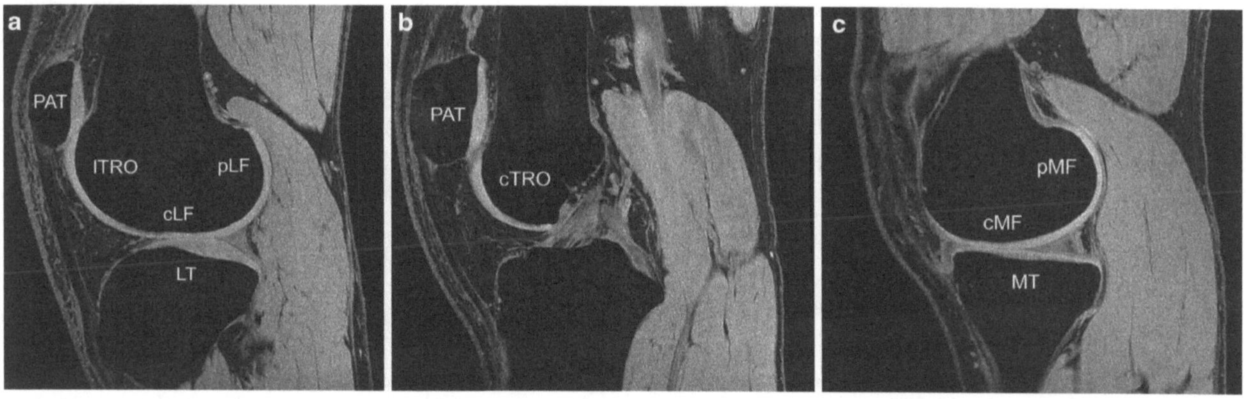

Fig. 12.1 Sagittal fat-suppressed spoiled gradient echo (SPGR) images of the articular cartilage compartments/subregions. (**a**) Patella (PAT), lateral tibia (LT), lateral trochlea (lTRO), central lateral femur (cLF), and posterior lateral femur (pLF). (**b**) Patella (PAT) and central trochlea (cTRO). (**c**) Medial tibia (MT), central medial femur (cMF), and posterior medial femur (pMF)

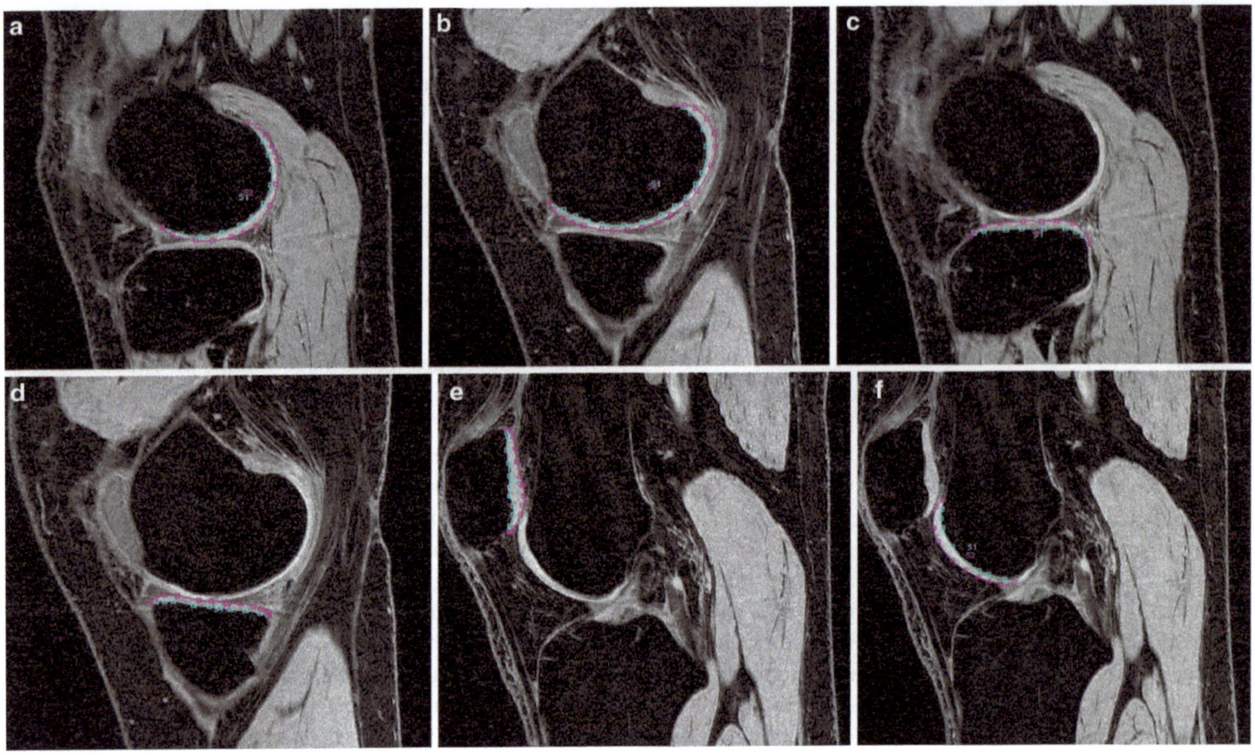

Fig. 12.2 Articular cartilage segmentation in sagittal fat-suppressed spoiled gradient recalled (SPGR) echo images using a semiautomatic technique based on Bezier splines and edge detection. (**a**) Lateral femur compartment; (**b**) medial femur compartment; (**c**) lateral tibia compartment; (**d**) medial tibia compartment; (**e**) patella compartment; and (**f**) trochlea compartment

allows direct segmentation in the T2 map (Fig. 12.4) [34]. It is a software program for the manual drawing of volumes of interest (VOI) delineating cartilage areas on the T2 maps. In order to exclude both fluid and chemical shift artifacts from the VOI, a technique was developed that allowed adjustment of the VOI simultaneously in the T2 map and first echo of the multiecho sequence by opening separate image panels at the same time with synchronized cursor, slice number, and zoom. Using this direct segmentation technique, segmentation time can be substantially reduced. Segmentation of the six standard compartments of the articular cartilage requires approximately 1 h, segmentation of the three compartments of one meniscus approximately 15 min [35–37]. Therefore, the direct segmentation technique is the first choice for cartilage T2 measurements in large sample sizes.

Calculation of T2 Relaxation Time Parameters

The standard parameter of T2 relaxation time measurements is the mean T2 value of all pixels included in the segmented compartment/subregion [14, 17, 24, 25, 34–37]. However, the mean T2 value does not provide information about the spatial distribution of pixels with particular low or high T2 values (Figs. 12.5 and 12.6). For articular cartilage, laminar and texture analysis were therefore introduced as additional parameters to assess spatial information.

Laminar analysis can be automatically performed and partitions the segmented compartment/subregion into a superficial and deeper cartilage layer (Fig. 12.7) [32, 33]. The superficial layer is orientated to the articular surface, the deeper layer to the bone–cartilage interface. Each cartilage pixel within the segmented compartment/subregion is assigned to one layer according to its closest distance to the bone–cartilage interface or the articular surface. With typical imaging parameters, matrix size, and resolution, there may only be three to seven pixels across the cartilage. Koff et al. alternatively divided the patellar cartilage into three layers, a superficial, intermediate, and deep zone [38]. Higher T2 values were reported in the superficial cartilage layer and recent studies suggested that laminar analysis might improve the sensitivity to detect longitudinal T2 changes as well as the classification between subjects with and without OA [32, 33].

Texture analysis based on gray level co-occurrence matrix (GLCM) was developed by Haralick et al. and is performed on a slice-by-slice basis in the T2 maps [39]. GLCM extracts information related to the spatial distribution of pixel intensities

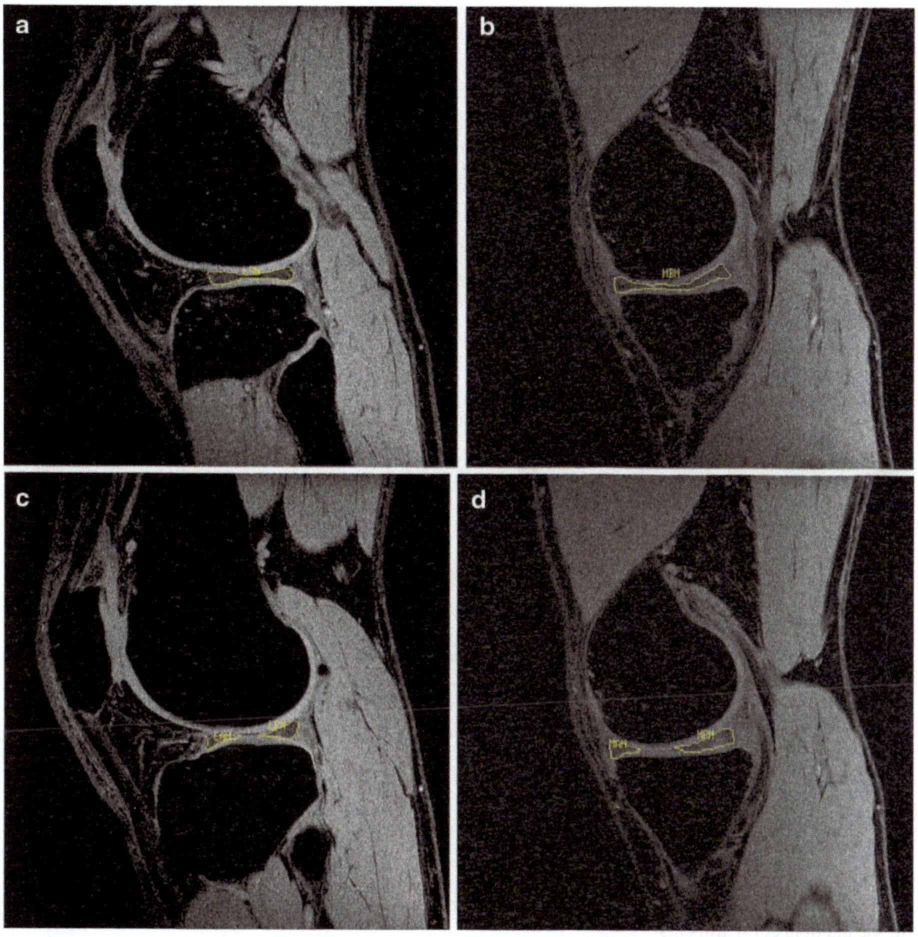

Fig. 12.3 Meniscus segmentation in sagittal fat-suppressed spoiled gradient echo (SPGR) images using a semiautomatic technique based on Bezier splines and edge detection. (**a**) Lateral meniscus body compartment; (**b**) medial meniscus body compartment; (**c**) lateral anterior and posterior meniscus compartments; and (**d**) medial anterior and posterior meniscus compartments

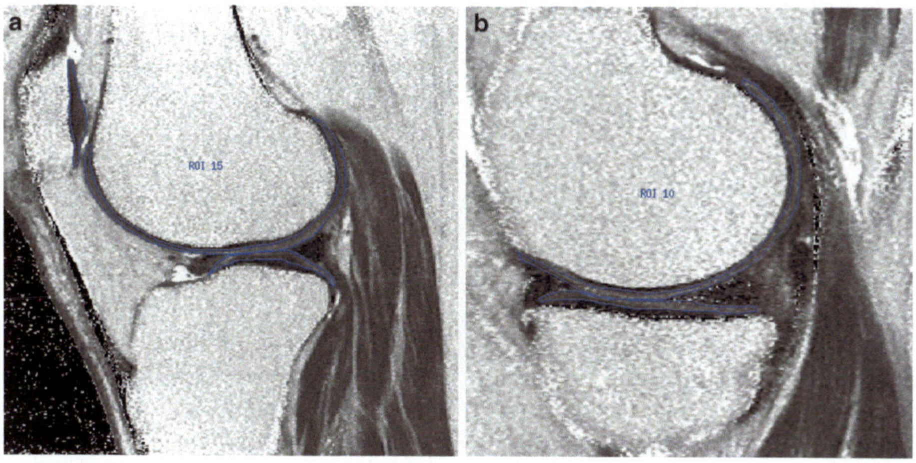

Fig. 12.4 Articular cartilage segmentation performed directly in the T2 map. (**a**) Patella, lateral femur, and lateral tibia compartments; and (**b**) medial femur and medial tibia compartments

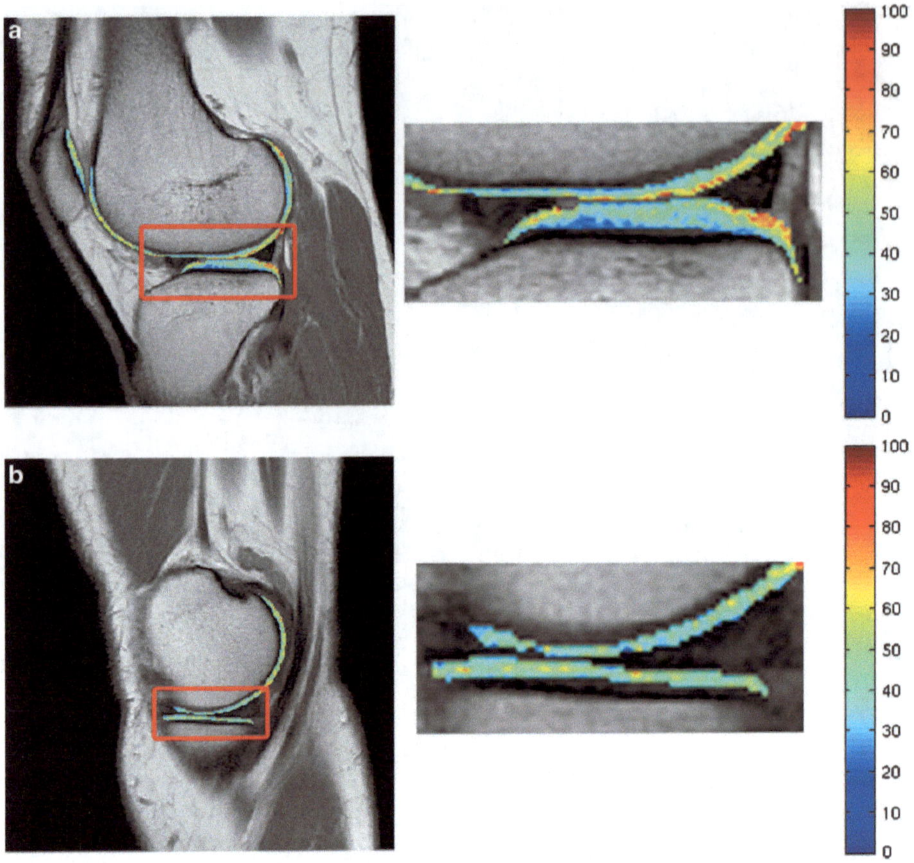

Fig. 12.5 Color-coded T2 maps in [ms] of articular cartilage compartments. (**a**) Patella, lateral femur and lateral tibia compartments; and (**b**) medial femur and medial tibia compartments

by analyzing their co-occurrences at a certain orientation and interpixel distance [31, 33, 40, 41]. Calculations are usually performed with the following four orientations: 0°–180°, 45°–225°, 90°–270°, and 135°–315°, where horizontal and vertical directions are in close correspondence to the anterior–posterior and superior–inferior anatomic directions. An interpixel distance of 1 is usually chosen (i.e., nearest neighbor pixel), but can also range from 1 to 3 as reported in a previous study [40]. Texture parameters are computed by creating matrices of pixel-intensity co-occurrences, converting the matrices into probabilities and combining the probabilities with different weight factors [33]. Two texture parameters from the contrast group (contrast and homogeneity), three from the orderliness group (angular second moment [ASM], energy, and entropy), and three from the stats group (mean, variance, and correlation) were calculated in previous studies [31, 33, 40, 41]. According to Haralick et al. [39], contrast is a measure of the amount of local variations present in the image. Angular second moment (ASM) is a measure of order, whereas entropy is a measure of disorder in the image. Correlation is a measure of gray-tone linear dependencies in the image. Texture analysis applied to T2 maps of OA patients and normal controls demonstrated that OA patients had higher entropy and contrast as well as significantly lower ASM than normal controls [40, 41]. The authors of these studies concluded that T2 values are not only elevated but also more heterogeneous in osteoarthritic cartilage. Therefore, texture analysis may provide additional information regarding cartilage degeneration.

Clinical Applications

Precision of T2 Measurements

T2 relaxation time measurements are only a discriminatory biomarker if the precision error of the T2 measurements is smaller than the T2 differences in healthy and diseased cartilage. The precision error of T2 relaxation time measurements depends on several crucial points. The operator dependency of the manual or (semi-)automatic segmentation techniques

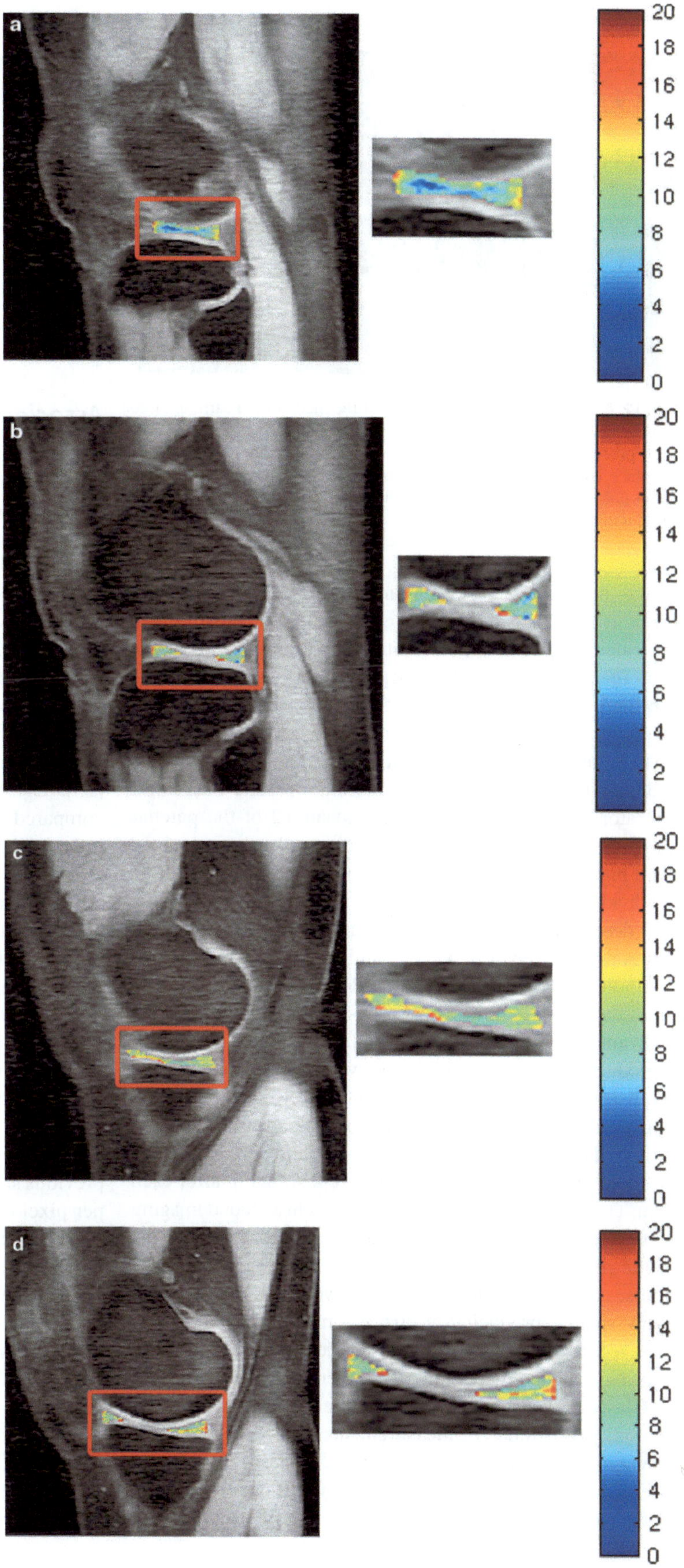

Fig. 12.6 Color-coded T2 maps in [ms] of the meniscal compartments. (**a**) Lateral meniscus body compartment; (**b**) lateral anterior and posterior meniscus compartments; (**c**) medial meniscus body compartment; and (**d**) medial anterior and posterior meniscus compartments

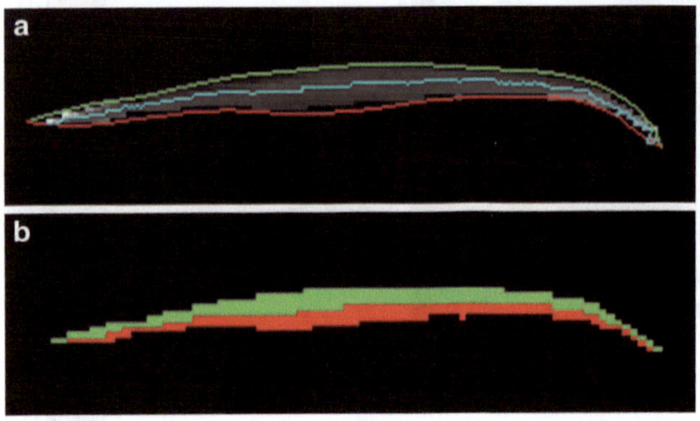

Fig. 12.7 Laminar analysis: Partition of the medial tibia cartilage into a superficial and deeper layer. (**a**) Partition is based on the proximity of each pixel to the articular surface (*green line*) and the bone–cartilage interface (*red line*), resulting in a borderline between the two layers (*blue line*). (**b**) Superficial layer is filled with *green*, deeper layer is filled with *red color*

is the first issue. Intra- and interoperator reproducibility errors for T2 measurements of each compartment/subregion are calculated as the coefficient of variation (CV) or as the root mean square (RMS) coefficient of variation of the repeated measurements, as outlined by Gluer et al. [42]. Intraoperator reproducibility errors for mean T2 amounted up to 5.70% for the standard articular cartilage compartments [15, 34]. Koff et al. reported higher interoperator than intraoperator reproducibility errors for mean T2 of the patellar cartilage (3.3% vs. 1.9%) [38]. Additionally, they obtained even higher reproducibility errors for mean T2 values of the subdivided patellar compartment, i.e., superficial, intermediate, and deep cartilage layer. The intraoperator reproducibility errors ranged from 1.8 to 3.1%, and the interoperator reproducibility errors from 3.2 to 5.0%. Reproducibility errors of meniscal T2 measurements were assessed by Rauscher et al. and amounted 4.55–13.71% [17]. All above-mentioned reproducibility errors were not derived from replicate image acquisitions, which is a limitation. Glaser et al. examined the reproducibility of mean T2 relaxation time measurements in the patella in replicate scans [43]. Four scans were performed in a first imaging session with knee repositioning after each scan. Three additional scans were acquired in a second imaging session after 1 week. The reproducibility error for mean T2 of the patella was 3–7%. No difference between intra- and intersession reproducibility was observed. Due to these relatively small reproducibility errors compared to changes in diseased cartilage, the authors concluded that T2 quantifications have a good discriminatory power.

Glaser et al. also observed no differences regarding reproducibility of patellar T2 measurements between 1.5 and 3 T scanners [44]. Significantly elevated T2 values were reported after 30 min of unloading the knee due to decompression of the cartilage and consequently increasing cartilage water content [45]. Loading and unloading the knee joint considerably affect the T2 values [46]. Therefore, physical activity before the scan and the time point of the T2 sequence within the MR protocol are important. Furthermore, an adequate MR scanner calibration is necessary to compare T2 maps acquired at different scanners, respectively at different time points to ensure reliable long-term follow-up examinations. All these potential error sources have to be taken into account when the clinical relevance of T2 relaxation time measurements is discussed.

Association of T2 Measurements with OA

Previous studies demonstrated that T2 relaxation times could differentiate OA patients and normal controls, which illustrates the clinical relevance of these measurements [23–25, 47]. Li et al. examined 16 healthy volunteers without clinical or radiological evidence of OA and 10 patients with early OA [24]. Mean T2 values were significantly higher in the early OA patients than in the healthy volunteers (averaged over all compartments 39.63 ± 2.69 vs. 34.74 ± 2.48 ms). Dunn et al. performed knee cartilage T2 measurements in 55 subjects who were categorized with radiography as healthy ($n = 7$) or as having mild OA ($n = 20$) or severe OA ($n = 28$) [23]. OA patients showed significantly higher T2 values compared to normal controls (Fig. 12.8). However, no significant difference was found between patients with mild and severe OA. Friedrich et al. analyzed T2 maps of 24 patients with clinical symptoms of medial knee OA, 12 with varus, and 12 with valgus alignment of the femorotibial joint [48]. Significantly higher T2 values were found in the medial compartments compared to the lateral compartments due to the medial knee OA. Additionally, they observed that patients with varus alignment had significantly higher T2 values than patients with valgus alignment suggesting an association of OA and joint alignment.

Z-score maps can be generated to better interpret T2 values of OA patients versus normal controls and were used in previous studies [23, 41]. T2 values are converted to z-scores per pixel on the basis of normal control T2 values for each compartment. With z-score maps, cartilage compartments can be visually graded and easily compared with different compartments as well as cartilage heterogeneity and variation from normal can be easily depicted. To assess the spatial distribution of T2 values in detail, texture analysis can be applied on T2 maps [33, 40, 41]. Blumenkrantz et al. examined eight mild OA patients and ten age-matched controls using T2 texture analysis [40]. In addition to elevated mean T2 values, significantly higher gray level co-occurrence matrix (GLCM) entropy (i.e., measure of disorder) was observed in the mild OA patients when compared to normal

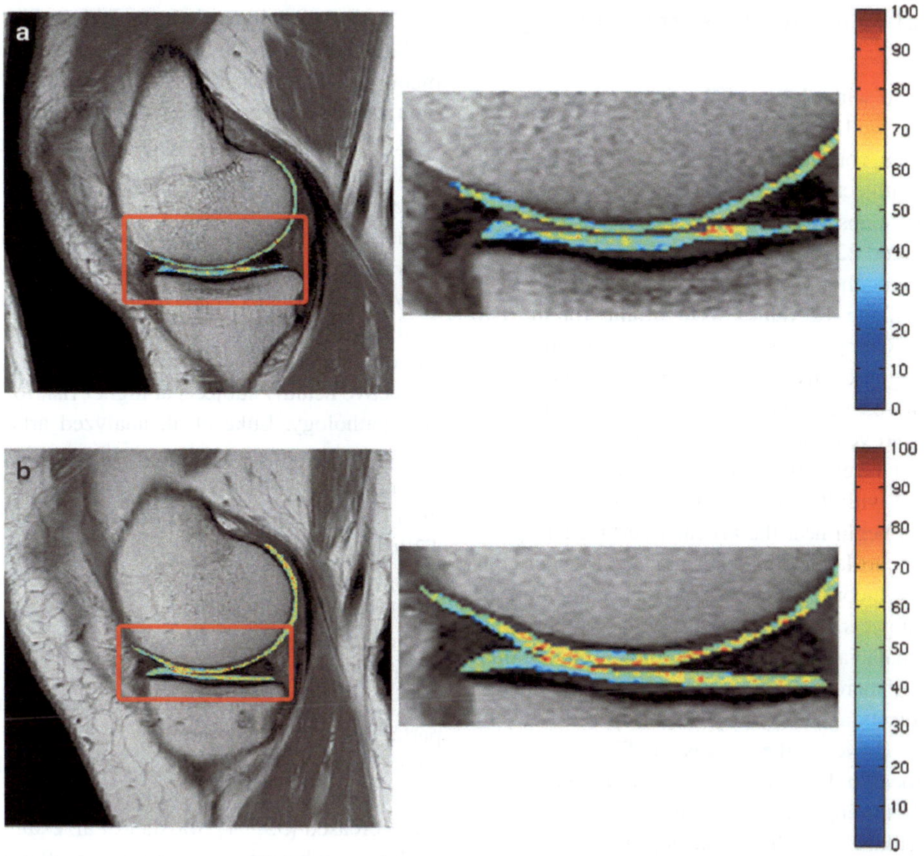

Fig. 12.8 Color-coded T2-maps in [ms] of normal control (**a**) and osteoarthritis (OA) patient (**b**) with significantly higher T2 values in the OA patient. (**a**) Medial femur and medial tibia compartments of normal control; and (**b**) medial femur and medial tibia compartments of OA patient

controls, suggesting more heterogeneous cartilage due to OA. Carballido-Gamio et al. compared 19 healthy controls and 17 subjects with mild OA [33]. They reported that healthy controls showed lower GLCM contrast, higher homogeneity, higher angular second moment, higher energy, lower entropy, lower mean, lower variance, and lower correlation in all compartments than the OA subjects. Texture analysis provides additional information regarding cartilage degeneration and can improve discrimination of subjects with and without OA beyond mean T2 values.

The sensitivity of T2 measurements can be also improved by using laminar analysis. Carballido-Gamio et al. examined longitudinal mean T2 changes in 13 OA patients over 2 years [32]. Significant longitudinal changes of mean T2 values were observed in the deep cartilage layer, but changes were nonsignificant in the superficial cartilage layer, suggesting that laminar analysis may improve the sensitivity to detect longitudinal T2 changes. Carballido-Gamio et al. also demonstrated that laminar analysis improves the classification between subjects with and without OA [33].

Meniscal T2 values correlate with clinical findings of OA and can be used to differentiate healthy subjects from patients with mild or severe OA [14, 17]. Rauscher et al. analyzed mensical T2 values of 60 subjects (23 healthy controls, 27 mild OA subjects, and 10 severe OA subjects) [17]. Averaged over all compartments, mean T2 values of healthy, mild OA, and severe OA subjects were significantly different (11.4 ± 3.9 vs. 13.5 ± 4.7 vs. 16.6 ± 8.2 ms). Zarins et al. reported that T2 measurements of the posterior horn of the medial meniscus and the medial tibia cartilage were higher in subjects having a meniscal tear (meniscal Whole-Organ Magnetic Resonance Imaging Score [WORMS] grade of 2–4) compared to subjects with meniscal WORMS grade of 0 or 1 [14]. Friedrich et al. graded meniscal signal and morphology qualitatively according to the Whole-Organ Magnetic Resonance Imaging Score (WORMS) and correlated the meniscal score with the T2 values of the articular cartilage [49]. Significantly increased T2 values were reported in the articular cartilage of patients with meniscal tears, suggesting that degeneration of meniscal and articular cartilage are intimately related.

Association of T2 Measurements with Aging

Aging is associated with elevated T2 values in articular and meniscal cartilage [7, 17, 50]. Rauscher et al. reported a statistically significant correlation of meniscal T2 values with age in 23 healthy subjects (34.1 ± 10.0 years old) [17]. Mosher et al. analyzed T2 maps of patellar cartilage from 30 asymptomatic women aged 22–86 years [50]. Subjects were stratified by age into four cohorts (18–30, 31–45, 46–65, and 66–86 years). Mean cartilage T2 values were similar for the two youngest cohorts. Compared with the 18–30-year-old group, T2 values were significantly higher in the superficial 40% of cartilage in the 46–65-year-old group and over the entire cartilage in the 66–86-year-old group. The authors concluded that the location of T2 elevations in women over the age of 45 years is consistent with the theory that senescent changes of cartilage collagen begin near the articular surface and progress to the deeper cartilage with advancing age. Mosher et al. strengthened this theory with a study that compared 25 asymptomatic subjects and 6 subjects with symptoms of patellar chondromalacia [7]. In the asymptomatic study population, a significant increase in T2 of the transitional zone was found in the subjects aged 46–60 years compared with the younger subjects. However, the increase in T2 was larger in magnitude and focal in distribution in the symptomatic study population. These findings suggest that diffuse increase in T2 in senescent cartilage is different in appearance than the focally increased T2 observed in damaged articular cartilage.

Association of T2 Measurements with Gender

Mosher et al. performed cartilage T2 measurements in a young healthy population consisting of seven male and ten female volunteers aged 22–29 years [51]. No differences in mean T2 values were found for males and females. Similarly, the spatial variation of T2 values showed the same pattern in both groups, with a minimum located in the radial zone and increasing T2 values toward the articular surface. The authors concluded that the magnitude and spatial dependency of cartilage T2 does not differ with gender at least in young, healthy subjects. Additional studies with T2 comparison of older males and females are required due to the fact that females are at increased risk for OA.

Association of T2 Measurements with Physical Activity

Generally, physical activity has a major impact on cartilage T2 values. Stehling et al. examined 120 subjects with risk factors for knee OA [34]. Physical activity was assessed by using the Physical Activity Scale for the Elderly (PASE). Significantly higher patellar T2 values, as well as prevalence and severity of meniscal and cartilage lesions, were found in subjects with high PASE scores compared to subjects with low PASE scores (Fig. 12.9). Stahl et al. compared 13 asymptomatic physically active subjects, 7 asymptomatic sedentary subjects, and 17 patients with mild OA [25]. T2 values were significantly higher in early OA patients compared to healthy subjects, but T2 values of active and sedentary subjects were not different. However, T2 values in active subjects with and without focal cartilage abnormalities differed significantly. Therefore, the authors suggested that T2 could be a parameter suited to identify active healthy subjects at higher risk for developing cartilage pathology. Luke et al. analyzed articular cartilage T2 measurements of ten asymptomatic marathon runners 2 weeks before, within 48 h after, and 3 months after running a marathon [52]. Postmarathon exams revealed significantly higher T2 values in all articular cartilage compartments of the knee except the lateral femur and tibia. T2 values recovered to baseline except in the medial femur compartment after 3 months. Stehling et al. observed similar results for meniscal T2 measurements [35]. T2 values increased significantly (from 11.1 to 13.6 ms) after competition in all mensical compartments of the 13 marathon runners. After 3 months, T2 values decreased again to baseline values (11.3 ms).

Interestingly, T2 values directly measured after running are decreased [53, 54]. Mosher et al. examined seven young healthy men before and immediately after 30 min of running [53]. They reported a statistically significant decrease in T2 of the superficial 40% of weight-bearing femoral cartilage after exercise. In a later study, Mosher et al. compared 22 marathon runners and 15 sedentary controls before and after 30 min of running [54]. Both groups, marathon runners and sedentary controls, revealed the same T2 response to running. T2 values decreased about 2–4 ms in the superficial femoral cartilage and about 1–3 ms in the superficial tibial cartilage. Smaller T2 decrease was observed in the intermediate cartilage layer, and no change was observed in the deep cartilage layer. Nishii et al. reported similar results with a mechanical loading system [46]. T2 maps were acquired from 22 healthy volunteers under static loading conditions by applying axial compression force of 50% of body weight during imaging. In the femur, a significant T2 decrease with loading was observed only at the region in direct contact with the opposing tibia cartilage, not covered by the meniscus. The T2 decrease in the medial femur amounted to 5.4%. In contrast, T2 decreased all over the medial and lateral tibia with loading (4.3–7.6%). All these observations may be explained by increased compression of the hyaline cartilage. The impact on the cartilage caused by running results in compression of the cartilage and efflux of water. Since the compressibility of the superficial cartilage layer is greater than the deeper layer, highest decrease in cartilage T2 after running was observed in the superficial cartilage.

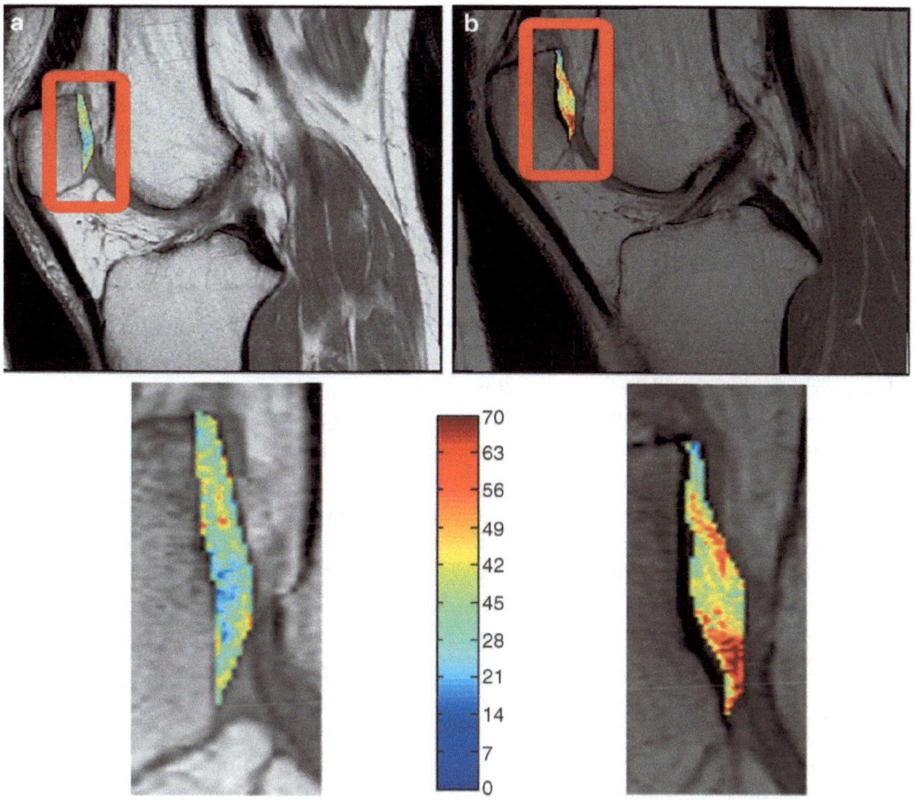

Fig. 12.9 Color-coded T2-maps in [ms] of the patella in subjects with low (**a**), respectively high (**b**) physical activity score. The subject with high physical activity (**b**) showed significantly higher patellar T2 values

Interrelationship of Cartilage T2 with the Underlying Bone

OA does not only affect the articular cartilage but also the underlying bone. An interrelationship between cartilage T2 and trabecular bone structure in the knee joint was demonstrated [55, 56]. Bolbos et al. examined 16 healthy controls and 16 patients with early OA [56]. Early OA patients had significantly higher T2 values and apparent trabecular separation (app.Tb.Sp) as well as lower apparent bone volume fraction (app.BV/TV) than normal controls. Trabecular bone structure correlated with articular cartilage T2 suggesting that loss of mineralized bone is associated with cartilage degeneration. Bining et al. investigated the association of cartilage T2 values with the presence of subchondral bone marrow edema [57]. They compared T2 values of 88 subjects with versus 60 subjects without subchondral bone marrow edema. Subjects with subchondral bone marrow edema pattern showed significantly increased T2 values in the adjacent articular cartilage. The authors concluded that cartilage T2 values and bone marrow edema are related and can both be used as markers for cartilage degeneration.

Association of T2 Measurements with OA-Related Knee Pain

As shown in a previous study, texture analysis based on T2 maps of the articular cartilage can be used for the prediction of longitudinal changes in Western Ontario and McMaster Universities (WOMAC) pain score [58]. OA patients with higher gray level co-occurrence matrix (GLCM) entropy at baseline showed higher increases in the rate-of-change in WOMAC pain scores after 2 years. Zarins et al. analyzed meniscal T2 maps from 19 controls and 44 OA patients [14]. They observed correlations upto $r = 0.55$ for meniscal T2 measurements and WOMAC scores. These studies suggest that T2 measurements as marker for cartilage degeneration are associated with OA-related pain.

Assessment of Cartilage Repair Tissue Using T2 Measurements

Assessment of cartilage repair tissue procedures can be performed with the magnetic resonance observation of cartilage repair tissue (MOCART) scoring system. Welsch et al. compared the clinical Lysholm score and the MOCART scoring system with T2 measurements and diffusion-weighted imaging in their ability to assess differences between cartilage repair tissue after microfracture therapy (MFX) and matrix-associated autologous chondrocyte transplantation (MACT) [59]. They evaluated 20 patients at different postoperative intervals from 12 to 63 months after MFX and 12–59 months after MACT. No differences were observed between MFX and MACT using the Lysholm and MOCART scoring systems. However, T2 measurements showed lower T2 values after MFX compared to MACT and diffusion-weighted imaging distinguished between healthy cartilage and cartilage repair tissue in both procedures. Therefore, the authors concluded that T2 relaxation time measurements and diffusion-weighted imaging may provide additional information about the outcome of cartilage repair procedures. Welsch et al. also examined the potential of zonal T2 mapping as a noninvasive tool in the longitudinal visualization of cartilage repair tissue maturation after MACT [60]. Fifteen patients were treated with MACT and underwent MRI 19.7 ± 12.1 and 31.7 ± 12.0 months after surgery. Healthy cartilage showed a significant T2 increase from the deep to superficial cartilage layer at both time points. Cartilage repair tissue after MACT showed no significant zonal increase from deep to superficial cartilage layer in the T2 maps acquired in the first MRI exam after surgery. However, a significant zonal stratification could be observed in the later MRI exam. Therefore the authors suggested that zonal T2 measurements may be sensitive enough to characterize the maturation of cartilage repair tissue. Further studies used T2 measurements as potential tool for the comparison of different cartilage repair techniques and their efficacy [61–63]. Welsch et al. compared T2 maps of ten patients who underwent MFX with T2 maps of ten patients who underwent MACT [62]. MRI was performed 28.6 ± 5.2 months after surgery in the MFX patient group and 27.4 ± 13.1 months after surgery in the MACT patient group. Healthy cartilage showed similar results for all patients with a significant T2 increase from deep to superficial cartilage. However, mean T2 values had statistically significant reduction in cartilage repair areas after MFX and showed no significant trend between the different cartilage layers. In contrast, mean T2 had no statistically significant decrease in cartilage repair areas after MACT and demonstrated a statistically significant increase from deep to superficial zones. The authors concluded that T2 relaxation time measurements seem to reflect differences in repair tissues formed after two surgical cartilage repair procedures. Salzmann et al. analyzed T2 maps of 18 patients who underwent MACT or osteochondral autograft transplantation (OCT) [61]. They reported significantly lower T2 values in the cartilage repair tissue after MACT compared to OCT. Welsch et al. evaluated different scaffolds for cartilage repair tissue by using T2 mapping [63]. All these studies demonstrated that T2 measurements may indicate different ultra-structural outcome of cartilage repair techniques, which are incompletely evaluated with clinical information.

Summary

Multiple studies have shown the potential and clinical relevance of cartilage T2 relaxation time measurements. Early detection of cartilage degeneration characterized by increase of T2 relaxation times can identify subjects with early OA or at increased risk for OA. Meniscal T2 values correlate with clinical findings of OA. T2 relaxation time measurements are associated with physical activity and may be helpful to detect active subjects at higher risk for developing cartilage pathology. Cartilage T2 values correlate with pain and are intimately related with bone changes due to OA. T2 measurements also emerged as a potential tool for the comparison of different cartilage repair techniques and their efficacy. The major limitation with bringing T2 measurements to clinical routine currently is the lack of a time-efficient and reliable segmentation algorithm. In the future, a fully automated segmentation algorithm for articular and meniscal cartilage will need to be developed. In addition, stable sequences with calibration algorithms are necessary to provide reproducible and precise data across different scanners.

References

1. Dijkgraaf LC, de Bont LG, Boering G, Liem RS. The structure, biochemistry, and metabolism of osteoarthritic cartilage: a review of the literature. J Oral Maxillofac Surg. 1995;53(10):1182–92.
2. Dijkgraaf LC, de Bont LG, Boering G, Liem RS. Normal cartilage structure, biochemistry, and metabolism: a review of the literature. J Oral Maxillofac Surg. 1995;53(8):924–9.
3. Blumenkrantz G, Majumdar S. Quantitative magnetic resonance imaging of articular cartilage in osteoarthritis. Eur Cell Mater. 2007;13:76–86.
4. Burstein D, Gray ML. Is MRI fulfilling its promise for molecular imaging of cartilage in arthritis? Osteoarthritis Cartilage. 2006; 14(11):1087–90.
5. Burstein D. Tracking longitudinal changes in knee degeneration and repair. J Bone Joint Surg Am. 2009;91 Suppl 1:51–3.
6. Dardzinski BJ, Mosher TJ, Li S, Van Slyke MA, Smith MB. Spatial variation of T2 in human articular cartilage. Radiology. 1997;205(2):546–50.
7. Mosher TJ, Dardzinski BJ, Smith MB. Human articular cartilage: influence of aging and early symptomatic degeneration on the spatial variation of T2 – preliminary findings at 3 T. Radiology. 2000;214(1):259–66.
8. Pai A, Li X, Majumdar S. A comparative study at 3 T of sequence dependence of T2 quantitation in the knee. Magn Reson Imaging. 2008;26(9):1215–20.

9. Peterfy CG, Schneider E, Nevitt M. The osteoarthritis initiative: report on the design rationale for the magnetic resonance imaging protocol for the knee. Osteoarthritis Cartilage. 2008;16(12):1433–41.
10. Maier CF, Tan SG, Hariharan H, Potter HG. T2 quantitation of articular cartilage at 1.5 T. J Magn Reson Imaging. 2003;17(3):358–64.
11. Watanabe A, Boesch C, Obata T, Anderson SE. Effect of multislice acquisition on T1 and T2 measurements of articular cartilage at 3T. J Magn Reson Imaging. 2007;26(1):109–17.
12. Smith HE, Mosher TJ, Dardzinski BJ, Collins BG, Collins CM, Yang QX, et al. Spatial variation in cartilage T2 of the knee. J Magn Reson Imaging. 2001;14(1):50–5.
13. Mosher TJ, Smith H, Dardzinski BJ, Schmithorst VJ, Smith MB. MR imaging and T2 mapping of femoral cartilage: in vivo determination of the magic angle effect. AJR Am J Roentgenol. 2001;177(3):665–9.
14. Zarins ZA, Bolbos RI, Pialat JB, Link TM, Li X, Souza RB, Majumdar S. Cartilage and meniscus assessment using T1rho and T2 measurements in healthy subjects and patients with osteoarthritis. Osteoarthritis Cartilage. 2010;18(11):1408–16.
15. Zuo J, Li X, Banerjee S, Han E, Majumdar S. Parallel imaging of knee cartilage at 3 Tesla. J Magn Reson Imaging. 2007;26(4):1001–9.
16. Welsch GH, Mamisch TC, Hughes T, Zilkens C, Quirbach S, Scheffler K, et al. In vivo biochemical 7.0 Tesla magnetic resonance: preliminary results of dGEMRIC, zonal T2, and T2* mapping of articular cartilage. Invest Radiol. 2008;43(9):619–26.
17. Rauscher I, Stahl R, Cheng J, Li X, Huber MB, Luke A, et al. Meniscal measurements of T1rho and T2 at MR imaging in healthy subjects and patients with osteoarthritis. Radiology. 2008;249(2):591–600.
18. Robson MD, Bydder GM. Clinical ultrashort echo time imaging of bone and other connective tissues. NMR Biomed. 2006;19(7):765–80.
19. Du J, Bydder M, Takahashi AM, Chung CB. Two-dimensional ultrashort echo time imaging using a spiral trajectory. Magn Reson Imaging. 2008;26(3):304–12.
20. Koff MF, Amrami KK, Felmlee JP, Kaufman KR. Bias of cartilage T2 values related to method of calculation. Magn Reson Imaging. 2008;26(9):1236–43.
21. Raya JG, Dietrich O, Horng A, Weber J, Reiser MF, Glaser C. T2 measurement in articular cartilage: impact of the fitting method on accuracy and precision at low SNR. Magn Reson Med. 2010;63(1):181–93.
22. Eckstein F, Ateshian G, Burgkart R, Burstein D, Cicuttini F, Dardzinski B, et al. Proposal for a nomenclature for magnetic resonance imaging based measures of articular cartilage in osteoarthritis. Osteoarthritis Cartilage. 2006;14(10):974–83.
23. Dunn TC, Lu Y, Jin H, Ries MD, Majumdar S. T2 relaxation time of cartilage at MR imaging: comparison with severity of knee osteoarthritis. Radiology. 2004;232(2):592–8.
24. Li X, Benjamin MC, Link TM, Castillo DD, Blumenkrantz G, Lozano J, et al. In vivo T(1rho) and T(2) mapping of articular cartilage in osteoarthritis of the knee using 3 T MRI. Osteoarthritis Cartilage. 2007;15(7):789–97.
25. Stahl R, Luke A, Li X, Carballido-Gamio J, Ma CB, Majumdar S, et al. T1rho, T2 and focal knee cartilage abnormalities in physically active and sedentary healthy subjects versus early OA patients – a 3.0-Tesla MRI study. Eur Radiol. 2009;19(1):132–43.
26. Bolbos RI, Link TM, Ma CB, Majumdar S, Li X. T1rho relaxation time of the meniscus and its relationship with T1rho of adjacent cartilage in knees with acute ACL injuries at 3 T. Osteoarthritis Cartilage. 2009;17(1):12–8.
27. Bae KT, Shim H, Tao C, Chang S, Wang JH, Boudreau R, et al. Intra- and inter-observer reproducibility of volume measurement of knee cartilage segmented from the OAI MR image set using a novel semi-automated segmentation method. Osteoarthritis Cartilage. 2009;17(12):1589–97.
28. Carballido-Gamio J, Bauer J, Lee KY, Krause S, Majumdar S. Combined image processing techniques for characterization of MRI cartilage of the knee. Conf Proc IEEE Eng Med Biol Soc. 2005;3:3043–6.
29. Duryea J, Neumann G, Brem MH, Koh W, Noorbakhsh F, Jackson RD, et al. Novel fast semi-automated software to segment cartilage for knee MR acquisitions. Osteoarthritis Cartilage. 2007;15(5):487–92.
30. Fripp J, Crozier S, Warfield SK, Ourselin S. Automatic segmentation of articular cartilage in magnetic resonance images of the knee. Med Image Comput Comput Assist Interv. 2007;10(Pt 2):186–94.
31. Carballido-Gamio J, Link TM, Majumdar S. New techniques for cartilage magnetic resonance imaging relaxation time analysis: texture analysis of flattened cartilage and localized intra- and inter-subject comparisons. Magn Reson Med. 2008;59(6):1472–7.
32. Carballido-Gamio J, Blumenkrantz G, Lynch JA, Link TM, Majumdar S. Longitudinal analysis of MRI T(2) knee cartilage laminar organization in a subset of patients from the osteoarthritis initiative. Magn Reson Med. 2010;63(2):465–72.
33. Carballido-Gamio J, Stahl R, Blumenkrantz G, Romero A, Majumdar S, Link TM. Spatial analysis of magnetic resonance T1rho and T2 relaxation times improves classification between subjects with and without osteoarthritis. Med Phys. 2009;36(9):4059–67.
34. Stehling C, Liebl H, Krug R, Lane NE, Nevitt MC, Lynch J, et al. Patellar cartilage: T2 values and morphologic abnormalities at 3.0-T MR imaging in relation to physical activity in asymptomatic subjects from the osteoarthritis initiative. Radiology. 2010;254(2):509–20.
35. Stehling C, Luke A, Stahl R, Baum T, Pan J, Link TM. Meniscal T1rho and T2 measured with 3.0T MRI increases after running a Marathon. [Oral Presentation at RSNA]. 2009. Chicago.
36. Stehling C, Müller-Höcker C, Schwaiger BJ, Lane NE, Krug R, Nevitt M, McCulloch CE, Lynch J, Link TM. Cartilage T2 and WORMS MR measurements predict changes in clinical parameters over a period of 2 years: Analysis of 217 non-symptomatic subjects from the Osteoarthritis Initiative. [Oral Presentation at ECR]. 2010. Vienna, Austria.
37. Stehling C, Schwaiger BJ, Müller-Höcker C, Kuo D, Lane NE, Lynch J, Nevitt M, McCulloch CE, Link TM. Changes of knee cartilage T2 under physical activity: 24-month follow-up analysis of 182 non-symptomatic subjects from the Osteoarthritis Initiative. [Oral Presentation at ECR]. 2010. Vienna, Austria.
38. Koff MF, Parratte S, Amrami KK, Kaufman KR. Examiner repeatability of patellar cartilage T2 values. Magn Reson Imaging. 2009;27(1):131–6.
39. Haralick R, Shanmugam K, Dinstein I. Textural features for image classification. IEEE Trans Syst Man Cybern. 1973;SMC-3(6):610–21.
40. Blumenkrantz G, Stahl R, Carballido-Gamio J, Zhao S, Lu Y, Munoz T, et al. The feasibility of characterizing the spatial distribution of cartilage T(2) using texture analysis. Osteoarthritis Cartilage. 2008;16(5):584–90.
41. Li X, Pai A, Blumenkrantz G, Carballido-Gamio J, Link T, Ma B, et al. Spatial distribution and relationship of T1rho and T2 relaxation times in knee cartilage with osteoarthritis. Magn Reson Med. 2009;61(6):1310–8.
42. Gluer CC, Blake G, Lu Y, Blunt BA, Jergas M, Genant HK. Accurate assessment of precision errors: how to measure the reproducibility of bone densitometry techniques. Osteoporos Int. 1995;5(4):262–70.
43. Glaser C, Mendlik T, Dinges J, Weber J, Stahl R, Trumm C, et al. Global and regional reproducibility of T2 relaxation time measurements in human patellar cartilage. Magn Reson Med. 2006; 56(3):527–34.
44. Glaser C, Horng A, Mendlik T, Weckbach S, Hoffmann RT, Wagner S, et al. T2 relaxation time in patellar cartilage – global and regional reproducibility at 1.5 tesla and 3 tesla. Rofo. 2007;179(2):146–52.
45. Trattnig S, Apprich S, Szomolanyi P, Mayerhoefer ME, Mamisch TC, Welsch GH. Detection of degenerative cartilage disease: Comparison of high resolution morphological MR and quantitative T2 mapping at 3.0 Tesla. [Oral Presentation ECR]. 2010. Vienna, Austria.
46. Nishii T, Kuroda K, Matsuoka Y, Sahara T, Yoshikawa H. Change in knee cartilage T2 in response to mechanical loading. J Magn Reson Imaging. 2008;28(1):175–80.

47. Yao W, Qu N, Lu Z, Yang S. The application of T1 and T2 relaxation time and magnetization transfer ratios to the early diagnosis of patellar cartilage osteoarthritis. Skeletal Radiol. 2009;38(11):1055–62.
48. Friedrich KM, Shepard T, Chang G, Wang L, Babb JS, Schweitzer M, et al. Does joint alignment affect the T2 values of cartilage in patients with knee osteoarthritis? Eur Radiol. 2010;20(6):1532–8.
49. Friedrich KM, Shepard T, de Oliveira VS, Wang L, Babb JS, Schweitzer M, et al. T2 measurements of cartilage in osteoarthritis patients with meniscal tears. AJR Am J Roentgenol. 2009;193(5):W411–5.
50. Mosher TJ, Liu Y, Yang QX, Yao J, Smith R, Dardzinski BJ, et al. Age dependency of cartilage magnetic resonance imaging T2 relaxation times in asymptomatic women. Arthritis Rheum. 2004;50(9):2820–8.
51. Mosher TJ, Collins CM, Smith HE, Moser LE, Sivarajah RT, Dardzinski BJ, et al. Effect of gender on in vivo cartilage magnetic resonance imaging T2 mapping. J Magn Reson Imaging. 2004;19(3):323–8.
52. Luke AC, Stehling C, Stahl R, Li X, Kay T, Takemoto S, et al. High-field magnetic resonance imaging assessment of articular cartilage before and after marathon running: does long-distance running lead to cartilage damage? Am J Sports Med. 2010;38:2273–80.
53. Mosher TJ, Smith HE, Collins C, Liu Y, Hancy J, Dardzinski BJ, et al. Change in knee cartilage T2 at MR imaging after running: a feasibility study. Radiology. 2005;234(1):245–9.
54. Mosher TJ, Liu Y, Torok CM. Functional cartilage MRI T2 mapping: evaluating the effect of age and training on knee cartilage response to running. Osteoarthritis Cartilage. 2010;18(3):358–64.
55. Blumenkrantz G, Lindsey CT, Dunn TC, Jin H, Ries MD, Link TM, et al. A pilot, two-year longitudinal study of the interrelationship between trabecular bone and articular cartilage in the osteoarthritic knee. Osteoarthritis Cartilage. 2004;12(12):997–1005.
56. Bolbos RI, Zuo J, Banerjee S, Link TM, Ma CB, Li X, et al. Relationship between trabecular bone structure and articular cartilage morphology and relaxation times in early OA of the knee joint using parallel MRI at 3 T. Osteoarthritis Cartilage. 2008;16(10):1150–9.
57. Bining HJ, Santos R, Andrews G, Forster BB. Can T2 relaxation values and color maps be used to detect chondral damage utilizing subchondral bone marrow edema as a marker? Skeletal Radiol. 2009;38(5):459–65.
58. Blumenkrantz G, Carballido-Gamio J, McCulloch CE, Lynch J, Link TM, Majumdar S. The relationship between the spatial distribution of cartilage MR T2 and longitudinal changes in pain: Data from the Osteoarthritis Initiative. [Poster ISMRM 2009]. 2009. Hawaii.
59. Welsch GH, Trattnig S, Domayer S, Marlovits S, White LM, Mamisch TC. Multimodal approach in the use of clinical scoring, morphological MRI and biochemical T2-mapping and diffusion-weighted imaging in their ability to assess differences between cartilage repair tissue after microfracture therapy and matrix-associated autologous chondrocyte transplantation: a pilot study. Osteoarthritis Cartilage. 2009;17(9):1219–27.
60. Welsch GH, Mamisch TC, Marlovits S, Glaser C, Friedrich K, Hennig FF, et al. Quantitative T2 mapping during follow-up after matrix-associated autologous chondrocyte transplantation (MACT): full-thickness and zonal evaluation to visualize the maturation of cartilage repair tissue. J Orthop Res. 2009;27(7):957–63.
61. Salzmann GM, Paul J, Bauer JS, Woertler K, Sauerschnig M, Landwehr S, et al. T2 assessment and clinical outcome following autologous matrix-assisted chondrocyte and osteochondral autograft transplantation. Osteoarthritis Cartilage. 2009;17(12): 1576–82.
62. Welsch GH, Mamisch TC, Domayer SE, Dorotka R, Kutscha-Lissberg F, Marlovits S, et al. Cartilage T2 assessment at 3-T MR imaging: in vivo differentiation of normal hyaline cartilage from reparative tissue after two cartilage repair procedures – initial experience. Radiology. 2008;247(1):154–61.
63. Welsch GH, Mamisch TC, Zak L, Blanke M, Olk A, Marlovits S, et al. Evaluation of cartilage repair tissue after matrix-associated autologous chondrocyte transplantation using a hyaluronic-based or a collagen-based scaffold with morphological MOCART scoring and biochemical T2 mapping: preliminary results. Am J Sports Med. 2010;38(5):934–42.

Chapter 13
MR $T_{1\rho}$ Relaxation Time Quantification in Cartilage

Xiaojuan Li

Keywords Cartilage • Osteoarthritis • MR $T_{1\rho}$ relaxation time • Quantification • Sequence development

Introduction

Osteoarthritis (OA) is characterized by the progressive loss of hyaline articular cartilage. MRI has been widely applied to visualize cartilage directly. However, conventional MRI is limited to showing cartilage morphological changes at a stage when cartilage is already irreversibly lost. Standard cartilage-dedicated MR techniques include fat-saturated T_2-weighted, proton density-weighted fast spin echo (FSE) sequences and T_1-weighted spoiled gradient echo (SPGR) sequences. These sequences are inconclusive in quantifying early degenerative changes of the cartilage matrix [1]. As discussed in detail in Chap. 1, hyaline articular cartilage is composed by few chondrocytes surrounded by a large extracellular matrix (ECM). The ECM is composed primarily by water and two groups of macromolecules: proteoglycan and collagen fibers. Early events in the development of cartilage matrix breakdown include the loss of proteoglycans, changes in water content, and molecular-level changes in collagen [2]. Early diagnosis of cartilage degeneration would require the ability to noninvasively detect changes in proteoglycan concentration and collagen integrity before gross morphologic changes occur. This capability of early diagnosis would be valuable for preventing the progression of disease and for therapeutic monitoring. MR $T_{1\rho}$ relaxation time quantification in cartilage has been proposed as a promising tool towards this goal, and $T_{1\rho}$ quantification techniques have been developed in the past decade for imaging early biochemical changes in cartilage matrix. The major clinical applications have been in osteoarthritis (OA) and acutely injured knees that have a high risk of developing OA. In this chapter, we will discuss the basic principles of $T_{1\rho}$ relaxation mechanism, technical development, and clinical applications of this novel technique.

Definition and Basic Principles of MR $T_{1\rho}$ Relaxation Time

The $T_{1\rho}$ parameter is defined as the time constant describing the spin-lattice relaxation in the rotating frame [3]. It probes the slow motion interactions between motionally restricted water molecules and their local macromolecular environment, and therefore provides unique biomedical information in the low-frequency regime. The frequency range is typically from a few hundred hertz to a few kilohertz. The macromolecules in articular cartilage ECM restrict the motion of water molecules. Changes to the ECM, such as PG loss, therefore, can be reflected in measurements of $T_{1\rho}$. The $T_{1\rho}$ is normally measured by the spin-lock (SL) technique. SL experiment was first described by Redfield in solid materials [4], which enabled the study of relaxation at very low fields without sacrificing the signal-to-noise ratio afforded by higher field strengths. In an SL experiment (Fig. 13.1), spins are flipped into the transverse plane along one axis, immediately followed by a SL pulse applied along the same axis. A SL pulse is an on-resonance, continuous wave radiofrequency (RF) pulse, normally with long duration and low energy. Since the magnetization and RF field are along the same direction, the magnetization is said to be "spin-locked" provided the locking condition is satisfied, i.e., the B_1 of locking pulses are much stronger than the local magnetic fields generated by, for example, magnetic moments of nuclei. Thus, the normal transverse relaxation (characterized by the relaxation time T_2) will not take place. Neither will the longitudinal relaxation (characterized by the relaxation time T_1) along B_0 occur because of the effect of the locking pulses. The spins will relax with a time constant $T_{1\rho}$ along B_1 of locking pulses in the transverse plane [3]. This is a situation similar to that of the longitudinal magnetization in the B_0

X. Li (✉)
Department of Radiology and Biomedical Imaging, University of California, 185 Berry Street, Suite 350, San Francisco, CA, USA
e-mail: xiaojuan.li@radiology.ucsf.edu

T.M. Link (ed.), *Cartilage Imaging: Significance, Techniques, and New Developments*, DOI 10.1007/978-1-4419-8438-8_13, © Springer Science+Business Media, LLC 2011

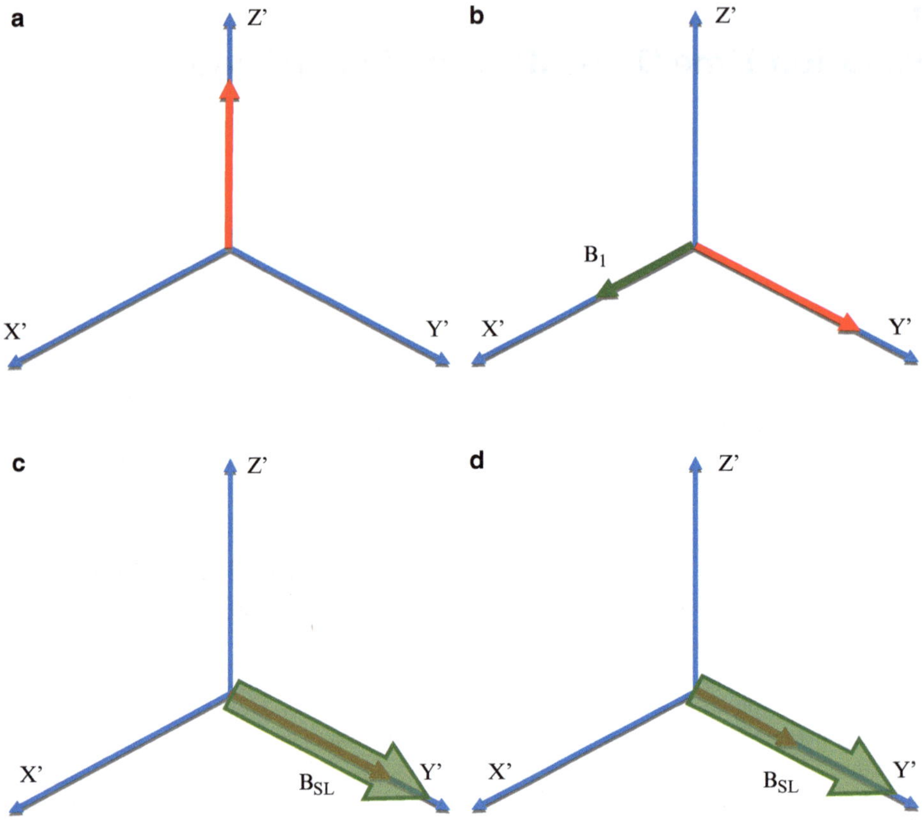

Fig. 13.1 The spin-lock experiment. The spins are flipped from the *Z*-axis (**a**) into the transverse along *Y′* with B_1 applied along *X′* (**b**), immediately followed by a spin-lock pulse (B_{SL}) applied along the same axis *Y′* (**c**). Under locking condition, the spins will relax with a time constant $T_{1\rho}$ along the locking pulses in the transverse plane (**d**). *X′–Y′–Z′* represents the rotating frame

field, but at a much lower strength of spin-lock B_1. $T_{1\rho}$ is always greater than T_2, but lower than T_1.

The amplitude of the SL pulse is commonly referenced in terms of the nutation frequency ($f = \gamma B_1$). The normal range of SL frequency is a few hundred hertz to a few kilohertz. $T_{1\rho}$ relaxation phenomena are sensitive to physicochemical processes with inverse correlation times on the order of the nutation frequency of the SL pulse. By setting the amplitude of the SL pulse to coincide with the frequency of the molecular processes of interest, the signal from the SL MRI sequence becomes heavily $T_{1\rho}$-weighted. $T_{1\rho}$ can be computed by acquiring a series of $T_{1\rho}$-weighted images at various SL pulse duration. $T_{1\rho}$ increases as the strength of the SL field increases, a phenomenon termed $T_{1\rho}$ dispersion. $T_{1\rho}$ dispersions may also have tissue specificity [3].

The mechanism of $T_{1\rho}$ relaxation time in biological tissues, particularly in cartilage, is not fully understood yet. Using native and immobilized protein solution, Makela et al. suggested that proton exchange between the protein side chain groups and bulk water contribute significantly to the $T_{1\rho}$ relaxation [5]. Based on spectroscopy experiments with peptide solutions, glycosaminoglycan (GAG) solutions, and bovine cartilage samples before and after proteoglycan (PG) degradation, Duvvuri et al. further suggested that cartilage hydrogen exchange from NH and OH groups to water may dominate the low-frequency (0–1.5 kHz) water $T_{1\rho}$ dispersion [6]. They speculated that increase of the low-frequency correlation rate with PG loss could be the result of increased proton exchange rates. Other evidence of a proton exchange pathway is the PH dependency of $T_{1\rho}$ values in the ischemic rat brain tissues [7]. Mlynarik et al., on the other hand, have suggested that the dominant relaxation mechanism in the rotating frame in cartilage at $B_0 \leq 3$ T seems to be dipolar interaction [8]. The contribution of scalar relaxation caused by proton exchange is only relevant at high fields such as 7 T. Clearly, further investigations are needed to better understand this relaxation mechanism.

Sequence Development of MR $T_{1\rho}$ in Cartilage

The $T_{1\rho}$-weighted imaging sequences are composed of two parts: magnetization preparation with $T_{1\rho}$ weight using spin-lock pulse cluster, and a following 2D or 3D data

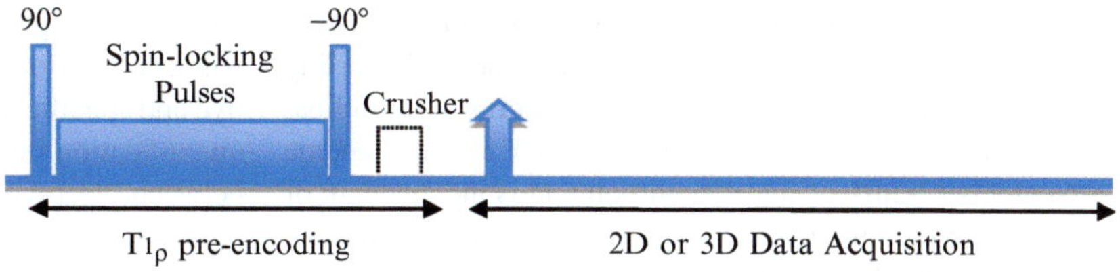

Fig. 13.2 The pulse sequence diagram of $T_{1\rho}$-weighted imaging. The sequence is composed of the $T_{1\rho}$ pre-encoding with spin-lock pulse cluster, followed by a 2D or 3D data acquisition

acquisition, as shown in Fig. 13.2. The spin-lock pulse cluster consists of a hard 90° pulse followed by a spin-lock pulse and a hard –90° pulse. The first 90° pulse applied along the *x*-axis flips the longitudinal magnetization into the transverse plane along the *y*-axis. Then, a long low-power pulse is applied along the *y*-axis to spin-lock the magnetization. The second 90° pulse flips this spin-locked magnetization back to the *z*-axis. Residual transverse magnetization is dephased by a crusher gradient. Magnetization stored along the *z*-axis is read out by the following sequences. Several modifications were performed in the SL pulse cluster in order to improve the robustness of spin locking to B0 and B1 inhomogeneity. Dixon et al. designed a composite SL pulse as 90 *y*–135 *x* – lock *x* – 135 *x*–90 *y* and showed the tolerance of this composite to shimming and frequency errors allows spin locking with relatively weak RF (low spin-lock frequency) and therefore low specific absorption rate (SAR) [9]. Charagundla et al. proposed a "self-compensated" SL pulse, the phase of the second half of the spin-lock pulse was shifted 180° from the first half, to reduce artifacts caused by B_1 inhomogeneity [10]. Witschey et al. from the same group further proposed an integrated spin echo and spin-lock pulses to eliminate banding artifact caused by B_0 and/or B_1 inhomogeneity [11].

Current $T_{1\rho}$ quantification techniques are based on either two-dimensional (2D) spin echo (SE), fast spin echo (FSE) [12], spiral imaging [13], echo planar imaging [14, 15] or three-dimensional (3D) gradient echo sequences [16–18]. These sequences have been implemented at both 1.5 T and 3 T on scanners from different manufactures.

The initial development of $T_{1\rho}$-weighted imaging was based on single-slice two-dimensional (2D) spin echo (SE) or fast spin echo (FSE) [12] sequences. $T_{1\rho}$-weighted images with varying TSLs were acquired and the $T_{1\rho}$ maps can be reconstructed pixel by pixel using the equation below:

$$S(\mathrm{TSL}) \propto e^{(-\mathrm{TSL}/\mathrm{T1\rho})}$$

The nonselective pulses (hard pulses) used in spin-lock experiment will saturate the longitudinal magnetization from nonexcited regions, thus making the implementation of the $T_{1\rho}$ sequence in multi-slice mode not straightforward. Wheaton et al. measured experimentally and theoretically modeled this longitudinal saturation as $T_{2\rho}$ decay [12]. The saturation data was used to correct the image data as a function of the SL pulse duration to make quantitative measurements of $T_{1\rho}$ using a multi-slice FSE sequence. The $T_{1\rho}$ quantification using this saturation-corrected multi-slice data was reported to be identical to that measured using single-slice spin-lock sequence [12]. Alternatively, an RF cycling technique was used to eliminate T_1 contamination in the $T_{1\rho}$-weighted images during multi-slice acquisition [13]. In this technique, as first described by Wright et al. [19], longitudinal magnetization is inverted immediately after alternate magnetization preparation. This technique needs no correction and modeling for longitudinal saturation, with a cost of increased scan time. The $T_{1\rho}$ measurement using RF cycling and 2D spiral multi-slice acquisition has been validated using MR spectroscopy method and single-slice acquisition [13]. Reproducibility was assessed using the average coefficient of variation of median $T_{1\rho}$ that was 0.68% in phantoms and 4.8% in healthy volunteers [13].

Compared with 2D methods, 3D imaging is free from artifacts caused by slice crosstalk. Therefore, 3D sequences can generally have a thinner slice thickness, and consequently may provide a more accurate assessment of cartilage degeneration. High-resolution MRI is particularly attractive in the context of OA where cartilage becomes very thin – on the order of, or less than, 1 mm. Furthermore, a 3D acquisition is desired due to the non-slice-selective nature of the $T_{1\rho}$ preparation pulses (spin-lock pulses).

Borthakur et al. have developed a 3D $T_{1\rho}$ mapping technique based on a steady-state spoiled gradient echo (SPGR) imaging sequence [16, 17, 20]. This method showed clinical promise at both 1.5 T and 3 T. However, using this method, the energy deposited by the sequence (as estimated by specific absorption rate, SAR) is intensive because $T_{1\rho}$ preparation pulses are applied every TR. Relatively long TRs (140 ms at 1.5 T and 175 ms at 3 T) are used in order to comply with the maximum SAR mandated by Food and Drug Administration (FDA). This long TR results in long acquisition times. In addition, this technique requires a prior knowledge of T_1 (or an assumption) for $T_{1\rho}$ quantification as T_1-dependent steady-state signals are used.

Recently, novel 3D acquisitions have been developed for in vivo knee $T_{1\rho}$ mapping based on SPGR [21] (referred as **M**agnetization-prepared **A**ngle-modulated **P**artitioned-k-space **S**poiled Gradient Echo **S**napshots, MAPSS) and balanced gradient echo (b-GRE) [18]. In both methods, transient signal evolving toward the steady state were acquired, which allows multiple TR acquisitions per spin-lock preencoding. Thus, these sequences are less SAR intensive than the previous 3D SPGR $T_{1\rho}$-weighted imaging using the steady-state signals. In MPASS, the acquisition was in an interleaved segmented elliptical centric phase encoding order immediately after a $T_{1\rho}$ magnetization preparation sequence. RF cycling was applied to eliminate the adverse impact of longitudinal relaxation on quantitative accuracy. This RF cycling scheme also yields a transient signal evolution that is independent of the prepared magnetization M_{prep}. However, the acquisition time was doubled because two acquisitions per phase encoding step were acquired. A variable flip angle train was then designed to provide a flat signal response to eliminate the filtering effect in k-space caused by transient signal evolution. Experiments in phantoms agreed well with results from simulation. Measurements in vivo using MAPSS agree well with previously developed 2D methods. The $T_{1\rho}$ values were 42.4 ± 5.2 ms in overall cartilage of healthy volunteers. The average coefficient of variation (CV) of mean $T_{1\rho}$ values ($n = 4$) for overall cartilage was 1.6%, with regional CV ranging from 1.7% to 8.7% [21].

In the method using b-GRE sequence, the transient signal decay during b-GRE image acquisition was corrected using a k-space filter. However, because the transient signal decay depended on the initial $T_{1\rho}$ preparation, the corresponding $T_{1\rho}$ map was altered by variations in the point spread function with TSL. Measurement of $T_{1\rho}$ using the $T_{1\rho}$-prepared b-GRE sequence matches standard $T_{1\rho}$-prepared SE in the medial patellar and lateral patellar cartilage compartments [18].

A technique challenge for $T_{1\rho}$-weighted imaging is the relatively high energy deposited to tissues during scans due to application of long duration of RF pulses. Previous studies have suggested $T_{1\rho}$ mapping sequences with reduced SAR using partial k-space acquisition approach [22] and "keyhole" acquisition [23]. $T_{1\rho}$ sequences have also been implemented using parallel imaging techniques [24, 25]. In these studies, no significant differences were found between parallel versus nonparallel $T_{1\rho}$ quantification.

MR $T_{1\rho}$ Quantification in Cartilage Specimens

In vitro studies have evaluated the relationship between $T_{1\rho}$ relaxation time and the biochemical composition of cartilage. Akella et al. have demonstrated that over 50% depletion of PG from bovine articular cartilage resulted in average $T_{1\rho}$ increases from 110 to 170 ms [26]. Regression analysis of the data showed a strong correlation ($R^2 = 0.987$) between changes in PG and $T_{1\rho}$. In another study on bovine cartilage at 4 T, $T_{1\rho}$ has been proposed as a more specific indicator of PG content than T_2 relaxation in trypsinized cartilage [27]. The authors reported that there was an excellent correlation ($R^2 = 0.89$) between $1/T_{1\rho}$ and GAG concentration while the correlation between $1/T_2$ and GAG concentration was rather poor ($R^2 = 0.01$). In $T_{1\rho}$ quantification experiments, the spin-lock techniques reduce dipolar interactions and therefore reduce the dependence of the relaxation time constant on collagen fiber orientation [28]. This may enable more sensitive and specific detection of changes in PG content using $T_{1\rho}$ quantification in cartilage. Wheaton et al. found correlations between $T_{1\rho}$ relaxation time, proteoglycan, and mechanical properties of bovine cartilage explants including aggregate modulus and hydraulic permeability [29]. Regatte et al. demonstrated $T_{1\rho}$ values in human cartilage specimens increased with increased clinical grades of degeneration [30], Fig. 13.3. More recently, Li et al. reported that in human OA cartilage obtained from patients who underwent total knee arthroplasty, $R_{1\rho}$ ($1/T_{1\rho}$) values had a significant, but moderate correlation with GAG contents ($R = 0.45$, $P = 0.002$) [31], Fig. 13.4. These studies form the experimental basis for using the $T_{1\rho}$ mapping techniques in studying cartilage pathology in OA.

Previous studies showed that collagen structure and orientation are dominating factors that affect T_2 relaxation in cartilage. This results in the "magic angle" effect and commonly seen laminar appearance in cartilage imaging [32, 33]. Similar to T_2, studies have demonstrated regional variations of cartilage $T_{1\rho}$. $T_{1\rho}$ values were highest at the superficial zone, decreased gradually in the middle zone, and increased in the region near the subchondral bone in bovine cartilage [26] and human cartilage specimens [30]. Although the trend of $T_{1\rho}$ and T_2 values are similar, $T_{1\rho}$ shows a larger dynamic range from the bone/cartilage interface to the cartilage surface, which may allow a higher sensitivity of distinguishing between healthy and degenerated cartilage. Furthermore, less laminar appearance was observed in $T_{1\rho}$-weighted images compared to T_2-weighted images due to reduced dipolar interaction during $T_{1\rho}$ relaxation [28]. Previous studies also investigated the correlation between T_2 and $T_{1\rho}$ values in cartilage. Mlyranik et al. [34] showed that the $T_{1\rho}$ relaxation times obtained were slightly longer than the corresponding T_2 values, but both parameters showed almost identical spatial distributions. Menezes et al. [35] have shown that $T_{1\rho}$ and T_2 changes in articular cartilage do not necessarily coincide, and might provide complimentary information. These studies suggested that $T_{1\rho}$ and T_2 reflect changes that may be associated with proteoglycan, collagen content and hydration and the true mechanism of $T_{1\rho}$ may arise from a weighted average of multiple biochemical changes occurring in cartilage in OA.

In Vivo MR $T_{1\rho}$ Quantification in Cartilage and Meniscus

In vivo studies show increased cartilage $T_{1\rho}$ values in OA subjects compared to controls [13, 17, 36, 37]. Figure 13.5 shows color-coded $T_{1\rho}$ maps overlaid on SPGR images for a

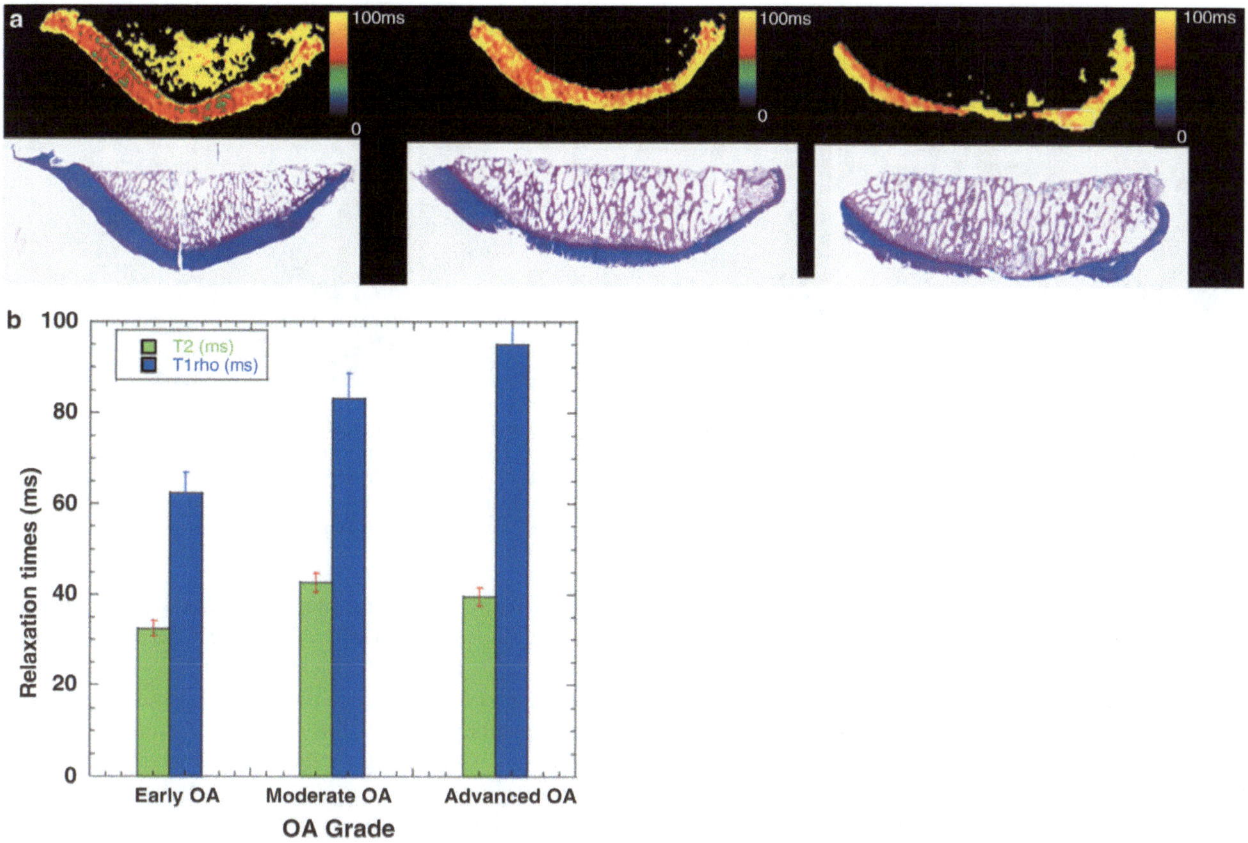

Fig. 13.3 (**a**) Representative $T_{1\rho}$ maps and histology of human cartilage with early OA (*left*), moderate OA (*middle*), and late OA (*right*). (**b**) Comparison of T_2 and $T_{1\rho}$ relaxation times as a function of various clinical grades of OA cartilage (early OA, moderate OA, and advanced OA) [30]

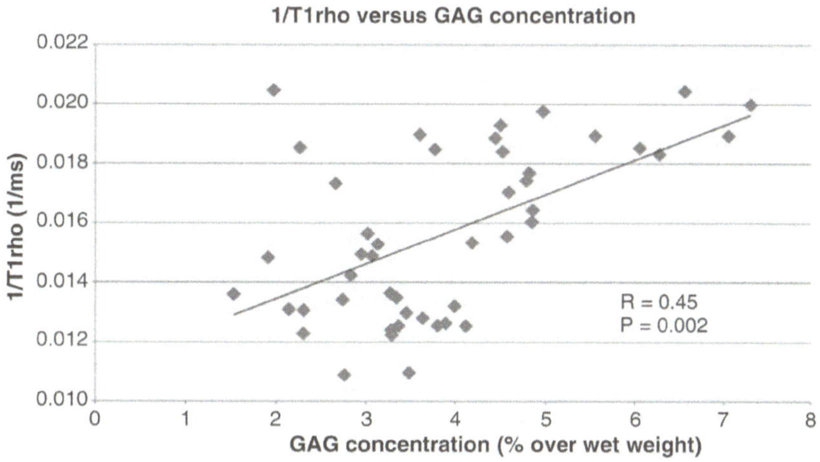

Fig. 13.4 Significant correlation was found between $R_{1\rho}$ relaxation rate ($1/T_{1\rho}$) and glycosaminoglycan (GAG) contents in human osteoarthritic cartilage [31]

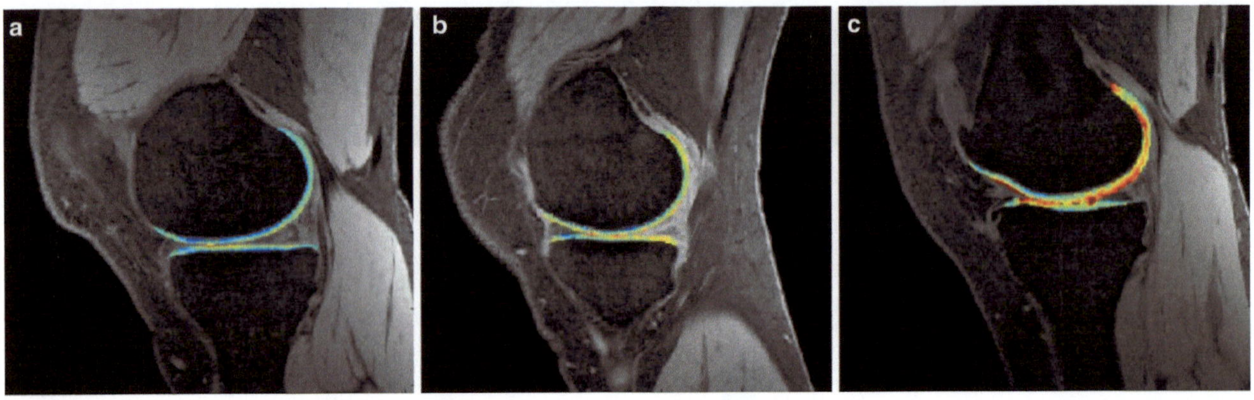

Fig. 13.5 $T_{1\rho}$ maps in knee cartilage. (**a**) A healthy control; (**b**) a patient with mild OA (KL = 1); (**c**) a patient with severe OA (KL = 3). The mean $T_{1\rho}$ in MFC was 32.9 ± 9.0 ms, 41.1 ± 11.0 ms, and 49.1 ± 14.2 ms in subject A, B, and C, respectively. The mean $T_{1\rho}$ in MT was 35.8 ± 11.4 ms, 39.3 ± 12.2 ms, and 43.6 ± 12.0 in subject **a**, **b**, and **c**, respectively. Data were acquired on a GE HDx 3 T MR scanner using an eight-channel phased-array knee coil. The $T_{1\rho}$ sequence was based on 3D SPGR acquisition (MAPSS, reference 21). Time of spin-lock = 0, 10, 40, 80 ms, frequency of spin-lock = 500, FOV = 14 cm, matrix = 256 × 192, slice thickness = 3 mm

healthy volunteer (a) and a patient with mild OA (b) and a patient with severe OA (c). Significant elevated $T_{1\rho}$ values in cartilage were observed in patients with OA. In a recent cohort study using 3 T MRI [37], the average $T_{1\rho}$ and T_2 values were significantly increased in OA patients compared with controls (52.04 ± 2.97 ms vs 45.53 ± 3.28 ms with P = 0.0002 for $T_{1\rho}$, and 39.63 ± 2.69 vs 34.74 ± 2.48 with P = 0.001 for T_2). Increased $T_{1\rho}$ and T_2 values were also correlated with increased severity in radiographic and MR grading of OA. $T_{1\rho}$ has a larger range and higher effect size than T_2, 3.7 versus 3.0. These studies reflect the potential for $T_{1\rho}$ imaging for noninvasive evaluation of diseased cartilage.

Another in vivo study applied T_2 and $T_{1\rho}$ measurements in physically active and sedentary healthy subjects as well as in patients with early OA [38]. Nine out of 13 active healthy subjects had focal cartilage abnormalities. $T_{1\rho}$ and T_2 values in active subjects with and without focal cartilage abnormalities differed significantly ($p < 0.05$, Fig. 13.6). $T_{1\rho}$ and T_2 values were significantly higher ($p < 0.05$) in early OA patients compared to healthy subjects. $T_{1\rho}$ measurements were superior to T_2 in differentiating OA patients from healthy subjects, yet $T_{1\rho}$ was moderately age-dependent. The authors suggested that $T_{1\rho}$ and T_2 could be a parameter suited to identify active healthy subjects at higher risk for developing cartilage pathology.

The spatial correlation between T_2 and $T_{1\rho}$ in cartilage has also been explored in vivo. A recent in vivo study quantified the pixel-by-pixel correlation of $T_{1\rho}$ and T_2 values in OA patients (n = 10) and healthy controls (n = 10) [39]. The investigators showed that, although the average $T_{1\rho}$ and T_2 values correlated significantly, the pixel-by-pixel correlation between $T_{1\rho}$ and T_2 showed a large range in both controls and OA patients (R = 0.522 ± 0.183, ranging from 0.221 to 0.763 in OA patients vs R = 0.624 ± 0.060, ranging from 0.547 to 0.726 in controls) [39]. Figure 13.7 shows $T_{1\rho}$ and T_2 maps from a control subject, a subject with mild OA, and a subject with severe OA. The differences between the $T_{1\rho}$ and T_2 maps are evident. These results suggested $T_{1\rho}$ and T_2 show different spatial distribution and may provide complementary information regarding cartilage degeneration in OA. Combining these two parameters may further improve our capability to diagnose early cartilage degeneration and injury.

As spatial variation was observed in a number of $T_{1\rho}$ and T_2 studies, texture analysis [40] has been applied to examine the spatial distribution of pixel values and quantify the heterogeneity in $T_{1\rho}$ and T_2 maps image [41–43]. The most commonly used texture analysis parameters are those extracted from the grey-level co-occurrence matrix (GLCM) as proposed by Haralick et al. [44]. The GLCM determines the frequency that neighboring grey-level values occur in an image. Parameters derived from GLCM provide information on the variation between neighboring pixels and directly quantify the distribution of the image signal. Blumenkrantz et al. demonstrated that mild OA patients (n = 8) had significantly elevated GLCM entropy and reduced ASM of cartilage T_2 values than controls (n = 14) [43]. Similarly, Li et al. reported that overall elevated contrast and entropy measurements and lower ASM and GLCM mean measurements of both $T_{1\rho}$ and T_2 values were observed in patients with OA (n = 10) when compared to controls (n = 10) [41]. These differences, however, appear more prevalent in $T_{1\rho}$ measurements in this cohort of patients [41]. The results from these studies indicate that $T_{1\rho}$ and T_2 relaxation time constants are not only increased but are also more heterogeneous in osteoarthritic cartilage.

Studies have also used $T_{1\rho}$ imaging to evaluate cartilage overlying bone marrow edema–like lesions (BMEL) in OA knees [45, 46]. In a 1-year longitudinal study with 23 OA patients, Zhao et al. have found that patients with BMEL

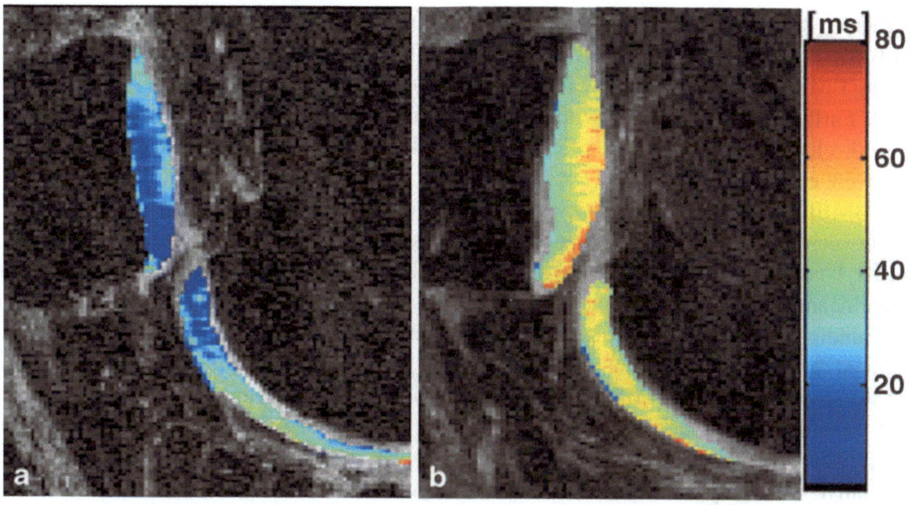

Fig. 13.6 Color-coded $T_{1\rho}$ maps overlaid on SPGR images (TR/TE: 20/7.5 ms) from a central section of the patello-femoral cartilage. (**a**) Demonstrates the $T_{1\rho}$ map of an asymptomatic active (25-year-old male) subject without focal cartilage abnormalities anywhere in the knee. The average $T_{1\rho}$ of the patello-femoral compartment was 33.7±0.73 ms. (**b**) Shows the $T_{1\rho}$ map of an asymptomatic (36-year-old female) active subject at the central femoro-patellar joint who had a cartilage lesion at the lateral patella. The average $T_{1\rho}$ of the patello-femoral compartment was 45.9±1.68 ms. Interestingly, compared to subject (**a**), the $T_{1\rho}$ values at the central patella and at the trochlea are globally increased, not only in the region of the defect, yet have a similar distribution [38]

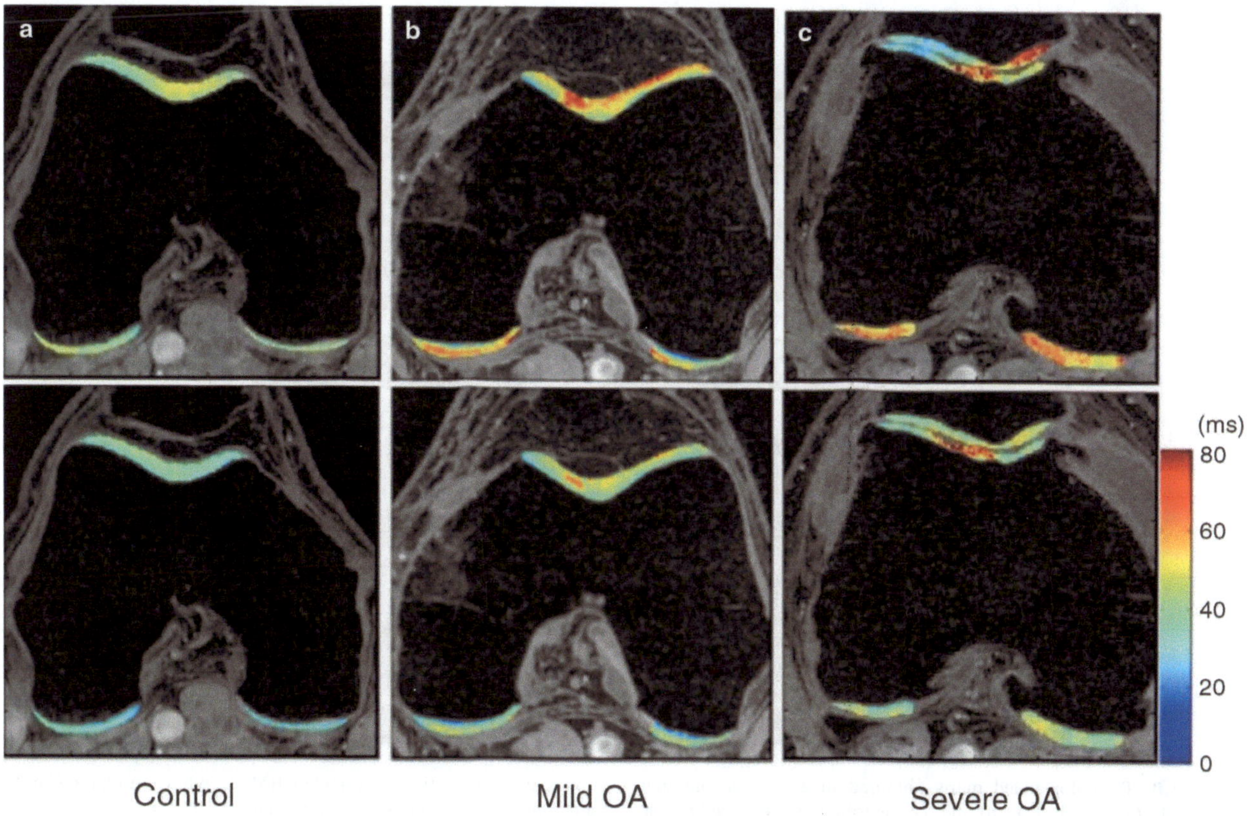

Fig. 13.7 $T_{1\rho}$ maps (*first row*) and T_2 maps (*second row*) for a healthy control (**a**), a patient with mild OA (**b**), and a patient with severe OA (**c**). (**a**) Control: The average $T_{1\rho}$ value was 40.1 ± 11.4 ms and T_2 value was 33.3 ± 10.5 ms in cartilage. (**b**) A patient with early OA (male, 66). The average $T_{1\rho}$ value was 45.5 ± 14.5 ms and T_2 value was 35.0 ± 10.9 ms in cartilage. (**c**) A patient with advanced OA (male, 46). The average $T_{1\rho}$ value was 55.4 ± 26.0 ms and T_2 value was 43.8 ± 11.1 ms in cartilage. The maps illustrate the differences between $T_{1\rho}$ and T_2 and demonstrate differences in cartilage heterogeneity between OA severity and between T_2 and $T_{1\rho}$ maps

showed overall higher $T_{1\rho}$ values in cartilage compared with those who had no BMEL (42.0 ± 3.7 ms vs 39.8 ± 1.4 ms, $P = 0.032$), suggesting BMEL may be correlated with disease severity of OA [46]. Furthermore, in patients with BMEL, both $T_{1\rho}$ values and clinical Whole-Organ MRI Score (WORMS) grading were elevated significantly ($P < 0.05$) in cartilage overlying BMEL (Fig. 13.8), suggesting a local spatial correlation between BMEL and more advanced cartilage degeneration. At 1-year follow-up, cartilage overlying BMEL showed a significantly higher $T_{1\rho}$ value increase compared with the surrounding cartilage, suggesting BMEL is indicative of accelerated cartilage degeneration. Interestingly, no such difference was found using WORMS scoring. This result suggests that quantitative cartilage imaging, such as $T_{1\rho}$, may be a more sensitive indicator of cartilage degeneration than semiquantitative scoring systems.

In addition to patients with OA, $T_{1\rho}$ quantification techniques have been applied to patients with acutely injured knees, who have a high risk of developing OA later in life. In patients with acute anterior cruciate ligament (ACL) tears, significantly increased $T_{1\rho}$ values were found in cartilage overlying bone marrow edema–like lesions (BMEL) when compared with surrounding cartilage at the lateral tibia (LT, $P < 0.05$), but no significant difference was found in the lateral femoral condyle [45, 47]. Two patients have been confirmed to have cartilage damage in regions with elevated $T_{1\rho}$ values using arthroscopic images, as shown in Fig. 13.9 [48].

One-year longitudinal follow-up on these ACL-injured knees [49, 50] showed that (1) in lateral sides, despite the resolution of BMEL, cartilage overlying the baseline BMEL still show significantly higher $T_{1\rho}$ compared to the surrounding cartilage, suggesting potential irreversible damage of cartilage in these regions, Fig. 13.10a and b; (2) in medial sides, $T_{1\rho}$ values in medial tibial and medial femoral condyles, especially the contact area, show significant elevation at as early as 1-year after ACL reconstruction compared to healthy controls, Fig. 13.10c and d. These results suggest cartilage damage after acute knee injuries that can be the risk factors for predisposing OA to these knees. Quantitative $T_{1\rho}$ can probe these degenerations at earlier time points than radiographs or conventional MRI. T_2 also showed increasing trend in these regions of cartilage, however it did not reach statistical significance. The authors speculated that $T_{1\rho}$ is more sensitive than T_2 in detecting cartilage damages and potential early

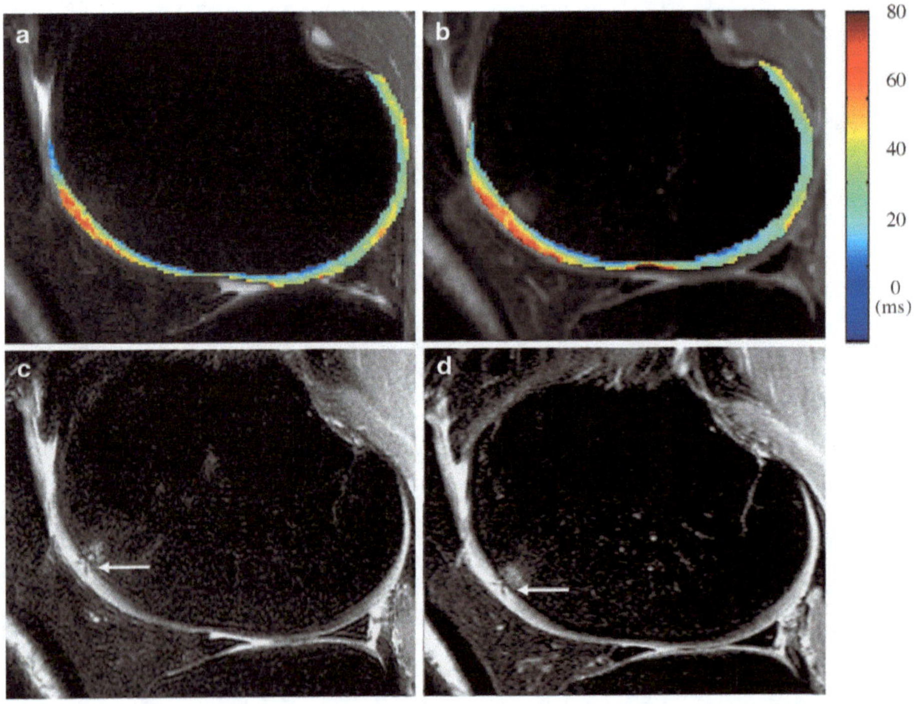

Fig. 13.8 $T_{1\rho}$ color-coded maps obtained in a 57-year-old man with mild OA at baseline (**a**) and 1-year follow-up (**b**). Sagittal fat-suppressed T2-weighted fast spin-echo image obtained in the same patient at baseline (**c**) and 1-year follow-up (**d**). $T_{1\rho}$ values of lateral femoral condyle were significantly higher in cartilage overlying (OC) the BMEL than surrounding cartilage (SC) at both baseline and 1-year follow-up. From baseline to 1-year follow-up, the $T_{1\rho}$ values increased significantly in cartilage overlying BMEL, while no change in $T_{1\rho}$ values in the surrounding cartilage. Sagittal FSE sequences demonstrate cartilage defects within cartilage overlying BMEL at the lateral femoral condyle (*arrows*). WORMS cartilage subscore grading was higher in OC than in SC both at baseline and 1-year follow-up. However, no significant changes in WORMS of cartilage overly BMEL from baseline to 1-year follow-up [46]

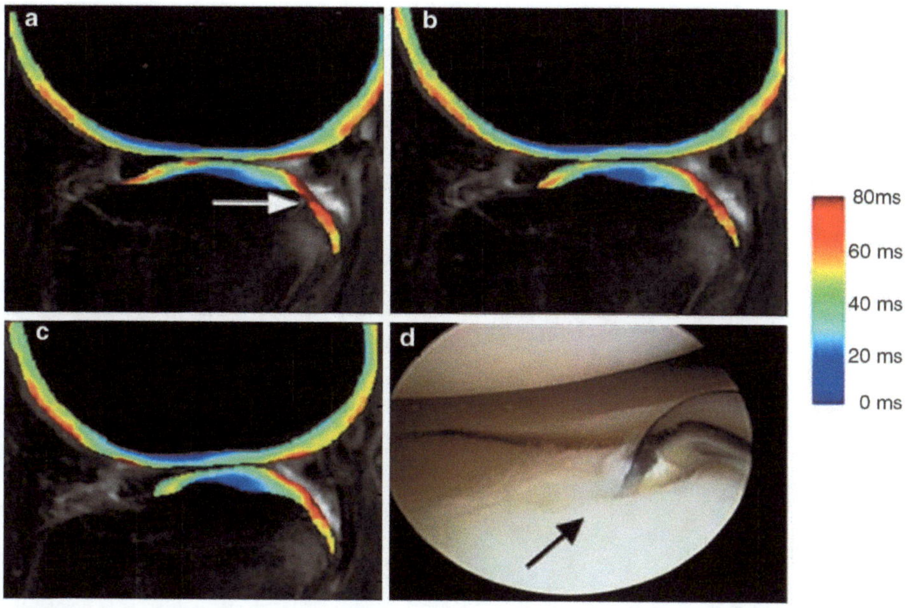

Fig. 13.9 (**a–c**) Color-coded $T_{1\rho}$ map overlaid on 3-T magnetic resonance images, demonstrating the increased $T_{1\rho}$ relaxation times along the posterolateral aspect of the tibial plateau, at the site of the tibial plateau bone bruise (white arrow). The mean $T_{1\rho}$ value of the cartilage directly over the bone bruise was 60.2 ± 13.7 ms, whereas the mean $T_{1\rho}$ value of the remaining cartilage was 37.5 ± 14.3 ms. (Of note, an area demonstrating increased $T_{1\rho}$ values also was observed in the region of the trochlea). (**d**) Arthroscopic image demonstrating Outerbridge grade-1 softening of the articular cartilage overlying the posterolateral aspect of the tibial plateau with a focal area of grade-2 fissures in the region of the bone bruise (*black arrow*) [48]

degeneration in ACL-injured knees. This may be explained by the fact that spin-lock techniques applied in $T_{1\rho}$ quantification reduce dipolar interactions and therefore reduce the dependence of $T_{1\rho}$ on collagen fiber, as compared to T_2, and increase the sensitivity for detecting proteoglycan loss. Loss of proteoglycan has been suggested as an initiating event during OA, when no changes occur in collagen contents or structure [2]. In fact, ACL-injured knees may serve as a valuable in vivo model for "early OA," and $T_{1\rho}$ can be an extremely valuable tool for evaluating and monitoring early degeneration in such joints due to its sensitivity to proteoglycan loss.

Furthermore, $T_{1\rho}$ quantification has been evaluated in meniscus in OA and ACL-injured knees [51, 52]. In vivo $T_{1\rho}$ measurements in the meniscus showed excellent reproducibility (coefficient of variation [CV] < 5%). Significant differences between three subject groups (controls $n = 27$; mild OA patient $n = 23$; severe OA patient $n = 10$) were found: Mean $T_{1\rho}$ values were 14.7 ± 5.5 ms for healthy controls ($n = 27$), 16.1 ± 6.6 ms for mild OA patients ($n = 23$), and 19.3 ± 7.6 ms for severe OA patients ($n = 10$), respectively. In acutely ACL-injured knees, significantly elevated $T_{1\rho}$ values were found in the lateral meniscus in patients compared with controls ($P < 0.01$). A significant correlation ($R^2 = 0.47$, $P = 0.007$) was found between $T_{1\rho}$ values of posterior horn of lateral meniscus and $T_{1\rho}$ values of posterior sub-compartment of lateral tibia cartilage in patients. This correlation suggested a strong injury-related relationship between meniscus and cartilage biochemical changes. However, because menisci have a much shorter $T_{1\rho}$ (~20 ms) compared to cartilage, acquisition sequences need to be optimized to quantify such a short relaxation time. The relationship between $T_{1\rho}$ values and biochemical composition (collagen, mainly type I, and proteoglycan) needs to be investigated.

Summary

$T_{1\rho}$ quantification in cartilage can provide valuable information related with biochemical changes in cartilage matrix. In particular, compared to more established T_2 relaxation time, $T_{1\rho}$ may provide more sensitive detection of proteoglycan loss at early stages of cartilage degeneration. Similar as T_2 quantification, $T_{1\rho}$ quantification requires no contrast agent inject and no special hardware. Technique challenges of $T_{1\rho}$ quantification include high SAR, especially at high and ultra high field strength, and relatively long acquisition time. Combined with new MR technique development, such as parallel imaging, $T_{1\rho}$ has great promise to serve as a diagnostic tool for early osteoarthritis.

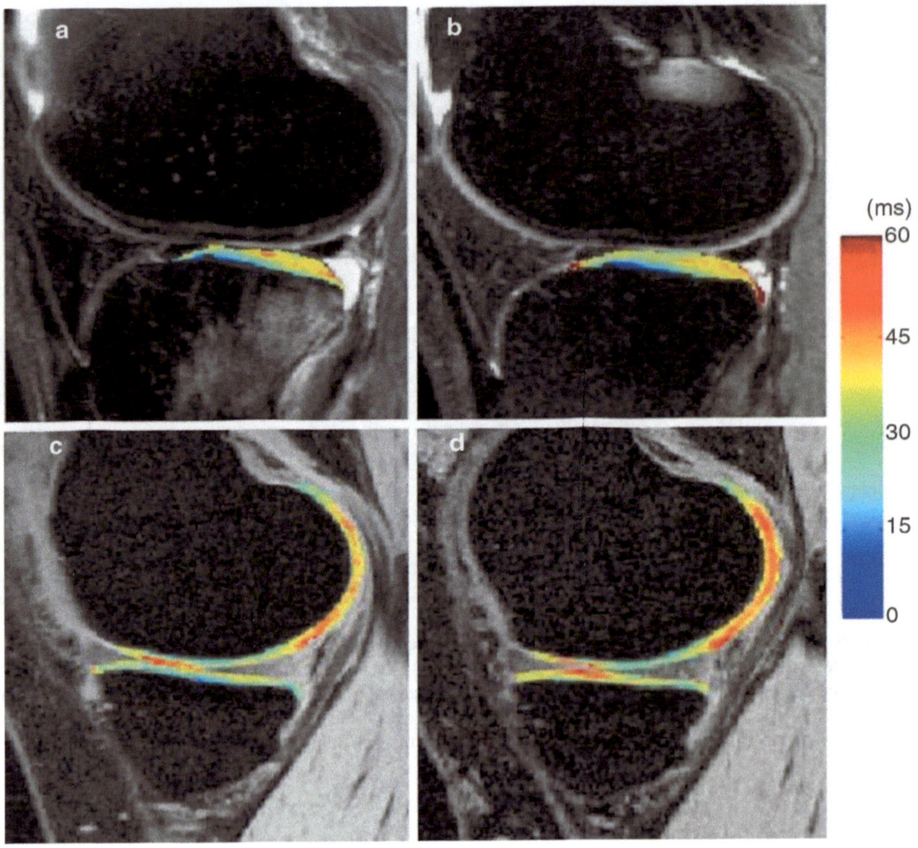

Fig. 13.10 $T_{1\rho}$ maps of the lateral side (**a** and **b**) and medial side (**c** and **d**) of an ACL-injured knee at baseline (**a** and **c**) and 1-year follow-up (**b** and **d**). $T_{1\rho}$ values in lateral-posterior tibia (LT-3) were elevated significantly in ACL-injured knees at baseline and remained high at 1-year follow-up despite resolution of bone bruise in LT. $T_{1\rho}$ values in the contacting area of MFC and MT were significantly elevated in ACL-injured knees at 1-year follow-up [50]

References

1. Gray ML, Eckstein F, Peterfy C, Dahlberg L, Kim YJ, Sorensen AG. Toward imaging biomarkers for osteoarthritis. Clin Orthop Relat Res. 2004;427:175–81.
2. Dijkgraaf LC, de Bont LG, Boering G, Liem RS. The structure, biochemistry, and metabolism of osteoarthritic cartilage: a review of the literature. J Oral Maxillofac Surg. 1995;53(10):1182–92.
3. Sepponen R. Rotating frame and magnetization transfer. In: Stark DD, Bradley WGJ, editors. Magnetic resonance imaging, vol. 1. St. Louis, MO: Mosby-Year Book; 1992. p. 204–18.
4. Redfield AG. Nucclear spin thermodynamics in the rotating frame. Science. 1969;164:1015–23.
5. Makela HI, Grohn OH, Kettunen MI, Kauppinen RA. Proton exchange as a relaxation mechanism for T1 in the rotating frame in native and immobilized protein solutions. Biochem Biophys Res Commun. 2001;289(4):813–8.
6. Duvvuri U, Goldberg AD, Kranz JK, Hoang L, Reddy R, Wehrli FW, et al. Water magnetic relaxation dispersion in biological systems: the contribution of proton exchange and implications for the noninvasive detection of cartilage degradation. Proc Natl Acad Sci USA. 2001;98(22):12479–84.
7. Kettunen M, Gröhn O, Silvennoinen M, Penttonen M, Kauppinen R. Effects of intracellular pH, blood, and tissue oxygen tension on T1rho relaxation in rat brain. Magn Reson Med. 2002;48(3):470–7.
8. Mlynarik V, Szomolanyi P, Toffanin R, Vittur F, Trattnig S. Transverse relaxation mechanisms in articular cartilage. J Magn Reson. 2004;169(2):300–7.
9. Dixon WT, Oshinski JN, Trudeau JD, Arnold BC, Pettigrew RI. Myocardial suppression in vivo by spin locking with composite pulses. Magn Reson Med. 1996;36(1):90–4.
10. Charagundla SR, Borthakur A, Leigh JS, Reddy R. Artifacts in T(1rho)-weighted imaging: correction with a self-compensating spin-locking pulse. J Magn Reson. 2003;162(1):113–21.
11. Witschey W, Borthakur A, Elliott M, Mellon E, Niyogi S, Wallman D, et al. Artifacts in T1 rho-weighted imaging: compensation for B(1) and B(0) field imperfections. J Magn Reson. 2007; 186(1):75–85.
12. Wheaton AJ, Borthakur A, Kneeland JB, Regatte RR, Akella SV, Reddy R. In vivo quantification of T1rho using a multislice spin-lock pulse sequence. Magn Reson Med. 2004;52(6):1453–8.
13. Li X, Han E, Ma C, Link T, Newitt D, Majumdar S. In vivo 3 T spiral imaging based multi-slice T(1rho) mapping of knee cartilage in osteoarthritis. Magn Reson Med. 2005;54(4):929–36.
14. Ristanis S, Stergiou N, Patras K, Tsepis E, Moraiti C, Georgoulis A. Follow-up evaluation 2 years after ACL reconstruction with bone-patellar tendon-bone graft shows that excessive tibial rotation persists. Clin J Sport Med. 2006;16(2):111–6.
15. Borthakur A, Hulvershorn J, Gualtieri E, Wheaton A, Charagundla S, Elliott M, et al. A pulse sequence for rapid in vivo spin-locked MRI. J Magn Reson Imaging. 2006;23(4):591–6.

16. Borthakur A, Wheaton A, Charagundla SR, Shapiro EM, Regatte RR, Akella SV, et al. Three-dimensional T1rho-weighted MRI at 1.5 Tesla. J Magn Reson Imaging. 2003;17(6):730–6.
17. Regatte RR, Akella SV, Wheaton AJ, Lech G, Borthakur A, Kneeland JB, et al. 3D-T1rho-relaxation mapping of articular cartilage: in vivo assessment of early degenerative changes in symptomatic osteoarthritic subjects. Acad Radiol. 2004;11(7):741–9.
18. Witschey W, Borthakur A, Elliott M, Fenty M, Sochor M, Wang C, et al. T1rho-prepared balanced gradient echo for rapid 3D T1rho MRI. J Magn Reson Imaging. 2008;28(3):744–54.
19. Wright GA, Brittain JH, Stainsby JA. Preserving T1 or T2 contrast in magnetization preparation sequences. ISMRM: New York; 1996, p. 1474.
20. Pakin S, Schweitzer M, Regatte R. 3D-T1rho quantitation of patellar cartilage at 3.0 T. J Magn Reson Imaging. 2006;24(6):1357–63.
21. Li X, Han E, Busse R, Majumdar S. In vivo T1rho mapping in cartilage using 3D magnetization-prepared angle-modulated partitioned k-space spoiled gradient echo snapshots (3D MAPSS). Magn Reson Med. 2008;59(2):298–307.
22. Wheaton A, Borthakur A, Corbo M, Charagundla S, Reddy R. Method for reduced SAR T1rho-weighted MRI. Magn Reson Med. 2004;51(6):1096–102.
23. Wheaton A, Borthakur A, Reddy R. Application of the keyhole technique to T1rho relaxation mapping. J Magn Reson Imaging. 2003;18(6):745–9.
24. Pakin S, Schweitzer M, Regatte R. Rapid 3D-T1rho mapping of the knee joint at 3.0 T with parallel imaging. Magn Reson Med. 2006;56(3):563–71.
25. Zuo J, Li X, Banerjee S, Han E, Majumdar S. Parallel imaging of knee cartilage at 3 Tesla. J Magn Reson Imaging. 2007;26(4):1001–9.
26. Akella SV, Regatte RR, Gougoutas AJ, Borthakur A, Shapiro EM, Kneeland JB, et al. Proteoglycan-induced changes in T1rho-relaxation of articular cartilage at 4 T. Magn Reson Med. 2001; 46(3):419–23.
27. Regatte RR, Akella SV, Borthakur A, Kneeland JB, Reddy R. Proteoglycan depletion-induced changes in transverse relaxation maps of cartilage: comparison of T2 and T1rho. Acad Radiol. 2002;9(12):1388–94.
28. Akella SV, Regatte RR, Wheaton AJ, Borthakur A, Reddy R. Reduction of residual dipolar interaction in cartilage by spin-lock technique. Magn Reson Med. 2004;52(5):1103–9.
29. Wheaton A, Dodge G, Elliott D, Nicoll S, Reddy R. Quantification of cartilage biomechanical and biochemical properties via T1rho magnetic resonance imaging. Magn Reson Med. 2005;54(5):1087–93.
30. Regatte R, Akella S, Lonner J, Kneeland J, Reddy R. T1rho relaxation mapping in human osteoarthritis (OA) cartilage: comparison of T1rho with T2. J Magn Reson Imaging. 2006;23(4):547–53.
31. Li X, Cheng J, Lin K, Saadat E, Bolbos R, Ries M, Horvai A, Link T, Majumdar S. Quantitative MRI using $T1\rho$ and T2 in human osteoarthritic cartilage specimens: correlation with biochemical measurements and histology. Magn Reson Imag. 2010 Dec 3. [Epub ahead of print].
32. Xia Y, Farquhar T, Burton-Wuster N, Ray E, Jelinski L. Diffusion and relaxation mapping of cartilage-bone plugs and excised disks using microscopic magnetic resonance imaging. Magn Reson Med. 1994;31:273–82.
33. David-Vaudey E, Ghosh S, Ries M, Majumdar S. T2 relaxation time measurements in osteoarthritis. Magn Reson Imaging. 2004;22(5):673–82.
34. Mlynarik V, Trattnig S, Huber M, Zembsch A, Imhof H. The role of relaxation times in monitoring proteoglycan depletion in articular cartilage. J Magn Reson Imaging. 1999;10(4):497–502.
35. Menezes NM, Gray ML, Hartke JR, Burstein D. T2 and T1rho MRI in articular cartilage systems. Magn Reson Med. 2004;51(3):503–9.
36. Duvvuri U, Charagundla SR, Kudchodkar SB, Kaufman JH, Kneeland JB, Rizi R, et al. Human knee: in vivo T1(rho)-weighted MR imaging at 1.5 T–preliminary experience. Radiology. 2001; 220(3):822–6.
37. Li X, Ma C, Link T, Castillo D, Blumenkrantz G, Lozano J, et al. In vivo T1rho and T2 mapping of articular cartilage in osteoarthritis of the knee using 3 Tesla MRI. Osteoarthritis Cartilage. 2007;15(7):789–97.
38. Stahl R, Luke A, Li X, Carballido-Gamio J, Ma C, Majumdar S, Link T. T1rho, T(2) and focal knee cartilage abnormalities in physically active and sedentary healthy subjects versus early OA patients-a 3.0-Tesla MRI study. Eur Radiol. 2008;Epub ahead of print.
39. Li X, Pai A, Blumenkrantz G, Carballido-Gamio J, Link T, Ma C, Ries M, Majumdar S. Spatial distribution and relationship of T1rho and T2 relaxation times in knee cartilage with osteoarthritis. Magn Reson Med. 2009;61(6):1310–8.
40. Petrou M, Sevilla PG. Dealing with texture. England: Wiley; 2006.
41. Li X, Pai A, Blumenkrantz G, Carballido-Gamio J, Link T, Ma C, et al. Spatial distribution and relationship of T1rho and T2 relaxation times in knee cartilage with osteoarthritis. Magn Reson Med. 2009;61(6):1310–8.
42. Carballido-Gamio J, Stahl R, Blumenkrantz G, Romero A, Majumdar S, Link T. Spatial analysis of magnetic resonance T1rho and T2 relaxation times improves classification between subjects with and without osteoarthritis. Med Phys. 2009;36(9):4059–67.
43. Blumenkrantz G, Stahl R, Carballido-Gamio J, Zhao S, Lu Y, Munoz T, et al. The feasibility of characterizing the spatial distribution of cartilage T(2) using texture analysis. Osteoarthritis Cartilage. 2008;16(5):584–90.
44. Haralick R, Shanmugam K, Dinstein I. Textural features for image classification. IEEE Trans Syst Man Cybern. 1973;3(6):610–8.
45. Li X, Ma C, Bolbos R, Stahl R, Lozano J, Zuo J, et al. Quantitative assessment of bone marrow edema pattern and overlying cartilage in knees with osteoarthritis and anterior cruciate ligament tear using MR imaging and spectroscopic imaging. J Magn Reson Imaging. 2008;28(2):453–61.
46. Zhao J, Li X, Bolbos R, Link T, Majumdar S. Longitudinal assessment of bone marrow edema-like lesions and cartilage degeneration in osteoarthritis using 3 T MR T1rho quantification. Skeletal Radiol. 2010;36(9):523–31.
47. Bolbos R, Ma C, Link T, Majumdar S, Li X. In vivo T1rho quantitative assessment of knee cartilage after anterior cruciate ligament injury using 3 Tesla magnetic resonance imaging. Invest Radiol. 2008;43(11):782–8.
48. Lozano J, Li X, Link T, Safran M, Majumdar S, Ma CB. Detection of posttraumatic cartilage injury using quantitative T1rho magnetic resonance imaging. A report of two cases with arthroscopic findings. J Bone Joint Surg Am. 2006;88(6):1349–52.
49. Theologis A, Kuo D, Cheng J, Bolbos R, Carballido-Gamio J, Ma C, Li X. Evaluation of bone bruises and associated cartilage in ACL inured knees using quantitative T1rho MRI: one-year cohort study. Arthroscopy. 2011;27(1):65–76.
50. Li X, Kuo D, Theologis A, Carballido-Gamio J, Stehling C, Link T, Ma C, Majumdar S. MRI T1rho and T2 of cartilage in anterior cruciate ligament reconstructed knees: initial experience with one-year follow-up. Radiology. 2011;258(2):505–14.
51. Rauscher I, Stahl R, Cheng J, Li X, Huber M, Luke A, et al. Meniscal measurements of T1rho and T2 at MR imaging in healthy subjects and patients with osteoarthritis. Radiology. 2008;249(2):591–600.
52. Bolbos R, Link T, Benjamin MC, Majumdar S, Li X. T1rho relaxation time of the meniscus and its relationship with T1rho of adjacent cartilage in knees with acute ACL injuries at 3 T. Osteoarthritis Cartilage. 2008; Epub ahead of print.

Chapter 14
Cartilage Matrix Assessment Using dGEMRIC

Martha L. Gray and Deborah Burstein

Keywords Assessment • Cartilage • dGEMRIC • Donnan Theory • Fixed charge density (FCD) • Glycosaminoglycans (GAG) • Matrix • Pathophysiological

Introduction

The functional integrity of cartilage is inextricably linked to the composition and architecture of the macromolecular network of cartilage. There has been much recent attention to developing nondestructive methods for imaging cartilage macromolecules. Over the next decade these should become sufficiently robust to serve as an important adjunct to the currently used destructive methods of microscopic and bulk biochemical analyses.

We focus here on an MRI technique called delayed Gadolinium-Enhanced MRI of Cartilage (dGEMRIC) for noninvasively imaging the glycosaminoglycan (GAG) concentration of articular cartilage. This technique is based on the concept of fixed charge in cartilage resulting from the glycosaminoglycans. Abundant evidence exists that diseased cartilage is lacking in GAG (and the associated charge) and that the mechanical properties of cartilage are strongly influenced by the concentration of GAG (or charge). The developments leading up to this imaging protocol, spanning nearly 50 years, have been recently reviewed in depth [1] and are summarized in the first part of this chapter. dGEMRIC is beginning to reveal interesting insights into cartilage physiology and pathology in vivo, and thus, the second half of this chapter is focused on providing examples that offer immediate opportunities to enhance our understanding of the etiopathology of cartilage degeneration, and possibly change the paradigm framing our approach to cartilage disease.

D. Burstein (✉)
Department of Radiology, Beth Israel Deaconess Medical Center, 330 Brookline Avenue, Boston, MA 02215, USA
e-mail: dburstei@bidmc.harvard.edu

Cartilage Fixed Charge Density (FCD) from Sulfated Glycosaminoglycans (S-GAG): Implications of FCD to Cartilage Pathophysiological and Functional States

Cartilage consists primarily of an aqueous electrolyte and a sparse population of cells that reside in a plentiful extracellular matrix comprising mainly collagen and glycosaminoglycan macromolecules. Collagen, which makes up about 20% of cartilage volume by weight (or 80% of the solid volume), forms an isoelectric fibrillar network. As such, collagen serves as the tissue's structural framework and its principal source of tensile and shear strength. GAG, which makes up about 5% of cartilage volume by weight (or 20% of solid volume), is a constituent of the proteoglycan macromolecule.

GAGs are repeating disaccharides with carboxyl and sulfate moieties that are charged under physiological conditions. These GAG chains are so densely packed that the concentration of negative charge can be as much as 150–300 mM in normal articular cartilage. Since these charges are integral elements of the GAG molecule, they are said to be "fixed" to the solid matrix, and the concentration of this fixed charge is called the fixed charge density (FCD). There are also abundant ions in the extracellular fluid. These ions are mobile within the fluid phase, and are therefore referred to as mobile ions.

A large body of work over the past 50 years provides considerable insight about the significance and biophysical mechanisms relating FCD or GAG and load-bearing properties [2]. For example, experiments in which the fixed charges were effectively "removed" (by degradation or ionic shielding) revealed a 50–80% decrease in compressive stiffness [3, 4]. The differences in GAG seen in the course of degenerative disease are similarly significant, varying from more than 50–80 mg/mL to nearly zero [5].

T.M. Link (ed.), *Cartilage Imaging: Significance, Techniques, and New Developments*,
DOI 10.1007/978-1-4419-8438-8_14, © Springer Science+Business Media, LLC 2011

Donnan Theory: The Basis for Imaging of Cartilage GAG

Nearly every method for measuring GAG is a measure of electrical charge of the extracellular matrix. These include the radiotracer method, histologic staining with cationic dyes (Fig. 14.1a), biochemical assays, and MRI-based methods. The MR-based strategy described in the next section is essentially an imaging version of the "radiotracer" method, invented in the 1970s by Maroudas and used to provide some of the first quantitative measurements of GAG (or equivalently FCD) distribution with depth from articular surface, with topological position, and with disease [6–9].

Donnan theory provides the theoretical basis for the radiotracer and imaging methods; it serves to relate the effect of fixed charge on the extracellular matrix by the concentration of mobile ions in the interstitial fluid ([2] and references therein). Qualitatively the Donnan relationship for cartilage can be described as follows. In order to maintain overall electroneutrality in cartilage, the negative fixed charge on the cartilage macromolecules is balanced by a relatively dilute concentration of anions (e.g., Cl^-), and more highly concentrated cations (e.g., Na^+), relative to blood or synovial fluid. The fixed charge in cartilage is significant, such that the mobile ion concentration in normal cartilage differs substantially from that in degenerated cartilage (Fig. 14.1 and Table 14.1). For instance, in tissue with normal [GAG], tissue [Na^+] is 150% greater than the sodium concentration in the blood, while the tissue [Cl^-] is more than 50% less than the concentration in the blood. In degenerated (GAG depleted) cartilage, the concentration of mobile ions in the blood and tissue are equal. Therefore, there is a substantial difference in the concentration of mobile ions in normal and GAG-depleted cartilage (Fig. 14.1 and Table 14.1).

MRI methods for measuring FCD, sodium MR, and delayed Gadolinium-Enhanced MRI of Cartilage (dGEMRIC), both

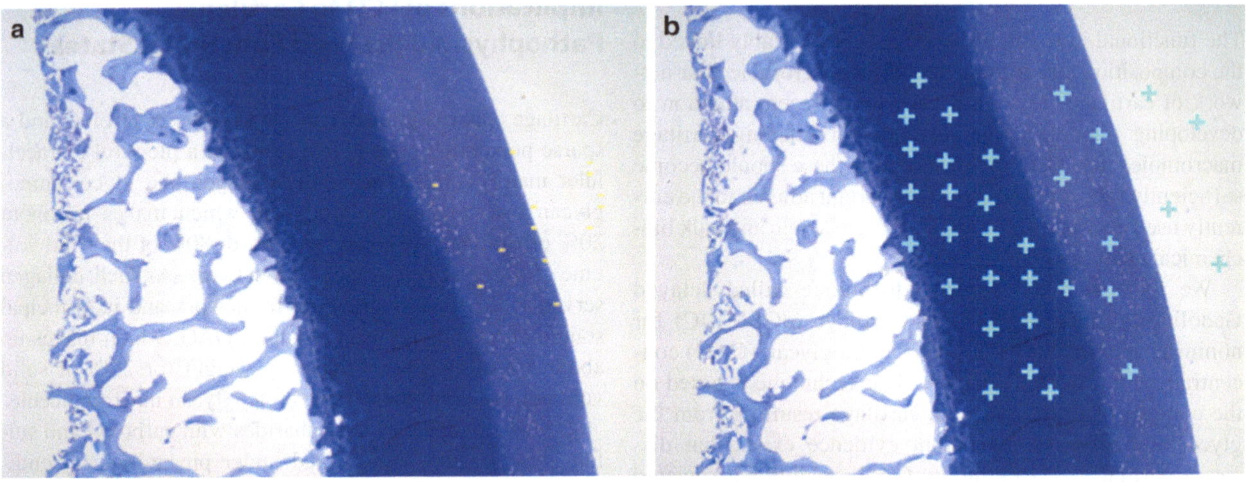

Fig. 14.1 (**a**) Toluidine blue, a cationic dye used to visualize GAG, reveals two dramatically different regions in this histological section: one staining light purple indicating low [GAG], and the other staining dark purple indicating "high" [GAG]. (**b**) Qualitative illustration of the relative distribution of mobile ions. Because of GAG's negative charge, mobile cations are more concentrated in cartilage than in the surrounding solution (e.g., bath, blood, synovial fluid), and are more concentrated in the high GAG versus the low GAG region. Conversely, the higher the GAG, the less concentrated the anions. Calculations (Table 14.1), assuming Donnan partitioning, predict a broad dynamic range when comparing mobile ion concentration in depleted versus normal tissue (Figure reprinted from [1])

Table 14.1 Donnan theory predictions for mobile ion concentrations in high and low GAG regions of cartilage

		Tissue state			
		Bath or synovial fluid	Fully depleted	Partially depleted	"Typical normal"
Fixed charge or GAG concentration	FCD (mM)		0	–50	–300
	[GAG] (mg/mL tissue water)		0	11	67
Mobile ion concentration (mM)	Na^+	150	150	177	362
	Cl^-	110	110	93	46
	$GdDTPA^{2-}$	1	1.00	0.72	0.17

In tissue with normal [GAG], the differences between tissue concentration and bathing concentrations of mobile ions are substantial: tissue [Na^+] is almost 1.5× and [Cl^-] less than half the bath concentration. This results in a substantial differential in mobile ion distributions between normal and GAG-depleted tissue. $GdDTPA^{2-}$ is of particular interest because it is an FDA approved MR contrast agent involve visualizing the distribution of a specific mobile ion (Na^+ and $Gd(DTPA)^{2-}$, respectively). $Gd(DTPA)^{2-}$ (Magnevist, Berlex, NJ) is a clinically approved MRI contrast agent.

To the extent that the concentration of the mobile ion probe can be measured, and the equilibrium conditions of Donnan can be achieved, in principal, these MR-based methods can provide a map or image reflecting GAG concentration. In cases where the equilibrating conditions are known (as is normally the case in vitro), Donnan theory can be used to convert the measurement of the ionic probe into a map of *absolute* GAG concentration. In cases where the equilibrating conditions are unknown (as is normally the case in vivo), the measurement can provide a map of *relative* GAG concentration. In either case, image contrast must be dominated by the mobile ion concentration (to provide the desired specificity), the mobile ion being measured must not bind to the matrix, and the mobile ion being measured must be in (quasi-) equilibrium with the bathing solution or synovial fluid/blood. These considerations ensure that the measurement or map reflects [GAG] rather than binding or transport of the mobile ion.

This approach has been demonstrated in vitro using MR measurements of the cation Na^+ by sodium MR spectroscopy and imaging [10–14] and of the divalent anion $Gd(DTPA)^{2-}$ using proton MR spectroscopy and imaging [15–18] (Fig. 14.2). The advantage to sodium is that it is a native, abundant, and MR-observable cation, that is essentially always in equilibrium with the synovial fluid/blood and is highly sensitive to changes in [GAG]. The disadvantages are that sodium MRI provides less resolution than a proton-based method, the fast relaxation of sodium confounds MR measurements of sodium concentration [11, 12], and sodium MRI is not generally available on standard clinical MRI instruments. Conversely, the advantages of $Gd(DTPA)^{2-}$ and proton MRI are the comparatively high resolution and sensitivity, with a reasonably straightforward implementation on standard MRI instruments. The disadvantages are the needs to introduce the contrast agent and ensure that it has fully penetrated the cartilage tissue before imaging and to convert the MRI measurement of T1 to $Gd(DTPA)^{2-}$ distribution, and hence GAG distribution.

In this chapter, we focus on the $Gd(DTPA)^{2-}$-based technique, known as dGEMRIC, given its wider availability and more extensively reported application studies in bench and clinical studies.

Assessing GAG by the dGEMRIC (Delayed Gadolinium-Enhanced MRI of Cartilage) Method

The underlying principle in using $Gd(DTPA)^{2-}$ as an indicator of [GAG] is the fact that the divalent anion will distribute within cartilage in inverse relation to the distribution of GAG (which itself has abundant negative charges). In the ex vivo version of this method, tissue is equilibrated in a solution containing $Gd(DTPA)^{2-}$. Then, a T1 image is used to compute tissue $[Gd(DTPA)^{2-}]$ according to the relation: $[Gd(DTPA)^{2-}]_{tissue} = (1/R)[(1/T1_{Gd}) - (1/T1_{no\text{-}Gd})]$, where $[Gd(DTPA)^{2-}]_{tissue}$ is the concentration of $Gd(DTPA)^{2-}$ in the tissue interstitial fluid, R is the relaxivity, $T1_{Gd}$ is the measured T1 in the presence of $Gd(DTPA)^{2-}$, and $T1_{no\text{-}Gd}$ is T1 in the absence of contrast agent. To first order at high fields, the relaxivity and T1 without contrast agent are independent of tissue composition [19, 20] and can be viewed as

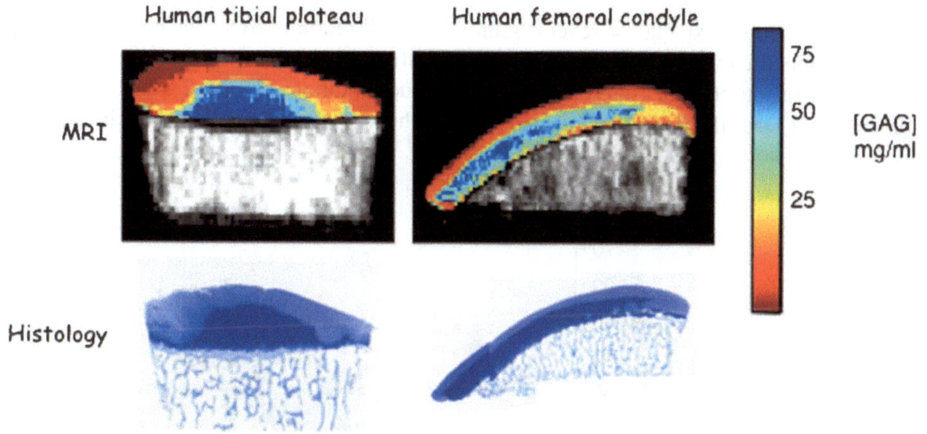

Fig. 14.2 MRI-based GAG maps and the corresponding toluidine-blue-stained histological section for two human osteochondral samples. The GAG maps were obtained using the dGEMRIC method for which tissue is equilibrated in $GdDTPA^{2-}$, then proton T1 measurements are made. The T1 is used to compute intra-tissue $[GdDTPA^{2-}]$ which in turn is used to compute [GAG] using a modified Donnan equation [15]. The close correspondence between histological staining and the MRI map support the interpretation of these dGEMRIC images as a metric of GAG (Figure reprinted from [1])

constants so that the conversion from T1 to $[Gd(DTPA)^{2-}]$ is straightforward. Then, using a modified Donnan theory, $[Gd(DTPA)^{2-}]$ in the tissue can be used, together with information about $[Gd(DTPA)^{2-}]$ in the equilibrating solution to compute tissue [GAG]. The assumption of a composition-independent R may not fully hold near the bone–cartilage interface [21] or at lower field strengths.

For in vivo assessment of cartilage [GAG], $Gd(DTPA)^{2-}$ needs to be introduced intravenously or intra-articularly, and given sufficient time to penetrate the cartilage. (Studies of uptake in the knee have indicated that 2 h following intravenous administration, including a 10-min period of passive motion immediately after the IV injection, permits full penetration of $Gd(DTPA)^{2-}$ into knee cartilages [16, 22, 23]). The intravenous administration provides more rapid cartilage penetration than does intra-articular [16], presumably because $Gd(DTPA)^{2-}$ can penetrate cartilage through both the articular surface and the bone/cartilage interface.

After this delay period, a series of T1-weighted images are obtained from which a quantitative T1 map can be computed. T1 measured in this way is referred to as the dGEMRIC index. The T1 map can be used directly or used to compute $[Gd(DTPA)^{2-}]$ as before, to provide a map of GAG distribution; however, more studies need to be done to determine whether the relaxivity varies as a function of depth [21] under in vivo conditions. (Presently we do not go further and quantify absolute [GAG] because the calculation requires knowledge of the effective equilibrating concentration).

Evidence that dGEMRIC Measures FCD and [GAG]

dGEMRIC has been validated in vitro against several standard methods [15, 19]. Specifically, [GAG] measured by dGEMRIC corresponds closely to that measured by sodium MR and by the biochemical DMMB assay for both human and bovine cartilage [15, 19, 24] (Fig. 14.3). In addition, abundant qualitative evidence exists that dGEMRIC images correspond closely to the corresponding histological images (Fig. 14.2). However, no gold standards exist against which to compare dGEMRIC in vivo. Instead, two strategies have been employed. The first validation strategy was to demonstrate that in vivo images taken before total joint arthroplasty were similar to the corresponding in vitro images and histology of tissue harvested during surgery [19] (Fig. 14.4). The second was to verify the essential role of charge in the measurement. Subjects were imaged twice using the dGEMRIC method, once using $Gd(DTPA)^{2-}$, the other using a similar sized nonionic contrast agent, Gadoteridol (Prohance). The nonionic contrast agent distributed uniformly in the joint cartilage, while the $Gd(DTPA)^{2-}$ did not, suggesting that the nonuniform distribution of $Gd(DTPA)^{2-}$ was a consequence of it being charged (and thus being sensitive to local fixed charge density) [16, 25] (Fig. 14.5). If the nonuniform distribution had been caused by, for example, nonuniform transport, then both $Gd(DTPA)^{2-}$ and Prohance would have shown nonuniformities.

These data support the overall conclusion that dGEMRIC can be a nondestructive measure of cartilage fixed charge density. For the most part, this translates to cartilage GAG, because many studies have shown that GAG accounts for most if not all the fixed charge density [2]. However, the conversion from the dGEMRIC measurement to a measure of [GAG] still depends on a number of assumptions, such as the number of charges per GAG disaccharide, the distribution of molecules that provide the fixed charge (i.e., GAG vs other molecules), ensuring that conditions include complete equilibrium with a known bathing concentration and known relaxivity of the contrast agent. Particularly for in vivo studies, these assumptions raise a number of methodological issues that still require further investigation. These include the possibility of altered contrast agent relaxivity under different tissue conditions [21, 26–28] and dosing and other factors such as the transport of contrast agent into cartilage with a variable

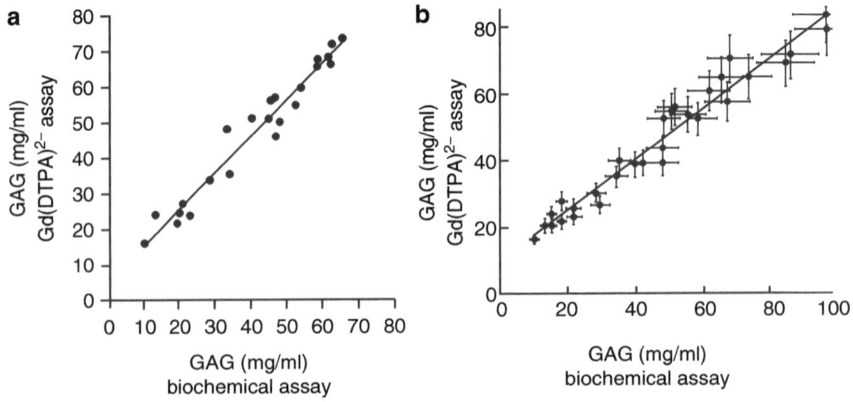

Fig. 14.3 Many studies have demonstrated that GAG determined by MRI in vitro (using the dGEMRIC method) corresponds well to that measured by the biochemical DMMB assay (Part a: Adapted from [15]; b: Adapted from [24])

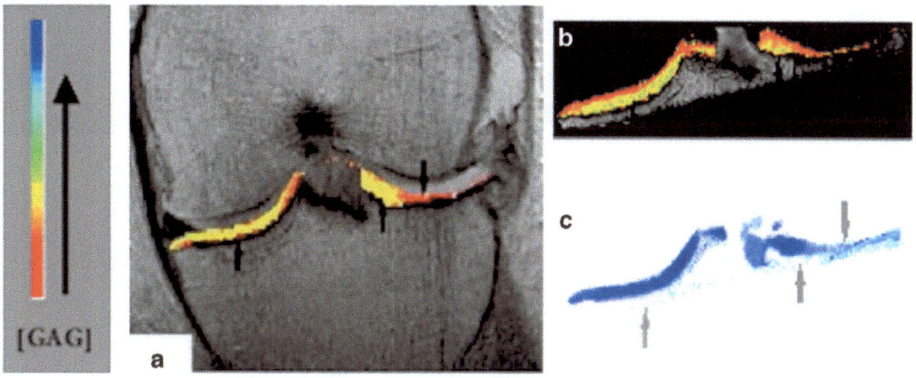

Fig. 14.4 Representative example from a study in which (**a**) in vivo dGEMRIC images were taken prior to total joint replacement, then compared with (**b**) in vitro dGEMRIC images, and (**c**) toluidine blue histology of tissue harvested during the surgery. The close correspondence between in vivo and in vitro images suggests that in vivo dGEMRIC is reflecting GAG distribution (Adapted from [19])

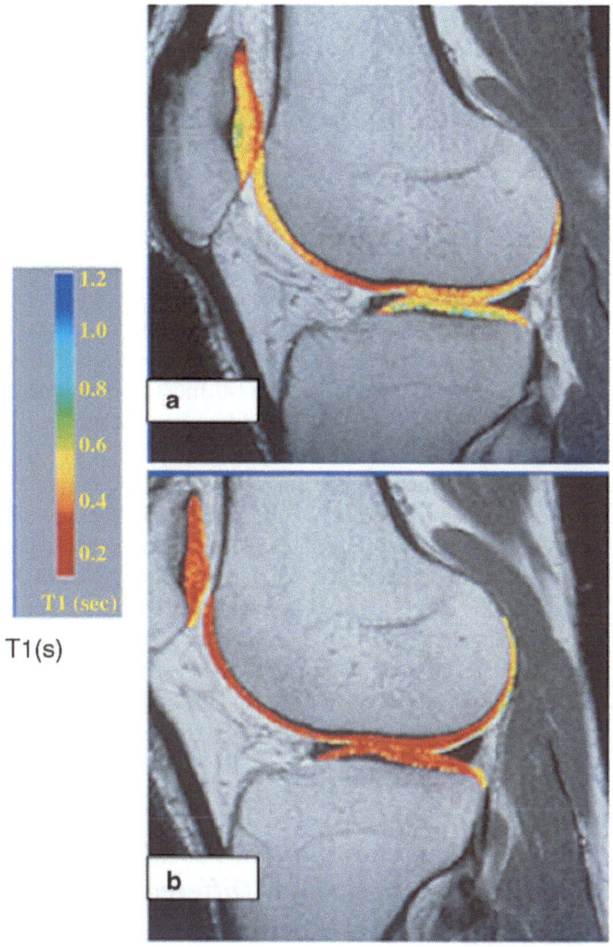

Fig. 14.5 Representative example from a study in which T1 imaging was done using (**a**) a charged contrast agent, $Gd(DTPA)^{2-}$, and (**b**) an uncharged contrast agent, Gd-HPDO3A. The uncharged agent distributed uniformly, suggesting that the distribution of the charged agent is related to tissue charge. (Adapted from [16])

blood concentration that might affect the equilibrating concentration of $Gd(DTPA)^{2-}$ in vivo [23, 28, 29].

Until these other factors are fully understood, in vivo studies of dGEMRIC report the T1 measurement directly as a "dGEMRIC Index". However, note that the effects of charge and transport generally are additive; for example, a faster penetration of contrast agent into degenerated cartilage and the higher concentration of contrast agent due to the lower fixed charge density of degenerated cartilage will both result in increased contrast agent concentration, therefore permitting a general assessment of cartilage status.

dGEMRIC Opportunities

The advent of methodology to measure FCD (and hence indirectly GAG) nondestructively on a spatially localized basis enables a number of in vitro and in vivo applications of dGEMRIC that are providing new insights into cartilage physiology, disease progression, and preventative or repair strategies.

In Vitro Monitoring of Cartilage Degradation, Development, and Repair

The dGEMRIC technique allows one to track the distribution of GAG across cartilage over time in culture with high resolution, thereby enabling long-term in vitro studies of the evolution of degradation, development, or repair and of factors that might be involved in these processes. For example, bovine cartilage plugs were monitored over time with the observation that chondrocytes could replenish GAG

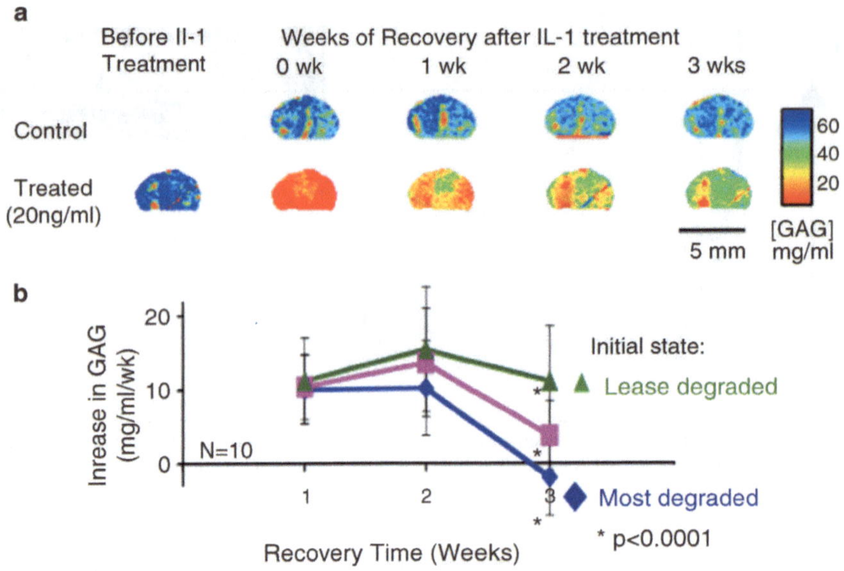

Fig. 14.6 (**a**) Representative in vitro dGEMRIC images of young bovine articular cartilage discs maintained in culture. After a 6–9 day exposure to IL-1ß, samples were cultured in basal medium. Treated samples recovered about 80% of their initial GAG. (**b**) IL-1 induces heterogeneous depletion of GAG. Image pixels were segmented into three groups according to the degree of initial loss. All regions replenished GAG at the same rate during the first 2 weeks. By week 3, differential recovery was seen, with the most degraded having no further increase. This differential recovery was not observed when GAGs were removed with trypsin, suggesting that IL-1 induced damage to other matrix components and limited the capacity for recovery (Adapted from [30])

within 5 weeks after trypsin depletion of GAG [17]. The characteristic stratification of GAG concentration (lower at the articular surface and higher in the deeper zones), although erased by the trypsin, was recapitulated. This differential recovery of GAG may be due to differences in the chondrocytes or in the collagen scaffold in the different tissue regions. The likely importance of the scaffold was also suggested by a study of GAG replenishment following interleukin-1 (IL-1) treatment. IL-1 induces chondrocytes to produce a variety of metalloproteinases against both GAG and collagen. The effect is heterogeneous, as revealed by the heterogeneous loss of GAG. Interestingly, while the initial rate of GAG recovery was similar through the tissue, during the third week, the region that had originally been most degraded showed no continued recovery, while the region that had been the least degraded continued to recover at the highest rate [30] (Fig. 14.6). This differential rate of recovery might be explained by IL-1-induced concomitant collagen damage that precluded full restoration of the GAG. MRI techniques to examine collagen could be used in conjunction with dGEMRIC to sort out such questions and better understand the conditions under which cartilage repair can occur. The noninvasiveness and spatial sensitivity of MRI is ideally suited for such longitudinal studies of cartilage in culture, and open the opportunity for monitoring more subtle changes than those which occur with trypsin and IL-1 degradation. Such observations are most convincing through changes monitored over time in individual samples rather than inferred from histological observations over a population of samples.

dGEMRIC as an Indicator of Functional State

The ability to map the biochemical composition of cartilage may provide a noninvasive means to determine its mechanical properties. Good correlations were noted between dGEMRIC and site-matched indentation stiffness measurements (Fig. 14.7) [21, 31–33]. However, differences in stiffness in different areas of the joint could not be explained by GAG measurements alone, suggesting the need for combined GAG/collagen studies [31, 32]. dGEMRIC can also provide information in line with mechanical information obtained at arthroscopy. In a clinical arthroscopic study, the dGEMRIC index was lower in diseased compartments than reference compartments [22]. These biomechanical properties may be measurable in vivo, as has recently been demonstrated by imaging individuals after exercise, and after loading the joint with a loading device during MRI [34].

In Vivo Studies: Changing the Paradigm: Improved Observation and Differentiation of Physiologic and Pathologic States and Response to Interventions in Pre-radiographic OA

Much of our understanding of osteoarthritis is limited because of the lack of a sensitive measure of early disease.

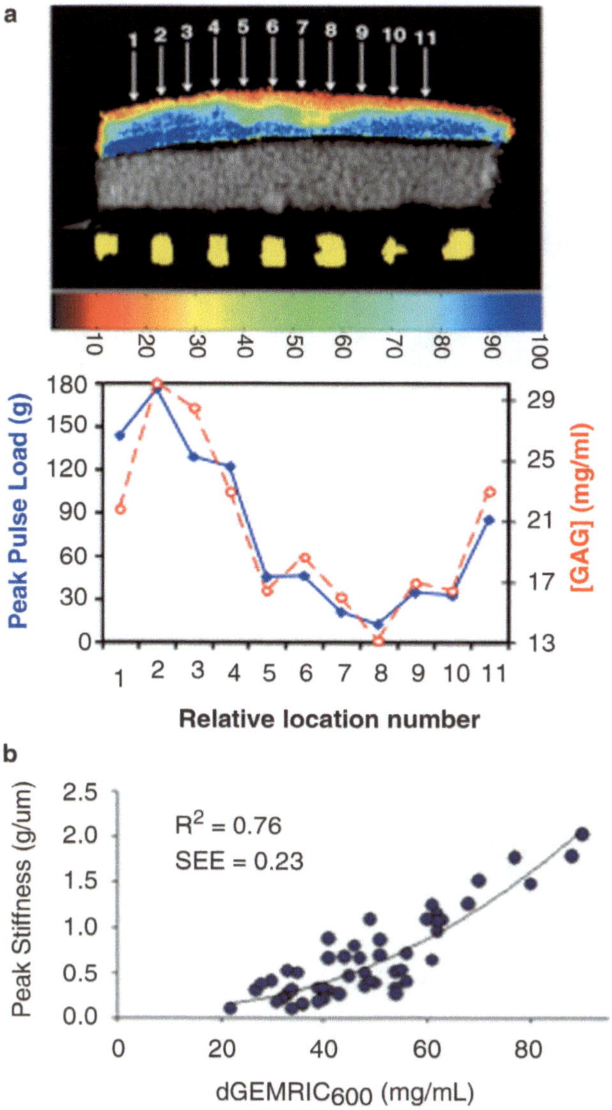

Fig. 14.7 (**a**) Representative example showing the relation between the dGEMRIC image of a human tibial plateau sample and the indentation stiffnesses at the positions corresponding to the arrows. The [GAG] in the lower plot is the average GAG for a volume comparable to the indentation volume (width 1.5 mm, depth 600 μm). If full depth averages are used, there is no correspondence between GAG and stiffness (Adapted from [31]). (**b**) Although the mechanical stiffness is not entirely due to GAG, there is a correspondence between the localized GAG measurement and peak indentation stiffness across many human tibial plateau samples (Figure adapted from [32])

The current gold standard is the radiograph, which is sensitive only in later stages of the disease (after tissue loss and bony changes have occurred). In many instances, large variation in dGEMRIC was observed even when no joint space narrowing was observed on radiographs [35], or when appearing grossly intact [36] (Fig. 14.8), presumably identifying areas of biochemical degradation preceding the actual loss of tissue. This observation was supported by data from a recent cross-sectional study [37], in which there was a broad distribution of dGEMRIC index in joints deemed "healthy" by radiography (KL Grade 0), and also in joints that had radiographic evidence of OA. This observation has important implications for studies aimed at evaluating therapeutic efficacy: vis, the radiographically "normal" group may include a large proportion of individuals with comparatively low GAG, perhaps reflecting early degeneration. Their inclusion within a "healthy control" group may ultimately mask what would otherwise be a good therapeutic effect. Although many more data are needed to know whether low dGEMRIC index has clinical significance, given our current understanding that loss of GAG is an early event in joint degeneration, these data should raise skepticism as to whether our current gold standard technologies of radiography are adequate for diagnosis and therapeutic evaluation.

The dGEMRIC index can also be used as a metric with which to evaluate what other clinical metrics correlate with cartilage degeneration. In the knee, the effects of alignment, age, and body mass index (BMI) have been investigated [36], in addition to knee extensor strength [38]. In hip dysplasia, age, severity of dysplasia, and the presence of a labral tear were identified as risk factors for OA [39].

Molecular differences within joints that had prior injuries also points to the potential to monitor pathologic changes in cartilage in response to injury before tissue loss occurs. As an example of this, cartilage in the medial compartment of knees with prior ACL injuries had lower dGEMRIC index than the lateral compartments, when compared with the contralateral knee [40]. Variations across patellar cartilage were found in individuals with recurrent patellar dislocation [41] (Fig. 14.9). Similarly, in the hip lower dGEMRIC was found in the medial compartment in individuals with femoroacetabular impingement [42] and Leg-Calve-Perthes disease [43].

Changing the Paradigm: Evidence that dGEMRIC May Provide Clinically Useful Predictive Information

Several studies evaluated whether dGEMRIC might provide some clinically relevant (as opposed to biologically relevant) information. One of the earliest was a study in which dGEMRIC images were taken of 17 knees in subjects with knee pain, but normal radiography. Consistent with the larger studies described above, there was a broad range of dGEMRIC index in this group. At follow-up 6 years later, 16 knees were evaluated; nine now had radiographic evidence of OA, with two of them having received a total joint replacement. The initial dGEMRIC index was significantly lower for those

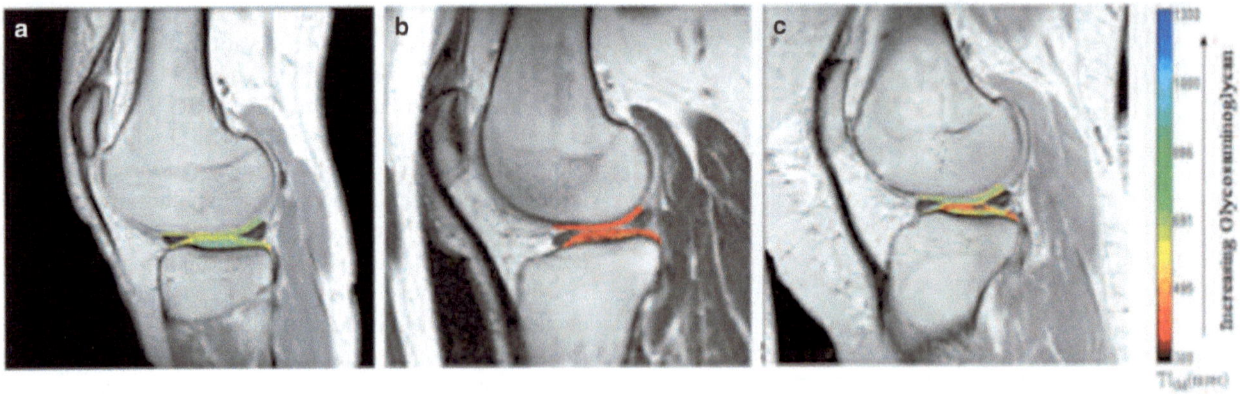

Fig. 14.8 The dGEMRIC index obtained after delayed gadolinium-enhanced MRI of cartilage for obese subjects who have no radiographic evidence of joint space narrowing. Representative examples include knees with (**a**) high global dGEMRIC index in cartilage; (**b**) low global dGEMRIC index in cartilage; and (**c**) focal areas of low uptake indicating selective GAG depletion. Longitudinal studies are needed to learn if there is an increased likelihood that the knees that appear to have lost GAG (e.g., **b** and **c**) have an increased rate or likelihood of joint deterioration (Figure from [36])

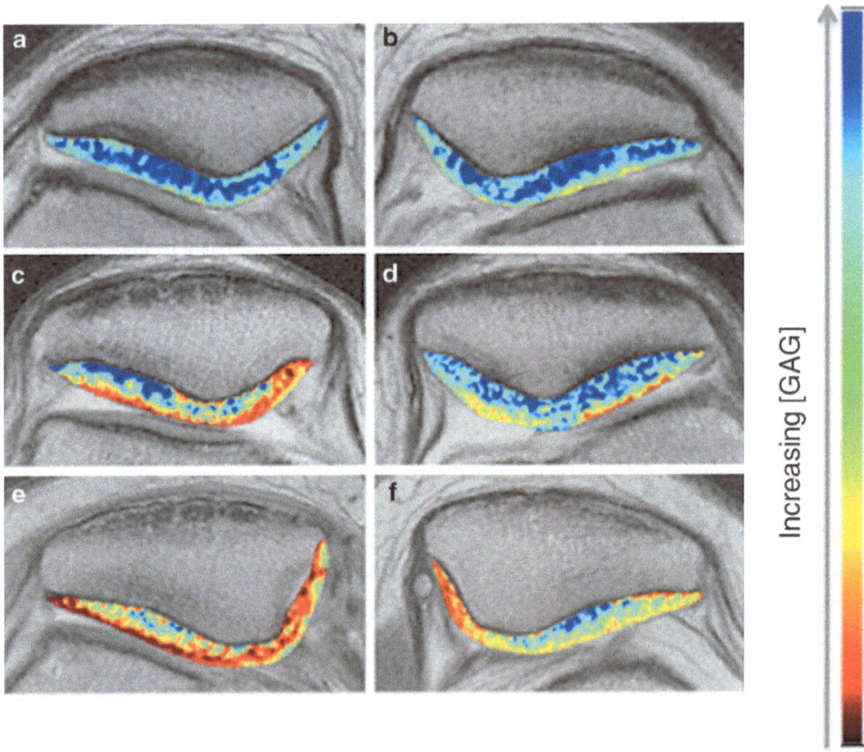

Fig. 14.9 dGEMRIC images of patella cartilage. (**a, b**) Right and left knees, respectively, in a healthy volunteer; (**c, d**) right dislocated knee and left nondislocated knee, respectively, in a patient with unilateral recurrent patellar dislocation (RPD); (**e, f**) right and left knees, respectively, in a patient with bilateral RPD. In knees of a healthy volunteer, cartilage at both medial and lateral facets of the patella had homogeneous dGEMRIC index throughout the cartilage (**a, b**). In the dislocated knee of a patient with unilateral RPD, the entire area of cartilage at the medial facet and the surface of cartilage at the lateral facet had shorter index (**c**), while in the nondislocated knee, only the surface of cartilage at the lateral facet had a shorter dGEMRIC index (**d**). In knees for a bilateral case, cartilage at both medial and lateral facets had shorter dGEMRIC index throughout the cartilage (**e, f**) (Figure from [41])

nine, suggesting that a low dGEMRIC index may, in fact, be predictive of progression to clinically evident OA [44].

The second study involved a population of subjects with hip dysplasia, a developmental malformation of the hip associated with a shallow acetabulum and early osteoarthritis. Comparison of dGEMRIC assessment with radiographic measures showed considerable variation in the dGEMRIC index, despite no apparent loss of tissue (Fig. 14.10a). dGEMRIC but not joint space width significantly correlated with the severity of dysplasia (Fig. 14.10b). These dGEMRIC data provided additional evidence that joint degeneration occurs early in young adulthood and suggested that the onset may be related to the severity of dysplasia. The study of dysplasia went further to investigate the possible role of dGEMRIC in outcome prediction: The present treatment for dysplastic hips is pelvic osteotomy to rotate the shallow acetabulum so that it covers the femoral head. The goals are to improve joint mechanics, relieve pain, and preserve the joint. Unfortunately, surgical results are variable and appear to depend upon the extent of preexisting arthritis [45]. A pilot study was conducted to explore whether dGEMRIC could provide a better measure to guide the decision and timing for osteotomy. In a prospective cohort study, patient age, radiographic severity of arthritis, severity of dysplasia, and dGEMRIC index were investigated as metrics to predict early failure after osteotomy. Nine of 52 osteotomies failed, with dGEMRIC index being the best predictor of failure ($p < 0.002$) [46] (Fig. 14.11). These data suggest that dGEMRIC may provide a more reliable basis on which surgeons can determine the timing for joint-preserving osteotomies.

Changing the Paradigm: Evidence that Cartilage Has the Capacity to Replenish Its Matrix

The prevailing clinical framework for osteoarthritis (OA), the most common degenerative disease of cartilage, is that OA is a progressive, irreversible destruction of cartilage, manifest by a reduction in joint space width. With radiographs as the mainstay for evaluating cartilage, and its associated inability to visualize the matrix, any processes that occur within the substance of the cartilage are simply invisible. Furthermore, there has been no way to evaluate preventative and therapeutic strategies that target cartilage during a period before there is frank loss of tissue. Methods such as dGEMRIC that permit an evaluation of the matrix itself offer

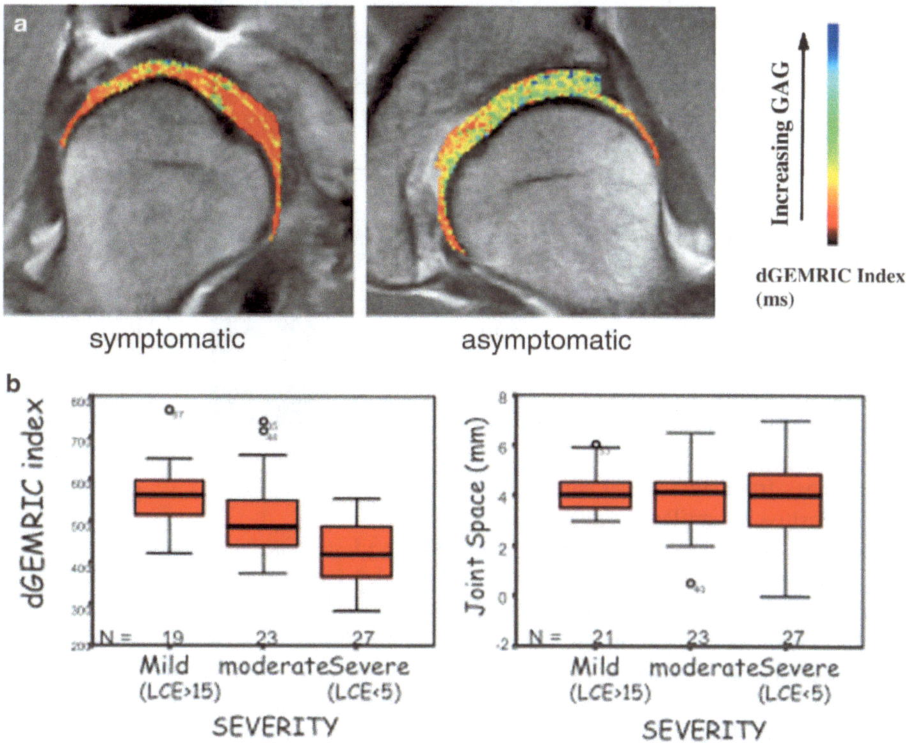

Fig. 14.10 (**a**) dGEMRIC images of the hips of a patient with unilateral hip dysplasia. The symptomatic hip has a much lower dGEMRIC index. (**b**) In this cross-sectional study, the dGEMRIC index correlated with the severity of dysplasia, while joint space width did not. *LCE* lateral center edge angle, a measure of dysplasia (Adapted from [50])

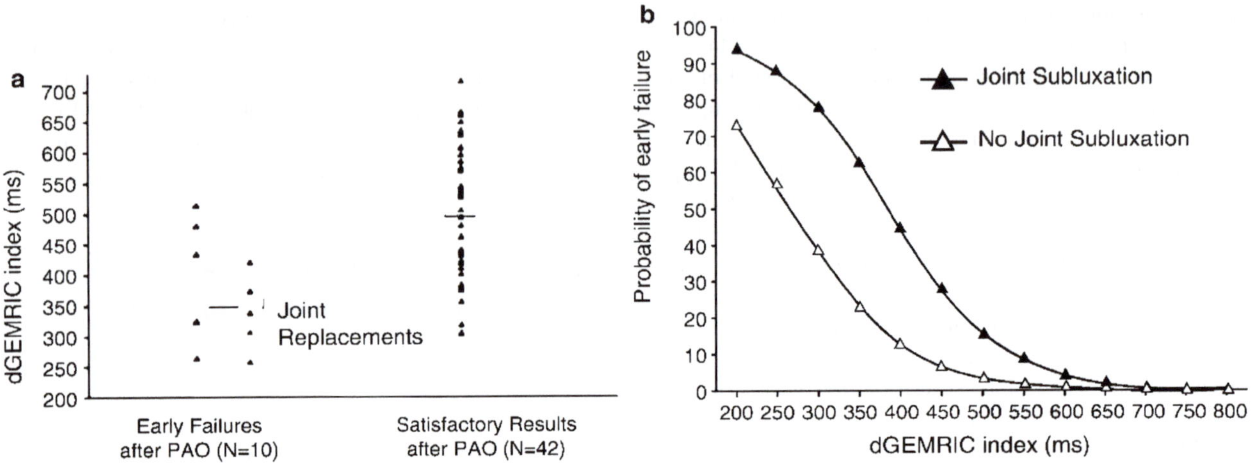

Fig. 14.11 (**a**) Distribution of dGEMRIC indices in hips with satisfactory results compared with those with unsatisfactory results after periacetabular osteotomy (PAO). Five hips that underwent total joint replacement had had lower dGEMRIC indices than the hips with worse pain and increased joint space narrowing after the osteotomy. (**b**) Calculated probability of failure after periacetabular osteotomy (PAO) according to the dGEMRIC index. A failed result is defined as a hip that underwent secondary arthroplasty, had increased pain, or had increased joint space narrowing (Figure adapted from [46])

the opportunity to visualize changes within the cartilage tissue itself, and so have the potential to shift the paradigm by recreating a framework that accounts for (patho)physiological changes within cartilage tissue. As noted in the examples above, in putatively healthy joints (showing no radiographic abnormalities), there is a wide variation in dGEMRIC index, possibly suggesting a wide variation in the functional integrity of the cartilage. A few studies are providing evidence that tissue with low dGEMRIC index can replenish its GAG, possibly "repairing" the matrix to a normal state.

For example, consider that the ultimate goal of joint-preserving surgery such as a pelvic osteotomy for hip dysplasia is to halt or even reverse the degenerative process. However, follow-up for a cohort of patients with successful osteotomies revealed that those with low dGEMRIC indexes prior to surgery had an increase in dGEMRIC index (Fig. 14.12) post-operatively [46], suggesting that cartilage injury may be reversible.

A second example comes from studies that suggest that the dGEMRIC index is sensitive to cartilage-modifying injuries. Individuals with a prior ACL injury have lower dGEMRIC values [47]. Although the temporal changes in dGEMRIC in those cases are unknown, one case study of a patient with a PCL injury revealed considerable changes in dGEMRIC in the months following the injury. Specifically, in the first few months after the injury, there was a dramatic drop in dGEMRIC index; by 6 months, the dGEMRIC index was near pre-injury levels (Fig. 14.13) [48].

Another final interesting example comes from work exploring whether exercise has an influence on dGEMRIC

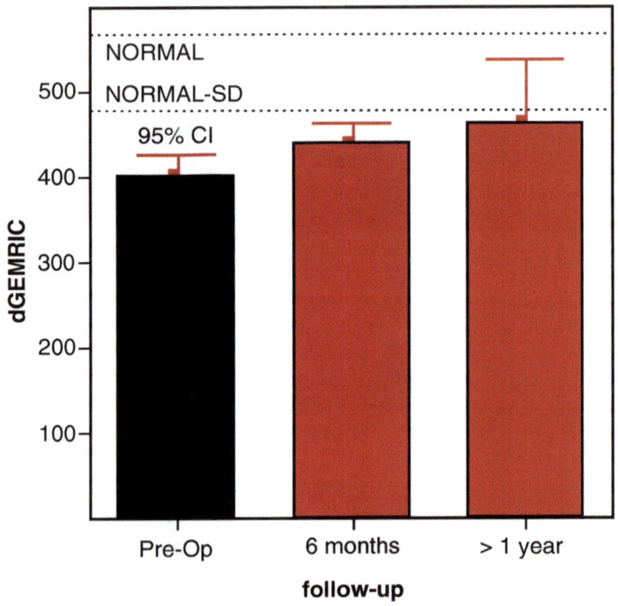

Fig. 14.12 dGEMRIC index before and after pelvic osteotomy. Of those with a low preoperative dGEMRIC index (<480 ms), there was a slight increase in the dGEMRIC Index after 1 year ($p = 0.08$) (From [1])

index. A cross-sectional study showed that the dGEMRIC index of knee cartilage in healthy volunteers correlated with the level of physical activity [49]. There are no data, as yet, showing whether a change in physical activity in healthy subjects is associated with a change in dGEMRIC index. However, there are some data for subjects who had suffered

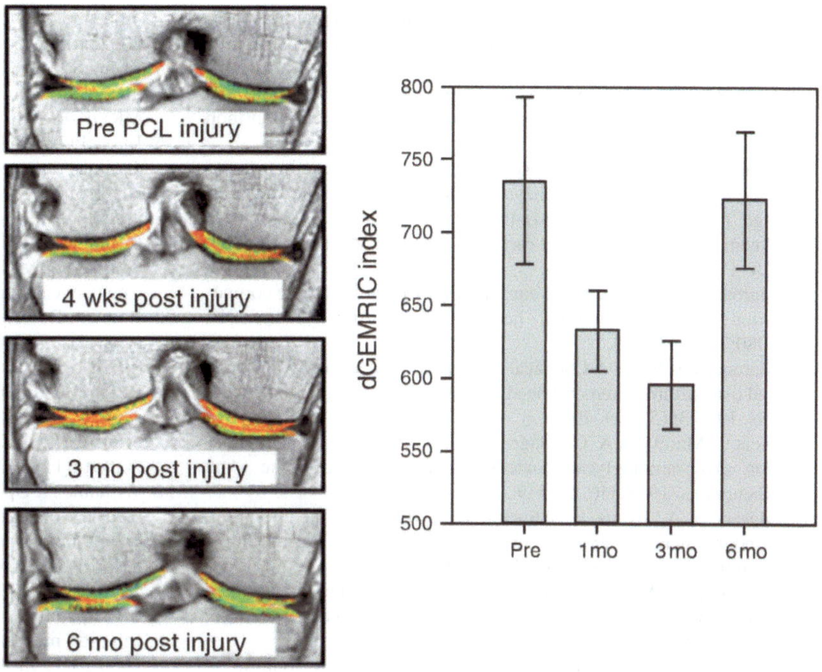

Fig. 14.13 Case study from an individual who had a PCL injury 1 week after a dGEMRIC image of the same knee. Repeat dGEMRIC imaging shows a substantially lower dGEMRIC index 1 and 3 months after the injury. By 6 months, the dGEMRIC index was at pre-injury levels (Adapted from [48])

a meniscal tear. Specifically, subjects who had meniscal tears were assigned to a 4-month exercise protocol. Those whose exercise following the tear was more intensive than baseline had an increase in dGEMRIC index, while those whose exercise was less intensive had a decrease in dGEMRIC index. These data provide the first in vivo evidence that exercise can, indeed, influence local GAG concentration, and support the appealing notion that exercise may be a therapeutic strategy.

These examples are encouraging in that they fit an appealing paradigm suggesting that relevant molecular changes can be monitored following an injury and in response to therapeutic measures (surgery and exercise), and, in particular, may suggest that matrix depleted of GAG can be restored. A word of caution is warranted, however, since (for all of the studies described in this section) long-term follow-up is needed to determine if the apparent increase in GAG concentration is sustained and if it is associated with an improvement in clinical outcome.

Summary

MRI has the potential to provide information regarding the molecular state of cartilage in both bench and clinical studies. The dGEMRIC technique demonstrates good correlations with known biochemical and biomechanical properties of the tissue. Furthermore, the dGEMRIC index has demonstrated measurable and reproducible changes with physiologic and pathologic processes in vitro and in vivo. With continued development of MRI pulse sequences to improve data acquisition speed, and with added insight from pilot clinical studies to define avenues of research, these and related methods may enter into standard use. Indeed, we appear to be on the leading edge of a paradigm shift, where rather than focusing on the late stage of disease with palliative therapy, we can recognize early degenerative changes and intervene with appropriate preventive and disease-reversing therapies.

Acknowledgments The authors deeply appreciate the dozens of collaborators, students, post-docs, and staff with whom we have worked over the last decades in developing and using the methods described here. We also deeply appreciate the essential support provided by numerous funding agencies, including: Proctor and Gamble Exploratory Research award, NIH-NIAMS, Arthritis Foundation, Pfizer, Orthopedic Research and Education Foundation (OREF), and Pharmacia. Finally, we thank the publisher and editors of the *Journal of Orthopaedic Research* who generously allowed us to use much of the text from an earlier review [1] in the preparation of this chapter.

References

1. Gray ML, Burstein D, Kim YJ, Maroudas A. Elizabeth Winston Lanier Award Winner. Magnetic resonance imaging of cartilage glycosaminoglycan: basic principles, imaging technique, and clinical applications. J Orthop Res. 2008;26(3):281–91.

2. Maroudas A. Physicochemical properties of articular cartilage. In: Freeman M, editor. Adult articular cartilage. 2nd ed. London, UK: Pitman Medical; 1979. p. 215–90.
3. Eisenberg SR, Grodzinsky AJ. Swelling of articular cartilage and other connective tissues: electromechanochemical forces. J Orthop Res. 1985;3(2):148–59.
4. Frank EH, Grodzinsky AJ, Koob TJ, Eyre DR. Streaming potentials: a sensitive index of enzymatic degradation in articular cartilage. J Orthop Res. 1987;5(4):497–508.
5. Freeman M. Adult articular cartilage. Freeman M, editor. London, UK: Pitman Medical; 1979.
6. Maroudas A, Bayliss MT, Venn MF. Further studies on the composition of human femoral head cartilage. Ann Rheum Dis. 1980;39(5):514–23.
7. Maroudas A, Venn M. Chemical composition and swelling of normal and osteoarthrotic femoral head cartilage. II Swelling. Ann Rheum Dis. 1977;36(5):399–406.
8. Ficat C, Maroudas A. Cartilage of the patella. Topographical variation glycosaminoglycan content normal fibrillated tissue. Ann Rheum Dis. 1975;34(6):515–9.
9. Maroudas A, Evans H, Almeida L. Cartilage of the hip joint. Topographical variation glycosaminoglycan content normal fibrillated tissue. Ann Rheum Dis. 1973;32(1):1–9.
10. Lesperance LM, Gray ML, Burstein D. Determination of fixed charge density in cartilage using nuclear magnetic resonance. J Orthop Res. 1992;10(1):1–13.
11. Jelicks LA, Paul PK, O'Byrne E, Gupta RK. Hydrogen-1, sodium-23, and carbon-13 MR spectroscopy of cartilage degradation in vitro. J Magn Reson Imaging. 1993;3(4):565–8.
12. Bashir A. Sodium NMR relaxation parameters in cartilage: implications for MR imaging [SM]. Cambridge: Massachusetts Institute of Technology; 1995. 134 p.
13. Insko EK, Reddy R, Leigh JS. High resolution, short echo time sodium imaging of articular cartilage. J Magn Reson Imaging. 1997;7(6):1056–9.
14. Shapiro EM, Borthakur A, Dandora R, Kriss A, Leigh JS, Reddy R. Sodium visibility and quantitation in intact bovine articular cartilage using high field (23)Na MRI and MRS. J Magn Reson. 2000;142(1):24–31.
15. Bashir A, Gray ML, Burstein D. Gd-DTPA2- as a measure of cartilage degradation. Magn Reson Med. 1996;36(5):665–73.
16. Bashir A, Gray ML, Boutin RD, Burstein D. Glycosaminoglycan in articular cartilage: in vivo assessment with delayed Gd(DTPA)(2-)-enhanced MR imaging. Radiology. 1997;205(2):551–8.
17. Allen RG, Burstein D, Gray ML. Monitoring glycosaminoglycan replenishment in cartilage explants with gadolinium-enhanced magnetic resonance imaging. J Orthop Res. 1999;17(3):430–6.
18. Trattnig S, Mlynarik V, Breitenseher M, Huber M, Zembsch A, Rand T, et al. MRI visualization of proteoglycan depletion in articular cartilage via intravenous administration of Gd-DTPA. Magn Reson Imaging. 1999;17(4):577–83.
19. Bashir A, Gray ML, Hartke J, Burstein D. Nondestructive imaging of human cartilage glycosaminoglycan concentration by MRI. Magn Reson Med. 1999;41(5):857–65.
20. Donahue KM, Burstein D, Manning WJ, Gray ML. Studies of Gd-DTPA relaxivity and proton exchange rates in tissue. Magn Reson Med. 1994;32(1):66–76.
21. Nieminen MT, Rieppo J, Silvennoinen J, Toyras J, Hakumaki JM, Hyttinen MM, et al. Spatial assessment of articular cartilage proteoglycans with Gd-DTPA-enhanced T1 imaging. Magn Reson Med. 2002;48(4):640–8.
22. Tiderius CJ, Olsson LE, Leander P, Ekberg O, Dahlberg L. Delayed gadolinium-enhanced MRI of cartilage (dGEMRIC) in early knee osteoarthritis. Magn Reson Med. 2003;49(3):488–92.
23. Tiderius C, Jessel R, Kim Y-J, Burstein D. Hip dGEMRIC in asymptomatic volunteers and patients with early osteoarthritis: the influence of timing after contrast injection. Magn Reson Imaging. 2007;57:803–5.
24. Zheng S, Xia Y. The impact of the relaxivity definition on the quantitative measurement of glycosaminoglycans in cartilage by the MRI dGEMRIC method. Magn Reson Med. 2010;63(1):25–32.
25. Burstein D, Bashir A, Gray ML. MRI techniques in early stages of cartilage disease. Invest Radiol. 2000;35(10):622–38.
26. Henkelman RM, Stanisz GJ, Menezes N, Burstein D. Can MTR be used to assess cartilage in the presence of Gd-DTPA2-? Magn Reson Med. 2002;48(6):1081–4.
27. Gillis A, Gray M, Burstein D. Relaxivity and diffusion of gadolinium agents in cartilage. Magn Reson Med. 2002;48(6):1068–71.
28. Burstein D, Velyvis J, Scott KT, Stock KW, Kim YJ, Jaramillo D, et al. Protocol issues for delayed Gd(DTPA)(2-)-enhanced MRI (dGEMRIC) for clinical evaluation of articular cartilage. Magn Reson Med. 2001;45(1):36–41.
29. Tiderius C, Hori M, Williams A, Sharma L, Prasad PV, Finnell M, et al. dGEMRIC as a function of BMI. Osteoarthritis Cartilage. 2006;14(11):1091–7.
30. Williams A, Oppenheimer RA, Gray ML, Burstein D. Differential recovery of glycosaminoglycan after IL-1-induced degradation of bovine articular cartilage depends on degree of degradation. Arthritis Res Ther. 2003;5(2):R97–105.
31. Samosky JT, Burstein D, Grimson WE, Howe R, Martin S, Gray ML. Spatially localized correlation dGEMRIC-measured GAG distribution mechanical stiffness human tibial plateau. J Orthop Res. 2005;23(1):93–101.
32. Baldassarri M, Goodwin JS, Farley ML, Bierbaum BE, Goldring SR, Goldring MB, et al. Relationship between cartilage stiffness and dGEMRIC index: correlation and prediction. J Orthop Res. 2007;25(7):904–12.
33. Juras V, Bittsansky M, Majdisova Z, Szomolanyi P, Sulzbacher I, Gabler S, et al. In vitro determination of biomechanical properties of human articular cartilage in osteoarthritis using multi-parametric MRI. J Magn Reson. 2009;197(1):40–7.
34. Mayerhoefer ME, Welsch GH, Mamisch TC, Kainberger F, Weber M, Nemec S, et al. The in vivo effects of unloading and compression on T1-Gd (dGEMRIC) relaxation times in healthy articular knee cartilage at 3.0 Tesla. Eur Radiol. 2010;20(2):443–9.
35. Williams A, Gillis A, McKenzie C, Po B, Sharma L, Micheli L, et al. Glycosaminoglycan distribution in cartilage as determined by delayed gadolinium-enhanced MRI of cartilage (dGEMRIC): potential clinical applications. AJR Am J Roentgenol. 2004;182(1):167–72.
36. Anandacoomarasamy A, Giuffre BM, Leibman S, Caterson ID, Smith GS, Fransen M, et al. Delayed gadolinium-enhanced magnetic resonance imaging of cartilage: clinical associations in obese adults. J Rheumatol. 2009;36(5):1056–62.
37. Burstein D, Eckstein F, Krishnan N. New strategies for clinical trials of OA: evidence from a longitudinal trail of radiography, MRI morphometry, and molecular MRI. Proceedings of the International Society for Magnetic Resonance in Medicine. Berkeley, CA; 2009.
38. Ericsson YB, Tjornstrand J, Tiderius CJ, Dahlberg LE. Relationship between cartilage glycosaminoglycan content (assessed with dGEMRIC) and OA risk factors in meniscectomized patients. Osteoarthritis Cartilage. 2009;17(5):565–70.
39. Jessel RH, Zurakowski D, Zilkens C, Burstein D, Gray ML, Kim YJ. Radiographic and patient factors associated with pre-radiographic osteoarthritis in hip dysplasia. J Bone Joint Surg Am. 2009;91(5):1120–9.
40. Fleming BC, Oksendahl HL, Mehan WA, Portnoy R, Fadale PD, Hulstyn MJ, et al. Delayed gadolinium-enhanced MR imaging of cartilage (dGEMRIC) following ACL injury. Osteoarthritis Cartilage. 2010;18(5):662–7.
41. Watanabe A, Obata T, Ikehira H, Ueda T, Moriya H, Wada Y. Degeneration of patellar cartilage in patients with recurrent patellar dislocation following conservative treatment: evaluation with

delayed gadolinium-enhanced magnetic resonance imaging of cartilage. Osteoarthritis Cartilage. 2009;17(12):1546–53.
42. Bittersohl B, Steppacher S, Haamberg T, Kim YJ, Werlen S, Beck M, et al. Cartilage damage in femoroacetabular impingement (FAI): preliminary results on comparison of standard diagnostic vs delayed gadolinium-enhanced magnetic resonance imaging of cartilage (dGEMRIC). Osteoarthritis Cartilage. 2009;17(10):1297–306.
43. Zilkens C, Holstein A, Bittersohl B, Jager M, Haamberg T, Miese F, et al. Delayed gadolinium-enhanced magnetic resonance imaging of cartilage in the long-term follow-up after Perthes disease. J Pediatr Orthop. 2010;30(2):147–53.
44. Owman H, Tiderius CJ, Neuman P, Nyquist F, Dahlberg LE. Association between findings on delayed gadolinium-enhanced magnetic resonance imaging of cartilage and future knee osteoarthritis. Arthritis Rheum. 2008;58:1727–30.
45. Minoda Y, Kadowaki T, Kim M. Total hip arthroplasty of dysplastic hip after previous Chiari pelvic osteotomy. Arch Orthop Trauma Surg. 2006;126:394–400.
46. Cunningham T, Jessel R, Zurakowski D, Millis MB, Kim YJ. Delayed gadolinium-enhanced magnetic resonance imaging of cartilage to predict early failure of Bernese periacetabular osteotomy for hip dysplasia. J Bone Joint Surg Am. 2006;88(7):1540–8.
47. Tiderius CJ, Olsson LE, Nyquist F, Dahlberg L. Cartilage glycosaminoglycan loss in the acute phase after an anterior cruciate ligament injury: delayed gadolinium-enhanced magnetic resonance imaging of cartilage and synovial fluid analysis. Arthritis Rheum. 2005;52(1):120–7.
48. Young AA, Stanwell P, Williams A, Rohrsheim JA, Parker DA, Giuffre B, et al. Glycosaminoglycan content of knee cartilage following posterior cruciate ligament rupture demonstrated by delayed gadolinium-enhanced magnetic resonance imaging of cartilage (dGEMRIC). J Bone Joint Surg Am. 2005;87(12):2763–7.
49. Tiderius CJ, Svensson J, Leander P, Ola T, Dahlberg L. dGEMRIC (delayed gadolinium-enhanced MRI of cartilage) indicates adaptive capacity of human knee cartilage. Magn Reson Med. 2004;51(2):286–90.
50. Kim YJ, Jaramillo D, Millis MB, Gray ML, Burstein D. Assessment of early osteoarthritis in hip dysplasia with delayed gadolinium-enhanced magnetic resonance imaging of cartilage. J Bone Joint Surg Am. 2003;85-A(10):1987–92.

Chapter 15
Imaging of Cartilage Repair

Goetz H. Welsch, Stephan Domayer, Vladimir Juras, Tallal C. Mamisch, and Siegfried Trattnig

Keywords Imaging • Cartilage • Repair • Morphological MR Assessment • Mosaicplasty • Microfracture • Diffusion-weighted imaging (DWI) • T1 rho • ACI techniques

Introduction

Articular cartilage lesions are a common pathology of the knee joint and many patients could benefit from cartilage repair. Such surgical treatment options may offer the possibility for patients with cartilage defects to avoid the development of osteoarthritis or delay its progression. Newly developed cartilage repair techniques, including arthroscopic or open surgical approaches, as well as marrow-stimulation techniques, osteochondral grafting, and chondrocyte implantation/transplantation, require knowledgeable and high-quality follow-up.

Morphological and biochemical magnetic resonance imaging (MRI) is now possible with high-field MR systems, advanced coil technology, and sophisticated sequence protocols capable of visualizing cartilage repair tissue, the adjacent articular cartilage, and the surrounding structures, in vivo, at high resolution, in clinically applicable scan times. Standard morphological approaches can demonstrate the constitution of cartilage repair tissue. Newer isotropic 3D sequences show great promise for improving cartilage imaging and also for the diagnosis of surrounding pathologies within the knee joint. Quantitative/biochemical MR approaches are able to provide a specific measure of the composition of cartilage. Cartilage physiology and ultrastructure can be determined, changes in cartilage macromolecules can be detected, and cartilage repair tissue can thus be assessed and potentially differentiated. In cartilage defects and following nonsurgical and surgical cartilage repair, morphological MRI provides the basis for diagnosis and follow-up evaluation, whereas biochemical MRI provides deeper insight into the composition of cartilage and cartilage repair tissue. A combination of both, together with clinical evaluation, may, in the future, represent a desirable multimodal approach to diagnosis, as well as for routine clinical follow-up after cartilage repair procedures. In addition to these advantages, the biomechanical properties of the repair tissue and the adjacent cartilage are of the utmost importance and these properties can be characterized using advanced MR techniques.

This chapter provides an overview of MRI of cartilage repair. The morphological depiction of cartilage on MRI is described, and emphasis is given to the Magnetic resonance Observation of Cartilage Repair Tissue (MOCART) scoring system. Furthermore, the use of biochemical MR methodologies for the visualization of cartilage repair tissue and the adjacent cartilage is illustrated. In the third section, a short overview is provided about MRI of the biomechanical properties of articular cartilage and cartilage repair tissue.

Morphological MR Assessment of Cartilage Repair

Morphological MR Sequences for Cartilage Repair Assessment

It has been demonstrated that in-plane spatial resolutions under 300 μm are required to reveal fraying of the articular surface of cartilage [1]. The introduction of high-field MRI units with 1.5, 3.0 T and beyond has provided the means to achieve such spatial resolutions while maintaining reasonable scan times using cartilage-sensitive sequences. To further decrease the scan time despite high-resolution parameters, new coil technology with multi-element design enables the use of parallel imaging, which can decrease scan time by a factor of 2–3. High-field MRI also increases the possibilities for 3D imaging; three-dimensional (3D) acquisitions yield even higher resolution and contrast-to-noise

S. Trattnig (✉)
Department of Radiology, MR Center, Medical University of Vienna, General Hospital of Vienna, Lazarettgasse 14, Vienna 1090, Austria
e-mail: siegfried.trattnig@meduniwien.ac.at

T.M. Link (ed.), *Cartilage Imaging: Significance, Techniques, and New Developments*,
DOI 10.1007/978-1-4419-8438-8_15, © Springer Science+Business Media, LLC 2011

ratio (CNR) than two-dimensional (2D) acquisitions. The 3D data set can be used to obtain slices in any plane. When an isotropic data set is obtained with the in-plane spatial resolution and the slice thickness in the same dimension, the voxel has the same length in every dimension, and additional planes can be reformatted from the original dataset with no loss in spatial resolution. In addition, with post-processing techniques, quantitative volume measurements can be added to cartilage assessment [2–4].

The most frequently used sequences for cartilage imaging are 3D gradient-echo (GRE) with fat suppression to visualize the thickness and surface of cartilage, and fluid-sensitive (mostly fat saturated) fast spin-echo (FSE) sequences for the assessment of internal cartilage structure [2, 5–7].

FSE imaging contrast is predominantly based on moderate T2 weighting and magnetization transfer effects, which results in low signal intensity of cartilage in contrast to the high signal intensity of joint fluid due to T2 weighting. The subchondral bone also demonstrates a high signal intensity due to fatty marrow, which remains relatively hyperintense on FSE T2 sequences, an effect called J-coupling. Cartilage is, therefore, outlined dark against bright synovial tissue and fluid as well as the subchondral plate [8, 9]. Intrachondral cartilage matrix damage and alterations of the cartilage surface can thus be readily assessed. Other advantages of FSE sequences are their inherent high resolution and low sensitivity to magnetic susceptibility artifacts, which are suppressed by the multiple refocusing 180° pulses of the FSE. This allows reliable MRI assessment after surgery. Figure 15.1 shows standard 2D MR sequences of a patient in the follow-up after cartilage repair using a matrix-associated chondrocyte transplantation (MACT) approach.

Standard T1-weighted, fat-suppressed, 3D spoiled gradient-echo (SPGR) sequences provide a high signal intensity for cartilage, while adjacent bone and synovial fluid remain dark. The 3D data set can be reformatted in any plane, allowing 3D visualization and volume measurements [9–11]. New isotropic 3D gradient-echo sequences comprise the DESS (Double-Echo Steady-State), True-FISP (Fast Imaging in Steady-state Precession), Balanced-FFE (Fast Field Echo), VIBE (Volume Interpolated Breath-hold Examination), MEDIC (Multi-Echo Data Image Combination). Furthermore, isotropic 3D fast spin-echo (FSE) sequences have recently become available (called PD [proton-density] SPACE [Sampling Perfection with Application optimized Contrasts using different flip angle Evolutions], or 3D Fast Spin-Echo [FSE] Extended Echo-Train Acquisition [XETA]), which may, in future applications, provide greater opportunity to characterize the constitution of cartilage, bone, menisci, ligaments, and the surrounding tissue within one clinically applicable sequence. A variety of results from the initial application of these sequences have been reported in the literature.

A fat-suppressed 3D FLASH (Fast Low-Angle Shot) sequence shows high contrast-to-noise ratios (CNR) and high reproducibility in the segmentation of articular cartilage, and facilitates accurate evaluation of total cartilage volume and regional distribution [12, 13]. Cartilage segmentation measurements could be established for quantitative MR evaluation, and cartilage thickness and volume could be used as sensitive image-based parameters for detecting and monitoring cartilage degeneration in OA [14].

The 3D DESS sequence has been shown to be valuable for the first stage of cartilage assessment [15, 16]. The sequence provides an intermediate cartilage signal, high

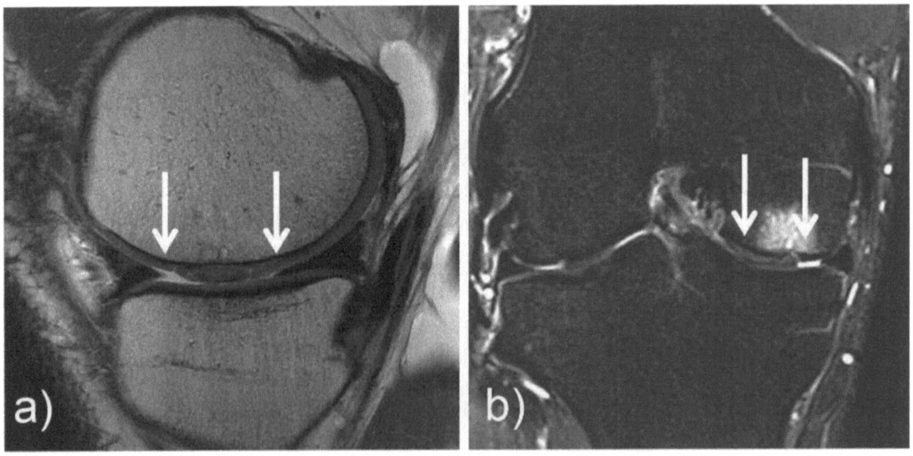

Fig. 15.1 Conventional high-resolution MRI of a 48-year-old male patient 24 months after matrix-associated chondrocyte transplantation (MACT) (*arrows*). (**a**) Sagittal PD-TSE (TR = 2,400 ms/TE = 28 ms; flip angle = 160°) with ultrahigh in-plane (0.23 × 0.23 mm) resolution (matrix = 512 × 512; FoV = 12 cm; slice thickness = 2 mm) and 34 slides achieved in 6 h 01 min; (**b**) coronal T1-weighted TIRM (7,690/41; flip angle 150°; TI = 220) with high-resolution (256 × 256; 15 cm; slice thickness = 3 mm) and 25 slices achieved in 2 h 19 min

cartilage-to-fluid contrast, and is suitable for quantitative volumetric measurements [17].

The 3D True-FISP sequence provides substantially higher SNR and CNR than the 3D FLASH sequence [18]. This advantage in signal might allow for higher spatial resolution, and thus, potential improvement in the accuracy of the segmentation process, especially at the articular surface [18]. With high-field MRI, this advantage might also be used to perform isotropic MR measurements in a minimal amount of time. Kornaat et al. [19] report that SSFP (Steady-State Free Precession)-based techniques have the highest increase in SNR and CNR efficiency at 3.0 T MRI. In recent articles by Duc et al. [20–22], the True-FISP sequence as an SSFP-based sequence was studied in detail at 1.5 T and also showed promising results. Compared to a 3D FLASH and a 3D DESS sequence, the preoperative detection of cartilage defects is possible with similar sensitivity, specificity, and accuracy for the water excitation True-FISP sequence; however, again, the SSFP-based sequences showed the highest SNR and CNR efficiency [22]. With the use of a dedicated, eight-channel knee coil, an isotropic (0.6 mm^3) 3D True-FISP dataset can be obtained in approximately 3 min. The potential to diagnose cartilage defects, anterior cruciate ligament abnormalities, and meniscal tears can be expected to be higher than with a set of standard 2D sequences [21]. Figure 15.2 visualizes an isotropic high-resolution 3D True-FISP data set of a patient 3 months after MACT.

Thus, 3D sequences have the potential to considerably improve cartilage defect assessment by reproducible, quantitative volumetric measurements in the submillimeter range.

Figures 15.3 and 15.4 demonstrate MR images of the knee obtained with a high-resolution isotropic 3D PD SPACE sequence in a patient 24 months after MACT of the medial femoral condyle. Whereas Fig. 15.3 gives an overview of the whole knee using multi-planar reconstruction (MPR) of the data set comprising an axial, sagittal, and coronal reconstruction, Fig. 15.4 gives a more specific detailed image of the cartilage repair tissue and provides the possibility for MR scoring.

MRI Scores

For the use of MRI in the evaluation of cartilage repair techniques in greater numbers of patients, an evaluation system that has low interobserver variability and is suited for statistical data analysis is necessary. It should have the potential to compare different cartilage surgery techniques and also to be used in multicenter studies [23, 24].

Roberts et al. [24] used four parameters to assess cartilage repair on MR images: surface integrity and contour; cartilage signal in the graft region; cartilage thickness; and changes in the underlying bone. The score is obtained by summing the values of the four parameters. The system assesses each parameter as normal or abnormal; still, there is no assessment of graft integration, degree of defect fill, or the presence of adhesions.

The Magnetic resonance Observation of Cartilage Repair Tissue (MOCART) scoring system was designed to systematically record observations that can be accurately and reproducibly determined [25]. The MOCART system has been shown to be reliable and has excellent interobserver reproducibility for the defined variables [25]. Correlation analyses of the MOCART system with the KOOS knee score demonstrated significant interrelations of the variables "filling of the defect," "structure of the repair tissue," "subchondral bone," and "signal intensity."

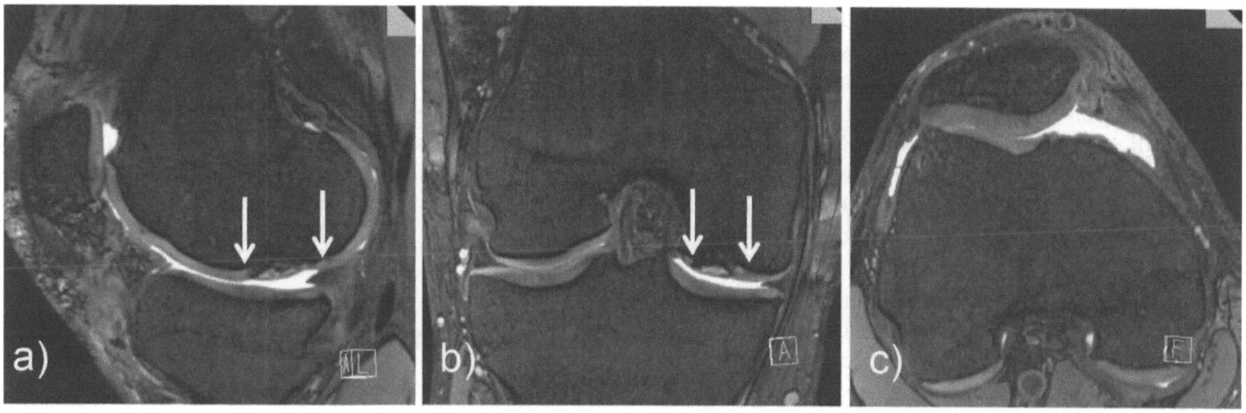

Fig. 15.2 Isotropic 0.4×0.4×0.4 mm 3D True-FISP sequence (8.9/3.8) with water excitation and high-resolution MR images reconstructed to visualize the cartilage repair tissue in a 22-year-old male patient, 3 months after MACT (*arrows*) in the sagittal (**a**) and coronal (**b**) planes. Additional axial (**c**) reconstructed images allow evaluation of the patellar cartilage. Three hundred and twenty slides were obtained in 6 min 46 sec (PAT 3). After the short follow-up interval, artifacts within the hyperintense repair tissue are still visible and cannot be clearly distinguished from possibly bony formation

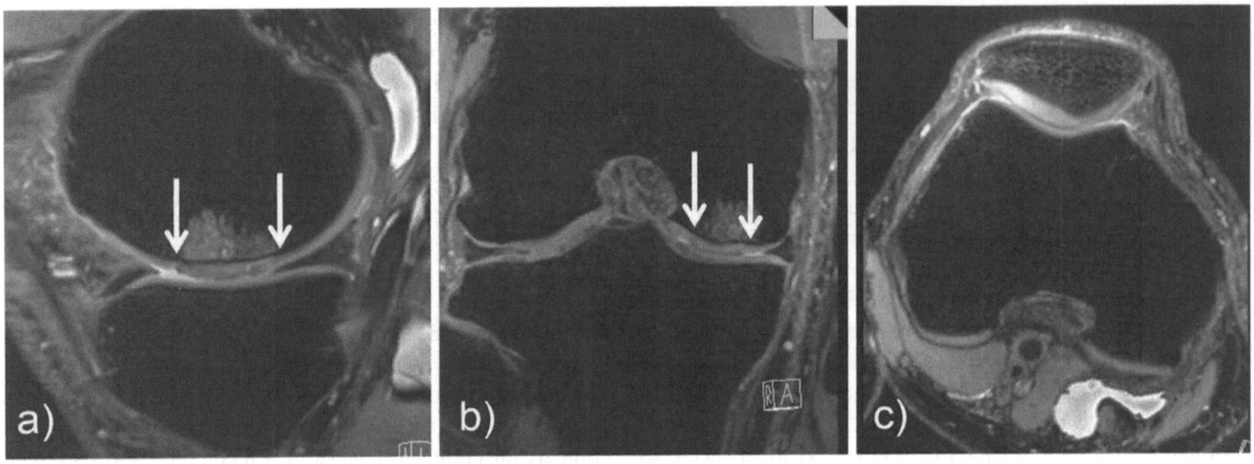

Fig. 15.3 High-resolution isotropic 0.5×0.5×0.6 mm fat-suppressed 3D PD SPACE sequence (1,500/34) of a patient 24 months after MACT (same patient as in Fig. 15.1) (*arrows*) and 192 sections obtained in 7 min 53 sec. Images reconstructed in the sagittal (**a**), coronal, (**b**) and transversal (**c**) planes

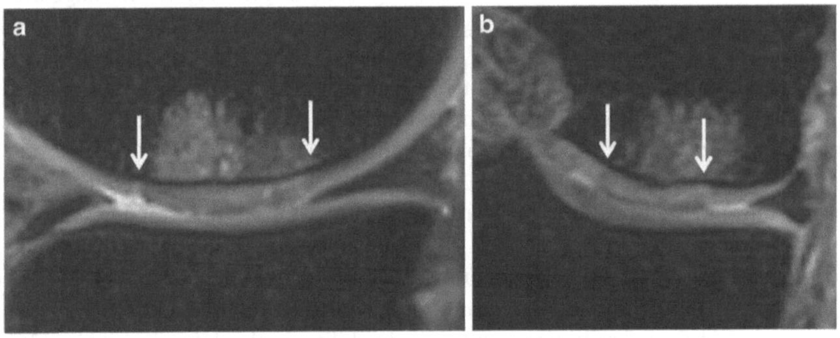

Fig. 15.4 Enlarged sagittal (**a**) and coronal (**b**) details of Fig. 15.3. According to the variables of the 3D MOCART score (Table 15.1), *variable 1* a slight hypertrophy of the repair tissue (~125°) is visualized in the coronal plane, *variable 2* the integration to the border zone shows in the sagittal plane a split-like lesion (*left arrow*), *variable 4* the surface of the repair tissue displays surface irregularity and fraying, *variable 5* a relatively homogeneous structure of the repair tissue, *variable 6* early normal signal intensity, *variable 7* an intact subchondral lamina, *variable 10* alterations in the subchondral bone, and *variable 11* no significant intra-articular effusion

The system is useful for longitudinal follow-up of patients after different cartilage repair techniques [25], and may facilitate multicenter studies that compare a particular cartilage repair technique.

The MR assessment of the MOCART score is based on standard MR sequences, also recommended by the International Cartilage Repair Society (ICRS) [26]. The MR evaluation of the cartilage repair tissue is performed on two-dimensional (2D) planes using high in plane resolution, together with a slice thickness of 2–4 mm. Following this current standard procedure, the MR sequences recommended by the ICRS and the recommended sequences for the MOCART scoring visualize the area of cartilage repair and the adjacent cartilage, as well as the surrounding structures in 2D.

The previously mentioned, new isotropic 3D sequences have the potential for high-resolution isotropic MR imaging and can be reformatted in arbitrary planes with no loss of spatial resolution. Building on the capabilities of multiplanar reconstruction (MPR), the cartilage repair tissue could be visualized in 3D, and its subsequent classification and grading by an MR-based scoring system might benefit.

Very recently, an improved MOCART scoring system, using the possibilities of 3D MPR in the postoperative evaluation of cartilage repair tissue, was presented as a 3D MOCART scoring system [27] (Table 15.1).

Monitoring of Various Cartilage Repair Techniques

Routine MR follow-up of cartilage repair tissue should be carried out at 3 months, 1 year, and 2 years. Imaging at 3 months verifies the adherence of repair tissue and discloses

Table 15.1 Three-dimensional (3D) Magnetic resonance Observation of Cartilage Repair Tissue (MOCART) score using an isotropic 3D MR sequence

Variables			
1. Defect fill (degree of defect repair and filling of the defect in relation to the adjacent cartilage)			
O	0%		
O	0–25%		
O	25–50%		
O	50–75%		
O	75–100%		
O	100%		
O	100–125%		
O	125–150%		
O	150–200%		
O	>200%		
Localization			
O Whole area of cartilage repair	O >50%	O <50%	
O Central	O Peripheral	O Weight-bearing	O Nonweight-bearing
2. Cartilage interface (integration with adjacent cartilage to border zone in two planes)			
Sagittal (femur, patella, trochlea, tibia)			
O	Complete		
O	Demarcating border visible (split-like)		
O	Defect visible <50%		
O	Defect visible >50%		
Coronal (femur, tibia); axial (patella, trochlea)			
O	Complete		
O	Demarcating border visible (split-like)		
O	Defect visible <50%		
O	Defect visible >50%		
Localization			
O Whole area of cartilage repair	O>50%	O<50%	
O Weight-bearing	O Nonweight-bearing		
3. Bone interface (integration of the transplant to the subchondral bone; integration of a possible periosteal flap)			
O	Complete		
O	Partial delamination		
O	Complete delamination		
O	Delamination of periosteal flap		
Localization			
O Weight-bearing	O Nonweight-bearing		
4. Surface (constitution of the surface of the repair tissue)			
O	Surface intact		
O	Surface damaged <50% of depth		
O	Surface damaged >50% of depth		
O	Adhesions		
Localization			
O Whole area of cartilage repair	O>50%	O<50%	
O Central	O Peripheral	O Weight-bearing	O Nonweight-bearing
5. Structure (constitution of the repair tissue)			
O	Homogeneous		
O	Inhomogeneous or cleft formation		
Localization			
O Whole area of cartilage repair	O>50%	O<50%	
O Central	O Peripheral	O Weight-bearing	O Nonweight-bearing
6. Signal intensity (intensity of MR signal in the repair tissue in comparison to the adjacent cartilage)			
O	Normal (identical to adjacent cartilage)		
O	Nearly normal (slight areas of signal alteration)		
O	Abnormal (large areas of signal alteration)		
Localization			
O Central	O Peripheral	O Weight-bearing	O Nonweight-bearing

(continued)

Table 15.1 (continued)

Variables			
7. Subchondral lamina (constitution of the subchondral lamina)			
O	Intact		
O	Not intact		
Localization			
O Whole area of cartilage repair	O >50%	O <50%	
O Central	O Peripheral	O Weight-bearing	O Nonweight-bearing
8. Chondral osteophytes (osteophytes within the cartilage repair area)			
O	Absent		
O	Osteophytes < 50% of the thickness of the cartilage transplant		
O	Osteophytes > 50% of the thickness of the cartilage transplant		
Localization			
Size: _______ mm (plane: _______) × _______ mm (plane: _______)			
O Central	O Peripheral	O Weight-bearing	O Nonweight-bearing
9. Bone marrow edema (maximum size and localization in relation to the cartilage repair tissue and other alterations assessed in the 3D MOCART score).			
O	Absent		
O	Small (<1 cm)		
O	Medium (<2 cm)		
O	Large (<4 cm)		
O	Diffuse		
Localization			
Size: _______ mm (plane: _______) × _______ mm (plane: _______)			
O Central	O Peripheral	O Weight-bearing	O Nonweight-bearing
O Relation to other alterations within this score of variable No. ________			
10. Subchondral bone (constitution of the subchondral bone)			
O	Intact		
O	Granulation tissue		
O	Cyst		
O	Sclerosis		
Localization			
O Whole area of cartilage repair	O >50%	O <50%	
O Central	O Peripheral	O Weight-bearing	O Nonweight-bearing
11. Effusion (approx. size of joint effusion visualized in all planes)			
O	Absent		
O	Small		
O	Medium		
O	Large		

early complications in the healing process, whereas imaging at 1 year assesses graft maturation and helps to guide patients with respect to the level of activity after cartilage surgery. Imaging after 2 years should help to disclose late complications of the graft.

Each surgical technique will show distinct features during follow-up that may occur in the course of the healing process or be associated with repair failure. The subsequent sections treat the current knowledge of cartilage repair tissue properties and the respective surgical techniques.

Microfracture

MRI is highly sensitive and specific to microfracture repair (MFX) tissue assessment. Arthroscopic evaluation of MRI at 1.0 T demonstrated specificity and sensitivity of 100% and 100% for defect filling and 80% and 82% for repair tissue quality, respectively [28]. MRI at 3.0 T certainly has the potential to further improve repair tissue quality assessment [29, 30].

Mithoefer et al. [31] evaluated 24 patients at 1.5 T at 12 ± 2 months after surgery, with the following parameters: repair cartilage signal; lesion morphology; defect filling; peripheral repair tissue integration; and subchondral edema.

With a cartilage-sensitive FSE sequence [5], repair tissue signal was hyperintense in 92%. Mild subchondral edema was observed in 71%. Repair tissue fill was graded 67–100% in most patients; still, the majority had depressed morphology compared to adjacent cartilage. Osseous overgrowth occurred in 25%. Persistent gap formation at the border to adjacent cartilage was reported in 92%.

Notably, clinical improvement correlated with the fill grade ($p < 0.05$). A subsequent decrease in clinical outcome at 24 months occurred in all patients with a poor fill grade, but three cases with good fill grades also decreased. Moderate, but significant, correlations were found between fill grade and the activities of daily living score and the SF-36 physical component score. A lower body-mass index was associated with a better fill grade on magnetic resonance imaging. Peripheral interfacing correlated well with the fill grade, but had no correlation with the outcome scores.

The filling grade of the defect is, thus, apparently, a major indicator for the outcome of MFX; again, 3D GRE imaging at high resolution may improve MRI assessment. Persisting gaps are considered adverse. Further investigation may clarify whether there is an association with repair tissue deterioration and subsequent failure. Mild subchondral edema apparently was not associated with clinical outcome; persistent alterations of the subchondral plate will also occur during long-term follow-up.

Mosaicplasty

Osteochondral autograft transfer (OAT) is usually performed at the knee and involves removing a healthy osteochondral core from a donor site (mostly trochlea) and implanting it at the usually weight-bearing portions of the femoral condyle, this procedure is also termed mosaicplasty. MRI evaluation of osteochondral grafts should include: (1) the number and size of the grafts; (2) bone and cartilage integration; (3) the cartilage surface contour; (4) an assessment of the signal in the graft, the adjacent bone marrow, and at the donor site; (v) details of any soft tissue abnormalities; and (vi) an assessment of the contrast enhancement patterns.

Cartilage and Bone Integration

Cartilage and bone integration should be considered separately. Cartilage of the OAT was reported by Link et al. [32] to be intact and with a regular surface in 85% of cases. Gaps between OAT and native cartilage were rarely visualized with standard MRI. However, in indirect MR arthrography, persistent fissure-like gaps between the implanted cartilage and native cartilage were demonstrated [33]. This finding corresponds well to OAT histology assessment and emphasizes the potential of contrast agent–enhanced MRI in challenging cases.

Regarding the integration of OAT bone, cystic cavities, with fluid-like signal intensity and/or a persistent edema-like signal within the subchondral bone, may be considered indicators for poor integration [32].

Cartilage and Bone Signal Intensity

OAT bone marrow signal intensities are reported to be consistent with edema within the first 12 months after implantation (hypointensity on T1-weighted images and hyperintensity on fat-suppressed PD-w or T2-weighted images). During the 12–24 month follow-up, the rate of edema-like signal intensities dropped to 17% [32]. Interestingly, in patients with OAT necrosis, T2 signal intensities varied depending on the morphologic type of necrosis (sclerotic or cystic degeneration). Clinical abnormalities were reported in only two of six patients with signs of OAT osteonecrosis [32]. Conversely, contrast-enhanced MRI was specific for necrosis. Sanders et al. [34] and Hangody and Fules [35] reported no cases of osteochondral necrosis in their patient groups. In OAT, cartilage signal intensity is similar to the surrounding cartilage in the vast majority of cases [32, 34, 35].

Graft and Adjacent Bone

The early postoperative period is dominated by subchondral bone marrow edema, which resolves with graft incorporation. A normal fatty marrow signal is seen within and around the plugs when solid bony incorporation occurs [32–34].

Bone marrow edema can be expected in and around the grafts in approximately 50% of the subjects during the first 12 months. After this period, a gradual decline will be observed in the majority of cases; still, edema may persist in a small number of cases for up to 3 years. Joint effusion and synovitis appear to follow a similar trend.

Incongruities at the bone–bone interface occur frequently due to the variation of OAT and native cartilage thickness. The focus of OAT surgery is the congruity of the joint cartilage surface, and therefore, is the main criterion in OAT integration assessment.

Complications assessed by MRI concern graft loosening or migration, incongruencies of the cartilage–cartilage interface, significant gaps between osteochondral plugs and adjacent native cartilage, and partial or complete graft necrosis. With respect to gaps, the postoperative period has to be considered, since surface congruity will improve over time due to fibrocartilaginous tissue formation between osteochondral plugs.

ACI Techniques

Assessment and interpretation of MR examinations for autologous chondrocyte implantation (ACI) and matrix-associated autologous chondrocyte implantation (MACI) patients should be performed in a systematic fashion. Careful attention should be paid to: (1) the degree of defect filling; (2) the integration of the graft to adjacent cartilage and underlying bone; (3) the internal structure and surface of the graft; (4) the signal intensity of the graft; and (5) any changes in the subchondral bone. Finally, the presence of adhesions to the graft or joint effusion should be noted. All categories are included in the MOCART score.

Defect Filling

ACI repair tissue is designed to have the same thickness as adjacent native cartilage to restore the joint surface and to stabilize native cartilage. Filling assessment, therefore, concerns the thickness of repair tissue in 2D slices. Still, with 3D techniques available, repair tissue interfaces to adjacent normal cartilage can be assessed accurately in all directions, and the volume of the repair tissue may also be quantified.

The ratio of cases with complete defect filling after ACI can be expected to be approximately 60–80% [24, 36–38].

Graft hypertrophy is considered one of the major adverse events of ACI, reportedly occurring in 2.4–20% of cases, and is associated with the use of a periosteal flap [39].

Graft hypertrophy is seen on MRI as the ACI graft protruding above the level of the native articular cartilage, and may involve part or the full width of the graft. Hypertrophy of grafts close to the intercondylar notch may cause impingement on the anterior cruciate ligament and requires arthroscopic debridement.

The incidence of graft hypertrophy after MACI is reported to be considerably lower, and, if present, may improve over time due to remodeling of the joint surface under weight-bearing [38, 40–42].

Integration

The interface between ACI and native cartilage should be indiscernible. Splits or fissures at the border zone are considered pathological [43, 44], and are indicated by fluid-like signal clefts or ill-defined high signal intensity at the interface on high-resolution MRI [43–47].

The clinical importance of gaps in the integration zone lies in the possible progress to graft delamination. A thin rim of fluid between the base of the graft and the subchondral bone plate, resembling a cartilage flap, may indicate a delaminated graft still in situ at the repair site. A dislocated delaminated graft may appear as a loose body in the joint [43, 44]. Clinical symptoms are often pain, swelling, and locking.

Structure and Surface

Irregularities of the graft surface on MR imaging have been described previously in up to 50% of implants, and thus, seem to be relatively common [10, 36, 43, 44, 48], especially in the early stages. At later stages, continuous smoothing of the graft surface has been observed, a finding that may be related to graft organization and remodeling. However, the development of surface defects over time is considered pathologic [38].

Graft tissue often has an inhomogeneous signal behavior at early stages that differs from the trilaminar appearance of native cartilage. During the maturation process, graft signal will become homogeneous in the majority of cases. Conversely, increasing inhomogeneity of the graft may indicate graft degeneration and beginning graft failure.

Signal Intensity

At 4 weeks after transplantation, the graft may have a fluid-like appearance, which could mimic graft delamination. However, on high-resolution imaging, the surface of the implant is seen as a thin dark line. This feature is more commonly seen with classic ACI [43].

During the first 6 months after implantation, repair tissue signal intensity will differ from native cartilage; with the T1-weighted GRE sequence, signal will increase, whereas a decrease is to be expected with the FSE sequence [38, 49].

At 12 months, the signal behavior of repair tissue is reported to resemble native cartilage [10, 43, 50, 51] in the majority of cases with both sequences. There have been reports of persisting hyperintensity in FSE up to 18 months [52], but the definite role of signal intensity has not been determined, as yet, and will likely be the subject of further studies.

Subchondral Lamina and Bone

The subchondral lamina should be kept intact in ACI and MACI; however, in patients after osteochondrosis dissecans, defects of the lamina will persist after implantation. It is important to differentiate these cases from cortical endplate damage that occurs after implantation by overuse or recurrent trauma. Subchondral edema is reported to occur regularly within the first 3–6 months after implantation [36, 37, 43, 52, 53], and is part of the healing process. Persistence of edema after this period, or even an increased intensity and size of subchondral edema, should be considered abnormal and be closely monitored [43, 44, 54]. Edema may be caused by abnormal joint loading due to overuse or joint malalignment. In contrast, there are also studies that consider the importance of bone marrow edema to be undetermined.

Cystic changes in the subchondral bone underneath the cartilage may indicate complications that require close clinical follow-up. Cyst formation has also been associated with a fibrocartilage – rather than hyaline-like repair tissue composition [37].

Adhesions

Symptomatic intra-articular adhesions that require arthroscopy occur in up to 10% of ACI patients. Aside from stiffness and pain, adhesions in connection with the Hoffa fat pad or the suprapatellar pouch can be a cause for graft dislocation by traction forces applied to the graft [45–47].

On MRI, adhesions appear as bands of intermediate-to-low signal intensity that traverse the joint and originate from the repair tissue.

Effusion

Reactive synovitis is a cause of pain in the early postoperative period, but normally resolves during follow-up. In cases of persisting effusion, alternate causes, such as meniscal tears, ligament injury, or the formation of new cartilage defects, must be excluded.

Regular Development of ACI/MACI Grafts

Serial MRI follow-up of MACI patients demonstrated a dynamic healing process over time. Significant milestones of ACI and MACI repair tissue formation within the first year are: (1) Bone marrow edema can be expected in the first 3 months after surgery, but should recede after that time. (2) The graft will have a fluid-like appearance 4 weeks after implantation, and then gradually approach the signal intensity of adjacent cartilage within 6–12 months. (3) Continuous graft remodeling, which may comprise a gradual defect filling, as well as intermittent graft hypertrophy, will result in a complete defect filling, with a smooth and intact surface after 12 months.

Biochemical MR Assessment of Cartilage Repair

Basics of Biochemical MRI of Healthy Cartilage and Cartilage Repair

To visualize the constitution of articular cartilage and cartilage repair tissue, a variety of different methodologies are available. When first looking at the composition of healthy hyaline articular cartilage, these methodologies can depict either one component of the cartilage or a combination of different components. More recent techniques, in particular, have not even been validated sufficiently; nevertheless, promising results during initial studies justify their use.

Basically, articular cartilage is complex, dense, connective tissue that relies on the diffusion of solutes for its nutrition [55]. Responsible for the biomechanical properties of articular cartilage is the extracellular matrix, mainly composed of water (~75%), collagen (~20%), and proteoglycan (PG) aggregates (~5%) [55, 56]. Water either freely moves throughout the matrix or is bound to macromolecules. Collagen in hyaline cartilage is largely type II, which creates a stable network throughout the cartilage. The negatively charged proteoglycans are composed of a central core protein to which glycosaminoglycans (GAG) are bound.

Articular cartilage is stratified primarily according to the orientation of collagen within a three-dimensional network [56, 57]. The superficial/tangential zone is characterized by flattened chondrocytes, relatively low quantities of proteoglycans, and high quantities of collagen fibrils arranged parallel to the articular surface. The middle/transitional zone has round chondrocytes, a high level of proteoglycans, and a random arrangement of collagen fibers. The deep/radial zone is characterized by low cell density, thick collagen fibrils that are perpendicular to the bone, and columns of chondrocytes. After the "tide mark," the underlying calcified layer is partly mineralized, and acts as the transition between cartilage and the subchondral bone.

The structure and the components of healthy hyaline cartilage formed the basis for (1) the different biochemical MR methodologies and (2) their use in the evaluation of articular cartilage. Hence, not only is the specific sequence essential, but also its ability to adapt to the zonal structure of articular cartilage, for example.

Within cartilage repair, generally all biochemical MR sequences can be used and (1) help to depict the ultrastructure of cartilage repair tissue; (2) help to judge the repair tissue as scar tissue, fibrocartilage, or hyaline-like cartilage; (3) help to define the maturation process of the repair tissue over time; (4) help to diagnose early as well as late failure; and (5) ideally, provide a predictive value for the performance of the repair tissue over time [16, 26, 37, 58–65].

Depending on the different cartilage repair techniques, the cartilage repair tissue in histological studies is seen to be hyaline-like cartilage, mixed hyaline-like and fibrocartilage, and fibrocartilage. Nevertheless, these histological studies show different results for these different cartilage repair procedures [35, 36, 40, 47, 66–72]. Thus, the depiction of the ultrastructure of the repair tissue using biochemical MRI is important. The significance of the quality of the cartilage repair tissue, and thus, the benefit of a biochemical MR evaluation, is illustrated when considering the results of one of the most widely recognized studies in this field by Knutsen et al., who compared ACT and MFX [71, 72]. Biopsies obtained from 67 patients showed no significant difference between the cartilage repair techniques (notwithstanding the trend toward a more hyaline-like structure after ACI). However, a comparison of the histological quality of the repair tissue in patients with and without treatment failure revealed that none of the patients with treatment failure in this study had hyaline-like cartilage. This finding suggests that repair cartilage, which is predominantly hyaline, may reduce the risk of subsequent failure [71]. In recent initial studies by our group [16, 60], a differentiation of cartilage repair tissue after MACT and MFX was possible using different biochemical MR methodologies, which demonstrate the feasibility of functional MR techniques as a "virtual biopsy."

Proteoglycan Sensitive

Although no MR sequence, perhaps, is really 100% specific for only proteoglycans or collagens, there are methodologies that reportedly focus mainly on one component of articular cartilage. The negatively charged proteoglycan, composed of a central core protein to which glycosaminoglycans (GAG) are bound, could be visualized (among others) by delayed gadolinium-enhanced MRI of cartilage (dGEMRIC) [73], sodium MR imaging [74, 75], and, very recently, chemical exchange–dependent saturation transfer (CEST) [76].

Delayed Gadolinium-Enhanced MRI of Cartilage

Glycosaminoglycans (GAG) are important to the cartilage tissue's biochemical and biomechanical functions. GAG are the main source of fixed charge density (FCD) in cartilage, and are often decreased in the early stages of cartilage degeneration [77], or in reparative cartilage after cartilage repair [62]. Intravenously administered gadolinium diethylenetriamine pentaacetate anion (Gd-DTPA^{2-}) penetrates the cartilage through both the articular surface and the subchondral bone. The contrast equilibrates in inverse relation to the FCD, which is, in turn, directly related to the GAG concentration. Therefore, T1, which is determined by the Gd-DTPA^{2-} concentration, becomes a specific measure of tissue GAG concentration, suggesting that Gd-DTPA^{2}-enhanced MRI has the potential to monitor the GAG content of cartilage in vivo [78]. Thus, T1 mapping, enhanced by delayed administration of Gd-DTPA^{2-} (T1 dGEMRIC), can be considered as a valuable methodology for detecting proteoglycan depletion in articular cartilage, and has shown promising results [79, 80].

As differences in pre-contrast values between cartilage repair tissue and normal hyaline cartilage are larger compared to early cartilage degeneration, in cartilage repair tissue, the pre-contrast T1 values must be calculated, as well [62]. The concentration of GAG is represented by delta ΔR1, i.e., the difference in relaxation rate ($R1 = 1/T1$) between $T1_{\text{pre-contrast}}$ and $T1_{\text{post-contrast.}}$ Thus, the sequence must be performed twice, for pre-contrast and delayed post-contrast T1 mapping. This increases the total scan time, and requires a break in between the two MR scans, where the contrast agent must be administered and a delay of at least 90 min after injection is needed for penetration of the contrast agent into the cartilage. Scan time reduction, compared to the standard inversion recovery (IR) evaluation, has been achieved with a new approach using fast T1 mapping [61]. Although the 90-minute delay is still required, this might increase the clinical applicability of the dGEMRIC technique.

Since GAG content is responsible for cartilage function, particularly its tensile strength, the monitoring of the development of GAG content in cartilage repair tissues may provide information about the quality of the repair tissue. A recent study by our group showed that dGEMRIC was able to differentiate between different cartilage repair tissues with higher delta ΔR1 values, and thus, lower GAG content, in cartilage repair tissue after MFX, compared to MACT [60]. The applicability of this technique has also been shown in regions other than the knee joint [81–83].

Figure 15.5 gives an example of the T1 dGEMRIC evaluation of cartilage repair tissue compared to the surrounding healthy seen control cartilage in a patient 24 months after MACT of the medial femoral condyle.

Sodium (^{23}Na) MR Imaging

Sodium MRI has been described as an in vivo technique for cartilage imaging, and is sensitive to proteoglycans [84, 85]. Due to the high effort with regard to the hard- and software requirements and a relative low signal-to-noise ratio, its clinical use is limited. However, as sodium MRI is seen to provide a direct measure of proteoglycans, its use as a standard of reference is highly promising. Similar to the principles described for dGEMRIC imaging, positive sodium ions are attracted by the negative fixed charged density (FCD) of the side chains of GAG. These electrostatic forces are responsible for a direct relationship between the local sodium concentration and FCD, and research has shown sodium imaging to be sensitive to small changes in GAG concentration [86, 87].

The MR sensitivity for ^{23}Na is only 9.2% of the 1H MR sensitivity, and the in vivo concentration is ~360 times lower than the in vivo water proton concentration. The combination of these factors results in a ^{23}Na signal that is approximately 4,000 times smaller than the ^{1}H signal. In addition, the very short T2 relaxation time of ^{23}Na leads to a further reduction in signal intensity.

Recent advances in magnet technology, improved gradient performance, and multi-coil technology may make sodium MRI feasible on high-field systems, and promising results have been demonstrated in vivo on pigs, in human wrists, and in the human knee joint [88–90].

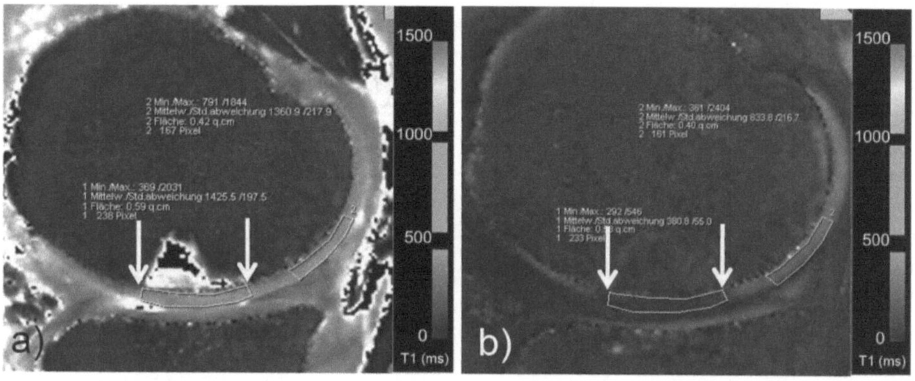

Fig. 15.5 Biochemical sagittal T1 dGEMRIC images of a patient 24 months after MACT of the medial femoral condyle. Whereas (**a**) shows the pre-contrast T1 map, (**b**) is showing the same plane for the post-contrast evaluation. For quantitative T1 mapping, a GRE sequence (15/3.15; flip angles 4.4° and 24.7°) with high resolution (448×448; 16 cm; slice thickness 3 mm) and 16 slides was obtained in 3 min 40 sec. The ROI evaluation was performed in the area of cartilage repair (TX) (*arrows*) and an area of control cartilage (2, REF). Pre-contrast (TX: 1,425 ms; Ref: 1,360 ms) and post-contrast (TX: 380 ms; Ref 833 ms) T1 values resulted in Delta T1-TX of 1.9 and a Delta T1-Ref of 0.47 (relative Delta-T1 of 4.04) indicating low GAG content of the repair tissue

Chemical Exchange Saturation Transfer Imaging

As the mapping of the GAG concentration is desirable in the follow-up of cartilage repair procedures, and because of the obvious limitations of sodium MRI, the presented dGEMRIC technique has the limitation of contrast agent administration and a time delay before post-contrast MRI. A recently described technique for the assessment of GAG concentration in vivo by chemical exchange–dependent saturation transfer (CEST) may have potential in future applications on articular cartilage [76].

Balaban and coworkers demonstrated that the chemical exchange between labile protons of low concentration solutes and bulk water protons provides a sensitivity enhancement scheme known as CEST [91–93]. When saturation is applied at a particular frequency far from the water resonance, this saturation is transferred rapidly between the solid-like matrix and free water. Notably, both proteoglycans and collagen macromolecules have exchangeable amide protons (~100 mM) that exchange with bulk water. In addition, each proteoglycan unit also has three –OH protons (~300 mM) that rapidly exchange with bulk water. Similarly, collagen has exchangeable amine protons ($-NH_2$). Recently, Ling et al. [76] extensively studied and identified the potential of the so-called gagCEST method in cartilage; however, this application is still in the very early stage, and more extensive studies and validation are required.

Collagen Sensitive

Although the differentiation of which components of articular cartilage are visualized by the specific sequence is not completely possible, the classic biochemical MR methodology that focuses on the collagen content of articular cartilage is T2 mapping [94]. In addition to the transverse relaxation time (T2) of articular cartilage, recently, T2* relaxation is being discussed for the depiction of the collagen matrix [95], and magnetization transfer contrast (MTC) might also play a more important role in future approaches [65].

T2 Relaxation Time Mapping

The transverse relaxation time (T2) of cartilage is a sensitive parameter for the evaluation of changes in water and collagen content and tissue anisotropy [94]. Cartilage T2 reflects the interaction of water and the extracellular matrix on a molecular level. The collagen fiber orientation defines the layers of articular cartilage. Thus, the three-dimensional organization and curvature of the collagen network, influenced by water mobility, the proteoglycan orientation, and the resulting magic angle at 55° (with respect to the main magnetic field (B0)), influence the appearance of T2 [57, 96]. In healthy articular cartilage, an increase in T2 values from deep to superficial cartilage layers can be observed based on the anisotropy of collagen fibers running perpendicular to cortical bone in the deep layer of cartilage [97]. Histologically validated animal studies have shown this zonal increase in T2 values as a marker of hyaline or hyaline-like cartilage structure after cartilage repair procedures in the knee [63, 98]. To visualize this zonal variation in vivo, high spatial resolution is essential, which can already be achieved at high-field MR, together with dedicated multichannel coils in clinical approaches. In cartilage repair tissue, global (bulk) T2 values, as well as line profiles, have shown an increase in the early postoperative follow-up, which might enable visualization of cartilage repair maturation [99]. Another study by our group further showed the ability of zonal T2 evaluation to differentiate cartilage repair tissue after MFX and MACT [16]. Whereas cartilage repair tissue after MFX, histologically seen as fibrocartilage, shows no zonal increase from deep to superficial cartilage aspects, repair tissue after MACT, histologically reported as hyaline-like, shows a significant stratification.

In osteoarthritis, however, T2 mapping has shown varying results [100–102] and the role of T2 as an absolute quantification parameter must be further analyzed. Nevertheless, T2 mapping seems to offer potential in this area as well. Conclusions would be more easily derived, however, from a longitudinal evaluation of the same subject, with MRI performed at the same time of day.

T2* Relaxation Time Mapping

In addition to standard 2D multi-echo spin-echo T2 relaxation, T2*-weighted 3D gradient-echo articular cartilage imaging has shown reliable results in the evaluation of chondromalacia of the knee [103]. In recent studies, T2* mapping, with its potentially short scan times, was correlated to standard T2, and showed information comparable to that obtained for articular cartilage in the knee, but with overall lower T2* values (ms) [104, 105]. Furthermore, also for T2*, a clear zonal variation between the deep and superficial cartilage layers was described for healthy cartilage. After cartilage repair using MFX, however, this stratification could not be found [104]. Thus, for standard T2, as well as for comparable techniques, zonal assessment of healthy and altered articular cartilage is crucial.

Thus, for T2*, the zonal variation between the subchondral border and the cartilage surface might have another explanation, due to the influence of local susceptibility fields on T2*. These local fields can operate at a macroscopic level, i.e., at the bone–cartilage interface or at the microscopic level, i.e., associated with the underlying microstructure of the cartilage. If these processes produce local changes in the macroscopic static field gradients, this might be more distinct in the deep cartilage zone. This problem in the evaluation of the cartilage near the subchondral bone plate might also account for the differences in the zonal stratification between T2 and T2*, with a clearer increase from the deep to superficial relaxation times in T2* compared to T2. Furthermore, T2* has not been sufficiently validated for its use in cartilage, and it could be that T2* visualizes different properties of articular cartilage in addition to collagen, and including, perhaps, proteoglycan aggregates. Thus, to describe the ultrastructure of articular cartilage, T2* relaxation might be a sensitive tool in addition to T2 relaxation. Problematic for both methodologies might be the fact that T2 or T2* values can increase or decrease when the structure of cartilage changes from healthy to pathological, or, when differences between control cartilage and cartilage repair tissue are reported. This is discussed for T2 in a review article by Burstein et al. [102], and might be a limitation for T2* as well.

Figure 15.6 displays a color-coded cropped T2 and T2* map of a patient 24 months after MACT of the lateral femoral condyle.

Hybrid Sequences

Future trends in T2 mapping might also include hybrid sequences that combine morphological and biochemical aspects in one sequence. With regard to the morphological assessment of articular cartilage, the fast Double-Echo Steady-State (DESS) sequence permits accurate and precise analysis [17, 106]. Based on the theory of Bruder et al. [107], the simultaneous acquisition of two separated Steady-State

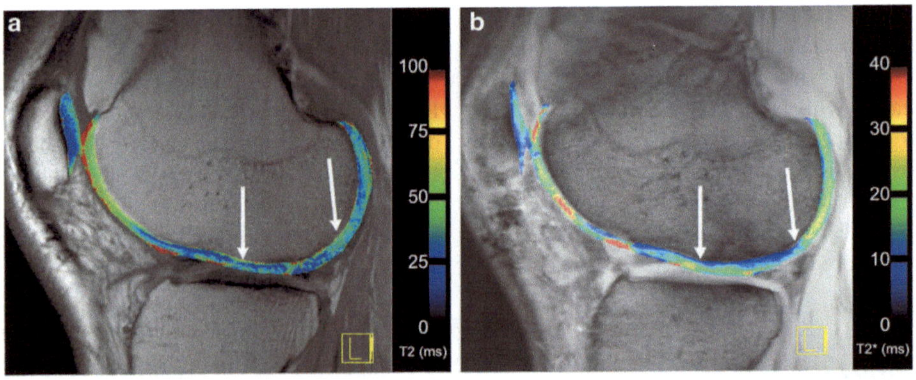

Fig. 15.6 Sagittal multi-echo (**a**) spin-echo T2 (1,650/12.9, 25.8, 38.7, 51.6, 65.5, 77.4; flip angle 180°) sequence and (**b**) GRE T2* (600/5.7, 9.8, 14.0, 18.1, 22.2, 26.4; flip angle 20°) sequence with identical high in-plane resolution (384×384; 16 cm; 3 mm slice thickness) obtained in a 27-year-old male patient 24 months after MACT (*arrows*) at the lateral femoral condyle of the knee. Six slices were obtained for T2 in 5 min 37 sec and T2* in 2 min 27 sec

Free Precession (SSFP) echoes within the DESS sequence allows the formation of two MR images with clearly different contrasts: S^+ = FISP (Fast Imaging Steady Precession) and S^- = PSIF (reversed FISP) . The PSIF part of the sequence leads to a high T2 contrast, whereas the FISP part provides representative morphological images with a contrast dominated by the T1/T2 ratio. In principle, the different T2 weightings of both echoes allow the calculation of quantitative T2 maps with a certain functional dependence on T1, depending on the chosen flip angle.

Magnetization Transfer Contrast

The use of MT imaging for articular cartilage was first described by Wolff et al. [108]. MT effects are based on the interaction of two different proton pools, the free (unbound) water pool, which is visible by MRI, and the bound proton pool, with protons bound to macromolecules. This reduces the mobility of these protons to such a degree that, with standard MRI, this bound proton pool is not visible. In certain tissues in the human body, such as the liver, the thyroid, muscle, and cartilage, however, the two proton pools are in equilibrium, biochemically and magnetically. After saturation of the magnetization of bound water molecules by off-resonance pulses, the equilibrium is shifted to the bound proton pool, which results in a reduction of the observable magnetization, and thus, in a reduction of the MR signal. Thus, MT is tissue-specific and may provide a quantitative method for tissue characterization of basic macromolecular dynamics and chemistry [108–113]. Nevertheless, to date, MT has been rarely used for the quantitative in vivo evaluation of articular cartilage. Initially, we found only one study with initial, but promising, results for cartilage repair [114]. In a study by our own group, based on the valuable work of Scheffler and Bieri [115] and their magnetization transfer–sensitized, Steady-State Free Precession (SSFP) MRI sequence, MTC was compared to T2 mapping in the assessment of global mean values, as well as zonal variations, of articular cartilage and cartilage repair tissue after MACT and MFX [65]. In this study, significant differences in global mean MT ratio (MTR) values between healthy cartilage sites and sites after cartilage repair were observed. Lower values for MTR were more pronounced in cartilage repair tissue after MFX compared to cartilage repair tissue after MACT. However, in contrast to T2 relaxation, MTC showed lower values for both MFX and MACT, whereas T2 showed lower values only for MFX, when comparing cartilage repair tissue to surrounding control cartilage. Hence, both biochemical methodologies do not measure exactly the same components of cartilage and cartilage repair tissue. Considering in vitro studies [116, 117], collagen concentration and collagen orientation may possibly play the most important role for both MTC and T2. T2 relaxation, nevertheless, might also be influenced by hydration, whereas MTC might be less influenced.

When using these (and other) biochemical MR techniques in cartilage repair, one of the most important things is to (1) either use an area of healthy cartilage as an internal control, or (2) perform longitudinal studies and compare the same subject at the same time of day. Furthermore, histologically validated studies might help to further clarify the impact of biomechanical MR techniques in the visualization of cartilage ultrastructure and specific components of articular cartilage.

Proteoglycan and/or Collagen Sensitive

The overview in this chapter about biochemical MR sequences leads to the next sequences that reflect a combination of all the components of articular cartilage, and their impact has been the subject of controversy. When considering diffusion-weighted imaging (DWI) of cartilage, which reflects its diffusivity, the articular cartilage or the repair tissue have to be seen as a complete system [118]. T1 rho relaxation might reflect a combination of cartilage macromolecules, and is sensitive to proteoglycans [88] and collagen [119].

Diffusion-Weighted Imaging

Diffusion-weighted imaging (DWI) is based on molecular motion that is influenced by intracellular and extracellular barriers. Consequently, it is possible to estimate the biochemical structure and architecture of the tissue by measuring molecular movement [118, 120]. When based on spin-echo (SE) sequences, DWI is relatively insensitive to susceptibility effects, but diffusion-weighted SE sequences require acquisition times that cannot be readily applied in clinical practice, and are very sensitive to bulk motion. Echo planar imaging (EPI)–based diffusion sequences are the current gold standard of DWI for neurological applications, but these suffer from image distortions (susceptibility artifacts) and from limitations in contrast and resolution (due to the long echo times required). Both these disadvantages render them impracticable for imaging tissues with short T2, such as cartilage and muscles. Alternatively, diffusion imaging can be performed using Steady-State Free Precession sequences (SSFP), which provide diffusion weighting at relatively short echo times [121]. This is achieved by the application of a monopolar diffusion-sensitizing gradient, which leads to a diffusion weighting of consecutive echoes (spin echoes, stimulated echoes, and higher order echoes) under steady-state conditions. For the assessment of diffusion-weighted images in articular cartilage, a three-dimensional steady-state diffusion technique, called PSIF, has been used.

In order to assess the diffusional behavior of the cartilage semiquantitatively, the diffusion sequence protocol should consist of two immediately consecutive measurements with zero (0), and 75 mT * ms * m^{-1} monopolar diffusion gradient moments for DWI, but identical imaging parameters. For evaluation, the quotient image (non-diffusion-weighted/diffusion-weighted image) is calculated on a pixel-by-pixel basis. The feasibility of diffusion-weighted PSIF imaging after matrix-associated chondrocyte transplantation has been demonstrated in vivo [122, 123]. The drawback of this technique is the semiquantitative character, since the *b*-values and diffusion weighting depend on several tissue and scanner parameters. Nevertheless, it remains – until now – the only approach for in vivo DWI in cartilage repair tissue, and might present one promising possibility for the depiction of the vital character of cartilage repair tissue on a non-contrast level.

Figure 15.7 visualizes a DWI approach in a patient 36 months after MACT of the patella.

T1 Rho

Relaxation time in the rotating frame (T1 rho) has been reported to be a sensitive marker of the loss of proteoglycans in articular cartilage [88, 124, 125]. T1 rho is a time constant that characterizes magnetic relaxation of spins under the influence of a radiofrequency field that is parallel to the spin magnetization. The resulting contrast is sensitive to the low-frequency interactions between water molecules and their local macromolecular environment, such as GAG and collagen, which are the main constituents of the extracellular matrix in cartilage. Changes in T1 rho were observed in cartilage plugs that were chemically or enzymatically depleted of GAG, but not in collagenase-treated tissue [125]. On the other hand, Menezes et al. found no correlation between the cartilage T1 rho and GAG concentration [126]. In addition, it was reported that the dominant T1 rho and T2 relaxation mechanism at $B_0 < 3$T is a dipolar interaction due to slow anisotropic motion of the water molecules in the collagen matrix.

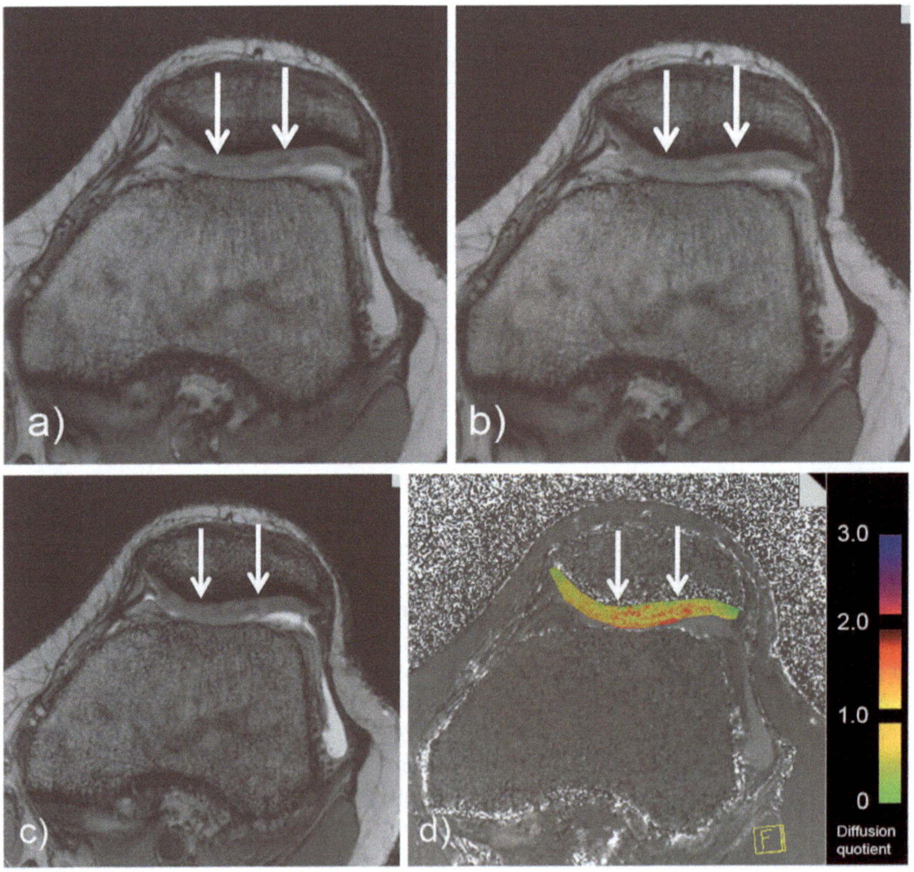

Fig. 15.7 Axial diffusion-weighted images of a patient 36 months after MACT (*arrows*) of the patella using a high-resolution, three-dimensional, balanced, steady-state gradient-echo pulse sequence (3D DW PSIF) with ((**a**) phase, (**b**) read) and without (**c**) a diffusion gradient of 75 mT * ms * m^{-1}. Images resulting in a semiquantitative diffusion map (**d**)

Summary/Discussion of Biochemical MRI of Cartilage Repair

As yet it is not well known which exact component of the repair tissue the new biochemical cartilage-sensitive MR methodologies are able to visualize. Moreover, due to the numerous cartilage repair procedures, the choice of a specific method in cartilage repair is challenging. Nevertheless, a number of studies emphasized the importance of biochemical MR imaging in the follow-up after cartilage repair and it seems that cartilage repair tissue maturation can be visualized by techniques like dGEMRIC or quantitative T2, for example [61, 64, 99, 127]. Furthermore, zonal assessment of cartilage repair tissue seems to be able to provide additional information about the constitution of the repair tissue, and is able to distinguish between repair tissues built by different cartilage repair procedures [16, 60]. Thus, if there is sufficient spatial resolution, the possible stratification of cartilage repair tissue, as a sign of hyaline-like structures [98], must be taken into consideration when analyzing cartilage repair tissue. Sufficient spatial resolution should be obtained not only for collagen-sensitive MR sequences, but also for all biochemical methodologies, because the proteoglycan concentration is also known to show different quantities from deep to superficial cartilage [128].

The promising results about the use of biochemical MRI in the depiction of cartilage repair tissue are, in part, based on the role model character of cartilage repair. Thus, in young patients with primarily healthy articular cartilage, a single cartilage defect is "repaired" by a procedure based on pluripotent bone marrow cells [129], or on different generations of cartilage transplantation techniques that are, in part, based on tissue engineering [130–133]. The goal should be twofold: (1) to optimize the diagnosis in the follow-up of cartilage repair to possibly provide a predictive value and (2) to use this role model to also optimize the biochemical MR techniques. In particular, the previously mentioned tissue-engineered scaffolds that are used in modern cartilage transplantation techniques could be evaluated in their performance by biochemical MRI.

Biomechanics of Articular Cartilage and Repair

Basics of Articular Cartilage Biomechanics

The articular cartilage can be thought of as a fiber-reinforced anisotropic composite material. The mechanical properties of articular cartilage are a function of the essential mechanical properties of the tissue components and the interplay of these components during loading. Collagen and proteoglycans (PGs) are the most important components that determine the mechanical integrity of cartilage. The interactions of these components with the tissue water determine the elasticity and stiffness of cartilage. Loading and deformation of cartilage will generate a combination of tensile, compressive, and shear stresses in the material. The dynamic mechanical properties of cartilage are strongly dependent on the collagen network integrity. Collagen lacks compressive properties, but demonstrates tensile viscoelastic and nonlinear behavior [134]. Under a static compression, cartilage settles into a mechanical equilibrium, which is determined primarily by the water-attracting PGs [135]. The relative high fixed charged density acts against the compressive stress, which induces osmotic swelling pressure, defined as the Donnan effect [136]. In case of continued loading application, there is a flow of interstitial water, which is controlled by tissue permeability. These changes support a rearrangement of the cartilage matrix [137]. The biomechanical properties of articular cartilage are depth dependent [138], and differ among particular cartilage layers [139] and anatomical locations [140].

Biomechanics of Degenerated Cartilage

Biomechanical studies of joints are based on the need to better understand their structure–function relationships in providing joint motion, and the pathomechanical processes involved in joint diseases, such as osteoarthritis. Cartilage degeneration is macroscopically manifested by the articular surface fibrillation, with the presence of cracks or fissures, and by partial or complete loss of the tissue [141]. Additional signs of OA include an increase in cartilage hydration, joint space narrowing, subchondral bone changes, osteophyte formation, evidence of altered cellular activity, and structural and compositional changes [142].

The tensile modulus (i.e., stiffness) of native human articular cartilage varies from 5 to 25 MPa, depending on the anatomical location on the joint surface, and the depth and orientation of the cartilage specimen relative to the joint surface [143, 144]. The tensile modulus can decrease by as much as 90%, reflecting significant damage to the OA cartilage solid network [143]. Decreases in the tensile stiffness and fracture stress of cartilage have been reported for human cartilage with OA [145]. These changes appear due to the disorganized and disrupted collagen fiber network, which has been observed macroscopically and histologically. Articular cartilage with surface fibrillation and erosion is more compliant, or deformable, in compression [146, 147]. Degenerated cartilage was found to be significantly more compliant in shear, which was attributed to fibrillation of the articular surface and loss of ground substance with OA.

Cartilage Biomechanics and MRI

Magnetic resonance imaging has been successfully used to predict the biomechanical properties of cartilage; however, the interpretation of the results is quite complex. Dynamic mechanical properties are related mainly to the PG content, i.e., the PG amount and volume distribution, which determine primarily the elastic modulus. However, the influence of collagen fibers must be considered. A significant correlation between T_{1Gd} (T_1 measured in the presence of contrast agent) and mechanical properties has been found in different anatomical locations (femoral and tibial human cartilage [148, 149], patellar and humeral animal cartilage [150, 151]), and engineered tissue [152]. Early changes in cartilage tissue degeneration (e.g., in osteoarthritis) are hardly detectable by morphological assessment, but, it has been shown that biomechanical properties of the cartilage tissue are altered, even in the early stages of degenerative processes [139]. MRI has great potential for the early diagnosis of these processes. A recent study by Juras et al. showed a statistically significant relationship between MR parameters (T_1, T_{1Gd}, and contrast agent concentration) and the instantaneous (*I*) and equilibrium (*Eq*) modulus [153] in degenerated cartilage. This relationship is valid in the whole spectrum of OA stages, i.e., from the mild to the advanced stage. Therefore, this could be used for early, in vivo diagnosis of articular cartilage degenerative diseases.

T2 may also successfully serve as a predictor of cartilage biomechanical properties. The stiffness and strength of AC tissue depend on the density and orientation of collagen fibers, and the type or amount of collagen cross-linking. A significant negative correlation between T2 and aggregate modulus H_A has been reported for patellar cartilage in a porcine model [154]. In the degenerated cartilage, the pre-stress of collagen fibrils is reduced, and subsequently, this greatly reduces shear stiffness of the solid matrix [155]. As T2 is mainly related to the collagen matrix, it may be used for the cartilage rigidity estimation [156]. MRI may be advantageous because of its noninvasive nature and the ability to provide prospective, in vivo assessment of cartilage biomechanical properties.

One of the main functions of the cartilage is to dissipate stress that is applied during physiological conditions. This is enabled by a typical three-layer anisotropy in cartilage, the presence of PG, and complex biochemical processes determined by water and dissolved solutes. Moreover, healthy cartilage requires compressive loading from physical activity to develop normally and maintain form and function. The structural and functional changes in cartilage after loading (e.g., after exercise) can be successfully detected by signal intensity changes in MR images. Eckstein et al. demonstrated a 5–6% decrease in patellar cartilage volume after compressive loading induced by performing 50 deep knee bends [157]. Mosher et al. found a statistically significant decrease in T2 of the superficial 40% of weight-bearing femoral cartilage after exercise [158].

Mechanical stress is an important modulator of cell physiology, and there is significant evidence that physical factors may be used to improve or accelerate tissue regeneration and repair. The mechanical properties of repair tissue are not identical to those of native tissue. MRI has an interesting ability to distinguish between native and transplant cartilage tissue, when there is an understanding of cartilage biomechanics. Loading applied onto the cartilage induces changes in water content and, to some extent, in collagen fiber orientation. The different response of cartilage tissue to the loading that appears in full knee extension, compared to 40° flexion, was exploit for the differentiation between native cartilage and MACT repair tissue in vivo [159]. The connection between biochemical MRI and cartilage biomechanics provides great potential for the monitoring of patients after surgical or pharmaceutical treatment of cartilage impairment.

Acknowledgments Funding for parts of this manuscript was provided by the concept "Vienna Advanced Clinical Imaging Center" (VIACLIC), based on the economic and scientific development program "Vienna Spots of Excellence": a collaboration of the Center of Excellence for Highfield MR and Siemens Austria.

References

1. Rubenstein JD, Li JG, Majumdar S, Henkelman RM. Image resolution and signal-to-noise ratio requirements for MR imaging of degenerative cartilage. AJR Am J Roentgenol. 1997;169: 1089–96.
2. Disler DG, McCauley TR, Kelman CG, Fuchs MD, Ratner LM, Wirth CR, et al. Fat-suppressed three-dimensional spoiled gradient-echo MR imaging of hyaline cartilage defects in the knee: comparison with standard MR imaging and arthroscop. AJR Am J Roentgenol. 1996;167:127–32.
3. Peterfy CG, van Dijke CF, Lu Y, Nguyen A, Connick TJ, Kneeland JB, et al. Quantification of the volume of articular cartilage in the metacarpophalangeal joints of the hand: accuracy and precision of three-dimensional MR imaging. AJR Am J Roentgenol. 1995;165: 371–5.
4. Recht MP, Piraino DW, Paletta GA, Schils JP, Belhobek GH. Accuracy of fat-suppressed three-dimensional spoiled gradient-echo FLASH MR imaging in the detection of patellofemoral articular cartilage abnormalities. Radiology. 1996;198:209–12.
5. Potter HG, Linklater JM, Allen AA, Hannafin JA, Haas SB. Magnetic resonance imaging of articular cartilage in the knee. An evaluation with use of fast-spin-echo imaging. J Bone Joint Surg Am. 1998;80:1276–84.
6. Recht M, Bobic V, Burstein D, Disler D, Gold G, Gray M, et al. Magnetic resonance imaging of articular cartilage. Clin Orthop Relat Res. 2001;391:S379–96.
7. Trattnig S. Overuse of hyaline cartilage and imaging. Eur J Radiol. 1997;25:188–98.

8. Constable RT, Anderson AW, Zhong J, Gore JC. Factors influencing contrast in fast spin-echo MR imaging. Magn Reson Imaging. 1992;10:497–511.
9. Yao L, Gentili A, Thomas A. Incidental magnetization transfer contrast in fast spin-echo imaging of cartilage. J Magn Reson Imaging. 1996;6:180–4.
10. Burkart A, Imhoff AB. Diagnostic imaging after autologous chondrocyte transplantation. Correlation of magnetic resonance tomography, histological and arthroscopic findings. Orthopade. 2000;29: 135–44.
11. Trattnig S, Huber M, Breitenseher MJ, Trnka HJ, Rand T, Kaider A, et al. Imaging articular cartilage defects with 3D fat-suppressed echo planar imaging: comparison with conventional 3D fat-suppressed gradient echo sequence and correlation with histology. J Comput Assist Tomogr. 1998;22:8–14.
12. Eckstein F, Sittek H, Milz S, Schulte E, Kiefer B, Reiser M, et al. The potential of magnetic resonance imaging (MRI) for quantifying articular cartilage thickness – a methodological study. Clin Biomech (Bristol, Avon). 1995;10:434–40.
13. Eckstein F, Winzheimer M, Westhoff J, Schnier M, Haubner M, Englmeier KH, et al. Quantitative relationships of normal cartilage volumes of the human knee joint – assessment by magnetic resonance imaging. Anat Embryol (Berl). 1998;197:383–90.
14. Gray ML, Eckstein F, Peterfy C, Dahlberg L, Kim YJ, Sorensen AG. Toward imaging biomarkers for osteoarthritis. Clin Orthop Relat Res. 2004;427:S175–81.
15. Domayer SE, Kutscha-Lissberg F, Welsch G, Dorotka R, Nehrer S, Gabler C, et al. T2 mapping in the knee after microfracture at 3.0 T: correlation of global T2 values and clinical outcome – preliminary results. Osteoarthritis Cartilage. 2008;16:903–8.
16. Welsch GH, Mamisch TC, Domayer SE, Dorotka R, Kutscha-Lissberg F, Marlovits S, et al. Cartilage T2 assessment at 3-T MR imaging: in vivo differentiation of normal hyaline cartilage from reparative tissue after two cartilage repair procedures – initial experience. Radiology. 2008;247:154–61.
17. Eckstein F, Hudelmaier M, Wirth W, Kiefer B, Jackson R, Yu J, et al. Double echo steady state magnetic resonance imaging of knee articular cartilage at 3 Tesla: a pilot study for the Osteoarthritis Initiative. Ann Rheum Dis. 2006;65:433–41.
18. Weckbach S, Mendlik T, Horger W, Wagner S, Reiser MF, Glaser C. Quantitative assessment of patellar cartilage volume and thickness at 3.0 tesla comparing a 3D-fast low angle shot versus a 3D-true fast imaging with steady-state precession sequence for reproducibility. Invest Radiol. 2006;41:189–97.
19. Kornaat PR, Reeder SB, Koo S, Brittain JH, Yu H, Andriacchi TP, et al. MR imaging of articular cartilage at 1.5T and 3.0T: comparison of SPGR and SSFP sequences. Osteoarthritis Cartilage. 2005;13:338–44.
20. Duc SR, Koch P, Schmid MR, Horger W, Hodler J, Pfirrmann CW. Diagnosis of articular cartilage abnormalities of the knee: prospective clinical evaluation of a 3D water-excitation true FISP sequence. Radiology. 2007;243:475–82.
21. Duc SR, Pfirrmann CW, Koch PP, Zanetti M, Hodler J. Internal knee derangement assessed with 3-minute three-dimensional isovoxel true FISP MR sequence: preliminary study. Radiology. 2008;246:526–35.
22. Duc SR, Pfirrmann CW, Schmid MR, Zanetti M, Koch PP, Kalberer F, et al. Articular cartilage defects detected with 3D water-excitation true FISP: prospective comparison with sequences commonly used for knee imaging. Radiology. 2007;245:216–23.
23. Marlovits S, Striessnig G, Resinger CT, et al. Definition of pertinent parameters for the evaluation of articular cartilage repair tissue with high-resolution magnetic resonance imaging. Eur J Radiol. 2004;52:310–19.
24. Roberts SMI, Darby AJ, Menage J, Evans H, Harrison PE, Richardson JB. Autologous chondrocyte implantation for cartilage repair: monitoring its success by magnetic resonance imaging and histology. Arthritis Res Ther. 2003;5:R60–73.
25. Marlovits S, Singer P, Zeller P, Mandl I, Haller J, Trattnig S. Magnetic resonance observation of cartilage repair tissue (MOCART) for the evaluation of autologous chondrocyte transplantation: determination of interobserver variability and correlation to clinical outcome after 2 years. Eur J Radiol. 2006;57: 16–23.
26. Brittberg M, Winalski CS. Evaluation of cartilage injuries and repair. J Bone Joint Surg Am. 2003;85-A(Suppl2):58–69.
27. Welsch GH, Zak L, Resinger C, Mamisch TC, Marlovits S, Trattnig S. Three-dimensional magnetic resonance observation of cartilage repair tissue (3D MOCART) score assessed with an isotropic 3D-True-FISP sequence at 3.0 Tesla. Miami: ICRS; 2009.
28. Ramappa AJ, Gill TJ, Bradford CH, Ho CP, Steadman JR. Magnetic resonance imaging to assess knee cartilage repair tissue after microfracture of chondral defects. J Knee Surg. 2007;20:228–34.
29. Link TM, Sell CA, Masi JN, Zanetti M, Koch PP, Kalberer F, et al. 3.0 vs 1.5 T MRI in the detection of focal cartilage pathology – ROC analysis in an experimental model. Osteoarthritis Cartilage. 2006;14:63–70.
30. Masi JN, Sell CA, Phan C, Han E, Newitt D, Steinbach L, et al. Cartilage MR imaging at 3.0 versus that at 1.5 T: preliminary results in a porcine model. Radiology. 2005;236:140–50.
31. Mithoefer K, Williams 3rd RJ, Warren RF, Potter HG, Spock CR, Jones EC, et al. The microfracture technique for the treatment of articular cartilage lesions in the knee A prospective cohort study. J Bone Joint Surg Am. 2005;87:1911–20.
32. Link TM, Mischung J, Wortler K, Burkart A, Rummeny EJ, Imhoff AB. Normal and pathological MR findings in osteochondral autografts with longitudinal follow-up. Eur Radiol. 2006;16: 88–96.
33. Herber S, Runkel M, Pitton MB, Kalden P, Thelen M, Kreitner KF. Indirect MR-arthrography in the follow up of autologous osteochondral transplantation. Rofo. 2003;175:226–33.
34. Sanders TG, Mentzer KD, Miller MD, Morrison WB, Campbell SE, Penrod BJ. Autogenous osteochondral "plug" transfer for the treatment of focal chondral defects: postoperative MR appearance with clinical correlation. Skeletal Radiol. 2001;30:570–8.
35. Hangody L, Fules P. Autologous osteochondral mosaicplasty for the treatment of full-thickness defects of weight-bearing joints: ten years of experimental and clinical experience. J Bone Joint Surg Am. 2003;85-A Suppl 2:25–32.
36. Henderson EJ, Tuy B, Connell D, Oakes B, Hettwer WH. Prospective clinical study of autologous chondrocyte implantation and correlation with MRI at three and 12 months. J Bone Joint Surg Br. 2003;85:1060–6.
37. Tins BJ, McCall IW, Takahashi T, Cassar-Pullicino V, Roberts S, Ashton B, et al. Autologous chondrocyte implantation in knee joint: MR imaging and histologic features at 1-year follow-up. Radiology. 2005;234:501–8.
38. Trattnig S, Pinker K, Krestan C, Plank C, Millington S, Marlovits S. Matrix-based autologous chondrocyte implantation for cartilage repair with HyalograftC: two-year follow-up by magnetic resonance imaging. Eur J Radiol. 2006;57:9–15.
39. Henderson I, Tuy B, Oakes B. Reoperation after autologous chondrocyte implantation. Indications and findings. J Bone Joint Surg Br. 2004;86:205–11.
40. Bartlett W, Skinner JA, Gooding CR, Carrington RW, Flanagan AM, Briggs TW, et al. Autologous chondrocyte implantation versus matrix-induced autologous chondrocyte implantation for osteochondral defects of the knee: a prospective, randomised study. J Bone Joint Surg Br. 2005;87:640–5.
41. Haddo O, Mahroof S, Higgs D, David L, Pringle J, Bayliss M, et al. The use of chondrogide membrane in autologous chondrocyte implantation. Knee. 2004;11:51–5.

42. Nehrer S, Domayer S, Dorotka R, Schatz K, Bindreiter U, Kotz R. Three-year clinical outcome after chondrocyte transplantation using a hyaluronan matrix for cartilage repair. Eur J Radiol. 2006;57:3–8.
43. Alparslan L, Minas T, Winalski CS. Magnetic resonance imaging of autologous chondrocyte implantation. Semin Ultrasound CT MR. 2001;22:341–51.
44. Alparslan L, Winalski CS, Boutin RD, Minas T. Postoperative magnetic resonance imaging of articular cartilage repair. Semin Musculoskelet Radiol. 2001;5:345–63.
45. Minas T, Chiu R. Autologous chondrocyte implantation. Am J Knee Surg. 2000;13:41–50.
46. Minas T, Peterson L. Advanced techniques in autologous chondrocyte transplantation. Clin Sports Med. 1999;18:13–44. v-vi.
47. Peterson L, Minas T, Brittberg M, Nilsson A, Sjogren-Jansson E, Lindahl A. Two- to 9-year outcome after autologous chondrocyte transplantation of the knee. Clin Orthop Relat Res. 2000;374:212–34.
48. Gold GE, Bergman AG, Pauly JM, Lang P, Butts RK, Beaulieu CF, et al. Magnetic resonance imaging of knee cartilage repair. Top Magn Reson Imaging. 1998;9:377–92.
49. James SL, Connell DA, Saifuddin A, Skinner JA, Briggs TW. MR imaging of autologous chondrocyte implantation of the knee. Eur Radiol. 2006;16:1022–30.
50. Henderson IJ, Tuy B, Connell D, Oakes B, Hettwer WH. Prospective clinical study of autologous chondrocyte implantation and correlation with MRI at three and 12 months. J Bone Joint Surg Br. 2003;85:1060–6.
51. Alparslan L, Winalski CS, Boutin RD, Minas T. Postoperative magnetic resonance imaging of articular cartilage repair. Semin Musculoskelet Radiol. 2001;5:345–63.
52. Brown WE, Potter HG, Marx RG, Wickiewicz TL, Warren RF. Magnetic resonance imaging appearance of cartilage repair in the knee. Clin Orthop Relat Res. 2004;422:214–23.
53. Gold GE, Hargreaves BA, Stevens KJ, Beaulieu CF. Advanced magnetic resonance imaging of articular cartilage. Orthop Clin North Am. 2006;37:331–47. vi.
54. Schweitzer ME, White LM. Does altered biomechanics cause marrow edema? Radiology. 1996;198:851–3.
55. Buckwalter JA, Mankin HJ. Articular cartilage: degeneration and osteoarthritis, repair, regeneration, and transplantation. Instr Course Lect. 1998;47:487–504.
56. Poole AR, Kojima T, Yasuda T, Mwale F, Kobayashi M, Laverty S. Composition and structure of articular cartilage: a template for tissue repair. Clin Orthop Relat Res. 2001;391:S26–33.
57. Goodwin DW, Zhu H, Dunn JF. In vitro MR imaging of hyaline cartilage: correlation with scanning electron microscopy. AJR Am J Roentgenol. 2000;174:405–9.
58. Potter HG, Black BR, le Chong R. New techniques in articular cartilage imaging. Clin Sports Med. 2009;28:77–94.
59. Potter HG, le Chong R, Sneag DB. Magnetic resonance imaging of cartilage repair. Sports Med Arthrosc. 2008;16:236–45.
60. Trattnig S, Mamisch TC, Pinker K, Domayer S, Szomolanyi P, Marlovits S, et al. Differentiating normal hyaline cartilage from post-surgical repair tissue using fast gradient echo imaging in delayed gadolinium-enhanced MRI (dGEMRIC) at 3 Tesla. Eur Radiol. 2008;18:1251–9.
61. Trattnig S, Marlovits S, Gebetsroither S, Szomolanyi P, Welsch GH, Salomonowitz E, et al. Three-dimensional delayed gadolinium-enhanced MRI of cartilage (dGEMRIC) for in vivo evaluation of reparative cartilage after matrix-associated autologous chondrocyte transplantation at 3.0T: Preliminary results. J Magn Reson Imaging. 2007;26:974–82.
62. Watanabe A, Wada Y, Obata T, Ueda T, Tamura M, Ikehira H, et al. Delayed gadolinium-enhanced MR to determine glycosaminoglycan concentration in reparative cartilage after autologous chondrocyte implantation: preliminary results. Radiology. 2006;239:201–8.
63. Watrin-Pinzano A, Ruaud JP, Cheli Y, Gonord P, Grossin L, Bettembourg-Brault I, et al. Evaluation of cartilage repair tissue after biomaterial implantation in rat patella by using T2 mapping. MAGMA. 2004;17:219–28.
64. Welsch GH, Mamisch TC, Marlovits S, Glaser C, Friedrich K, Hennig FF, et al. Quantitative T2 mapping during follow-up after matrix-associated autologous chondrocyte transplantation (MACT): full-thickness and zonal evaluation to visualize the maturation of cartilage repair tissue. J Orthop Res. 2009;27:957–63.
65. Welsch GH, Trattnig S, Scheffler K, Szomonanyi P, Quirbach S, Marlovits S, et al. Magnetization transfer contrast and T2 mapping in the evaluation of cartilage repair tissue with 3T MRI. J Magn Reson Imaging. 2008;28:979–86.
66. Bachmann G, Basad E, Lommel D, Steinmeyer J. MRI in the follow-up of matrix-supported autologous chondrocyte transplantation (MACI) and microfracture. Radiologe. 2004;44:773–82.
67. Bentley G, Biant LC, Carrington RW, Akmal M, Goldberg A, Williams AM, et al. A prospective, randomised comparison of autologous chondrocyte implantation versus mosaicplasty for osteochondral defects in the knee. J Bone Joint Surg Br. 2003;85:223–30.
68. Brittberg M, Lindahl A, Nilsson A, Ohlsson C, Isaksson O, Peterson L. Treatment of deep cartilage defects in the knee with autologous chondrocyte transplantation. N Engl J Med. 1994;331:889–95.
69. Gudas R, Kalesinskas RJ, Kimtys V, Stankevicius E, Toliusis V, Bernotavicius G, et al. A prospective randomized clinical study of mosaic osteochondral autologous transplantation versus microfracture for the treatment of osteochondral defects in the knee joint in young athletes. Arthroscopy. 2005;21:1066–75.
70. Gudas R, Stankevicius E, Monastyreckiene E, Pranys D, Kalesinskas RJ. Osteochondral autologous transplantation versus microfracture for the treatment of articular cartilage defects in the knee joint in athletes. Knee Surg Sports Traumatol Arthrosc. 2006;14:834–42.
71. Knutsen G, Drogset JO, Engebretsen L, Grontvedt T, Isaksen V, Ludvigsen TC, et al. A randomized trial comparing autologous chondrocyte implantation with microfracture Findings at five years. J Bone Joint Surg Am. 2007;89:2105–12.
72. Knutsen G, Engebretsen L, Ludvigsen TC, Drogset JO, Grontvedt T, Solheim E, et al. Autologous chondrocyte implantation compared with microfracture in the knee. A randomized trial. J Bone Joint Surg Am. 2004;86-A:455–64.
73. Burstein D, Velyvis J, Scott KT, Stock KW, Kim YJ, Jaramillo D, et al. Protocol issues for delayed Gd(DTPA)(2-)-enhanced MRI: (dGEMRIC) for clinical evaluation of articular cartilage. Magn Reson Med. 2001;45:36–41.
74. Bashir A, Gray ML, Burstein D. Gd-DTPA2- as a measure of cartilage degradation. Magn Reson Med. 1996;36:665–73.
75. Borthakur A, Shapiro EM, Beers J, Kudchodkar S, Kneeland JB, Reddy R. Sensitivity of MRI to proteoglycan depletion in cartilage: comparison of sodium and proton MRI. Osteoarthritis Cartilage. 2000;8:288–93.
76. Ling W, Regatte RR, Navon G, Jerschow A. Assessment of glycosaminoglycan concentration in vivo by chemical exchange-dependent saturation transfer (gagCEST). Proc Natl Acad Sci USA. 2008;105:2266–70.
77. Burstein D, Bashir A, Gray ML. MRI techniques in early stages of cartilage disease. Invest Radiol. 2000;35:622–38.
78. Bashir A, Gray ML, Boutin RD, Burstein D. Glycosaminoglycan in articular cartilage: in vivo assessment with delayed Gd(DTPA)(2-)-enhanced MR imaging. Radiology. 1997;205:551–8.
79. Tiderius CJ, Olsson LE, Leander P, Ekberg O, Dahlberg L. Delayed gadolinium-enhanced MRI of cartilage (dGEMRIC) in early knee osteoarthritis. Magn Reson Med. 2003;49:488–92.

80. Williams A, Gillis A, McKenzie C, Po B, Sharma L, Micheli L, et al. Glycosaminoglycan distribution in cartilage as determined by delayed gadolinium-enhanced MRI of cartilage (dGEMRIC): potential clinical applications. Am J Roentgenol. 2004;182: 167–72.
81. Kim YJ, Jaramillo D, Millis MB, Gray ML, Burstein D. Assessment of early osteoarthritis in hip dysplasia with delayed gadolinium-enhanced magnetic resonance imaging of cartilage. J Bone Joint Surg Am. 2003;85A:1987–92.
82. Vaga S, Raimondi MT, Caiani EG, Costa F, Giordano C, Perona F, et al. Quantitative assessment of intervertebral disc glycosaminoglycan distribution by gadolinium-enhanced MRI in orthopedic patients. Magn Reson Med. 2008;59:85–95.
83. Williams A, Shetty SK, Burstein D, Day CS, McKenzie C. Delayed gadolinium enhanced MRI of cartilage (dGEMRIC) of the first carpometacarpal (1CMC) joint: a feasibility study. Osteoarthritis Cartilage. 2008;16(4):530–2.
84. Reddy R, Li S, Noyszewski EA, Kneeland JB, Leigh JS. In vivo sodium multiple quantum spectroscopy of human articular cartilage. Magn Reson Med. 1997;38:207–14.
85. Reddy R, Shinnar M, Wang Z, Leigh JS. Multiple-quantum filters of spin-3/2 with pulses of arbitrary flip angle. J Magn Reson B. 1994;104:148–52.
86. Ling W, Regatte RR, Schweitzer ME, Jerschow A. Behavior of ordered sodium in enzymatically depleted cartilage tissue. Magn Reson Med. 2006;56:1151–5.
87. Navon G, Werrmann JG, Maron R, Cohen SM. 31P NMR and triple quantum filtered 23Na NMR studies of the effects of inhibition of Na+/H+exchange on intracellular sodium and pH in working and ischemic hearts. Magn Reson Med. 1994;32:556–64.
88. Borthakur A, Mellon E, Niyogi S, Witschey W, Kneeland JB, Reddy R. Sodium and T1rho MRI for molecular and diagnostic imaging of articular cartilage. NMR Biomed. 2006;19:781–821.
89. Shapiro EM, Borthakur A, Dandora R, Kriss A, Leigh JS, Reddy R. Sodium visibility and quantitation in intact bovine articular cartilage using high field (23)Na MRI and MRS. J Magn Reson. 2000;142:24–31.
90. Wheaton AJ, Casey FL, Gougoutas AJ, Dodge GR, Borthakur A, Lonner JH, et al. Correlation of T1rho with fixed charge density in cartilage. J Magn Reson Imaging. 2004;20:519–25.
91. Guivel-Scharen V, Sinnwell T, Wolff SD, Balaban RS. Detection of proton chemical exchange between metabolites and water in biological tissues. J Magn Reson. 1998;133:36–45.
92. Ward KM, Aletras AH, Balaban RS. A new class of contrast agents for MRI based on proton chemical exchange dependent saturation transfer (CEST). J Magn Reson. 2000;143:79–87.
93. Ward KM, Balaban RS. Determination of pH using water protons and chemical exchange dependent saturation transfer (CEST). Magn Reson Med. 2000;44:799–802.
94. Mosher TJ, Dardzinski BJ. Cartilage MRI T2 relaxation time mapping: overview and applications. Semin Musculoskelet Radiol. 2004;8:355–68.
95. Welsch GH, Mamisch TC, Hughes T, Zilkens C, Quirbach S, Scheffler K, et al. In vivo biochemical 7.0 Tesla magnetic resonance: preliminary results of dGEMRIC, zonal T2, and T2* mapping of articular cartilage. Invest Radiol. 2008;43:619–26.
96. Goodwin DW, Wadghiri YZ, Dunn JF. Micro-imaging of articular cartilage: T2, proton density, and the magic angle effect. Acad Radiol. 1998;5:790–8.
97. Smith HE, Mosher TJ, Dardzinski BJ, Collins BG, Collins CM, Yang QX, et al. Spatial variation in cartilage T2 of the knee. J Magn Reson Imaging. 2001;14:50–5.
98. White LM, Sussman MS, Hurtig M, Probyn L, Tomlinson G, Kandel R. Cartilage T2 assessment: differentiation of normal hyaline cartilage and reparative tissue after arthroscopic cartilage repair in equine subjects. Radiology. 2006;241:407–14.
99. Trattnig S, Mamisch TC, Welsch GH, Glaser C, Szomolanyi P, Gebetsroither S, et al. Quantitative T2 mapping of matrix-associated autologous chondrocyte transplantation at 3 Tesla: an in vivo cross-sectional study. Invest Radiol. 2007;42:442–8.
100. David-Vaudey E, Ghosh S, Ries M, Majumdar S. T2 relaxation time measurements in osteoarthritis. Magn Reson Imaging. 2004;22:673–82.
101. Dunn TC, Lu Y, Jin H, Ries MD, Majumdar S. T2 relaxation time of cartilage at MR imaging: comparison with severity of knee osteoarthritis. Radiology. 2004;232:592–8.
102. Burstein D, Gray ML. Is MRI fulfilling its promise for molecular imaging of cartilage in arthritis? Osteoarthritis Cartilage. 2006;14:1087–90.
103. Murphy BJ. Evaluation of grades 3 and 4 chondromalacia of the knee using T2*-weighted 3D gradient-echo articular cartilage imaging. Skeletal Radiol. 2001;30:305–11.
104. Hughes T, Welsch GH, Trattnig S, Brandi L, Domayer S, Mamisch TC. T2-star relaxation as a means to diffrentiatie cartilage repair tissue after microfracturing therapy. Intern Soc Magn Reson Med. 2007;15:183.
105. Wietek B, Martirosian P, Machann J, Mueller-Horvath C, Claussen CD, Schick F. T2 and T2* mapping of the human femoral-tibial cartilage at 1.5 and 3 tesla. Intern Soc Magn Reson Med. 2007;15:516.
106. Eckstein F, Kunz M, Schutzer M, Hudelmaier M, Jackson RD, Yu J, et al. Two year longitudinal change and test–retest-precision of knee cartilage morphology in a pilot study for the osteoarthritis initiative. Osteoarthritis Cartilage. 2007;15:1326–32.
107. Bruder H, Fischer H, Graumann R, Deimling M. A new steady-state imaging sequence for simultaneous acquisition of two MR images with clearly different contrasts. Magn Reson Med. 1988;7:35–42.
108. Wolff SD, Chesnick S, Frank JA, Lim KO, Balaban RS. Magnetization transfer contrast: MR imaging of the knee. Radiology. 1991;179:623–8.
109. Gray ML, Burstein D, Lesperance LM, Gehrke L. Magnetization transfer in cartilage and its constituent macromolecules. Magn Reson Med. 1995;34:319–25.
110. Kim DK, Ceckler TL, Hascall VC, Calabro A, Balaban RS. Analysis of water-macromolecule proton magnetization transfer in articular cartilage. Magn Reson Med. 1993;29:211–15.
111. Seo GS, Aoki J, Moriya H, Karakida O, Sone S, Hidaka H, et al. Hyaline cartilage: in vivo and in vitro assessment with magnetization transfer imaging. Radiology. 1996;201:525–30.
112. Wolff SD, Balaban RS. Magnetization transfer contrast (MTC) and tissue water proton relaxation in vivo. Magn Reson Med. 1989;10:135–44.
113. Wolff SD, Eng J, Balaban RS. Magnetization transfer contrast: method for improving contrast in gradient-recalled-echo images. Radiology. 1991;179:133–7.
114. Palmieri F, De Keyzer F, Maes F, Van Breuseghem I. Magnetization transfer analysis of cartilage repair tissue: a preliminary study. Skeletal Radiol. 2006;35:903–8.
115. Bieri O, Scheffler K. Optimized balanced steady-state free precession magnetization transfer imaging. Magn Reson Med. 2007;58:511–18.
116. Potter K, Butler JJ, Horton WE, Spencer RG. Response of engineered cartilage tissue to biochemical agents as studied by proton magnetic resonance microscopy. Arthritis Rheum. 2000;43:1580–90.
117. Vahlensieck M, Dombrowski F, Leutner C, Wagner U, Reiser M. Magnetization transfer contrast (MTC) and MTC-subtraction: enhancement of cartilage lesions and intracartilaginous degeneration in vitro. Skeletal Radiol. 1994;23:535–9.
118. Miller KL, Hargreaves BA, Gold GE, Pauly JM. Steady-state diffusion-weighted imaging of in vivo knee cartilage. Magn Reson Med. 2004;51:394–8.
119. Mlynarik V, Szomolanyi P, Toffanin R, Vittur F, Trattnig S. Transverse relaxation mechanisms in articular cartilage. J Magn Reson. 2004;169:300–7.

120. Glaser C. New techniques for cartilage imaging: T2 relaxation time and diffusion-weighted MR imaging. Radiol Clin North Am. 2005;43:641–53. vii.
121. Deoni SC, Peters TM, Rutt BK. Quantitative diffusion imaging with steady-state free precession. Magn Reson Med. 2004;51:428–33.
122. Friedrich KM, Mamisch TC, Plank C, Langs G, Marlovits S, Salomonowitz E, et al. Diffusion-weighted imaging for the follow-up of patients after matrix-associated autologous chondrocyte transplantation. Eur J Radiol. 2010;73(3):622–8. Epub 2009 Jan 31.
123. Mamisch TC, Menzel MI, Welsch GH, Bittersohl B, Salomonowitz E, Szomolanyi P, et al. Steady-state diffusion imaging for MR in-vivo evaluation of reparative cartilage after matrix-associated autologous chondrocyte transplantation at 3 tesla-Preliminary results. Eur J Radiol. 2008;65:72–9.
124. Regatte RR, Akella SV, Lonner JH, Kneeland JB, Reddy R. T1rho relaxation mapping in human osteoarthritis (OA) cartilage: comparison of T1rho with T2. J Magn Reson Imaging. 2006;23:547–53.
125. Regatte RR, Akella SV, Wheaton AJ, Borthakur A, Kneeland JB, Reddy R. T 1 rho-relaxation mapping of human femoral-tibial cartilage in vivo. J Magn Reson Imaging. 2003;18:336–41.
126. Menezes NM, Gray ML, Hartke JR, Burstein D. T2 and T1rho MRI in articular cartilage systems. Magn Reson Med. 2004;51:503–9.
127. Pinker K, Szomolanyi P, Welsch GC, Mamisch TC, Marlovits S, Stadlbauer A, et al. Longitudinal evaluation of cartilage composition of matrix-associated autologous chondrocyte transplants with 3-T delayed gadolinium-enhanced MRI of cartilage. AJR Am J Roentgenol. 2008;191:1391–6.
128. Maroudas A, Bayliss MT, Venn MF. Further studies on the composition of human femoral head cartilage. Ann Rheum Dis. 1980;39:514–23.
129. Steadman JR, Rodkey WG, Rodrigo JJ. Microfracture: surgical technique and rehabilitation to treat chondral defects. Clin Orthop Relat Res. 2001;391:S362–9.
130. Marlovits S, Zeller P, Singer P, Resinger C, Vecsei V. Cartilage repair: generations of autologous chondrocyte transplantation. Eur J Radiol. 2006;57:24–31.
131. Hettrich CM, Crawford D, Rodeo SA. Cartilage repair: third-generation cell-based technologies–basic science, surgical techniques, clinical outcomes. Sports Med Arthrosc. 2008;16:230–5.
132. Kon E, Delcogliano M, Filardo G, Montaperto C, Marcacci M. Second generation issues in cartilage repair. Sports Med Arthrosc. 2008;16:221–9.
133. McNickle AG, Provencher MT, Cole BJ. Overview of existing cartilage repair technology. Sports Med Arthrosc. 2008;16:196–201.
134. Julkunen P, Kiviranta P, Wilson W, Jurvelin JS, Korhonen RK. Characterization of articular cartilage by combining microscopic analysis with a fibril-reinforced finite-element model. J Biomech. 2007;40:1862–70.
135. Korhonen RK, Laasanen MS, Toyras J, Lappalainen R, Helminen HJ, Jurvelin JS. Fibril reinforced poroelastic model predicts specifically mechanical behavior of normal, proteoglycan depleted and collagen degraded articular cartilage. J Biomech. 2003;36:1373–9.
136. Hasler EM, Herzog W, Wu JZ, Muller W, Wyss U. Articular cartilage biomechanics: theoretical models, material properties, and biosynthetic response. Crit Rev Biomed Eng. 1999;27:415–88.
137. Briant P, Bevill S, Andriacchi TP. Quantifying variations in collagen matrix deformation in loaded articular cartilage. Proceeding of the ASME Summer Bioengineering Conference, Keystone, CO. 2007;47:931–2.
138. Laasanen MS, Toyras J, Korhonen RK, Rieppo J, Saarakkala S, Nieminen MT, et al. Biomechanical properties of knee articular cartilage. Biorheology. 2003;40:133–40.
139. Appleyard RC, Burkhardt D, Ghosh P, Read R, Cake M, Swain MV, et al. Topographical analysis of the structural, biochemical and dynamic biomechanical properties of cartilage in an ovine model of osteoarthritis. Osteoarthritis Cartilage. 2003;11:65–77.
140. Arokoski JPA, Hyttinen MM, Helminen HJ, Jurvelin JS. Biomechanical and structural characteristics of canine femoral and tibial cartilage. J Biomed Mater Res. 1999;48:99–107.
141. Sokoloff L. Biology of degenerative joint disease. Perspect Biol Med. 1963;7:94–106.
142. Maroudas A. Physicochemical properties of cartilage in light of ion exchange theory. Biophys J. 1968;8:575–95.
143. Akizuki S, Mow VC, Muller F, Pita JC, Howell DS, Manicourt DH. Tensile properties of human knee-joint cartilage. 1. Influence of ionic conditions, weight bearing, and fibrillation on the tensile modulus. J Orthop Res. 1986;4:379–92.
144. Kempson GE, Muir H, Pollard C, Tuke M. Tensile properties of cartilage of human femoral condyles related to content of collagen and glycosaminoglycans. Biochim Biophys Acta. 1973;297:456–72.
145. Kempson GE, Freeman MAR, Swanson SAV. Tensile properties of articular cartilage. Nature. 1968;220:1127–8.
146. Hayes WC, Mockros LF. Viscoelastic properties of human articular cartilage. J Appl Physiol. 1971;31:562–8.
147. Kempson GE, Swanson SAV, Spivey CJ, Freeman MAR. Patterns of cartilage stiffness on normal and degenerate human femoral heads. J Biomech. 1971;4:597–609.
148. Kurkijarvi JE, Nissi MJ, Kiviranta I, Jurvelin JS, Nieminen MT. Delayed gadolinium-enhanced MRI of cartilage (dGEMRIC) and T-2 characteristics of human knee articular cartilage: topographical variation and relationships to mechanical properties. Magn Reson Med. 2004;52:41–6.
149. Samosky JT, Burstein D, Grimson WE, Howe R, Martin S, Gray ML. Spatially-localized correlation of dGEMRIC-measured GAG distribution and mechanical stiffness in the human tibial plateau. J Orthop Res. 2005;23:93–101.
150. Nieminen MT, Toyras J, Laasanen MS, Silvennoinen J, Helminen HJ, Jurvelin JS. Prediction of biomechanical properties of articular cartilage with quantitative magnetic resonance imaging. J Biomech. 2004;37:321–8.
151. Nissi MJ, Toyras J, Laasanen MS, Rieppo J, Saarakkala S, Lappalainen R, et al. Proteoglycan and collagen sensitive MRI evaluation of normal and degenerated articular cartilage. J Orthop Res. 2004;22:557–64.
152. Nieminen MT, Rieppo J, Silvennoinen J, Toyras J, Hakumaki JM, Hyttinen MM, et al. Spatial assessment of articular cartilage proteoglycans with Gd-DTPA-Enhanced T1 imaging. Magn Reson Med. 2002;48:640–8.
153. Juras V, Bittsansky M, Majdisova Z, Szomolanyi P, Sulzbacher I, Gabler S, et al. In vitro determination of biomechanical properties of human articular cartilage in osteoarthritis using multi-parametric MRI. J Magn Reson. 2009;197:40–7.
154. Wayne JS, Kraft KA, Shields KJ, Yin C, Owen JR, Disler DG. MR imaging of normal and matrix-depleted cartilage: correlation with biomechanical function and biochemical composition. Radiology. 2003;228:493–9.
155. Zhu WB, Mow VC, Koob TJ, Eyre DR. Viscoelastic shear properties of articular-cartilage and the effects of glycosidase treatments. J Orthop Res. 1993;11:771–81.
156. Nieminen MT, Toyras J, Rieppo J, Hakumaki JM, Silvennoinen J, Helminen HJ, et al. Quantitative MR microscopy of enzymatically degraded articular cartilage. Magn Reson Med. 2000;43:676–81.
157. Eckstein F, Tieschky M, Faber SC, Haubner M, Kolem H, Englmeier KH, et al. Effect of physical exercise on cartilage volume and thickness in vivo: MR imaging study. Radiology. 1998;207:243–8.
158. Mosher TJ, Smith HE, Collins C, Liu Y, Hancy J, Dardzinski BJ, et al. Change in knee cartilage T2 at MR imaging after running: a feasibility study. Radiology. 2005;234:245–9.
159. Juras V, Welsch GH, Millington S, Szomolanyi P, Mamisch TC, Pinker K, et al. Kinematic biomechanical assessment of human articular cartilage transplants in the knee using 3-T MRI: an in vivo reproducibility study. Eur Radiol. 2009;19(5):1246–52.

Chapter 16
Cartilage as a Biomarker

Thomas M. Link

Keywords Biomarker • Cartilage • Cartilage volume measurements • dGEMRIC • Imaging • Joint space width (JSW) • MRI gradings • Radiographs

Introduction

Traditionally biomarkers have been defined as biochemical substances that in addition to disease diagnosis allow classification of disease severity, risk of onset and progression, as well as assessment of the efficacy of a treatment [1]. The meaning of the generic term biomarkers, however, has been greatly expanded and applied to all detection methods used in the life sciences and may be defined as any detectable biologic parameter, whether biochemical, genetic, histologic, anatomic, physical, functional, or metabolic [2]. Development of biomarkers has been a major focus of the National Institutes of Health (NIH), in particular during the American Recovery and Reinvestment Act of 2009, and biomarkers were defined as measurements that define early biochemical and structural changes of a disease process such as osteoarthritis that may be applied as markers during longitudinal studies and provide information on disease progression. Eventually, these could be used for both preventive intervention and as preliminary indications for pathways of disease pathogenesis to guide therapeutic development (J. McGowan in http://orwh.od.nih.gov/recovery/). According to the US Food and Drug Administration (FDA), biomarkers ideally would serve as surrogate markers synonymous with primary outcome measures in definitive effectiveness trials of new therapeutic agents [3].

Imaging biomarkers have been defined as any anatomic, physiologic, biochemical, or molecular parameter detectable with one or more imaging methods used to help establish the presence and/or severity of disease [2]. Clearly, semiquantitative or quantitative measures obtained through cartilage imaging can serve as biomarkers, in particular to characterize osteoarthritis. The goal of this chapter is to discuss imaging techniques that can or have the potential to provide imaging-derived measures of cartilage in particular with respect to defining and grading osteoarthritis as well as quantifying the risk of progression and the effect of therapeutic intervention. The classification of the different roles of imaging biomarkers is based on a previous article published by the Osteoarthritis Biomarkers Network, which is a consortium of five sites, funded by the National Institutes of Health/ National Institute of Arthritis, Musculoskeletal, and Skin Disease (NIH/NIAMS) to develop and characterize new biomarkers and refine existing OA biomarkers [1]. According to this publication, a biomarker classification scheme is proposed that includes five categories: diagnostic, burden of disease, prognostic, efficacy of intervention, and investigative [1]. In this chapter, we first define the different biomarkers and then outline basic requirements for imaging biomarkers. We finally apply the proposed biomarker classification system [1] to the individual imaging-based cartilage biomarkers.

Imaging-Based Cartilage Biomarkers

For many years, *semiquantitative grading of radiographs* has been used as a standard imaging biomarker. The Kellgren–Lawrence scale has been first described in 1957 [4] and has been established as a standard of reference for OA. In fact, the World Health Organization (WHO) adopted these criteria for the radiological classification of OA as the standard for epidemiological studies and an atlas was published in 1963 [5]. Also, joint space width (JSW) derived from radiographs has served as an imaging biomarker [6], it should be noted, however, that JSW is affected by both menisci and cartilage and is therefore a very limited cartilage imaging biomarker.

Given the inherent limitations of radiographs, however, MRI-derived measures have been increasingly used as

T.M. Link (✉)
Department of Radiology and Biomedical Imaging, University of California at San Francisco, 400 Parnassus Ave, A-367, San Francisco, CA 94131, USA
e-mail: Thomas.Link@radiology.ucsf.edu

T.M. Link (ed.), *Cartilage Imaging: Significance, Techniques, and New Developments*,
DOI 10.1007/978-1-4419-8438-8_16, © Springer Science+Business Media, LLC 2011

biomarkers for OA and cartilage. *Semiquantitative MRI gradings* are based on standard MR imaging sequences and include the WORMS [7], BLOKS [8], and KOSS [9] classifications; of these, currently the WORMS classification is most frequently used. These scores are whole organ classifications and include evaluation of cartilage, menisci, bone marrow, synovitis, joint effusion, osteophytes, and ligaments. Semiquantitative markers focusing only on cartilage, based on the arthroscopic Outerbridge and Noyes and Stabler classifications [10, 11] have also been used. In addition, a quantitative cartilage lesion marker (UCSF score) has been described to better assess early cartilage lesions [12].

Since cartilage is of major significance for the evaluation of OA *MR-derived cartilage volume measurements* have been developed as biomarkers, with the goal to provide outcome measurements, which could be used to assess therapy effects of disease-modifying drugs faster than standard radiographic measurements. Though development of effective OA drugs has not been as successful as initially anticipated, fairly standardized volumetric measurements are currently in place [13]. The newest set of biomarkers focus on the *biochemical composition of the cartilage*, with the most frequently used techniques being T1rho, T2 relaxation time measurements and dGEMRIC (delayed gadolinium-enhanced MR of cartilage). Though these biomarkers hold significant promise in diagnosing cartilage degeneration at the earliest stages, before actual cartilage loss occurs, they are not well standardized and more work is required to establish these measurements in a clinical setting. It has been hypothesized that anatomic MRI of cartilage providing information on volume and morphological defects will not provide sufficient assessment of the anabolic and catabolic activities of joint structures and that MR-based measurements of biochemical cartilage composition will eventually be more helpful as biomarkers [14].

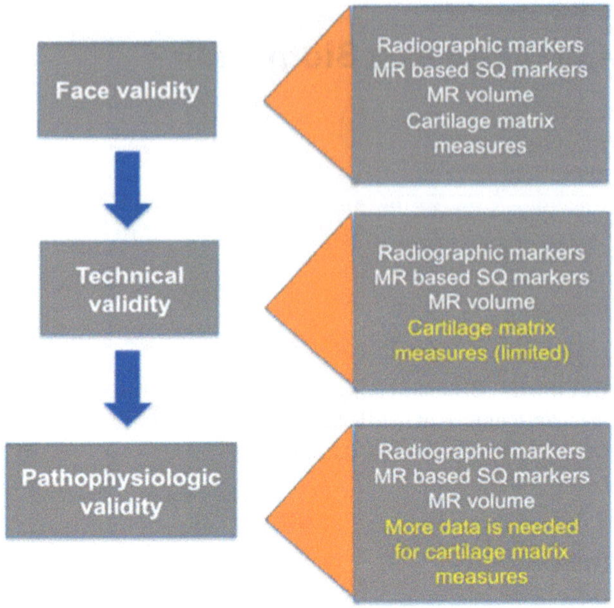

Fig. 16.1 Imaging biomarkers in relation to face validity, technical validity, and pathophysiologic validity. While face validity and technical validity have been established for most of the listed biomarkers, pathophysiologic validity is under investigation in particular for cartilage matrix biomarkers; more longitudinal studies are required to better understand the role of cartilage matrix biomarkers. *SQ* semiquantitative

Requirements for Imaging Biomarkers: Validity and Reliability

Before new parameters are defined as biomarkers, they need to be rigorously tested both in terms of validity and reliability. Validity includes face, technical and pathophysiologic validity [15] (Fig. 16.1). Face validity is the first step in the process of developing a biomarker; common sense rules are applied to test that it actually measures what it is intended to measure. For example, if cartilage and glycosaminoglycans are important entities for joint biomechanics and deteriorate during OA, parameters measuring these two entities would be considered as valuable to assess OA. If face validity is given, technical validity is the next step in establishing a biomarker; this requires demonstration that the measurement is accurate ("true") and precise ("repeatable") [15]. A large number of previous studies using animal models, histology, and arthroscopy as a standard of reference have shown that semiquantitative cartilage scores are accurate with reported sensitivities and specificities of around 70–90% [16–22]. Also, studies have been performed validating MR-based measures of cartilage volume [23, 24]. However, validation of cartilage matrix measurements has limitations and neither dGEMRIC nor T1rho nor T2 have provided full evidence, that what they are exactly measuring what they are assumed to measure, that is, glycosaminoglycans, water content, and collagen integrity [15]. Previous validation studies were mostly performed in cartilage specimens and showed variable correlations with a variety of standards of reference [25–28]. Precision with respect to reproducibility of the previously listed biomarkers has been analyzed extensively and was found to be satisfactory to excellent for semiquantitative cartilage gradings, volume and cartilage matrix measurements. After establishing face and technical validity, the ultimate utility is to establish pathophysiologic validity [15]. This requires large clinical cross-sectional and longitudinal studies validating the biomarkers in their potential to determine the risk for OA or to monitor the disease process. With the extensive imaging data available from Osteoarthritis Initiative and other trials, investigations on these issues are emerging and will provide information on disease etiology and the relationship of the biomarkers with clinical outcomes [15].

Proposed Biomarker Classification System for OA According to Bauer et al.

Role of Cartilage Imaging Biomarkers in Diagnosing OA

Diagnostic markers need to be able to classify individuals as diseased or non-diseased (Table 16.1) [1]. The current, accepted gold standard for diagnosing OA has been the Kellgren–Lawrence (K-L) score [4] with a K-L score of ≥2 being defined as diseased. While a number of previous studies using semiquantitative and quantitative MR-based measurements have been able to differentiate individuals with and without OA with good results [29–32], it is not entirely clear which threshold or cutoff level should be used to define OA. MR Studies using semiquantitative grading to differentiate normals and OA subjects frequently have used a grade 1 (cartilage inhomogeneity and swelling in WORMS and in the modified Noyes and Stabler classification) and higher to identify cartilage degeneration and early OA [33, 34]; it should be noted, however, that cartilage inhomogeneity and swelling have limited validity as shown by a previous study which compared MR findings with histological findings [21]. Alternatively, a threshold of >1 could be used to differentiate individuals with and without degenerative disease or osteoarthritis, yet given the number of normal healthy individuals without pain, who have >grade 1 lesions, this threshold would be very (probably overly) sensitive in identifying diseased subjects. Previous studies have identified cartilage and meniscal lesions in a high percentage (45–54%) of individuals without signs or symptoms of OA [12, 33–35].

Issues are even more complex for quantitative measures, which are currently mostly research tools and would need a substantial amount of standardization and validation before they can be used. Clearly, currently there is no "numerical value," be it an absolute value or T-score, in place, which would allow differentiation of healthy and diseased patients. Ideally, cartilage matrix measurements derived from T1rho, T2 relaxation time, or dGEMRIC techniques would provide values, T- or Z-scores, that would allow disease classification such as dual energy X-ray absorptiometry (DXA) measurements allow it for osteoporosis [36].

Classification of Disease Burden with Cartilage Imaging Biomarkers

While current imaging biomarkers, except for radiographs, are limited in differentiating diseased and non-diseased individuals, they have been found to be very useful in classifying disease burden in a number of studies [12, 31, 33, 34, 37]. Cross-sectional studies have been performed [29, 31, 38] correlating the current standard of reference, radiographic KL-scores, with MR-based imaging markers and it has been demonstrated that MR findings well correspond with the individual KL-scores. However, it should be noted that given its unique visualization of cartilage and other joint tissues, MRI is far superior to radiography in characterizing disease burden, which in turn questions the role of the current standard of reference.

Also, it should be noted that while several semiquantitative scores are available (WORMS, BLOKS, KOSS), it is not well standardized which score or subcomponent of a score should be used in defining the overall disease burden. In previous studies, both maximum scores and summary scores have been used [29, 31, 33, 34], but the number of studies performed in this field is still limited and overall standardization would be required to better compare results from different studies or have a unique measurement for disease burden. The same applies for cartilage volume and biochemical matrix measurements; global joint measurements may be less sensitive than those obtained in compartments and joint areas which are more prone to disease (such as the medial compartment of the knee).

Table 16.1 Role of imaging as biomarkers for OA, classification of biomarkers according to Osteoarthritis Biomarkers Network as published by Bauer et al. [1]

Biomarker	Radiographs	Semiquantitative techniques	Quantitative assessment
Diagnostic marker	KL-score	Cartilage (WORMS) grade >1? Not defined	Not defined
Burden of disease	KL-score, JSW	WORMS, BLOKS, KOSS	Cartilage volume T1rho, T2, dGEMRIC
Prognostic marker	JSW	Limited information	T2? Volume-based measurements?
Efficacy of intervention	KL-score, JSW	Limited information	Cartilage volume dGEMRIC?

To date most information is available on burden of disease biomarkers, while studies on prognostic markers are emerging (OAI, MOST). Data on efficacy of intervention are limited, *JSW* joint space width

Imaging Biomarkers and Their Role in Assessing the Prognosis of OA

Ideally an imaging biomarker should clearly define the risk and prognosis of a certain measurement or finding to develop a disease such as OA or to characterize the risk for progression of disease. However, since OA and cartilage degeneration are slowly progressing, this requires long-term longitudinal studies over many years, which allow characterization of the disease course in relationship to baseline findings. Currently, information in this field is limited and large multicenter trials such as the OAI are required to better characterize the role of MR-based imaging biomarkers in this field. Also, there are a wide variety of outcome measures or findings, which have been used as surrogates for OA progression, including joint replacement, pain (determined using questionnaires), change in KL-scores, cartilage volume loss, or cartilage structural changes. There is overlap between biomarkers used to assess progression and risk and outcome measures defining disease progression, which makes understanding this field quite complex. Also parameters may be used as outcome markers, which are not suitable such as bone marrow edema pattern respectively bone marrow lesions. The latter findings suggest bone remodeling or necrosis and may increase or decrease with the progression of OA.

The analytic approach to a prognostic marker is different from a disease burden marker, as they intend to measure the risk of future conditions. For dichotomous or categorical outcomes (e.g., joint replacement, change in KL-score), analyses are performed using relative risk (RR) or odds ratios (OR), while for continuous outcome markers the RR or OR per SD increase or decrease in the marker or the area under curve from Receiver Operator Characteristics (ROC) analysis are accepted biostatistical approaches [1].

Previous studies have been performed that analyzed imaging biomarkers with different outcome measures as a standard of reference. In a meta-analysis, Emarani et al. investigated joint space narrowing as a biomarker with change in KL-grade serving as a standard of reference [39]. These investigators found that the overall mean risk of K-L progression was associated with increased joint space narrowing and risk of progression was related with shorter study duration, OA definition (K-L > or = 2 versus K-L > or = 1) and cohorts composed of subjects with both incident and prevalent OA [39]. Felson et al. found that increasing bone marrow edema pattern (biomarker) was associated with development of knee pain (outcome) [40] and Dam et al. used progressive radiographic joint space narrowing as a reference (outcome) and found cartilage-based texture measures (biomarker) to be associated with progressive disease [41]. Currently, limited information on cartilage matrix measurements in predicting progression of disease are available; initial studies suggested that baseline cartilage T2 measurements (biomarker) are associated with progressive loss of physical activity (measured with the physical activity scale for the elderly) [42] and progression of pain scores (measured with WOMAC) [43].

It should be noted that while in OA we are currently just beginning to understand the role of radiological cartilage markers for risk of disease progression and defining clinical outcomes versus biomarkers, in osteoporosis issues are better standardized. The standard outcome variable in osteoporosis is occurrence of fragility fractures, and biomarkers are in place to effectively characterize the risk of fractures. The FRAX tool is a good example how risk can be determined based on constitutional findings, clinical history, and quantitative biomarkers (femoral neck DXA T-score) [44].

Classifying the Efficacy of Intervention with Imaging Biomarkers

Assessing the role of a biomarker in classifying the efficacy of an intervention requires endpoints, which are used as a standard of reference and effective interventions. While those biomarkers and interventions are available in osteoporosis for many years, the field is substantially less advanced in OA. Longitudinal, randomized controlled trials are required that assess the effect of interventions/therapies versus a control group that did not receive the same intervention. Biomarkers that assess the efficacy of intervention will be mostly continuous and analyses will be performed with regression models relating the change in biomarker (per SD) to change in the outcome variable [1]. Typical outcome variables would be change in pain scores, radiographic grading, or cartilage volume. The biomarker must not only correlate with the clinical outcome but also must capture the net effect of treatment on clinical outcome, which is often very difficult for a biomarker to satisfy [14].

Given the limited interventions that are currently available in treating cartilage degeneration, only a relatively limited number of clinical trials have been performed using cartilage imaging biomarkers. These trials focused on analyzing the effects of medications [45, 46] and other interventions such as physical exercise [47] and whole body vibration [48] on cartilage. Most of these studies used MR-based cartilage volume measurements as a biomarker for cartilage loss [45, 46, 48] and one of these studies used dGEMRIC [47].

Raynauld et al. analyzed the effect of Celecoxib using cartilage volume loss in the medial compartment of the knee (femoral condyle and tibial plateau) assessed by MRI as an outcome in subjects receiving continuous treatment daily for 12 months [45]. The 95% confidence intervals for the mean observed celecoxib cohort joint medial compartment cartilage volume loss (6.81% [6.01; 7.60]) and mean predicted loss (modelized historical cohort) (5.65% [5.10; 6.19]) indicated no significant difference and hence no effect of celecoxib on the medial compartment cartilage volume loss. In another study, the same investigators explored the effects of licofelone as a disease-modifying osteoarthritis drug in comparison with naproxen in patients with knee OA using quantitative MRI [46]. They found that cartilage volume loss in the global joint and medial and lateral compartments was significantly less in the licofelone than in the naproxen group at 12 and 24 months [46]. Roos et al. used dGEMRIC as a biomarker to study GAG concentrations in patients at risk of knee OA who start moderate exercise regimens [47]. They found an improvement in the T1(Gd) in the exercise group compared with the control group ($n = 14$) (15 ms versus −15 ms; $P = 0.036$) and concluded that adult human articular cartilage has a potential to adapt to loading change [47].

Investigative Cartilage Imaging Biomarkers

Investigative markers are those which have been newly developed and lack of sufficient scientific investigations does not allow classification into one of the previously mentioned categories [1]. The purpose of creating this category was to facilitate and encourage codification of potential OA biomarkers and support further research development to establish a role for the biomarker in one or more of the other categories [1]. Potential cartilage imaging biomarkers, which are currently investigated, include sodium MRI [49] and chemical exchange-dependent saturation transfer (gagCEST) MRI [50]. Both of these techniques have potential for assessing cartilage glycosaminoglycan content in vivo.

Summary and Conclusion

Cartilage imaging biomarkers have gained a significant role in various aspects of OA. Radiographs are used to define and diagnose OA, yet MR-based morphological cartilage biomarkers are superior in characterizing disease burden. The role of MR-based (both semiquantitative and quantitative) biomarkers in characterizing prognosis and risk of OA is under investigation with a number of studies showing great promise. In terms of measuring effect of therapy and intervention, experiences are limited but MR-based measurements of cartilage volume have found to be useful. Finally it should be stressed that biomarkers need to have face, technical, and pathophysiologic validity. Currently pathophysiologic validity for quantitative cartilage matrix techniques such as dGEMRIC, T2, and T1rho needs further investigation. Also we need to be aware of the fact that overall barriers for validating and using OA biomarkers are significant, OA is a complex disease affecting different joints as well as different regions and structures within a joint in different individuals [14]. However, with large multicenter, longitudinal trials (such as the OAI) and focused hypotheses, proof may eventually be provided for the utility of a number of cartilage imaging biomarkers.

References

1. Bauer DC, Hunter DJ, Abramson SB, Attur M, Corr M, Felson D, et al. Classification of osteoarthritis biomarkers: a proposed approach. Osteoarthritis Cartilage. 2006;14(8):723–7.
2. Smith JJ, Sorensen AG, Thrall JH. Biomarkers in imaging: realizing radiology's future. Radiology. 2003;227(3):633–8.
3. Katz R. Biomarkers and surrogate markers: an FDA perspective. NeuroRx. 2004;1(2):189–95.
4. Kellgren J, Lawrence J. Radiological assessment of osteoarthritis. Ann Rheum Dis. 1957;16:494–501.
5. Kellgren J, Jeffrey M, Ball J. The epidemiology of chronic rheumatism: atlas of standard radiographs of arthritis. Oxford, UK: Blackwell; 1963.
6. Kothari M, Guermazi A, von Ingersleben G, Miaux Y, Sieffert M, Block JE, et al. Fixed-flexion radiography of the knee provides reproducible joint space width measurements in osteoarthritis. Eur Radiol. 2004;14(9):1568–73.
7. Peterfy CG, Guermazi A, Zaim S, Tirman PF, Miaux Y, White D, et al. Whole-Organ Magnetic Resonance Imaging Score (WORMS) of the knee in osteoarthritis. Osteoarthritis Cartilage. 2004; 12(3):177–90.
8. Hunter DJ, Lo GH, Gale D, Grainger AJ, Guermazi A, Conaghan PG. The reliability of a new scoring system for knee osteoarthritis MRI and the validity of bone marrow lesion assessment: BLOKS (Boston Leeds Osteoarthritis Knee Score). Ann Rheum Dis. 2008;67(2):206–11.
9. Kornaat PR, Ceulemans RY, Kroon HM, Riyazi N, Kloppenburg M, Carter WO, et al. MRI assessment of knee osteoarthritis: Knee Osteoarthritis Scoring System (KOSS)–inter-observer and intra-observer reproducibility of a compartment-based scoring system. Skeletal Radiol. 2005;34(2):95–102.
10. Recht M, Kramer J, Marcelis S, Pathria M, Trudell D, Haghigi P, et al. Abnormalities of articular cartilage in the knee: analysis of available MR techniques. Radiology. 1993;187:473–8.
11. Recht M, Piraino D, Paletta G, Schils J, Belhobek G. Accuracy of fat-suppressed three-dimensional spoiled gradient-echo FLASH MR Imaging in the detection of patellofemoral articular cartilage abnormalities. Radiology. 1996;198:209–12.
12. Stahl R, Luke A, Ma CB, Krug R, Steinbach L, Majumdar S, et al. Prevalence of pathologic findings in asymptomatic knees of marathon runners before and after a competition in comparison with physically active subjects-a 3.0 T magnetic resonance imaging study. Skeletal Radiol. 2008;37(7):627–38.
13. Eckstein F, Ateshian G, Burgkart R, Burstein D, Cicuttini F, Dardzinski B, et al. Proposal for a nomenclature for magnetic resonance imaging based measures of articular cartilage in osteoarthritis. Osteoarthritis Cartilage. 2006;14(10):974–83.
14. Felson DT, Lohmander LS. Whither osteoarthritis biomarkers? Osteoarthritis Cartilage. 2009;17(4):419–22.
15. Gray ML. Toward imaging biomarkers for glycosaminoglycans. J Bone Joint Surg Am. 2009;91 Suppl 1:44–9.

16. Bredella MA, Tirman PF, Peterfy CG, Zarlingo M, Feller JF, Bost FW, et al. Accuracy of T2-weighted fast spin-echo MR imaging with fat saturation in detecting cartilage defects in the knee: comparison with arthroscopy in 130 patients. AJR Am J Roentgenol. 1999;172(4):1073–80.
17. Kijowski R, Blankenbaker DG, Davis KW, Shinki K, Kaplan LD, De Smet AA. Comparison of 1.5- and 3.0-T MR imaging for evaluating the articular cartilage of the knee joint. Radiology. 2009;250(3):839–48.
18. Link T, Majumdar S, Peterfy C, Daldrup H, Uffmann M, Dowling C, et al. High resolution MRI of small joints: impact of spatial resolution on diagnostic performance and SNR. Magn Reson Imaging. 1998;16:147–55.
19. Link TM, Sell CA, Masi JN, Phan C, Newitt D, Lu Y, et al. 3.0 vs 1.5 T MRI in the detection of focal cartilage pathology–ROC analysis in an experimental model. Osteoarthritis Cartilage. 2006;14(1):63–70.
20. Ristow O, Steinbach L, Sabo G, Krug R, Huber M, Rauscher I, et al. Isotropic 3D fast spin-echo imaging versus standard 2D imaging at 3.0 T of the knee-image quality and diagnostic performance. Eur Radiol. 2009;19:1263–72.
21. Saadat E, Jobke B, Chu B, Lu Y, Cheng J, Li X, et al. Diagnostic performance of in vivo 3T Fast Spin Echo MRI for articular cartilage abnormalities in human osteoarthritic knees using histology as standard of reference. Eur Radiol. 2008;18:2292–302.
22. Potter HG, Linklater JM, Allen AA, Hannafin JA, Haas SB. Magnetic resonance imaging of articular cartilage in the knee. An evaluation with use of fast-spin-echo imaging. J Bone Joint Surg Am. 1998;80(9):1276–84.
23. Bauer JS, Krause S, Ross C, Mueller D, Majumdar S, Link TM. Accuracy of volumetric cartilage measurements of the knee at 1.5T and 3.0T. RSNA, Chicago; 2005. p. 305.
24. Peterfy CG, van Dijke CF, Lu Y, Nguyen A, Connick TJ, Kneeland JB, et al. Quantification of the volume of articular cartilage in the metacarpophalangeal joints of the hand: accuracy and precision of three-dimensional MR imaging. AJR Am J Roentgenol. 1995;165(2):371–5.
25. Bashir A, Gray ML, Hartke J, Burstein D. Nondestructive imaging of human cartilage glycosaminoglycan concentration by MRI. Magn Reson Med. 1999;41(5):857–65.
26. Cheng J, Saadat E, Bolbos R, Jobke B, Siddiqui S, Ries M, et al. Detection of proteoglycan content in human osteoarthritic cartilage samples with magnetic resonance T1rho imaging. Toronto: ISMRM; 2008.
27. David-Vaudey E, Ghosh S, Ries M, Majumdar S. T2 relaxation time measurements in osteoarthritis. Magn Reson Imaging. 2004;22(5):673–82.
28. Mlynarik V, Trattnig S, Huber M, Zembsch A, Imhof H. The role of relaxation times in monitoring proteoglycan depletion in articular cartilage. J Magn Reson Imaging. 1999;10(4):497–502.
29. Kornaat PR, Bloem JL, Ceulemans RY, Riyazi N, Rosendaal FR, Nelissen RG, et al. Osteoarthritis of the knee: association between clinical features and MR imaging findings. Radiology. 2006; 239(3):811–7.
30. Li X, Ma BC, Link TM, Castillo DD, Blumenkrantz G, Lozano J, et al. In vivoT(1rho) and T(2) mapping of articular cartilage in osteoarthritis of the knee using 3T MRI. Osteoarthritis Cartilage. 2007;15:789–97.
31. Link TM, Steinbach LS, Ghosh S, Ries M, Lu Y, Lane N, et al. Osteoarthritis: MR imaging findings in different stages of disease and correlation with clinical findings. Radiology. 2003;226(2):373–81.
32. Williams A, Sharma L, McKenzie CA, Prasad PV, Burstein D. Delayed gadolinium-enhanced magnetic resonance imaging of cartilage in knee osteoarthritis: findings at different radiographic stages of disease and relationship to malalignment. Arthritis Rheum. 2005;52(11):3528–35.
33. Stehling C, Lane NE, Nevitt MC, Lynch J, McCulloch CE, Link TM. Subjects with higher physical activity levels have more severe focal knee lesions diagnosed with 3T MRI: analysis of a non-symptomatic cohort of the osteoarthritis initiative. Osteoarthritis Cartilage. 2010;18(6):776–86.
34. Stehling C, Liebl H, Krug R, Lane NE, Nevitt MC, Lynch J, et al. Patellar cartilage: T2 values and morphologic abnormalities at 3.0-T MR imaging in relation to physical activity in asymptomatic subjects from the osteoarthritis initiative. Radiology. 2010;254(2):509–20.
35. Stahl R, Luke A, Li X, Carballido-Gamio J, Ma CB, Majumdar S, et al. T1rho, T(2) and focal knee cartilage abnormalities in physically active and sedentary healthy subjects versus early OA patients-a 3.0-Tesla MRI study. Eur Radiol. 2009;19:132–43.
36. Writing group for the ISCD Position Development Conference. Diagnosis of osteoporosis in men, premenopausal women, and children. J Clin Densitom. 2004;7(1):17–26.
37. Roemer FW, Guermazi A, Javaid MK, Lynch JA, Niu J, Zhang Y, et al. Change in MRI-detected subchondral bone marrow lesions is associated with cartilage loss – the MOST study A longitudinal multicenter study of knee osteoarthritis. Ann Rheum Dis. 2008;68:1461–5.
38. Phan CM, Link TM, Blumenkrantz G, Dunn TC, Ries MD, Steinbach LS, et al. MR imaging findings in the follow-up of patients with different stages of knee osteoarthritis and the correlation with clinical symptoms. Eur Radiol. 2006;16:608–18.
39. Emrani PS, Katz JN, Kessler CL, Reichmann WM, Wright EA, McAlindon TE, et al. Joint space narrowing and Kellgren-Lawrence progression in knee osteoarthritis: an analytic literature synthesis. Osteoarthritis Cartilage. 2008;16(8):873–82.
40. Felson DT, Niu J, Guermazi A, Roemer F, Aliabadi P, Clancy M, et al. Correlation of the development of knee pain with enlarging bone marrow lesions on magnetic resonance imaging. Arthritis Rheum. 2007;56(9):2986–92.
41. Dam EB, Loog M, Christiansen C, Byrjalsen I, Folkesson J, Nielsen M, et al. Identification of progressors in osteoarthritis by combining biochemical and MRI-based markers. Arthritis Res Ther. 2009; 11(4):R115.
42. Stehling C, Mueller-Hoecker C, Schwaiger BJ, Lane NE, Krug R, Nevitt MC, et al. Cartilage T2 and WORMS MR measurements predict changes in clinical parameters over a period of 2 years: analysis of 217 nonsymptomatic subjects from the osteoarthritis initiative. ECR scientific program 2010, Vienna; 2010. p. S133.
43. Blumenkrantz G, Carballido-Gamio J, McCulloch C, Lynch J, Link T, Majumdar S. The relationship between the spatial distribution of cartilage MR T2 and longitudinal changes in pain: data from the osteoarthritis initiative. Honolulu, Hawaii: ISMRM; 2009.
44. Kanis JA, Oden A, Johansson H, Borgstrom F, Strom O, McCloskey E. FRAX and its applications to clinical practice. Bone. 2009; 44(5):734–43.
45. Raynauld JP, Martel-Pelletier J, Beaulieu A, Bessette L, Morin F, Choquette D, et al. An open-label pilot study evaluating by magnetic resonance imaging the potential for a disease-modifying effect of celecoxib compared to a modelized historical control cohort in the treatment of knee osteoarthritis. Semin Arthritis Rheum. 2010;40(3):185–92.
46. Raynauld JP, Martel-Pelletier J, Bias P, Laufer S, Haraoui B, Choquette D, et al. Protective effects of licofelone, a 5-lipoxygenase and cyclo-oxygenase inhibitor, versus naproxen on cartilage loss in knee osteoarthritis: a first multicentre clinical trial using quantitative MRI. Ann Rheum Dis. 2009;68(6):938–47.
47. Roos EM, Dahlberg L. Positive effects of moderate exercise on glycosaminoglycan content in knee cartilage: a four-month, randomized, controlled trial in patients at risk of osteoarthritis. Arthritis Rheum. 2005;52(11):3507–14.
48. Liphardt AM, Mundermann A, Koo S, Backer N, Andriacchi TP, Zange J, et al. Vibration training intervention to maintain cartilage thickness and serum concentrations of cartilage oligometric matrix protein (COMP) during immobilization. Osteoarthritis Cartilage. 2009;17(12):1598–603.

49. Borthakur A, Mellon E, Niyogi S, Witschey W, Kneeland JB, Reddy R. Sodium and T1rho MRI for molecular and diagnostic imaging of articular cartilage. NMR Biomed. 2006;19(7):781–821.

50. Ling W, Regatte RR, Navon G, Jerschow A. Assessment of glycosaminoglycan concentration in vivo by chemical exchange-dependent saturation transfer (gagCEST). Proc Natl Acad Sci USA. 2008;105(7):2266–70.

Chapter 17
Frontiers in Molecular Imaging of Cartilage: Future Developments

Ravinder Reddy, Arijitt Borthakur, Walter R. T. Witschey, and J. Bruce Kneeland

Keywords Biomarkers • Cartilage • Chemical exchange saturation transfer (CEST) • Developments • Future • Frontiers • Imaging pulse sequences • Molecular imaging

The Need for Imaging Biomarkers

Recent research has led to the development of drugs that, in animal models, have shown the potential of protecting against the breakdown of macromolecules in cartilage, effectively halting the progression of OA. Because of the long natural history of OA (10–20 years in humans), validating the efficacy of these drugs over the natural course of the disease is not feasible. Instead, what is needed is a validated *noninvasive* imaging biomarker that can directly assess their effect on molecular changes associated with early stages of cartilage degeneration that precede morphological changes.

The current lack of adequate methods to quantify these changes has hampered research in the development of these drugs and other potential disease-modifying agents for early OA. Current imaging methods for assessing cartilage include radiography, computed tomography (CT), and magnetic resonance imaging (MRI), and arthrography performed in conjunction with any of these imaging techniques.

Joint space narrowing determined from conventional radiographs has been the mainstay of detecting and following the course of OA. However, it can only detect OA at a rather late stage when a significant amount of cartilage has already been lost and cannot yield any information on molecular changes that precede morphological changes. The latest generation of multi-slice CT scanners probably have sufficient resolution to image cartilage directly to some extent, but have only been used in conjunction with arthrography and cannot give any information about the molecular structure of cartilage.

R. Reddy (✉)
Department of Radiology, School of Medicine, University of Pennsylvania, 422 Curie Blvd, B1-Stellar-Chance Laboratory, Philadelphia, PA 19104-6100, USA
e-mail: krr@upenn.edu

Conventional MRI permits the direct visualization of cartilage at high resolution and can detect morphologic changes with high levels of accuracy. However, it has not proven either sensitive or specific for the detection of early molecular changes. Arthrography, which describes the intra-articular injection of a contrast agent prior to imaging, can be performed with all of the above modalities and will probably increase the accuracy of any of them for the detection of morphologic changes, but it is mildly invasive and painful and is not practical for longitudinal studies. Furthermore, it will not increase the accuracy of any of these modalities for the detection of changes at the molecular level.

Several MRI methods have been advanced to detect and quantify the early molecular changes in OA. These techniques include T_2 relaxation mapping [2–14], delayed gadolinium-enhanced magnetic resonance imaging contrast (dGEMRIC) [15–17], $T_{1\rho}$ relaxation mapping [18–22], glycosaminoglycans (GAG) measurement using chemical exchange saturation transfer (gagCEST) [23], and the direct MRI of sodium [24–28]. T_2 is predominantly affected by changes in collagen content and to a smaller extent in PG in the tissue. Since the dominant contribution to T_2 relaxation is the dipolar interaction of protons of water associated with collagen, it is primarily useful in quantifying changes associated with the collagen component of the cartilage. dGEMRIC relies on the diffusion of gadolinium contrast agent into cartilage and has been shown to be useful in quantifying changes in PG. T_2 mapping and dGEMRIC have been used in concert in a number of trials for the assessment of regenerated cartilage following injury and their properties are discussed at length in recent review articles [7, 29–32]. Recent advances in MRI of cartilage in general have been reviewed extensively [6, 7, 29, 31–51] and a complete review of MRI of cartilage is beyond the scope of this chapter.

In this chapter, we will focus on three promising imaging-based biomarkers, namely, sodium, $T_{1\rho}$, and CEST MRI that exploit endogenous PG as contrast and hence enable quantitative assessment of PG macromolecular integrity of cartilage. Brief background of these techniques, current status, and potential future developments are discussed.

T.M. Link (ed.), *Cartilage Imaging: Significance, Techniques, and New Developments*, DOI 10.1007/978-1-4419-8438-8_17, © Springer Science+Business Media, LLC 2011

Sodium NMR

Sodium is one of the most "NMR-visible" nuclei in living systems. It is a spin 3/2 nucleus and possesses a quadrupole moment (Q), which interacts with the electric field gradient (EFG) generated by the electronic distribution around the nucleus [52]. The NMR relaxation properties of a nucleus depend on its immediate environment and its interactions that perturb the dominant Zeeman Hamiltonian in a significant manner. The most important interaction experienced by sodium nuclei is that between the nonspherically symmetric nucleus and surrounding electric field gradients. This is called the quadrupolar interaction. In general, sodium in solids experiences most of these interactions, while in liquids the static quadrupolar interaction is averaged to zero because of rapid rotational motion. In the intermediate regimes, for example, in biological tissues, where the spin dynamics are outside motional narrowing regime, the quadrupolar interaction is averaged to a residual value, termed as residual quadrupolar coupling (RQC), and the spin dynamics result in bi-exponential relaxation rates. Multiple quantum-filtered (MQF) ^{23}Na NMR can be used to analyze spectra from such systems [52, 53].

Sodium NMR of Cartilage

Due to the sparse cellular content (~2% by volume) and highly ordered nature of cartilage, most of the sodium in the ECM of cartilage is in the slow-motion regime and exhibits bi-exponential relaxation-induced multiple quantum coherences.

Single Quantum (SQ) Signal Expression

Consider a spin 3/2 nucleus in biological tissues with bi-exponential relaxation and nonzero RQC in a magnetic field. Immediately following the application of a nonselective 90° pulse, the longitudinal magnetization is flipped into the transverse plane and then evolves under the influence of bi-exponential relaxation rates and RQC during the acquisition period t. Dropping the factors representing temperature, the signal expression following a 90° pulse is given by [54, 55]

$$S(t) \sim M_0 \left[\frac{1}{5} \left(\frac{3}{2} e^{-\left(R_S^{(1)} - i\omega_Q\right)} + 2e^{-R_C^{(1)}t} + \frac{3}{2} e^{-\left(R_S^{(1)} + i\omega_Q\right)} \right) \right] \quad (17.1)$$

where M_0 is the thermal equilibrium magnetization, $R_s^{(1)}$ and $R_c^{(1)}$ are relaxation rates of satellite and central transitions, respectively, and ω_Q is the residual quadrupolar frequency. Here, for ease of illustration, it is assumed that the nonzero quadrupole interaction is large enough to create line splittings.

As illustrated by the above equation, the sodium NMR signal from cartilage and other biological tissues is governed by, M_0, $R_s^{(1)}$, $R_c^{(1)}$ and ω_Q. It should be noted here that 40% of total sodium is observed through the central transition, which decays with longer time constant ($1/R_c^{(1)}$) compared to 60% of the total sodium contributing to the satellite transitions, which decay with a faster relaxation time ($1/R_s^{(1)}$). Therefore, in order to quantify absolute sodium concentration from biological tissues, one has to use ultrashort RF pulses, shorter receiver dead times, and shorter echo times, typically from a few 100 μs to 1 ms. Otherwise, a significant amount of the fast-decaying signal is lost before detection, which leads to lower signal and an underestimation of [Na].

Sodium MQF Spectroscopy and Imaging

MQ-filtered spectroscopy via even-ranked double quantum coherence ($T_{\pm 2}^{2}$) and triple quantum coherence ($T_{\pm 3}^{3}$) and imaging with ultrashort duration RF pulses enables the measurement of all the parameters that govern sodium spin dynamics in cartilage. Therefore, MQF sodium NMR studies are indispensable in the quantification of critical parameters (such as relaxation rates and ω_Q) that characterize sodium dynamics in biological tissues [25]. However, due to an order of magnitude lower signal-to-noise ratio (SNR) of MQF signals compared to SQ signals, their utility in the diagnostic imaging of cartilage is limited.

Sodium MRI of Cartilage Fixed-Charge Density (FCD)

As discussed in the introduction, loss of PG is the initiating event in OA. The ability to quantify these molecular changes will provide a handle on early diagnosis and treatment monitoring. Based on the fact that Donnan equilibrium holds for cartilage equilibrated in very dilute solutions, Maroudas et al. have shown that FCD of cartilage is correlated with glycosaminoglycans (GAG) content of cartilage [56]. Since the FCD is counterbalanced by the Na+ ions, loss of PG (hence GAG and FCD) due to cartilage degeneration results in the loss of sodium ions from the tissue. The loss of the negatively charged PG lowers the FCD in the tissue, thereby releasing positively charged sodium ions. Using ideal Donnan equilibrium conditions FCD can be related to tissue sodium concentration according to the following equation:

$$\mathrm{FCD(mM)} = \frac{\left[\mathrm{Na}_{\mathrm{SF}}^{+}\right]^2}{\left[\mathrm{Na}_{\mathrm{tissue}}^{+}\right]} - \left[\mathrm{Na}_{\mathrm{tissue}}^{+}\right] \quad (17.2)$$

where $\left[\mathrm{Na}_{\mathrm{SF}}^{+}\right]$ is the sodium concentration in the synovial fluid and $\left[\mathrm{Na}_{\mathrm{tissue}}^{+}\right]$ is the sodium concentration in the tissue [57].

$\left[Na_{SF}^{+}\right]$ is typically in the range of 140–150 mM, while in phosphate-buffered saline (PBS) it is 154 mM.

Depending on the age and location in the tissue [57], healthy human cartilage FCD ranges from –50 to –250 mM. FCD from [GAG] can be calculated with the following equation by assuming 2 mol of negative charge per mole of chondroitin sulfate (one from sulfate and one from carboxylate) and a molecular weight of chondroitin sulfate of 502.5 g/mol [57]:

$$FCD(mM) = -2 \times \frac{GAG(mg/L)}{502.5(mg/mmol)} \tag{17.3}$$

Because of the very short relaxation time of the outer (satellite) transitions, one has to perform spectroscopic and imaging experiments with ultrashort echo times, typically in the range of 200–1,000 μs. Since invariably NMR and MRI experiments involve finite pulse lengths, some of the fast-decaying components are lost and the signal detected following an RF pulse underestimates the true sodium content. In spite of this, as long as the observed signal is calibrated with appropriate relaxation-matched reference sodium phantoms, it is possible to measure absolute sodium content of the tissue.

Sodium spectroscopy work has been performed at varying field strengths ranging from 2T to 9.4T. Most MQF spectroscopy to date has been carried out at magnetic fields greater than 4T. After early biochemical and sodium single and MQF NMR spectroscopy studies of cartilage, low-resolution sodium MRI was acquired from human knee in vivo [58] at 1.5T. The majority of sodium MRI experiments, however, were performed at 3 and 4T. Reddy et al. [24], for the first time, demonstrated the feasibility of acquiring a high-resolution (voxel size of 6.25 μL) 3D data set of sodium images of the knee of healthy human volunteers with excellent SNR (16:1) at 4T. Sodium images were also compared to corresponding proton images to demonstrate the differences in tissue contrast. In these studies, 3D sodium MRI of 16 slices in the knee joint was performed with volume RF coils in less than a half hour with a voxel size of 6 μL with an SNR of 12:1. The echo times employed in these experiments was ~2 ms. However, by exploiting the increased sensitivity of surface coils, it was possible to improve the SNR to 16:1 and the imaging time was reduced to less than 20 min. Sodium imaging at 4T clearly demonstrated feasibility of measuring cartilage FCD in vivo in healthy as well as osteoarthritic patients.

The feasibility of quantitative imaging of sodium at 3T and 4T scanners on humans and animal models has been demonstrated [24, 28, 59–61] [62]. Further, its utility in measuring FCD changes in animal model of OA has been described [63].

Recently, the feasibility of high-quality 3D sodium MRI of human knee at 7T has been demonstrated [62, 64, 65].

Advantages and Drawbacks

The major advantages of sodium MRI, especially in the case of cartilage, is that it is highly specific to PG content and since the sodium from surrounding structures in the joint is low (<50 mM), cartilage can be visualized with very high contrast without the requirement of any exogenous contrast agent such as that in dGEMRIC [15]. It can be used to quantify early molecular changes associated with PG loss in OA.

The disadvantages of sodium MRI are that it requires field strengths ≥3T to obtain quality sodium images that enable accurate quantification of cartilage FCD. Since the T_{2f} of cartilage lies in the range of 1–2 ms, substantial signal is lost before acquisition. This as well as the low sodium concentration are the major contributors to the low SNR of sodium compared to conventional proton MRI. Furthermore, due to the limitations of gradient strengths and other hardware requirements such as tuned transmit receive switches, most of the sodium imaging experiments reviewed here employed echo times of ≥2 ms. Additionally, the sodium gyromagnetic ratio, $\gamma \sim 0.25$ of that of proton, means that sodium MRI requires four times stronger gradients to obtain images with identical resolution to that of proton MRI. With the exception of MQF-prepared twisted projection imaging (TPI) [66], sodium MQF imaging is currently not clinically feasible due to the low sensitivity of the technique and has therefore been relegated to spectroscopic methods to study spin physics of quadrupolar nuclei, and to quantify structures of materials and specimens.

Future Perspectives

While the specificity of sodium MRI may not be critical for diagnosis of the disease, it plays an important role in the development and evaluation of disease-modifying therapies that target the loss of PG.

Although the current sodium imaging methods quantify the tissue [Na] in healthy cartilage accurately, in degenerated cartilage care should be taken in interpreting the results for the following reasons: In degenerated cartilage, the increased water content dilutes the sodium content and potentially may underestimate the actual [Na] to a small degree, and thereby erroneously amplify the GAG loss.

Recent advances in gradient technology (with a gradient strength of >4 G/cm) may enable one to achieve ultrashort TE (<200 μs) acquisitions that can significantly improve SNR. Radiofrequency coil technology (multiple channel capability) and tuned preamplifiers would further contribute to high SNR. These advances may potentially make the clinical sodium MRI feasible at 3T scanners, but still with limited SNR.

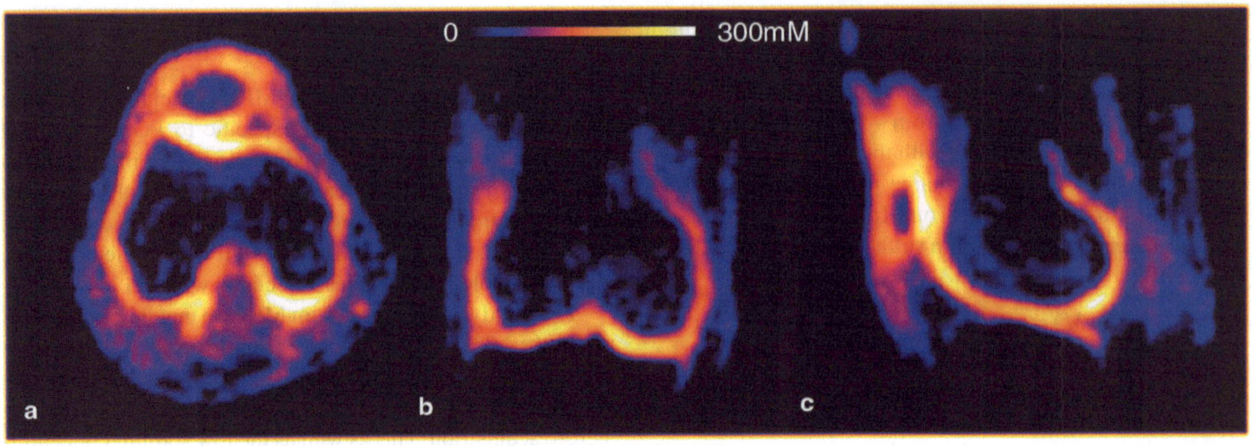

Fig. 17.1 Sodium MRI of healthy human knee at 7T obtained with a home-built birdcage RF coil. Representative axial (**a**), coronal (**b**), and sagittal (**c**) views from a 3D data set of knee of a healthy volunteer. Nominal resolution is 2 mm isotropic. SNR of sodium in cartilage in these images is ~25. After a hard 90° RF pulse (~300 μs) and a short delay (~50 μs), the free induction signal was sampled during the ramp-up time of readout gradient. This is an ultra short echo radial pulse sequence with a TE ~200 μs and the following imaging parameters used: TR = 5 ms, TE ~ 200 μs, and N_{acq} = 10, BW = 500 Hz/pixel, matrix size = 128 × 128 × 128, flip angle =15° (author's own work)

Further, the recent proliferation of 7T whole-body MRI scanners in clinical research centers could have a significant impact on sodium MRI and its potential for clinical use [62, 64, 65]. Since the SNR of low gamma nuclei such as sodium scales as $B_0^{7/2}$ [67–69] and the lack of B_1 penetration and B_0 susceptibility issues due to shorter wavelength that plague the high-field proton imaging, sodium MRI can be particularly advantageous at higher fields. Further, unlike proton T1, which increases with field strength, the T_1 of sodium is predominantly due to quadrupolar interaction and may not change appreciably at higher field. This retains the rapid averaging capability of sodium MRI even at high fields. The low γ of sodium will also mean significantly lower power deposition compared to proton imaging. It is therefore likely that with the improved SNR, sodium MRI at 7T (Fig. 17.1) and higher fields would emerge as a robust tool for quantitative imaging of PG content of cartilage.

$T_{1\rho}$ MRI

One method of probing the nuclear spectrum of spin relaxation mechanisms is to perform an NMR "dispersion" experiment, which measures relaxation times at different static field strengths using the field cycling approach [70]. Although this method provided insights into relaxation phenomena of tissues, it is limited by the need to measure T_1 at different static field strengths. With this method, study of slow motions on the order of kHz is difficult as they have to be performed at low static fields (on the order of kHz) and as a result suffer from poor SNR. On the other hand, $T_{1\rho}$ (spin lattice relaxation in rotating frame) experiments can be performed at high fields and have the potential to provide information about the low-frequency motions in biological systems with high SNR.

In $T_{1\rho}$ MRI (Fig. 17.2), a long-duration, low-power radiofrequency (RF) referred to as "spin-lock" (SL) pulse is applied to the magnetization in the transverse plane. The magnetization is spin-locked and undergoes relaxation in the presence of a B_1 field in the rotating frame, a situation similar to that of the longitudinal magnetization in the B_0 field. The spin-locked magnetization will relax with a time constant $T_{1\rho}$, the spin-lattice relaxation in the rotating frame, during the RF field. Depending on the B_1 field strength, the spin-lock pulse attenuates the effect of dipolar relaxation, static dipolar coupling, chemical exchange, and background gradients on the signal to a varying degree. Therefore $T_{1\rho}$ is always greater than T_2. In a typical $T_{1\rho}$ mapping experiment, the duration of the SL pulse is incremented, while the amplitude of SL pulse ($\omega_1 = (\gamma B_1) \sim$ 0.1-few kHz) is fixed. Alternatively, the measurement of $T_{1\rho}$ as a function of the B_1 amplitude, for a fixed spin-lock length (TSL) is also possible. The "$T_{1\rho}$-dispersion" curve obtained in this case is governed by the spectral density components of the sample on the order of ω_1.

Measurement of the MR signal following the SL pulse is ideal for spectroscopic measurement of $T_{1\rho}$ of a sample. However, for imaging applications, it is often more convenient to prepare the magnetization using a pulse cluster, shown in Fig. 17.3. Evolution of the magnetization during the pulse cluster is illustrated in Fig. 17.4. The thermal equilibrium magnetization vector (M_0), initially along z-axis

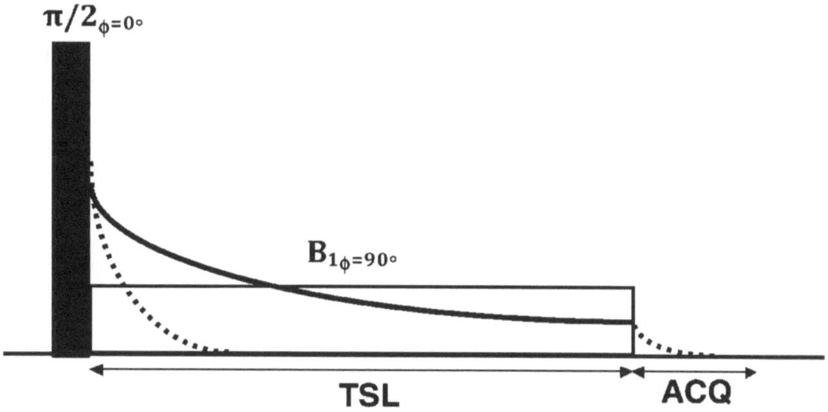

Fig. 17.2 Pulse sequence for spin-locking magnetization in the transverse plane. Initially, a $\pi/2$ pulse flips the longitudinal magnetization into the transverse plane. The open rectangle pulse represents the spin-lock (SL) pulse and TSL and B_1 are its duration and amplitude, respectively. The *dotted line* represents the decay magnetization in the absence of spin-locking and is governed by the time constant, T_2*. However, if the magnetization is spin-locked, it decays according to $T_{1\rho}$ (*solid line*) for the time TSL. But after the SL pulse, the decay is again T_2* during which time the signal may be acquired [111]

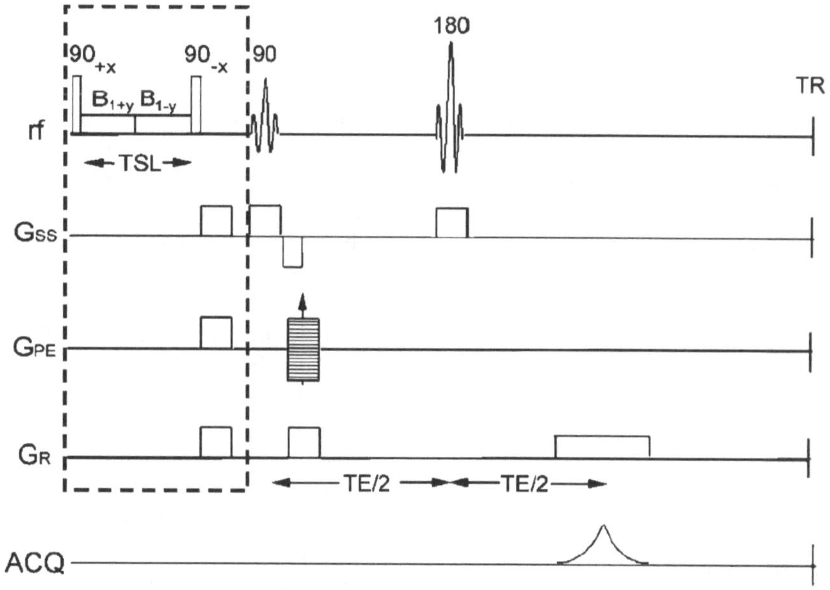

Fig. 17.3 A four-pulse cluster and crusher gradients for $T_{1\rho}$ pre-encoding (outlined by the *dashed box*) preceding a pin-echo readout pulse sequence. TSL and B_1 are the duration and amplitude of the spin-lock pulses, respectively

(panel a), is nutated by the first hard 90° pulse which is applied along the *x*-axis in the rotating frame of reference, into the transverse plane (panel b). The magnetization, now along the *y*-axis, is immediately spin-locked by the SL pulse (shown in red in panel c). For the duration of the TSL period, the magnetization decays with a time constant $T_{1\rho}$ (panel d). The magnetization becomes " $T_{1\rho}$-prepared" and results in a $T_{1\rho}$-weighted signal as a function of TSL. This $T_{1\rho}$-prepared magnetization is then restored to the longitudinal axis by the second hard 90° applied along the negative *x*-axis (panel e) and can be spatially encoded by appending any imaging pulse sequence to this $T_{1\rho}$ pulse cluster. A typical image data set containing four or five images acquired at different TSL times can be fit to the following expression to generate a pixel-by-pixel $T_{1\rho}$ map:

$$S(\mathrm{TSL}) = S_0 e^{\frac{-\mathrm{TSL}}{T_{1\rho}}} + C \tag{17.4}$$

where S(TSL), S_0, TSL, and C are transverse magnetization, thermal equilibrium magnetization, length of the spin-lock

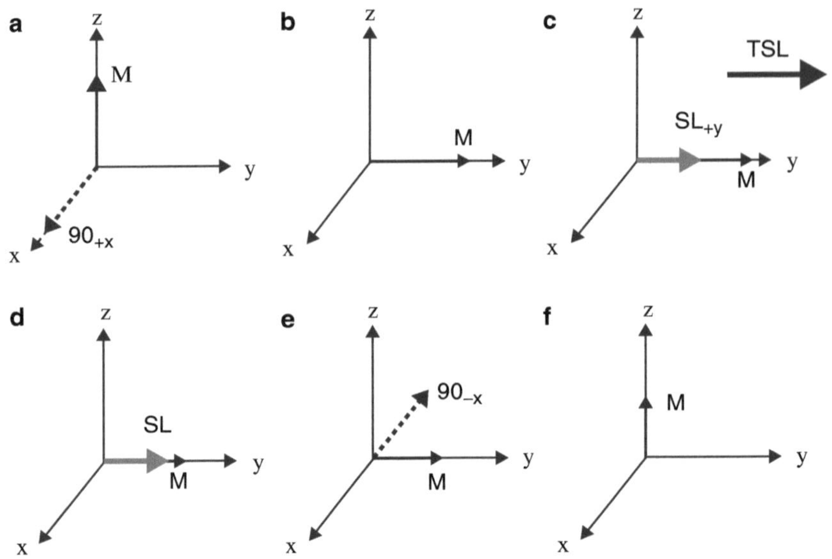

Fig. 17.4 Vector diagram of the evolution of the magnetization during a spin-lock pulse cluster

pulse, and a constant, respectively. In the above description, the on-resonance condition is assumed.

The $T_{1\rho}$ experiment can also be performed in the off-resonance condition to quantify $T_{1\rho}^{off}$, where the magnetization is spin-locked at an effective field given by:

$$\omega_{eff} = \sqrt{\omega_1 + \Delta\omega} \tag{17.5}$$

where $\Delta\omega$ is the resonance offset.

In biological tissues, off-resonance RF irradiation, in addition to spin-locking, also leads to a "magnetization transfer (MT)" effect and it complicates the analysis of $T_{1\rho}^{off}$. The details of off-resonance continuous wave as well as frequency swept experiments can be found in ([1, 71–73]). However, for the rest of the sections we restrict ourselves to describing $T_{1\rho}$ in the on-resonance condition.

Mechanism of T1ρ Relaxation in Cartilage

Redfield first demonstrated the spin-lock phenomenon in solid materials and presented his relaxation theory in the presence of a time-dependent Hamiltonian [74, 75]. The spin interactions with different internal Hamiltonians (J-coupling, chemical shift, dipole–dipole interaction, chemical exchange, etc.) will take place in the presence of a continuous RF field of SL pulse, thereby imparting time dependence to the interaction Hamiltonians. Thus the RF field not only introduces time dependence into the Hamiltonian, but also changes the axis of quantization of the spins and modifies other characteristics that determine the relaxation behavior. Later, several investigators developed the theory for applications in liquid state in different conditions [76].

The interactions that are studied using this methodology can be broadly categorized into (a) scalar coupling, (b) dipole–dipole, and (c) chemical exchange processes. In NMR, in the case of the spin-lattice relaxation in the laboratory frame or rotating frame, the dynamical information is contained in spectral density functions. Although there is abundant literature on studies of T_1 and T_2 relaxation times in biological systems, there are relatively few studies on $T_{1\rho}$ mechanisms in biological tissues at high static fields.

In biological tissues, the $T_{1\rho}$ relaxation may have contributions from several interactions. Depending upon the tissue type, several mechanisms operative simultaneously but with different relative contributions. In what follows, a brief description of individual relaxation mechanisms that may be operative in biological tissues is provided.

Depending upon the limiting case that is applicable for a given tissue, one has to include the appropriate $R_{1\rho}$ (=1/ $T_{1\rho}$) in the expression observed in biological tissues. As long as ω_1 is less than or on the order of a few kHz, dipolar relaxation due to molecular rotational processes (fluctuating dipolar fields $R_{1\rho}^{FD}$) and diffusion ($R_{1\rho}^{Diff}$) do not contribute to the $T_{1\rho}$ dispersion, but they add as constants to the overall value of $T_{1\rho}$. Indeed, it has been shown that, in biological tissues, diffusion (rotational and translational) contributions to all relaxation rates are constant (C) and independent of frequency [77].

The T_1 contribution can be calculated either by standard methods or treated as a constant. The remaining terms are due to the exchange processes ($R_{1\rho}^{Ex}$) that are associated with water protons and other exchangeable protons on macromolecules (such as –OH and –NH), and residual static dipolar coupling ($R_{1\rho}^{RDI}$). As discussed above, depending upon the tissue type and limiting cases, appropriate contributions due to the dominant exchange mechanism and static dipolar interaction terms should be included in the total expression for $T_{1\rho}$. Therefore, the observed $R_{1\rho}$ in biological tissues can be expressed as:

$$R_{1\rho}(\omega_1) = R_{1\rho}^{FD}(\omega_1) + R_{1\rho}^{Diff}(\omega_1) + R_{1\rho}^{Ex}(\omega_1) + R_{1\rho}^{RDI}(\omega_1) \quad (17.6)$$

$T_{1\rho}$ MRI of Cartilage

Contrast in $T_{1\rho}$ MRI is based on proton relaxation rates that are influenced by multiple intrinsic spin parameters, which can be manipulated by the SL pulse length and amplitude. T2 and $T_{1\rho}$ relaxation rate in cartilage is influenced by proton exchange from –OH groups on the GAG chains, fluctuating dipolar relaxation, static dipole–dipole interaction of spins on the oriented collagen macromolecule, spin diffusion, etc. Of all these interactions, the dipole–dipole interaction due to oriented collagen and diffusion dominates the T2 relaxation and masks any contributions to relaxation from spin exchange due to loss of PG. Because of these reasons, T2 mapping is interpreted as being primarily sensitive to collagen. On the other hand, the spin-lock pulse in the $T_{1\rho}$ mapping sequence attenuates the diffusion and dipole–dipole contributions to relaxation significantly, and leads to the greatly enhanced dynamic range and makes the measurement sensitive to spin exchange-mediated relaxation due to GAG.

When the GAG is lost from the tissue, there will be a small increase in the water content of the tissue and the combined effect results in increased $T_{1\rho}$ relaxation time. The degree of attenuation of the dipole–dipole interaction and diffusion depends on the magnitude of the spin-lock pulse amplitude. In general, as long as $\omega_1 > \omega_d$ (residual dipolar interaction), the static dipolar interaction is attenuated. However, in practice this condition is rarely satisfied in vivo on human cartilage due to specific absorption rate (SAR) constraints. Therefore, the measured $T_{1\rho}$ predominantly will have contributions from GAG, the attenuated static dipole–dipole interactions, and the time-dependent dipole–dipole interaction.

Current Status

Although early $T_{1\rho}$ experiments on cartilage were in spectroscopic experiments, later on these were extended to single-slice imaging and then followed by the development of 3D and multi-slice imaging methods. Studies on phantoms and isolated matrix components have shown that both PG and collagen contribute to $T_{1\rho}$. Ex vivo studies on bovine specimens subjected to sequential PG depletion have shown a strong correlation between $1/T_{1\rho}$ and [GAG] although correlation between $1/T_2$ and [GAG] was found to be rather poor [20]. Ex vivo bovine studies and in vivo studies on animal models have shown that treatment with the cytokine IL-1β elevated the $T_{1\rho}$ [78]. In osteoarthritic human specimens, there was a strong correlation between percentage change in FCD measured from sodium MR and percentage change in $1/T_{1\rho}$ [61]. The $T_{1\rho}$ relaxation rate also strongly correlates with mechanical properties of tissue [79]. However, in studies on a small number of human specimens at 8.5T, conflicting results were observed: in some specimens elevated $T_{1\rho}$ was observed in the GAG-depleted region and in some other specimens it remained almost unchanged [80]. Similarly, in studies (at 8.5T) on a small group of bovine specimens subjected to IL-1β, $T_{1\rho}$ was found to be unchanged [81].

Existing results to date suggest that the contributions to $T_{1\rho}$ dispersion is predominantly due to the dipolar interaction of water molecules associated with collagen and it is influenced by the orientation of cartilage. Although proton exchange between amide and hydroxyl protons on GAG molecules and bulk water may also contribute to the dispersion, its contribution is relatively small at lower fields.

Based on data in bovine cartilage, it appears that the strong correlation between [GAG] and $1/T_{1\rho}$ is predominantly due to PG. The fact that a similar trend is observed in IL-1β-treated specimens, and in human OA specimens, in which some collagen changes are expected, suggests that in addition to the proteoglycan contribution there may be a small contribution from collagen as well to the observed $T_{1\rho}$. In other words, $T_{1\rho}$, in addition to measuring PG changes, may also be affected by collagen structural and content changes (if any) present in early OA. Since $T_{1\rho}$ dispersion in cartilage is predominantly due to the static residual dipolar interaction of water protons associated with oriented collagen, a dispersion map computed from images obtained as a function of SL pulse amplitude, B_1, at a constant SL length may reflect the changes in collagen structure and content.

In human studies, elevated levels of $T_{1\rho}$ were observed in OA subjects (without radiographic OA) compared to healthy subjects [82, 83]. $T_{1\rho}$ was found to have stronger correlation between OA disease severity measured in vivo, whereas correlation between changes in T_2 is not statistically significant [84]. Compared to the healthy subjects, in patients with arthroscopically confirmed grade I chondromalacia (without radiographic OA), significantly elevated $T_{1\rho}$ was observed [85] (Figs. 17.5 and 17.6). $T_{1\rho}$ detection of posttraumatic cartilage injury correlated with arthroscopic findings [86] and elevated $T_{1\rho}$ relaxation times were found in cartilage matrix in patients with ACL injuries [87–89]. Significantly elevated

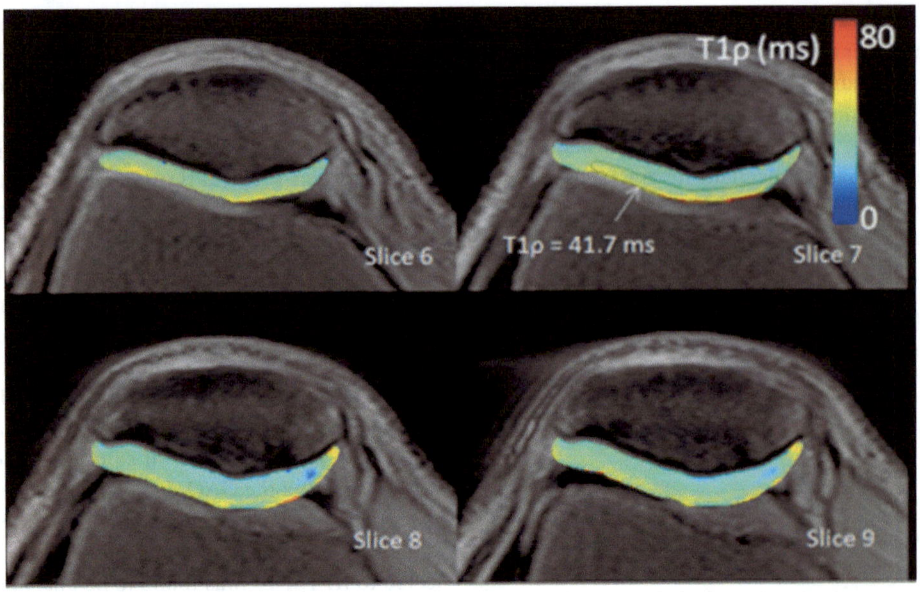

Fig. 17.5 T1ρ relaxation maps from a 30-year-old male with no previous history of knee injury and no knee pain. Patellar cartilage is homogeneously, smoothly varying and has a characteristic increase in relaxation time from the deep cartilage adjacent to the sub-chondral bone to the superficial cartilage adjacent to the synovium. At an ROI drawn at the cartilage surface, T1ρ = 41.7 ms [85]

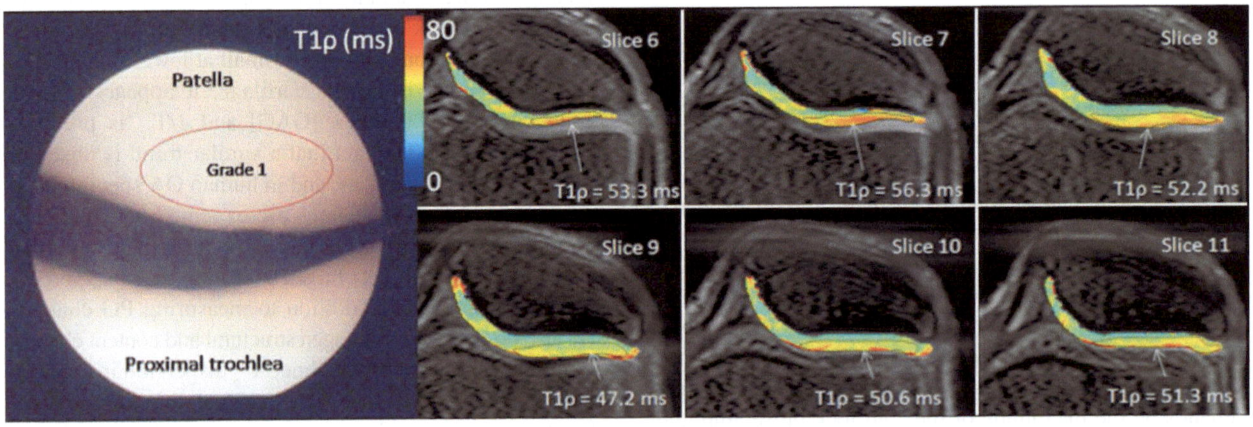

Fig. 17.6 Arthroscopic photographs and T1ρ relaxation maps from a 40-year-old male (patient 1). The patient was observed at arthroscopy to have diffuse grade 1 chondromalacia throughout the entire knee joint. No focal defects or thinning was observed in either patellar or femorotibial compartments on MRI; however, a heterogeneous T1ρ distribution was observed, as well as local elevated T1ρ and cartilage thinning was observed in the lateral patellar superficial compartment and elevated T1ρ = 47–56 ms across six slices. Diffuse, low femoral condyle compartment T1ρ ~ 38 ms was observed [85]

$T_{1\rho}$ values were found in the femoral non-weight-bearing portions when compared with weight-bearing portions both in anterior cruciate ligament-injured patients and controls [90]. Recent study results demonstrate that $T_{1\rho}$, T_2, and contrast-enhanced techniques may provide complementary information about the molecular environment in cartilage during the evolution of OA [91]. These in vivo data clearly indicate that $T_{1\rho}$ may serve as a surrogate marker for pre-radiographic molecular changes in cartilage and may be useful in longitudinal studies.

Imaging Pulse Sequences

Initial $T_{1\rho}$ imaging experiments were performed on articular cartilage using a $T_{1\rho}$ sequence based on a spin echo or SE [19] and fast spin echo or FSE [18]. Recently, a $T_{1\rho}$-prepared 3D gradient-echo (GRE)-based pulse sequence was developed and implemented using either adiabatic pulses [92] or hard pulses [93] in the $T_{1\rho}$ preparation period. Like most 3D GE-based sequences, the 3D $T_{1\rho}$ sequence enables rapid data collection but produces images with a reduced SNR compared

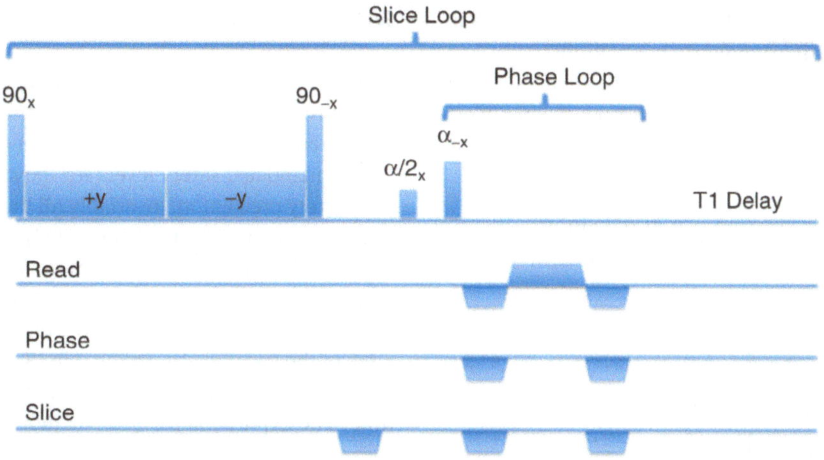

Fig. 17.7 The 3D-balanced gradient-echo (b-GRE) version of the $T_{1\rho}$ pulse sequence. The $T_{1\rho}$-prepared magnetization is followed by the b-GRE sequence in which echoes are read out in each "phase loop" during the approach to the steady state. A delay time for T_1 recovery is inserted before reapplying $T_{1\rho}$ pre-encoding for the second phase encode loop in the slice direction, labeled "slice loop" (Adapted from Witschey et al. [98]

to SE-based images. Further, to accelerate the acquisition, a short TR is typically employed, which introduces significant T_1 weighting in the resulting image and may obscure $T_{1\rho}$-based contrast. Advantages of this sequence are that it provides volumetric $T_{1\rho}$ maps and one of the early data set can be used to compute cartilage volume.

To overcome the limitations, such as low SNR and poor $T_{1\rho}$ contrast, associated with volumetric data acquisition with a 3D $T_{1\rho}$ prepared sequence, a 2D multi-slice spin-lock (MS-SL) pulse sequence was developed [94]. In this sequence, saturation of longitudinal magnetization by the application of nonselective SL pulses is experimentally measured and theoretically modeled as $T_{2\rho}$ decay. The saturation data was used to correct the image data as a function of the SL pulse duration to make quantitative measurements of $T_{1\rho}$. It was found that $T_{1\rho}$ measured using saturation-corrected MS-SL data is identical to that measured using SS-SL sequence [95].

A multi-slice $T_{1\rho}$ mapping with spiral readout was also implemented at 3T [84]. In this sequence, $T_{1\rho}$-prepared magnetization was read out by multi-slice spiral readout. Acquiring a second image that has an inverted longitudinal magnetization compensated T_1 weighting. The total imaging time was ~13 min for a 3D data set of 16 slices. Acquisition of data with this sequence is limited to an axial orientation because spiral acquisition does not allow the use of an anti-aliasing filter that is necessary for sagittal or coronal plane acquisition with a knee coil.

A method for acquiring $T_{1\rho}$-weighted images in a time-efficient manner was demonstrated in a new pulse sequence [96] called SLEPI (spin-locked echo planar imaging). It was shown that the SLEPI sequence could significantly reduce susceptibility-induced artifacts during EPI acquisition, while maintaining image contrast similar to long echo time (TE) images. However, the low resolution of EPI images restricts the application of this pulse sequence to mapping $T_{1\rho}$ in large structures with relatively long T_2. Although the 3D fast GRE sequence and multi-slice sequences described above have been implemented without exceeding SAR limits, they typically require 20–25 min for gathering a 3D $T_{1\rho}$ map. As it is too time consuming (24 min for 4 TSL time points) to collect isotropic 3D maps, typical 3D $T_{1\rho}$ maps are collected with 2–4 mm slice thickness, thereby making it difficult to use a single 3D $T_{1\rho}$ map to visualize different cross sections. This necessitates collection of 3D maps in at least two views.

To accomplish this, recently a balanced gradient-echo (b-GRE) $T_{1\rho}$ pulse sequence (Fig. 17.7) was developed by combining the time-efficient 3D-balanced steady state free precision (b-SSFP) sequence [96] with appropriate modifications [98]. The performance of this sequence was verified by comparing $T_{1\rho}$ relaxation maps obtained with this sequence with that of a standard single-slice $T_{1\rho}$-turbo-spin-echo (TSE) sequence. The difference in average $T_{1\rho}$ of cartilage was minimal (39.4 and 38.4 ms, respectively), while the total acquisition time for the b-GRE sequence for 30 slices was ~10 min. Integrating this sequence with SENSE imaging [99] is expected to further improve its temporal resolution, but at the expense of some SNR.

Extension to Ultrahigh Fields

Effect of Chemical Exchange on $T_{1\rho}$ Sensitivity at Ultrahigh Fields

In the context of cartilage imaging, considering the orders of magnitude differences in the concentrations of GAG and water, the exchange between –OH groups of GAG chains with the protons of water molecules can be considered as a two-site exchange with asymmetric populations.

Expressions for $R_{1\rho}(=1/T_{1\rho})$ for chemical exchange between two sites, A and B, that have distinct magnetic environments, Larmor frequencies, and have asymmetric populations can be written as [100]:

$$R_{1\rho} = R_1 \cos^2\theta + R_2 \sin^2\theta + \frac{p_a p_b \delta^2 k \sin^2\theta}{\omega_{eff}^2 + k^2} \quad (17.7)$$

where

$$\begin{aligned} \delta &= \delta_a - \delta_b \\ \omega_{aeff}^2 &= \delta_a^2 + \omega_1^2 \\ \omega_{beff}^2 &= \delta_b^2 + \omega_1^2 \end{aligned} \quad (17.8)$$

and R_1 and R_2 are the intrinsic longitudinal and transverse relaxation rates, respectively, resulting from processes other than chemical exchange, δ_a, δ_b are the chemical-shift frequency offset from resonance of nuclei in sites A and B, θ is the flip angle of the excitation pulse, $k = k_a + k_b$ is the exchange rate, and the site populations are $p_a = k_b/k$ and $p_b = k_a/k$. If one of the sites is much more populated than the other, then in the asymmetric populations limit, $p_a >> p_b$; $\delta \sim \delta_a$ and $\omega_{eff} \sim \omega_{aeff}$.

If R_1 and R_2 are assumed to be population averages, then The effect of differences between the intrinsic relaxation rates for species in sites A and B on $R_{1\rho}$ is negligible. When θ is 90°, that is, the on-resonance condition, Eq. 7 simplifies to the more familiar expression with R_2 representing the "exchange free" transverse relaxation rate:

$$R_{1\rho} = R_2 + \frac{p_a p_b \delta^2 k}{\omega_1^2 + k^2} \quad (17.9)$$

These results are accurate provided that the spin relaxation decay is dominated by a single exponential damping constant. These $R_{1\rho}$ expressions would be useful in analyzing experimental data when exchange is not fast and site populations are unequal. Since this expression involves a chemical-shift difference term that is field dependent, there would be an increase in $R_{1\rho}$ with field strength. This exchange model has been used to analyze $T_{1\rho}$ dispersion in cartilage [101].

Given that the chemical shift is proportional to the static field, the exchange-mediated $T_{1\rho}$ relaxivity is expected to increase as a square of the B_0 field. Thus, $T_{1\rho}$ studies at 7T would have substantially higher sensitivity for GAG changes compared to lower fields such as 1.5 or 3T and enable the detection of smaller changes in macromolecular content at very early stages of OA. Despite the above advantages, the $T_{1\rho}$ imaging at 7T would certainly face SAR issues that have to be mitigated with clever spin manipulation strategies.

SAR Considerations

During MRI, the power of the applied RF pulses has to be monitored at all times to ensure that the energy deposited in the patient remains below US Food and Drug Administration (FDA) mandated safety levels for the specific absorption rate. As a safety precaution, invariably all the clinical scanners have built-in mechanisms to continuously monitor and halt MRI scans if the FDA-mandated power level is exceeded at any point. While the most accurate method would be to measure the power output to the RF coil in real time, *a priori* knowledge of the specific absorption rate (SAR) of a pulse sequence can provide additional safety and save valuable experiment time. The expression for SAR includes the following [112]:

$$\text{SAR} \propto B_0^2 \times \theta^2 \times \text{RF}_{\text{dutycycle}} \times \text{Patient}_{\text{size}} \quad (17.10)$$

Since the SAR increases as the square of the flip angle (θ) of RF pulse and B_0 field, usable spin-lock amplitudes at 7T will be severely limited and may lead to suboptimal contrast that may not allow the gains of higher $R_{1\rho}$ relaxivity. Following are some of the approaches that can be used to address the issue of SAR at ultrahigh fields.

Low SAR Approaches

Keyhole approach: This method exploits a partial k-space acquisition approach in which a full-power spin-lock pulse is applied only to the central phase-encode lines of k-space, while the remaining phase-encode lines receive a low-power (50% amplitude of the maximum) spin-lock pulse. Acquisition of high- and low-power phase-encode lines are interleaved temporally to minimize average power deposition. This strategy ensures that the majority of signal energy in the central portion of k-space is fully $T_{1\rho}$ weighted, while at the same time the overall SAR of the acquisition is lower, and consequently, total imaging time is reduced. This "keyhole" acquisition approach was exploited in reducing the overall imaging time by 40% for $T_{1\rho}$ mapping in human knee [102]. These approaches can be combined with any of the acquisition sequences described above to reduce SAR and/or improve temporal resolution.

Difference image approach: In this approach, instead of a series of spin-lock-weighted images, one acquires two images one with low ω_1 (<100 Hz) and the other with a high ω_1 (~500 Hz) of spin-lock pulse. From Eq. 17.9, signal acquired with a low ω_1 (~100 Hz) spin-lock pulse retains the exchange effect, while the signal acquired with a high ω_1 (provided $\omega_1 > k$) is unaffected by exchange. A simple logarithmic difference of these two images will provide a quantitative $T_{1\rho}$ map. While this strategy may be advantageous over the full $T_{1\rho}$-mapping approach due to a shorter image acquisition time, it still is not optimal, as one of the images has to be acquired with a spin-lock pulse with high-peak B_1, which may be problematic at ultrahigh fields due to SAR limits. But a trade-off can be made with the time-savings by using a larger TR to reduce the time average SAR.

The Spin-Locked Steady State Free Precision (SL-SSFP): In this method, an SL pulse is integrated with the SSFP sequence in such a way that spin-locking is performed while the magnetization processes around the *z*-axis on a cone by incrementing the phase of the SL pulses [103]. In this experiment, the magnetization is spatially encoded between successive spin-lock pulses, thus obviating the need for preparatory pulse cluster especially the high SAR 90° pulses. The difference imaging approach can be utilized to obtain a $T_{1\rho}$ map. Compared to a conventional bSSFP acquisition, the advantage of this sequence is that image contrast is determined primarily by the effective field orientation and not the choice of flip angle of the RF pulse. An undesirable characteristic of this approach is the high sensitivity of b-SSFP sequences to B_0 field inhomogeneity.

Summary

$T_{1\rho}$ MRI exploits contrast due to endogenous proteins in tissue and provides color-coded quantitative relaxation maps (in terms of ms scale), which are potentially independent of scanner type, and eliminates the subjectivity of diagnosis and longitudinal monitoring. It provides an index of overall molecular changes in cartilage without the requirement of any exogenous contrast agent. It can be performed on any low field strength MRI scanners including the widely popular 1.5T clinical scanner and has the potential to detect changes in macromolecular content as early as a year.

One of the issues that potentially hampers the progress in using $T_{1\rho}$ technology widely is its non-availability on clinical as well as on the research scanners. So far, the $T_{1\rho}$ studies have been mostly of a "demonstration of feasibility" nature on a very limited number of healthy and OA subjects. $T_{1\rho}$ studies on a large group of OA subjects with mild to moderate OA (with a different degree of radiographic OA) and age-matched healthy subjects are needed to address the issues about precision of the measurement, effect of age, severity of the disease, and longitudinal changes in OA.

Chemical Exchange Saturation Transfer (CEST)

In cartilage imaging, CEST [23, 104–108] exploits the –OH or hydroxyl proton group on the GAG side chains of PG molecule. In general, these exchangeable protons are invisible to conventional MRS as they are constantly exchanging with water (H_2O) protons and thus "share their magnetization" with that of water. The exchange rate of these protons depends on pH and temperature and at neutral pH it is 1000 s^{-1}. On the NMR timescale, if this exchange is on the slow-to-intermediate level, then saturating the –OH protons with a long RF pulse at its chemical shift will terminate the "sharing of magnetization" between the –OH protons and water. Concomitantly, the water resonance signal is reduced in proportion to the concentration of –OH protons. This reduction in water proton signal could be imaged with a variety of MR imaging approaches in order to directly detect the concentration of proton exchanging functional groups.

In order for the CEST effect to be efficiently observed, the slow-to-intermediate exchange condition must be fulfilled, that is, chemical shift between exchanging spins, $\Delta\omega > k$, the exchange rate of solute spin. There are two issues that have to be addressed while implementing this method in vivo: the direct saturation of water and the background magnetization transfer effect in biological tissues. To account for these effects, in CEST MRI typically two images are required, one with a saturation pulse applied at the resonance frequency of interest and the other acquired with an equal frequency offset but applied on the other side of the bulk water peak. Then a difference image provides the CEST effect from those spins:

$$\mathrm{CEST_{asym}}(\Delta\omega) = \frac{M_{\mathrm{sat}}(-\Delta\omega) - M_{\mathrm{sat}}(\Delta\omega)}{M_0} \qquad (17.11)$$

where M_0 is the equilibrium magnetization, M_{sat} ($\pm\Delta\omega$) are the magnetizations obtained with saturation at a "+" and "–" offset to the water resonance with a $\Delta\omega$ equivalent to the resonance offset of the exchanging spins.

In interpreting the CEST effect, other factors that play a role are the suboptimal amplitude and duration of the saturation pulse. These effects can be incorporated into a general solution obtainable from theoretical analysis of a two-site exchange model in the presence of RF saturation [108–110]:

$$\mathrm{CEST_{asym}}(\Delta\omega) = \frac{k \cdot \alpha \cdot f}{\mathrm{R_{1w}} + k \cdot f}\left[1 - e^{-(\mathrm{R_{1w}} + k \cdot f)t_{\mathrm{sat}}}\right] \qquad (17.12)$$

where *k* is the exchange rate (s^{-1}); *a* is the factor that accounts for suboptimal saturation with 1 describing complete saturation (at high enough B_1 power of saturation pulse); $f = n$ [metabolite]/2[H_2O] is the fraction of exchangeable protons on the metabolite ("*n*" is number exchangeable protons, n = 1 for –OH); R_{1w} (=1/T_{1w}) is the longitudinal relaxation rate of water protons; and t_{sat} is the length of the saturation pulse.

Current Status

While some initial experiments on phantoms and preliminary in vivo data on knee cartilage [23] have been reported, more work is needed to completely characterize this method in terms of its applicability in imaging GAG changes in cartilage during OA process.

Advantages and Drawbacks

While the major advantages of the CEST method are that it has high specificity to the changes in the GAG, does not require exogenous contrast agent, and benefits from imaging at ultrahigh fields, it comes with several parameters that potentially may confound the results. Since it depends on the exchange rate of –OH protons on GAG, it is highly specific to pH and any pH changes during the cartilage degeneration process would confound the results. Further, this method is also potentially influenced by any changes in the exchange rate of –OH protons due to increase in water content as well as changes in the other macromolecules such as collagen of cartilage. Since this method depends on the exchange-mediated reduction in the water signal, it provides negative contrast.

Further, as this method is based on the difference of two images, it is highly susceptible to water line shape changes of cartilage in vivo, and exchange rate is not favorable to observe optimal CEST at 3T since the chemical-shift difference is not greater than the exchange rate ($\Delta\omega < k$). Owing to the relatively small chemical-shift difference of –OH protons from water (1.00 ppm, ~129Hz at 3T), there will be a significant direct saturation of water and any asymmetry in the line shape due to susceptibility-induced artifacts would significantly confound the results from this method.

However, CEST imaging will benefit substantially from the use of ultrahigh fields for the following reasons: First, the chemical-shift difference of –OH at 7T is 300 Hz, which satisfies the slow-to-intermediate exchange rate condition ($\Delta\omega > k$). Second, the larger chemical-shift difference leads to reduced direct water saturation and makes it less susceptible to the asymmetry in water line shape due to susceptibility effects. Also, 7T would provide overall more than two times higher SNR compared to 3T field.

Future Developments

While sodium imaging is highly suited to compute PG with high specificity, as it comes with low resolution and lacks the morphological details, without proton MRI as such it may not be usable to diagnose or evaluate the efficacy of potential therapies. Further, at present, its sensitivity at 3T is not optimal and needs further improvements in RF coils and pulse sequences to obtain additional SNR that enable it to be useful for clinical studies. Hence in order to obtain quality sodium scans, it has to be performed at high static fields such as 7T. Due to the small chemical-shift difference and inadequate sensitivity at low fields (1.5T, 3T), CEST MRI is also a technique that is optimal for use at 7T. However, as it depends on the difference image, a uniform line shape is essential to obtain quantitative information. Thus, although both of these methods have high specificity for PG and are expected to play important roles in evaluation of potential therapies that target PG loss, they need high fields and cannot be used for diagnosis without supplementing with morphological proton MRI.

$T_{1\rho}$ MRI, on the other hand, provides positive contrast, is sensitive to both PG and collagen changes, can be performed at 1.5T and 3T fields with excellent sensitivity, provides morphological details such as cartilage volume, does not require any exogenous contrast agent, and thus serves as an excellent tool for both diagnosis, longitudinal monitoring, and evaluation of therapeutic efficacy. While its sensitivity is expected to increase at high fields (7T) SAR issues potentially may nullify the sensitivity gains achievable at high fields. However, as discussed in Section "$T_{1\rho}$ MRI", with further technical developments it may be possible to design low SAR versions of the method that would enable integration of the three methods and realization of the advantages of $T_{1\rho}$ MRI as well as PG-specific sodium and CEST MRI at ultrahigh fields.

Given the above, ideally, performing sodium, CEST and $T_{1\rho}$ MRI at ultrahigh fields would improve sensitivity as well as specificity of these methods in assessing cartilage integrity. Therefore, a double-tuned coil array that enables the computation of $T_{1\rho}$ and sodium maps at ultrahigh fields is highly desirable. Using such a coil, it may be possible to obtain information on cartilage volume that provide morphological changes and total tissue loss, as well as changes specific to PG, and integrated molecular changes (water content and macromolecular (PG + collagen)) in a single scan session.

An alternate approach that may be considered is to perform $T_{1\rho}$ MRI at low fields (1.5T or 3T) and sodium and CEST MRI at 7T to obtain comprehensive information about cartilage integrity. However, this requires two separate RF coils and two separate scan sessions that doubles the cost of the scan and creates subject scheduling problems. Further, a robust co-registration of proton images obtained at 1.5T or 3T and sodium/CEST images obtained at 7T is a critical step for the success of this approach. Since the target of these molecular imaging tools is early changes in the tissue, one of the advantages of this approach is that low-field $T_{1\rho}$ MRI may help to screen patients that have morphologically intact cartilage and early OA and need high-field sodium/CEST scans. Advanced OA populations may not require sodium/CEST scans and hence all the subjects may not have to go through two separate scans. However, further work is needed to determine the advantages and potential drawbacks of this approach over an integrated approach at ultrahigh field.

These advances potentially lead to a protocol of quantitative imaging biomarkers that enables the determination of integrated molecular and morphological changes in cartilage degeneration and contributes to the development of disease-modifying drugs, disease management, and hence to patient care. Because of the long natural history of OA (10–20 years in humans), these sensitive imaging biomarkers are expected to significantly accelerate the drug development process by assessing the therapeutic potential in terms of efficacy at the early stages of the disease and thereby lowering the cost and duration of clinical trials. While the discussion in this chapter dealt with cartilage imaging, the same tools are expected to be applicable to other cartilage-like tissues such as intervertebral discs and menisci.

References

1. Liimatainen T, Sorce DJ, Connell R, Garwood M, Michacli S. MRI Contrast from relaxation along fictitious field (RAFF). Magn Reson Med. 2010;64: 983–994.
2. Mosher TJ, Smith H, Dardzinski BJ, Schmithorst VJ, Smith MB. MR imaging and T2 mapping of femoral cartilage: in vivo determination of the magic angle effect. AJR Am J Roentgenol. 2001;177(3):665–9.
3. Smith HE, Mosher TJ, Dardzinski BJ, Collins BG, Collins CM, Yang QX, et al. Spatial variation in cartilage T2 of the knee. J Magn Reson Imaging. 2001;14(1):50–5.
4. Dardzinski BJ, Mosher TJ, Li S, Van Slyke MA, Smith MB. Spatial variation of T2 in human articular cartilage. Radiology. 1997;205(2):546–50.
5. David-Vaudey E, Ghosh S, Ries M, Majumdar S. T2 relaxation time measurements in osteoarthritis. Magn Reson Imaging. 2004;22(5):673–82.
6. Glaser C. New techniques for cartilage imaging: T2 relaxation time and diffusion-weighted MR imaging. Radiol Clin North Am. 2005;43(4):641–53. vii.
7. Mosher TJ, Dardzinski BJ. Cartilage MRI T2 relaxation time mapping: overview and applications. Semin Musculoskelet Radiol. 2004;8(4):355–68.
8. Mosher TJ, Smith HE, Collins C, Liu Y, Hancy J, Dardzinski BJ, et al. Change in knee cartilage T2 at MR imaging after running: a feasibility study. Radiology. 2005;234(1):245–9.
9. Van Breuseghem I, Bosmans HT, Elst LV, Maes F, Pans SD, Brys PP, et al. T2 mapping of human femorotibial cartilage with turbo mixed MR imaging at 1.5 T: feasibility. Radiology. 2004; 233(2):609–14.
10. Dunn TC, Lu Y, Jin H, Ries MD, Majumdar S. T2 relaxation time of cartilage at MR imaging: comparison with severity of knee osteoarthritis. Radiology. 2004;232(2):592–8.
11. Nieminen MT, Menezes NM, Williams A, Burstein D. T2 of articular cartilage in the presence of Gd-DTPA2. Magn Reson Med. 2004;51(6):1147–52.
12. Nieminen MT, Rieppo J, Toyras J, Hakumaki JM, Silvennoinen J, Hyttinen MM, et al. T2 relaxation reveals spatial collagen architecture in articular cartilage: a comparative quantitative MRI and polarized light microscopic study. Magn Reson Med. 2001; 46(3):487–93.
13. Van Breuseghem I, Palmieri F, Peeters RR, Maes F, Bosmans HT, Marchal GJ. Combined T1-T2 mapping of human femoro-tibial cartilage with turbo-mixed imaging at 1.5T. J Magn Reson Imaging. 2005;22(3):368–72.
14. Watrin-Pinzano A, Ruaud JP, Olivier P, Grossin L, Gonord P, Blum A, et al. Effect of proteoglycan depletion on T2 mapping in rat patellar cartilage. Radiology. 2005;234(1):162–70.
15. Burstein D, Velyvis J, Scott KT, Stock KW, Kim YJ, Jaramillo D, et al. Protocol issues for delayed Gd(DTPA)2–enhanced MRI (dGEMRIC) for clinical evaluation of articular cartilage. Magn Reson Med. 2001;45(1):36–41.
16. Bashir A, Gray ML, Boutin RD, Burstein D. Glycosaminoglycan in articular cartilage: in vivo assessment with delayed Gd(DTPA)(2-)-enhanced MR imaging. Radiology. 1997;205(2):551–8.
17. Bashir A, Gray ML, Burstein D. Gd-DTPA2– as a measure of cartilage degradation. Magn Reson Med. 1996;36(5):665–73.
18. Duvvuri U, Charagundla SR, Kudchodkar SB, Kaufman JH, Kneeland JB, Rizi R, et al. Human knee: in vivo T1(rho)-weighted MR imaging at 1.5 T–preliminary experience. Radiology. 2001;220(3):822–6.
19. Duvvuri U, Reddy R, Patel SD, Kaufman JH, Kneeland JB, Leigh JS. T_{1r}-relaxation in articular cartilage: effects of enzymatic degradation. Magn Reson Med. 1997;38(6):863–7.
20. Regatte RR, Akella SV, Borthakur A, Kneeland JB, Reddy R. Proteoglycan depletion-induced changes in transverse relaxation maps of cartilage: comparison of T2 and T1rho. Acad Radiol. 2002;9(12):1388–94.
21. Akella SV, Regatte RR, Gougoutas AJ, Borthakur A, Shapiro EM, Kneeland JB, et al. Proteoglycan-induced changes in T1rho-relaxation of articular cartilage at 4T. Magn Reson Med. 2001;46(3):419–23.
22. Reddy R, Insko EK, Kaufman JH, Bolinger L, Kneeland JB, Leigh JS. MR imaging of cartilage under spin-locking. Proceedings of the International Society of Magnetic Resonance, 3rd Scientific Meeting. Nice, France; 1995, p. 1535.
23. Ling W, Regatte RR, Navon G, Jerschow A. Assessment of glycosaminoglycan concentration in vivo by chemical exchange-dependent saturation transfer (gagCEST). Proc Natl Acad Sci USA. 2008;105(7):2266–70.
24. Reddy R, Insko EK, Noyszewski EA, Dandora R, Kneeland JB, Leigh JS. Sodium MRI of human articular cartilage *in vivo*. Magn Reson Med. 1998;39(5):697–701.
25. Borthakur A. Sodium NMR: an noninvasive probe for proteoglycan macromolecules. Philadelphia, PA: University of Pennsylvania; 2000. p. 104.
26. Reddy R, Shuchun L, Noyszewski EA, Kneeland JB, Leigh JSf. In vivo sodium multiple quantum spectroscopy of human articular cartilage. Magn Reson Med. 1997;38(2):207.
27. Shapiro E. Multi-nuclear magnetic resonance methods for evaluating cartilage degeneration. Philadelphia, PA: University of Pennsylvania; 2001. p. 139.
28. Wheaton AJ, Borthakur A, Shapiro EM, Regatte RR, Akella SV, Kneeland JB, et al. Proteoglycan loss in human knee cartilage: quantitation with sodium MR Imaging–Feasibility Study. Radiology. 2004;231(3):900–5.
29. Burstein D, Gray M. New MRI techniques for imaging cartilage. J Bone Joint Surg Am. 2003;85-A Suppl 2:70–7.
30. Goodwin DW, Dunn JF. MR imaging and T2 mapping of femoral cartilage. AJR Am J Roentgenol 2002;178(6):1568–69; author reply 1569–70.
31. Gray ML, Burstein D. Molecular (and functional) imaging of articular cartilage. J Musculoskelet Neuronal Interact. 2004;4(4):365–8.

32. Gray ML, Eckstein F, Peterfy C, Dahlberg L, Kim YJ, Sorensen AG. Toward imaging biomarkers for osteoarthritis. Clin Orthop Relat Res. 2004(427 Suppl):S175–81.
33. Gatehouse PD, Thomas RW, Robson MD, Hamilton G, Herlihy AH, Bydder GM. Magnetic resonance imaging of the knee with ultrashort TE pulse sequences. Magn Reson Imaging. 2004;22(8):1061–7.
34. Gold GE, Hargreaves BA, Reeder SB, Vasanawala SS, Beaulieu CF. Controversies in protocol selection in the imaging of articular cartilage. Semin Musculoskelet Radiol. 2005;9(2):161–72.
35. Gold GE, McCauley TR, Gray ML, Disler DG. What's new in cartilage? Radiographics. 2003;23(5):1227–42.
36. Hall LD. Magnetic resonance imaging as a noninvasive means for quantitating the dimensions of articular cartilage in the human knee. Arthritis Rheum. 2004;50(1):5–9.
37. Lang P, Noorbakhsh F, Yoshioka H. MR imaging of articular cartilage: current state and recent developments. Radiol Clin North Am. 2005;43(4):629–39. Vii.
38. Manaster BJ, Johnson T, Narahari U. Imaging of cartilage in the athlete. Clin Sports Med. 2005;24(1):13–37.
39. Nishimura K. Magnetic resonance imaging in rheumatoid arthritis. Nippon Rinsho. 2005;63 Suppl 1:405–9.
40. O'Byrne E, Pellas T, Laurent D. Qualitative and quantitative in vivo assessment of articular cartilage using magnetic resonance imaging. Novartis Found Symp. 2003;249:190–8. discussion 198–202, 234–198, 239–141.
41. Peterfy CG. Imaging of the disease process. Curr Opin Rheumatol. 2002;14(5):590–6.
42. Potter HG, Ho ST, Altchek DW. Magnetic resonance imaging of the elbow. Semin Musculoskelet Radiol. 2004;8(1):5–16.
43. Raynauld JP. Quantitative magnetic resonance imaging of articular cartilage in knee osteoarthritis. Curr Opin Rheumatol. 2003; 15(5):647–50.
44. Recht MP, Goodwin DW, Winalski CS, White LM. MRI of articular cartilage: revisiting current status and future directions. AJR Am J Roentgenol. 2005;185(4):899–914.
45. Schmitt F, Grosu D, Mohr C, Purdy D, Salem K, Scott KT, et al. 3 Tesla MRI: successful results with higher field strengths. Radiologe. 2004;44(1):31–47.
46. Trattnig S, Plank C, Pinker K, Striessnig G, Mlynarik V, Nobauer I, et al. Diagnostic imaging of cartilage replacement therapy. Radiologe. 2004;44(8):748–55.
47. Tsou IY, Yegappan M, Ong WS, Goh PO, Tan JL, Chee TS. Cartilage injury and repair: assessment with magnetic resonance imaging. Singapore Med J. 2006;47(1):80–7. quiz 88.
48. Van Breuseghem I. Ultrastructural MR imaging techniques of the knee articular cartilage: problems for routine clinical application. Eur Radiol. 2004;14(2):184–92.
49. Verstraete KL, Almqvist F, Verdonk P, Vanderschueren G, Huysse W, Verdonk R, et al. Magnetic resonance imaging of cartilage and cartilage repair. Clin Radiol. 2004;59(8):674–89.
50. Winalski CS, Gupta KB. Magnetic resonance imaging of focal articular cartilage lesions. Top Magn Reson Imaging. 2003;14(2):131–44.
51. Young IR, Bydder GM. Magnetic resonance: new approaches to imaging of the musculoskeletal system. Physiol Meas. 2003; 24(4):R1–23.
52. Slichter CP. Principles of magnetic resonance. Berlin; New York: Springer; 1996. xi, 655 p.
53. Jaccard G, Wimperis S, Bodenhausen G. Multiple quantum NMR spectroscopy of S =3/2 spins in isotropic phase: a new probe for multiexponential relaxation. J Chem Phys. 1986;85(11):6282–93.
54. Johan RCvdM. Thermal relaxation and coherence dynamics of spin 3/2. I. Static and fluctuating quadrupolar interactions in the multipole basis. Concepts in Magnetic Resonance Part A. 2003;19A(2):97–116.
55. Van Der Maarel JRC. Relaxation of spin 3/2 in a nonzero average electric field gradient. Chem Phys Lett. 1989;155(3):288.
56. Maroudas A, Muir H, Wingham J. The correlation of fixed negative charge with glycosaminoglycan content of human articular cartilage. Biochim Biophys Acta. 1969;177(3):492–500.
57. Lesperance LM, Gray ML, Burstein D. Determination of fixed charge-density in cartilage using nuclear-magnetic-resonance. J Orthop Res. 1992;10(1):1–13.
58. Granot J. Sodium imaging of human body organs and extremities in vivo. Radiology. 1988;167:547–50.
59. Shapiro EM, Borthakur A, Dandora R, Kriss A, Leigh JS, Reddy R. Sodium visibility and quantitation in intact bovine articular cartilage using high field ^{23}Na MRI and MRS. J Magn Reson. 2000;142(1):24–31.
60. Shapiro EM, Borthakur A, Gougoutas A, Reddy R. ^{23}Na MRI accurately measures FCD in articular cartilage. Magn Reson Med. 2002;47(2):284–91.
61. Wheaton AJ, Casey FL, Gougoutas AJ, Dodge GR, Borthakur A, Lonner JH, et al. Correlation of T1rho with fixed charge density in cartilage. J Magn Reson Imaging. 2004;20(3):519–25.
62. Staroswiecki E, Bangerter NK, Gurney PT, Grafendorfer T, Gold GE, Hargreaves BA. In vivo sodium imaging of human patellar cartilage with a 3D cones sequence at 3 T and 7 T. J Magn Reson Imaging. 2010;32(2):446–51.
63. Wheaton AJ, Borthakur A, Dodge GR, Kneeland JB, Schumacher HR, Reddy R. Sodium magnetic resonance imaging of proteoglycan depletion in an in vivo model of osteoarthritis. Acad Radiol. 2004;11(1):21–8.
64. Madelin G, Lee JS, Inati S, Jerschow A, Regatte RR. Sodium inversion recovery MRI of the knee joint in vivo at 7T. J Magn Reson. 2010;494(4–6):331–6.
65. Wang L, Wu Y, Chang G, Oesingmann N, Schweitzer ME, Jerschow A, et al. Rapid isotropic 3D-sodium MRI of the knee joint in vivo at 7T. J Magn Reson Imaging. 2009;30(3):606–14.
66. Borthakur A, Hancu I, Boada FE, Shen GX, Shapiro EM, Reddy R. *In vivo* triple quantum filtered twisted projection sodium MRI of human articular cartilage. J Magn Reson. 1999;146:286–90.
67. Chen CN, Sank VJ, Cohen SM, Hoult DI. The field dependence of NMR imaging. I. Laboratory assessment of signal-to-noise ratio and power deposition. Magn Reson Med. 1986;3(5):722–9.
68. Wen H, Chesnick AS, Balaban RS. The design and test of a new volume coil for high field imaging. Magn Reson Med. 1994;32(4):492–8.
69. Ugurbil K, Adriany G, Andersen P, Chen W, Garwood M, Gruetter R, et al. Ultrahigh field magnetic resonance imaging and spectroscopy. Magn Reson Imaging. 2003;21(10):1263–81.
70. Koenig SH, Brown III RD. Field-cycling relaxometry of protein solutions and tissues: implications for MRI. Prog NMR Spectrosc. 1990;22:487–567.
71. Rommel E, Kimmich R, Korperich H, Kunze C, Gersonde K, et al. T1r dispersion imaging and localized T1r dispersion relaxometry: applications in vivo to mouse adenocarcinoma. Magn Reson Med. 1992;24:149–57.
72. Santyr GE, Fairbanks EJ, Kelcz F, Sorenson JA. Off-resonance spin locking for MR imaging. Magn Reson Med. 1994;32(1): 43–51.
73. Charagundla SR, Stolpen AH, Leigh JS, Reddy R. Off-resonance proton T_{1r} dispersion imaging of ^{17}O-enriched tissue phantoms. Magn Reson Med. 1998;39(4):588–95.
74. Redfield AG. Nuclear magnetic resonance saturation and rotary saturation in solids. Phys Rev. 1955;98(6):1787.
75. Redfield AG. Nuclear spin thermodynamics in the rotating frame. Science. 1969;164(3883):1015.
76. Bull TE. Relaxation in the rotating frame in liquids. Prog Nucl Magn Reson Spectrosc. 1992;24:377.
77. Knispel RR. NMR study of the two-phase equilibrium in cysteine hydrochloride monohydrate. II. J Chem Phys. 1974;61(3):1125.

78. Wheaton AJ, Dodge GR, Borthakur A, Kneeland JB, Schumacher HR, Reddy R. Detection of changes in articular cartilage proteoglycan by T(1rho) magnetic resonance imaging. J Orthop Res. 2005;23(1):102–8.
79. Wheaton AJ, Dodge GR, Elliott DM, Nicoll SB, Reddy R. Quantification of cartilage biomechanical and biochemical properties via T1rho magnetic resonance imaging. Magn Reson Med. 2005;54(5):1087–93.
80. Mlynarik V, Trattnig S, Huber M, Zembsch A, Imhof H. The role of relaxation times in monitoring proteoglycan depletion in articular cartilage. J Magn Reson Imag. 1999;10(4):497–502.
81. Menezes NM, Gray ML, Hartke JR, Burstein D. T2 and T1rho MRI in articular cartilage systems. Magn Reson Med. 2004;51(3):503–9.
82. Regatte RR, Akella SV, Borthakur A, Kneeland JB, Reddy R. In vivo proton MR three-dimensional T1rho mapping of human articular cartilage: initial experience. Radiology. 2003;229(1):269–74.
83. Regatte RR, Akella SV, Wheaton AJ, Lech G, Borthakur A, Kneeland JB, et al. 3D-T1rho-relaxation mapping of articular cartilage: in vivo assessment of early degenerative changes in symptomatic osteoarthritic subjects. Acad Radiol. 2004;11(7):741–9.
84. Li X, Han ET, Ma CB, Link TM, Newitt DC, Majumdar S. In vivo 3T spiral imaging based multi-slice T(1rho) mapping of knee cartilage in osteoarthritis. Magn Reson Med. 2005;54(4):929–36.
85. Witschey WR, Borthakur A, Fenty M, Kneeland BJ, Lonner JH, McArdle EL, et al. T1rho MRI quantification of arthroscopically confirmed cartilage degeneration. Magn Reson Med. 2010; 63(5):1376–82.
86. Lozano J, Li X, Link TM, Safran M, Majumdar S, Ma CB. Detection of posttraumatic cartilage injury using quantitative T1rho magnetic resonance imaging. A report of two cases with arthroscopic findings. J Bone Joint Surg Am. 2006;88(6):1349–52.
87. Stahl R, Luke A, Li X, Carballido-Gamio J, Ma CB, Majumdar S, et al. T1rho, T2 and focal knee cartilage abnormalities in physically active and sedentary healthy subjects versus early OA patients–a 3.0-Tesla MRI study. Eur Radiol. 2009;19(1):132–43.
88. Li X, Ma CB, Link TM, Castillo DD, Blumenkrantz G, Lozano J, et al. In vivo T(1rho) and T(2) mapping of articular cartilage in osteoarthritis of the knee using 3 T MRI. Osteoarthritis Cartilage. 2007;15(7):789–97.
89. Bolbos RI, Link TM, Ma CB, Majumdar S, Li X. T1rho relaxation time of the meniscus and its relationship with T1rho of adjacent cartilage in knees with acute ACL injuries at 3 T. Osteoarthritis Cartilage. 2009;17(1):12–8.
90. Bolbos RI, Ma CB, Link TM, Majumdar S, Li X. In vivo T1rho quantitative assessment of knee cartilage after anterior cruciate ligament injury using 3 Tesla magnetic resonance imaging. Invest Radiol. 2008;43(11):782–8.
91. Taylor C, Carballido-Gamio J, Majumdar S, Li X. Comparison of quantitative imaging of cartilage for osteoarthritis: T2, T1rho, dGEMRIC and contrast-enhanced computed tomography. Magn Reson Imaging. 2009;27(6):779–84.
92. Aronen HJ, Ramadan UA, Peltonen TK, Markkola AT, Tanttu JI, Jaaskelainen J, et al. 3D spin-lock imaging of human gliomas. Magn Reson Imaging. 1999;17(7):1001–10.
93. Borthakur A, Wheaton AJ, Charagundla SR, Shapiro EM, Regatte RR, Akella SVS, et al. Three-dimensional T_{1r}-weighted MRI at 1.5 Tesla. J Magn Reson Imaging. 2003;17:730–6.
94. Wheaton AJ, Borthakur A, Charagundla SR, Reddy R. Pulse sequence for multislice T1rho-weighted MRI. Magn Reson Med. 2004;51(2):362–9.
95. Wheaton AJ. Quantitative spin-lock magnetic resonance imaging: technical development and biomedical applications. Philadelphia, PA: University of Pennsylvania; 2005. p. 188.
96. Borthakur A, Hulvershorn J, Gualtieri E, Wheaton AJ, Charagundla S, Elliott MA, et al. A pulse sequence for rapid in vivo spin-locked MRI. J Magn Reson Imaging. 2006;23(4):591–6.
97. Schmitz B, Hagen T, Reith W. Three-dimensional true FISP for high-resolution imaging of the whole brain. Eur Radiol. 2003;13(7):1577–82.
98. Witschey WR, Borthakur A, Elliott MA, Fenty M, Sochor MA, Wang C, et al. T1rho-prepared balanced gradient echo for rapid 3D T1rho MRI. J Magn Reson Imaging. 2008;28(3):744–54.
99. Pruessmann KP, Weiger M, Scheidegger MB, Boesiger P. SENSE: sensitivity encoding for fast MRI. Magn Reson Med. 1999; 42(5):952–62.
100. Trott O, Palmer III AG. R1rho relaxation outside of the fast-exchange limit. J Magn Reson. 2002;154(1):157.
101. Mlynarik V, Szomolanyi P, Toffanin R, Vittur F, Trattnig S. Transverse relaxation mechanisms in articular cartilage. J Magn Reson. 2004;169(2):300–7.
102. Wheaton AJ, Borthakur A, Reddy R. Application of the keyhole technique to T1rho relaxation mapping. J Magn Reson Imag. 2003;18(6):745–9.
103. Witschey WR, Borthakur A, Elliott MA, Magland J, McArdle EL, Wheaton A, et al. Spin-locked balanced steady-state free-precession (slSSFP). Magn Reson Med. 2009;62(4):993–1001.
104. Forsen S, Hoffman RA. Study of moderately rapid chemical exchange reactions by means of nuclear magnetic double resonance. J Chem Phys. 1963;39(11):2892–901.
105. Sherry AD, Woods M. Chemical exchange saturation transfer contrast agents for magnetic resonance imaging. Annu Rev Biomed Eng. 2008;10:391–411.
106. Ward KM, Aletras AH, Balaban RS. A new class of contrast agents for MRI based on proton chemical exchange dependent saturation transfer (CEST). J Magn Reson. 2000;143(1):79–87.
107. Zhou J, van Zijl PC. Chemcial exchange saturation transfer imaging and spectroscopy. Prog NMR Spectrosc. 2006;48:109–36.
108. Woessner DE, Zhang S, Merritt ME, Sherry AD. Numerical solution of the Bloch equations provides insights into the optimum design of PARACEST agents for MRI. Magn Reson Med. 2005;53(4):790–9.
109. van Zijl PC, Jones CK, Ren J, Malloy CR, Sherry AD. MRI detection of glycogen in vivo by using chemical exchange saturation transfer imaging (glycoCEST). Proc Natl Acad Sci USA. 2007;104(11):4359–64.
110. Zhou J, Wilson DA, Sun PZ, Klaus JA, Van Zijl PC. Quantitative description of proton exchange processes between water and endogenous and exogenous agents for WEX, CEST, and APT experiments. Magn Reson Med. 2004;51(5):945–52.
111. Borthakur A, Mellon E, Niyogi S, Witschey W, Kneeland JB, Reddy R. Sodium and T1rho MRI for molecular and diagnostic imaging of articular cartilage. NMR Biomed. 2006;19(7):781–821.
112. McRobbie DW. MRI from picture to proton. Cambridge, UK; New York: Cambridge University Press; 2007. xii, 397 p.

Chapter 18
Future Perspective and Significance of Cartilage Imaging and Quantification

Thomas M. Link and Sharmila Majumdar

Keywords Biochemical MR techniques • Cartilage imaging • Future • Morphological MR techniques • Perspective • Pharmacotherapies • Quantification • Significance • Volumetric cartilage quantification

Introduction

Cartilage is one of the most significant structures for joint function and is compromised in degenerative and traumatic joint disease. MR imaging has been established as the standard cartilage imaging modality, and techniques have been developed and optimized to visualize cartilage morphology, to quantify its volume and to analyze its biochemical composition. The substantial amount of research that is invested in the development of these morphologic and quantitative imaging techniques is geared at preventing and treating traumatic and degenerative cartilage disease at the earliest stages.

Prevention

Prevention is achieved by modifying risk factors, which include obesity, knee injury, [1, 2] and excessive physical exercise [3–6]. Vigorous physical exercise is in particular a substantial risk factor in subjects who may not have adequate cartilage quality or other structural limitations of the joint that may lead to accelerated degenerative disease [7]. We are increasingly confronted with joint injury and degeneration in individuals with high levels of physical activity, not infrequently already in young and middle-aged adults. In order to prevent cartilage injury, it is of vital importance to tailor physical activity at early stages and/or institute injury prevention programs [8–11]. In particular, individuals with higher susceptibility to cartilage damage need to be educated on how to prevent joint injury. With modification of physical activities, joint injury, degeneration, and long-term disability may potentially be prevented. Injury prevention programs have been successfully used in athletes and are currently used at some institutions in recreational runners. Structured functional biomechanics programs have reported 88% reduction in noncontact anterior cruciate ligament tears in soccer players [10], and a 43% reduction in knee and ankle injuries in a cohort of young athletes in a variety of sports [12]. Another risk factor that may be modified is obesity and a large number of preventive efforts are targeted at weight loss.

Treatment

Unfortunately *pharmacotherapies* for the treatment of osteoarthritis have limitations and effective medications are desperately needed [13]. A number of medications have been applied such as licofelone, which was shown to significantly reduce cartilage volume loss over time, thus suggesting a protective effect in patients with knee OA [14]. Also, a previous study using chondroitins 4 and 6 sulfate demonstrated that radiographic progression of knee osteoarthritis was significantly reduced in the chondroitins 4 and 6 sulfate group compared with the placebo group (28% versus 41% [$P <$ 0.0005]) [15]. Other studies, however, found less positive results for glucosamine and chondroitin sulfate [16–18] and none of the pharmacotherapies developed to date has been effectively shown to regenerate cartilage.

Cartilage repair procedures are also challenging and have controversial success rates [19]. Microfracture, drilling procedures, autologous chondrocyte implantation, and osteochondral autograft transfer systems have been used with various success rates [20–22]. *Mosaicplasty*, also termed osteochondral autograft transplantation (OAT) or autologous osteochondral transplantation [23, 24], is used most frequently at the knee and ankle joints, but has also been advocated in other joints such as the elbow to treat focal chondral or osteochondral defects due to injury, degeneration,

S. Majumdar (✉)
Department of Radiology and Biomedical Imaging,
University of California at San Francisco, 1700 4th St., Suite 203,
San Francisco, CA, 94158, USA
e-mail: Sharmila.Majumdar@ucsf.edu

T.M. Link (ed.), *Cartilage Imaging: Significance, Techniques, and New Developments*,
DOI 10.1007/978-1-4419-8438-8_18, © Springer Science+Business Media, LLC 2011

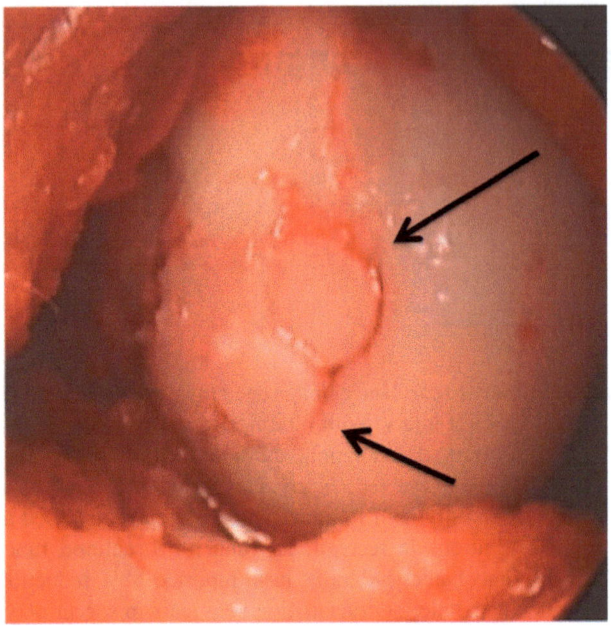

Fig. 18.1 Arthroscopic image of a patient who underwent mosaicplasty of the knee. Multiple round osteochondral plugs are shown (*arrows*)

osteochondritis dissecans, or osteonecrosis (Fig. 18.1). Using the *microfracture technique*, small perforations are created in the subchondral bone plate after debridement of a cartilage defect. *Drilling procedures* are applied in osteochondritis dissecans if the cartilage surface is intact, but they are frequently only successful if patients are skeletally immature [25]. *Chondrocyte implantation* has been performed with autologous chondrocytes and allografts. The cartilage defect is debrided and filled with a suspension of cultured chondrocytes and covered by a periosteal flap or the defect is filled with chondrocyte-impregnated scaffolds [26]. Results are somewhat controversial [27, 28] with one study indicating that cartilage repair tissue was of varying morphology ranging from predominantly hyaline in 22% of biopsy specimens, mixed in 48%, to predominantly fibrocartilage, in 30% [28]. A study [29] comparing mosaicplasty and autologous chondrocyte implantation showed that both treatments resulted in a decrease in patient symptoms. However, the morphological and histological improvement provided by the autologous chondrocyte implantation lagged behind that provided by mosaicplasty. Histologically, the defects treated with autologous chondrocyte implantation were primarily filled with fibrocartilage, whereas the osteochondral cylinder transplants retained their hyaline character. In summary, however, there is limited evidence that any of these interventions significantly alters the natural history of cartilage degeneration [30].

It should also be noted that these techniques are not suited for older individuals and those with extensive cartilage defects, such as osteoarthritis patients. Cartilage repair is tailored for younger subjects with focal osteochondral pathology and otherwise relatively healthy cartilage. Studies on the evolution of these osteochondral lesions and their significance are limited. A previous study [31] following these defects in a small number of patients (n = 12, age range: 9–46 years) for an average period of 11 years found that after skeletal maturity these individuals developed OA while in individuals under the age of 18 the lesions healed or were not visualized any more. The results of this study suggest that younger adults with smaller cartilage lesions may be good candidates for cartilage repair.

Significance of Cartilage Imaging and Quantification

Cartilage imaging and quantification impact management both in treating and preventing degeneration and disability; requirements for imaging techniques are dependent on clinical indications:

1. High-resolution imaging of cartilage is indispensible to plan cartilage repair, that is, select the correct repair technique and plan the intervention knowing the exact size and depth of the defect. This is particularly important for younger individuals and high-level athletes. The most important pathological conditions that require high-resolution imaging are cartilage injury and osteochondritis dissecans.
2. Volumetric cartilage imaging, which sensitively monitors cartilage loss, is a reproducible test which has the potential to monitor the natural evolution of osteoarthritis and to assess the effects of new therapies. Subregional analysis of cartilage volume as well as loading and unloading studies may provide additional tools to enhance monitoring of the disease process. A significant fund of knowledge has been obtained using volumetric cartilage quantification in multiple clinical studies.
3. Given that prevention currently appears to be the most effective method to manage osteoarthritis, it is crucial to identify individuals at risk for cartilage degeneration and those with very early degenerative changes. In fact, prevention of osteoarthritis and disability is one of the most significant tasks and research objectives in our aging society. The socioeconomical impact of osteoarthritis-induced disability on our society is tremendous. Our preventive efforts must aim already at the young and middle-aged active subjects, where preventive interventions and therapies may potentially prove most effective. New MR-based biomarkers may have a substantial impact on preventive efforts (Fig. 18.2). While standard morphological MR techniques visualize cartilage defects and volumetric MRI sensitively assesses volume loss both of which are

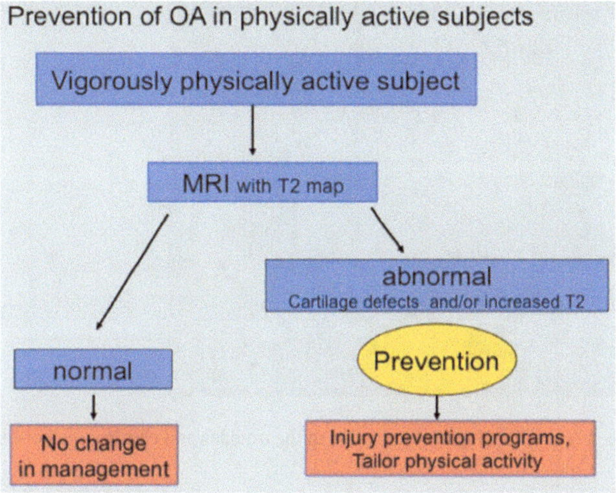

Fig. 18.2 Potential effect of T2 relaxation time measurements on preventive management of individuals performing vigorous physical activity

irreversible, it would be more beneficial to characterize the biochemical composition of cartilage before cartilage is lost and identify individuals with potentially reversible changes or those who would benefit most from preventive management [32]. Ideally those techniques would allow cartilage quality assessment before cartilage is irreversibly lost such as bone densitometry measurements currently allow assessment of fracture risk before actual fractures have occurred.

Future Requirements for Cartilage Imaging

Morphological MR Techniques

In order to optimize preoperative planning, in particular of cartilage repair, MR imaging techniques need to be optimized in terms of spatial resolution to best possibly visualize cartilage defects. Previous studies have established the benefit of 3 T imaging [33–35], and new sequences have been proposed to better visualize cartilage structure and morphology including balanced SSFP imaging, 3D fast spin echo (FSE) sequences, and ultrashort TE imaging [36–38].

In the future 7 T MRI may be introduced as a new technique to enhance both morphological and biochemical imaging. Early studies have shown the potential of in vivo cartilage imaging at 7.0 T [39, 40] (Fig. 18.3), but in order to achieve a clinically viable performance dedicated coils and new sequences need to be developed. It should be noted that standard FSE imaging used for cartilage is not feasible at 7.0 T given specific absorption rate (SAR) issues and that gradient echo sequences may be more viable.

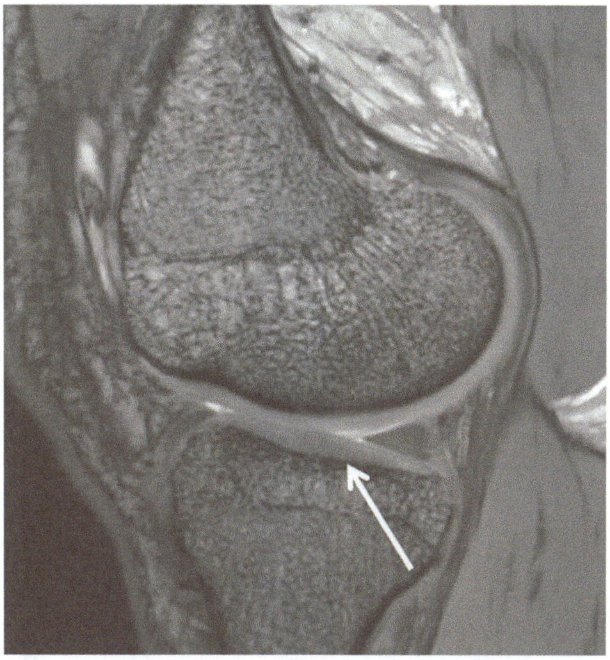

Fig. 18.3 Sagittal MR image of the knee obtained at 7 T using a FIESTA (fast imaging employing steady state acquisition) sequence. Note high anatomic detail and visualization of the cartilage radial zone with parallel-oriented collagen fibrils at the tibia (*arrow*)

In terms of new imaging sequences, an increasing trend is noted to move from 2D to 3D sequences. Three-dimensional FSE sequences have been used and promising studies have been performed, showing similar performance in diagnosing cartilage lesions with 2D and 3D FSE sequences [41, 42] (Fig. 18.4). Potentially these sequences would allow shortening imaging time by eliminating acquisition in multiple imaging planes and with decreased slice thickness they would allow visualization of smaller defects.

In addition to 3D FSE sequences, gradient echo sequences are investigated, which include balanced steady-state free precession (SSFP) imaging [37, 43]. These sequences have been named differently depending on the manufacturer and are called true fast imaging with steady-state free precession (true-FISP, Siemens Healthcare) [44], fast imaging employing steady-state acquisition (FIESTA, GE Healthcare), and balanced fast-field echo imaging (Philips Heathcare) [38]. Using these sequences, fluid is bright and cartilage is intermediate in signal. Results of recent studies are promising but to date these sequences are not considered part of the standard cartilage imaging protocol (Fig. 18.5).

Ultrashort TE (UTE) MR imaging has been investigated [36, 45] to better analyze pathologies of the cartilage–bone interface; cadaver studies have been performed and showed that the high signal intensity on UTE images of human articular joints originates from the calcified cartilage and the deepest layer of the uncalcified cartilage, without a definite

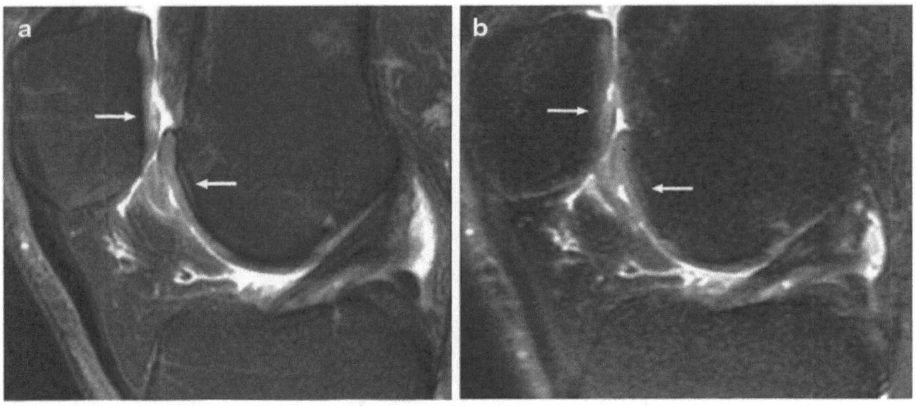

Fig. 18.4 Fat saturated, sagittal 2D (**a**) and 3D-FSE (**b**) images of the knee showing cartilage delamination at the trochlea and cartilage defects at the patella (*arrow*). Comparable demonstration of these focal defects

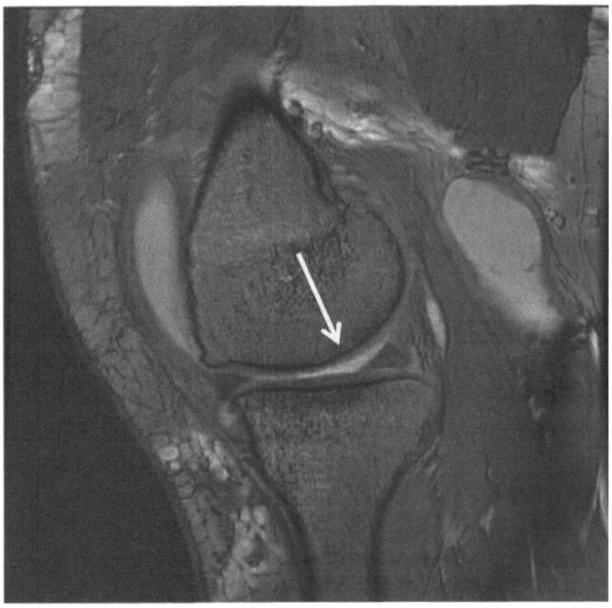

Fig. 18.5 Sagittal 3D FIESTA sequence of the medial knee joint compartment obtained at 3 T shows extensive cartilage fibrillation at the femoral condyle (*arrow*). In addition, moderate joint effusion and large popliteal cyst are also shown

contribution from subchondral bone. These data suggest that UTE sequences may provide a way of better assessing abnormalities at or near the osteochondral junction [36]. In the future, in vivo studies will be required to better understand the clinical significance of these findings.

Another new technique to morphologically characterize cartilage is diffusion-weighted imaging and diffusion tensor imaging (DTI), which to date has mostly been used in neuroimaging. Given the fact that cartilage also has a defined anisotropic collagen architecture, diffusion-weighted imaging and DTI may be used to visualize structural changes in the alignment of the collagen network during simulated function and loading conditions, which may indicate early disease processes [46]. Initial specimen studies have been performed confirming the potential of this new technique and although these data are still preliminary [47–50], DTI may become a powerful tool in the noninvasive study of cartilage structure and function and may provide insight into changes observed as a result of degradation in the setting of osteoarthritis or traumatic chondral injury [46]. As in UTE imaging, however, clinical feasibility with standard MR systems needs to be demonstrated and patient studies are required.

Volumetric Cartilage Quantification

Sensitive quantification of cartilage loss is the major goal of this technique and accurate cartilage segmentation is the key ingredient. Considerable effort has been spent on optimizing cartilage volume measurements to assess the natural evolution of OA and to serve as potential outcome marker in pharmaceutical trials. The MR sequences that have been almost exclusively used for cartilage morphology quantification are thin section fat-saturated T1-weighted spoiled gradient (SPGR) echo or fast low angle shot (FLASH) sequences. With these images, cartilage displays higher signal in comparison with adjacent tissues (bone and joint fluid) facilitating segmentation of the cartilage. Several semiautomated techniques have been described to optimize cartilage segmentation including active shape models, edge detection, fitting B-splines to manually segmented points, and B-spline Snake (active contours) [51–53], but to date most large-scale studies have relied on manual segmentation (Fig. 18.6).

It should be noted, however, that cartilage segmentation using current techniques takes too long to be established as a routine clinical tool. Segmentation needs to be automatic, quick, and highly reproducible in order to be of clinical

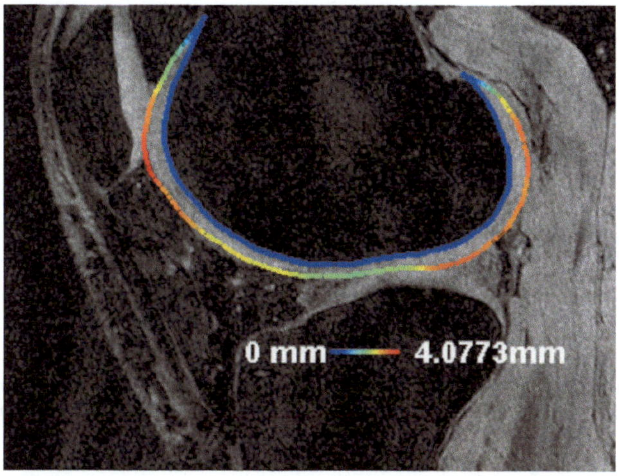

Fig. 18.6 Cartilage segmentation of the lateral femoral condyle obtained with semiautomatic spline technique overlaid on fat-saturated SPGR (spoiled gradient echo) sequence. Color map of the peripheral spline provides color map indicating cartilage thickness

significance. If this goal is not achieved, it is highly unlikely that cartilage volume measurements will lose their stigma as a pure research tool.

Biochemical MR Techniques

In the last years, significant interest focused on imaging cartilage biochemical composition as a potential early marker for degenerative joint disease. Cartilage consists of approximately 70% water and the remainder predominantly of type II collagen fibers and glycosaminoglycans (GAG). Several techniques have been developed to assess the composition of the cartilage matrix. The major techniques are (a) delayed gadolinium-enhanced MR imaging of cartilage (dGEMRIC), (b) T2 relaxation time measurements, and (c) T1rho. Recently, sodium ((23)Na) [54] and chemical exchange-dependent saturation transfer (gagCEST) techniques [55] have been suggested as alternative techniques, but clinical application is far more challenging than this of the previously mentioned techniques.

Initial studies have shown that the dGEMRIC measurement of GAG corresponds to the true GAG concentration as measured with biochemistry and histology [56, 57]. This technique has also been used in a number of clinical studies and variations of this measurement have been shown in patients with osteoarthritis, trials of autologous chondrocyte implants, and subjects with sedentary lifestyle versus those with regular exercise [58–61]. With the event of nephrogenic systemic fibrosis, there have been some concerns about using gadolinium in older osteoarthritis patients who may have potential renal dysfunction.

Another approach that has been used to measure cartilage composition is T2 mapping. It was shown that increasing T2 relaxation time was proportional to the distribution of cartilage water and is sensitive to small water content changes [62]. In an early study, Dardzinski et al. examined the spatial variation of in vivo cartilage T2 in young asymptomatic adults and found a reproducible pattern of increasing T2 that was proportional to the known spatial variation in cartilage water and was inversely proportional to the distribution of proteoglycans [63]. These authors postulated that the regional T2 differences were secondary to the restricted mobility of cartilage water within an anisotropic solid matrix. T2 measurements are used in the NIH-funded Osteoarthritis Initiative (OAI) Multicenter Trial, and initial research has shown promise in quantifying early degenerative changes of cartilage [6]. Stehling et al. [6] showed in middle-aged asymptomatic individuals with risk factors for knee osteoarthritis using 3.0 T MRI that physically active individuals had more knee abnormalities and higher patellar T2 values than those that were less physically active. The rich dataset from the OAI will eventually provide an excellent source to evaluate the role of T2 relaxation times in predicting osteoarthritis and monitoring its natural evolution (Fig. 18.7).

The third parameter that has been proposed to measure cartilage composition is 3D-T1rho-relaxation mapping. T1rho describes the spin-lattice relaxation in the rotating frame and changes in the extracellular matrix of cartilage, like loss of GAG, may be reflected in measurements of T1rho due to less restricted motion of water protons. Preliminary results demonstrated the in vivo feasibility of quantifying early biochemical changes in symptomatic osteoarthritis subjects employing T1rho-weighted MR imaging on a 1.5 T clinical scanner [64, 65]. A number of clinical studies [66–68] have shown the potential of the technique to predict early degenerative hyaline cartilage disease and suggested that this parameter may be superior to T2 relaxation time in assessing hyaline cartilage degeneration.

Though these techniques have shown promise in measuring cartilage composition and disease burden, the number of longitudinal studies is limited and it is not yet clear whether these biomarkers will be able to predict osteoarthritis development and progression. Also it is not yet well known whether these parameters will be sensitive in monitoring the natural evolution of osteoarthritis and the response of cartilage to therapy. In addition, a number of technical issues have to be resolved before these techniques are used in multiple centers with comparable results. These include standardized imaging and optimizing reproducibility of image acquisition and analysis. This again includes fast, precise and reproducible cartilage segmentation, which to date has not been achieved. Ideally, these techniques should be as standardized and as simple to use as dual X-ray absorptiometry (DXA) to quantify bone mineral density. Unfortunately,

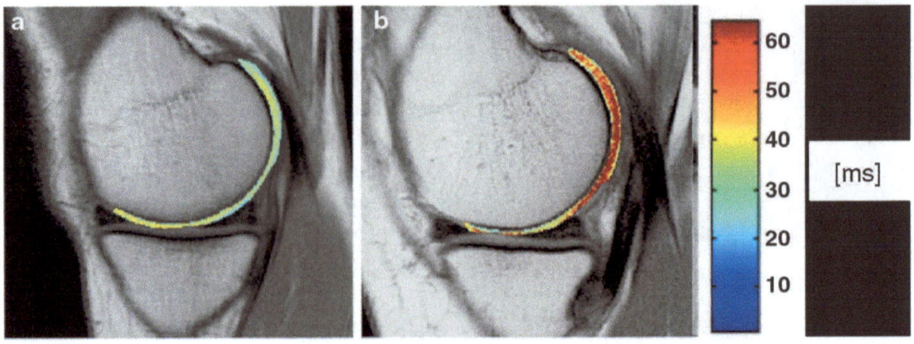

Fig. 18.7 T2 relaxation time maps overlaid on sagittal FSE images of the medial knee compartment. Low T2 values in (**a**) indicating low water content and suggesting integrity of collagen fibrils, while high T2 values in (**b**) indicate higher water content with cartilage degeneration, though cartilage volume appears to be maintained

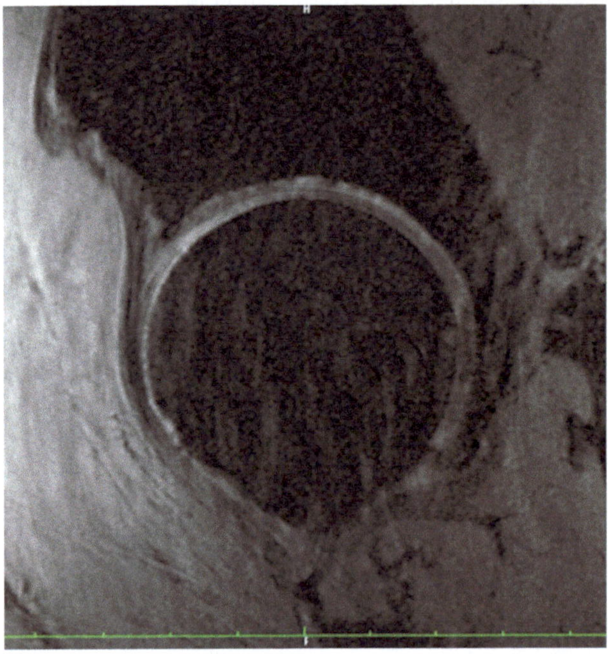

Fig. 18.8 Sagittal high-resolution fat-saturated SPGR sequence of the hip showing cartilage with intermediate to high signal and allowing differentiation of superior and anterior acetabular and femoral cartilage

we are currently far away from anything, which would be similarly simple and easy to use as DXA for quantification of hyaline cartilage.

Imaging of Hip, Ankle, and Other Joints

It should be noted that most of our efforts so far have focused on optimizing cartilage imaging for the knee, however, sensitive assessment of hip joint cartilage and of other joints is becoming increasingly clinically relevant. The relatively thin cartilage of the hip joint, as well as its complex geometry, poses challenges for standardized, reproducible assessment of cartilage; but with appropriate pulse sequence parameters, dedicated surface coils (such as the cardiac coil for single hip imaging) and high-field systems (3.0 T) accurate, reproducible morphological assessment of cartilage and the labrum may be mastered [69] (Fig. 18.8). Initial studies have shown feasibility of volumetric measurements, T1rho, T2 relaxation time, and dGEMRIC at the hip joint to evaluate early degenerative disease and to monitor cartilage loss [70–72]. But it should be noted that compared to the knee, hip imaging is far more demanding and a number of challenges have to be mastered before quantitative volumetric and matrix measurements are clinically applicable. These include the difficulty in differentiating femoral and acetabular cartilage as well as challenges in segmenting cartilage reproducibly in a reasonable amount of time. Imaging of the cartilage of the ankle, wrist, elbow, and shoulder is currently clinically less relevant and has similar challenges given that cartilage in these joints is thin and the anatomy is complex. Initial studies have shown the feasibility of assessing cartilage repair at the ankle using dGEMRIC techniques [73].

Imaging of Joint Function and Loading

A number of cartilage abnormalities may only be explained and detected during joint motion and loading. MRI performed during loading or kinematic MRI may better visualize early joint and cartilage abnormalities leading to osteoarthritis. Abnormal patellofemoral joint motion is one of these conditions and a possible cause of patellofemoral pain and accelerated joint degeneration. A recent study investigated patellofemoral joint kinematics during dynamic, weight-bearing knee extension and assessed the effects of knee braces on patellofemoral motion [74]. The results of this study suggested that some subjects with patellofemoral pain exhibit

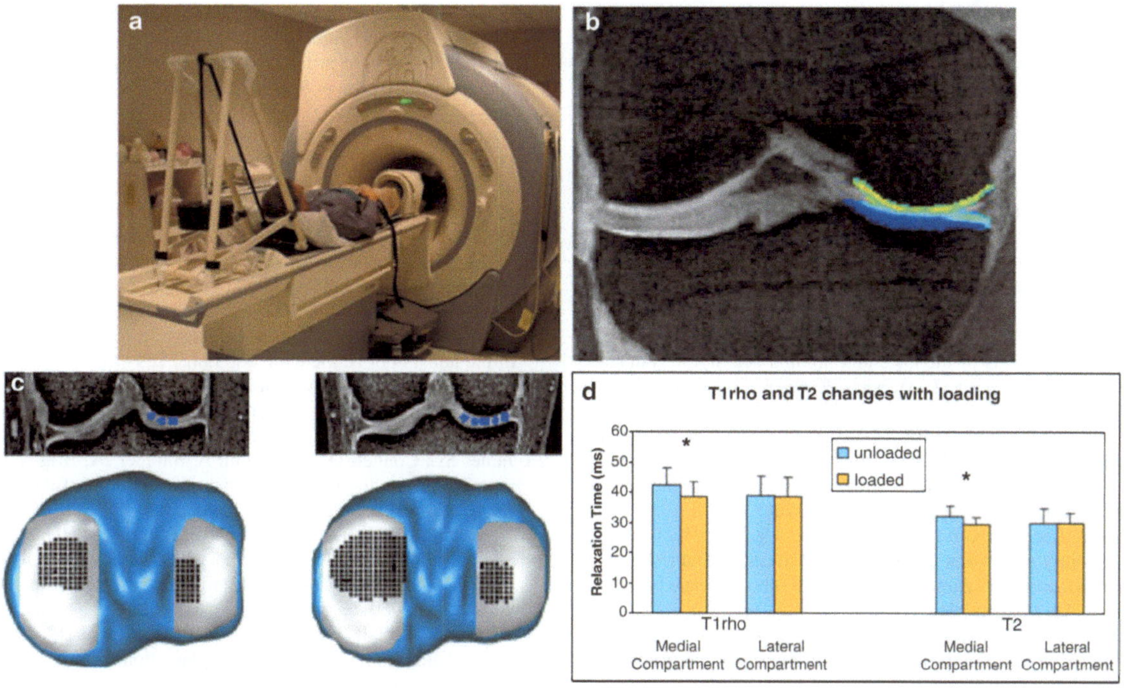

Fig. 18.9 Cartilage in vivo loading: (**a**) setup during MRI, (**b**) representative coronal MR image with color map at medial knee compartment, (**c**) regions with most pronounced changes highlighted, and (**d**) T1rho and T2 values at the medial and lateral knee compartment with and without mechanical loading. Note significant changes in T1rho and T2 during loading, which are only found in the medial joint compartment

abnormal weight-bearing joint kinematics and that braces may be effective in reducing patellar maltracking in these subjects. Initial studies have also investigated cartilage matrix changes due to mechanical loading using T2 relaxation time measurements [75] and dGEMRIC [76]. In addition, investigators have also focused on measuring T1rho and T2 changes due to loading in individuals with and without osteoarthritis and found more pronounced changes in patients with early degenerative changes in the medial joint compartment [77, 78] (Fig. 18.9). Clearly, however, more work is needed to better understand the response of abnormal cartilage to kinematic and loaded joint MRI and how these techniques would potentially affect patient management.

Summary and Conclusion

New operative and pharmacological therapeutic modalities, as well as vigorous preventive efforts targeted at osteoarthritis and related disability, have made cartilage imaging an important area of research with increasing clinical significance. Though morphological imaging is of tremendous importance to plan therapies (such as cartilage repair), quantitative, biochemical imaging has gained increasing relevance in detecting the earliest degenerative changes as well as in analyzing cartilage quality, which may predict development of osteoarthritis. These new imaging techniques may together with new pharmacological therapies and vigorous preventive efforts revolutionize management of osteoarthritis and could have a tremendous impact on population health. The future goals of cartilage imaging will be (a) to improve morphological evaluation of cartilage also in joints which so far have been less accessible (such as the hip), (b) to standardize the new biochemical, cartilage matrix techniques, (c) to make analysis clinically feasible, (d) to understand whether these new techniques can predict the development of osteoarthritis, and (e) to provide evidence that they can effectively monitor new therapies.

References

1. Felson DT. An update on the pathogenesis and epidemiology of osteoarthritis. Radiol Clin North Am. 2004;42(1):1–9. v.
2. Niu J, Zhang YQ, Torner J, Nevitt M, Lewis CE, Aliabadi P, et al. Is obesity a risk factor for progressive radiographic knee osteoarthritis? Arthritis Rheum. 2009;61(3):329–35.
3. Major NM, Helms CA. MR imaging of the knee: findings in asymptomatic collegiate basketball players. AJR Am J Roentgenol. 2002;179(3):641–4.
4. Stahl R, Luke A, Ma CB, Krug R, Steinbach L, Majumdar S, et al. Prevalence of pathologic findings in asymptomatic knees of

marathon runners before and after a competition in comparison with physically active subjects – a 3.0 T magnetic resonance imaging study. Skeletal Radiol. 2008;37(7):627–38.
5. Stehling C, Lane NE, Nevitt MC, Lynch J, McCulloch CE, Link TM. Subjects with higher physical activity levels have more severe focal knee lesions diagnosed with 3T MRI: analysis of a non-symptomatic cohort of the osteoarthritis initiative. Osteoarthritis Cartilage. 2010;18(6):776–86.
6. Stehling C, Liebl H, Krug R, Lane NE, Nevitt MC, Lynch J, et al. Patellar cartilage: T2 values and morphologic abnormalities at 3.0-T MR imaging in relation to physical activity in asymptomatic subjects from the osteoarthritis initiative. Radiology. 2010;254(2): 509–20.
7. Vignon E, Valat JP, Rossignol M, Avouac B, Rozenberg S, Thoumie P, et al. Osteoarthritis of the knee and hip and activity: a systematic international review and synthesis (OASIS). Joint Bone Spine. 2006;73(4):442–55.
8. Gilchrist J, Mandelbaum BR, Melancon H, Ryan GW, Silvers HJ, Griffin LY, et al. A randomized controlled trial to prevent noncontact anterior cruciate ligament injury in female collegiate soccer players. Am J Sports Med. 2008;36(8):1476–83.
9. Lim BO, Lee YS, Kim JG, An KO, Yoo J, Kwon YH. Effects of sports injury prevention training on the biomechanical risk factors of anterior cruciate ligament injury in high school female basketball players. Am J Sports Med. 2009;37(9):1728–34.
10. Mandelbaum BR, Silvers HJ, Watanabe DS, Knarr JF, Thomas SD, Griffin LY, et al. Effectiveness of a neuromuscular and proprioceptive training program in preventing anterior cruciate ligament injuries in female athletes: 2-year follow-up. Am J Sports Med. 2005;33(7):1003–10.
11. Silvers HJ, Mandelbaum BR. Prevention of anterior cruciate ligament injury in the female athlete. Br J Sports Med. 2007;41 Suppl 1:i52–9.
12. Olsen L, Scanlan A, MacKay M, Babul S, Reid D, Clark M, et al. Strategies for prevention of soccer related injuries: a systematic review. Br J Sports Med. 2004;38(1):89–94.
13. Abramson SB, Attur M, Yazici Y. Prospects for disease modification in osteoarthritis. Nat Clin Pract Rheumatol. 2006;2(6):304–12.
14. Raynauld JP, Martel-Pelletier J, Bias P, Laufer S, Haraoui B, Choquette D, et al. Protective effects of licofelone, a 5-lipoxygenase and cyclo-oxygenase inhibitor, versus naproxen on cartilage loss in knee osteoarthritis: a first multicentre clinical trial using quantitative MRI. Ann Rheum Dis. 2009;68(6):938–47.
15. Kahan A, Uebelhart D, De Vathaire F, Delmas PD, Reginster JY. Long-term effects of chondroitins 4 and 6 sulfate on knee osteoarthritis: the study on osteoarthritis progression prevention, a two-year, randomized, double-blind, placebo-controlled trial. Arthritis Rheum. 2009;60(2):524–33.
16. Clegg DO, Reda DJ, Harris CL, Klein MA, O'Dell JR, Hooper MM, et al. Glucosamine, chondroitin sulfate, and the two in combination for painful knee osteoarthritis. N Engl J Med. 2006;354(8):795–808.
17. Sawitzke AD, Shi H, Finco MF, Dunlop DD, Bingham 3rd CO, Harris CL, et al. The effect of glucosamine and/or chondroitin sulfate on the progression of knee osteoarthritis: a report from the glucosamine/chondroitin arthritis intervention trial. Arthritis Rheum. 2008;58(10):3183–91.
18. Sawitzke AD, Shi H, Finco MF, Dunlop DD, Harris CL, Singer NG, et al. Clinical efficacy and safety of glucosamine, chondroitin sulphate, their combination, celecoxib or placebo taken to treat osteoarthritis of the knee: 2-year results from GAIT. Ann Rheum Dis. 2010;69(8):1459–64.
19. Richter W. Cell-based cartilage repair: illusion or solution for osteoarthritis. Curr Opin Rheumatol. 2007;19(5):451–6.
20. Bedi A, Feeley BT, Williams 3rd RJ. Management of articular cartilage defects of the knee. J Bone Joint Surg Am. 2010;92(4): 994–1009.
21. Gudas R, Stankevicius E, Monastyreckiene E, Pranys D, Kalesinskas RJ. Osteochondral autologous transplantation versus microfracture for the treatment of articular cartilage defects in the knee joint in athletes. Knee Surg Sports Traumatol Arthrosc. 2006;14(9): 834–42.
22. Zaslav K, Cole B, Brewster R, DeBerardino T, Farr J, Fowler P, et al. A prospective study of autologous chondrocyte implantation in patients with failed prior treatment for articular cartilage defect of the knee: results of the Study of the Treatment of Articular Repair (STAR) Clinical Trial. Am J Sports Med. 2009;37(1):42–55.
23. Imhoff AB, Oettl GM. Arthroscopic and open techniques for transplantation of osteochondral autografts and allografts in various joints. Surg Technol Int. 2000;8:249–52.
24. Hangody L. The mosaicplasty technique for osteochondral lesions of the talus. Foot Ankle Clin. 2003;8(2):259–73.
25. Kawasaki K, Uchio Y, Adachi N, Iwasa J, Ochi M. Drilling from the intercondylar area for treatment of osteochondritis dissecans of the knee joint. Knee. 2003;10(3):257–63.
26. James SL, Connell DA, Saifuddin A, Skinner JA, Briggs TW. MR imaging of autologous chondrocyte implantation of the knee. Eur Radiol. 2006;16(5):1022–30.
27. Henderson IJ, Tuy B, Connell D, Oakes B, Hettwer WH. Prospective clinical study of autologous chondrocyte implantation and correlation with MRI at three and 12 months. J Bone Joint Surg Br. 2003;85(7):1060–6.
28. Roberts S, McCall IW, Darby AJ, Menage J, Evans H, Harrison PE, et al. Autologous chondrocyte implantation for cartilage repair: monitoring its success by magnetic resonance imaging and histology. Arthritis Res Ther. 2003;5(1):R60–73.
29. Horas U, Pelinkovic D, Herr G, Aigner T, Schnettler R. Autologous chondrocyte implantation and osteochondral cylinder transplantation in cartilage repair of the knee joint A prospective, comparative trial. J Bone Joint Surg Am. 2003;85-A(2):185–92.
30. Safran MR, Seiber K. The evidence for surgical repair of articular cartilage in the knee. J Am Acad Orthop Surg. 2010;18(5):259–66.
31. Prakash D, Learmonth D. Natural progression of osteo-chondral defect in the femoral condyle. Knee. 2002;9(1):7–10.
32. Felson DT, Lohmander LS. Whither osteoarthritis biomarkers? Osteoarthritis Cartilage. 2009;17(4):419–22.
33. Kijowski R, Blankenbaker DG, Davis KW, Shinki K, Kaplan LD, De Smet AA. Comparison of 1.5- and 3.0-T MR imaging for evaluating the articular cartilage of the knee joint. Radiology. 2009;250: 839–48.
34. Link TM, Sell CA, Masi JN, Phan C, Newitt D, Lu Y, et al. 3.0 vs 1.5 T MRI in the detection of focal cartilage pathology – ROC analysis in an experimental model. Osteoarthritis Cartilage. 2006;14(1): 63–70.
35. Wong S, Steinbach L, Zhao J, Stehling C, Ma CB, Link TM. Comparative study of imaging at 3.0 T versus 1.5 T of the knee. Skeletal Radiol. 2009;38(8):761–9.
36. Bae WC, Dwek JR, Znamirowski R, Statum SM, Hermida JC, D'Lima DD, et al. Ultrashort echo time MR imaging of osteochondral junction of the knee at 3 T: identification of anatomic structures contributing to signal intensity. Radiology. 2010;254(3):837–45.
37. Chen CA, Kijowski R, Shapiro LM, Tuite MJ, Davis KW, Klaers JL, et al. Cartilage morphology at 3.0T: assessment of three-dimensional magnetic resonance imaging techniques. J Magn Reson Imaging. 2010;32(1):173–83.
38. Gold GE, Chen CA, Koo S, Hargreaves BA, Bangerter NK. Recent advances in MRI of articular cartilage. AJR Am J Roentgenol. 2009;193(3):628–38.
39. Stahl R, Krug R, Kelley DA, Zuo J, Ma CB, Majumdar S, et al. Assessment of cartilage-dedicated sequences at ultra-high-field MRI: comparison of imaging performance and diagnostic confidence between 3.0 and 7.0 T with respect to osteoarthritis-induced changes at the knee joint. Skeletal Radiol. 2009;38(8):771–83.

40. Wang L, Wu Y, Chang G, Oesingmann N, Schweitzer ME, Jerschow A, et al. Rapid isotropic 3D-sodium MRI of the knee joint in vivo at 7T. J Magn Reson Imaging. 2009;30(3):606–14.
41. Kijowski R, Davis KW, Woods MA, Lindstrom MJ, De Smet AA, Gold GE, et al. Knee joint: comprehensive assessment with 3D isotropic resolution fast spin-echo MR imaging – diagnostic performance compared with that of conventional MR imaging at 3.0 T. Radiology. 2009;252(2):486–95.
42. Ristow O, Steinbach L, Sabo G, Krug R, Huber M, Rauscher I, et al. Isotropic 3D fast spin-echo imaging versus standard 2D imaging at 3.0 T of the knee-image quality and diagnostic performance. Eur Radiol. 2009;19:1263–72.
43. Gold GE, Reeder SB, Yu H, Kornaat P, Shimakawa AS, Johnson JW, et al. Articular cartilage of the knee: rapid three-dimensional MR imaging at 3.0 T with IDEAL balanced steady-state free precession–initial experience. Radiology. 2006;240(2):546–51.
44. Duc SR, Pfirrmann CW, Koch PP, Zanetti M, Hodler J. Internal knee derangement assessed with 3-minute three-dimensional isovoxel true FISP MR sequence: preliminary study. Radiology. 2008;246(2):526–35.
45. Koff MF, Potter HG. Noncontrast MR techniques and imaging of cartilage. Radiol Clin North Am. 2009;47(3):495–504.
46. Potter HG, Black BR, le Chong R. New techniques in articular cartilage imaging. Clin Sports Med. 2009;28(1):77–94.
47. de Visser SK, Bowden JC, Wentrup-Byrne E, Rintoul L, Bostrom T, Pope JM, et al. Anisotropy of collagen fibre alignment in bovine cartilage: comparison of polarised light microscopy and spatially resolved diffusion-tensor measurements. Osteoarthritis Cartilage. 2008;16(6):689–97.
48. de Visser SK, Crawford RW, Pope JM. Structural adaptations in compressed articular cartilage measured by diffusion tensor imaging. Osteoarthritis Cartilage. 2008;16(1):83–9.
49. Filidoro L, Dietrich O, Weber J, Rauch E, Oerther T, Wick M, et al. High-resolution diffusion tensor imaging of human patellar cartilage: feasibility and preliminary findings. Magn Reson Med. 2005;53(5):993–8.
50. Meder R, de Visser SK, Bowden JC, Bostrom T, Pope JM. Diffusion tensor imaging of articular cartilage as a measure of tissue microstructure. Osteoarthritis Cartilage. 2006;14(9):875–81.
51. Ghosh S, Ries M, Lane N, Ghajar C, Majumdar S. Segmentation of high resolution articular cartilage MR images. Trans Orthopedic Res Soc (ORS). 2000:246.
52. Solloway S, Hutchinson CE, Waterton JC, Taylor CJ. The use of active shape models for making thickness measurements of articular cartilage from MR images. Magn Reson Med. 1997;37(6):943–52.
53. Stammberger T, Eckstein F, Michaelis M, Englmeier KH, Reiser M. Interobserver reproducibility of quantitative cartilage measurements: comparison of B-spline snakes and manual segmentation. Magn Reson Imaging. 1999;17(7):1033–42.
54. Borthakur A, Mellon E, Niyogi S, Witschey W, Kneeland JB, Reddy R. Sodium and T1rho MRI for molecular and diagnostic imaging of articular cartilage. NMR Biomed. 2006;19(7):781–821.
55. Ling W, Regatte RR, Navon G, Jerschow A. Assessment of glycosaminoglycan concentration in vivo by chemical exchange-dependent saturation transfer (gagCEST). Proc Natl Acad Sci USA. 2008;105(7):2266–70.
56. Trattnig S, Mlynarik V, Breitenseher M, Huber M, Zembsch A, Rand T, et al. MRI visualization of proteoglycan depletion in articular cartilage via intravenous administration of Gd-DTPA. Magn Reson Imaging. 1999;17(4):577–83.
57. Bashir A, Gray ML, Hartke J, Burstein D. Nondestructive imaging of human cartilage glycosaminoglycan concentration by MRI. Magn Reson Med. 1999;41(5):857–65.
58. Burstein D, Gray M. New MRI techniques for imaging cartilage. J Bone Joint Surg Am. 2003;85-A Suppl 2:70–7.
59. Gillis A, Bashir A, McKeon B, Scheller A, Gray ML, Burstein D. Magnetic resonance imaging of relative glycosaminoglycan distribution in patients with autologous chondrocyte transplants. Invest Radiol. 2001;36(12):743–8.
60. Williams A, Gillis A, McKenzie C, Po B, Sharma L, Micheli L, et al. Glycosaminoglycan distribution in cartilage as determined by delayed gadolinium-enhanced MRI of cartilage (dGEMRIC): potential clinical applications. AJR Am J Roentgenol. 2004;182(1):167–72.
61. Williams A, Sharma L, McKenzie CA, Prasad PV, Burstein D. Delayed gadolinium-enhanced magnetic resonance imaging of cartilage in knee osteoarthritis: findings at different radiographic stages of disease and relationship to malalignment. Arthritis Rheum. 2005;52(11):3528–35.
62. Liess C, Lusse S, Karger N, Heller M, Gluer CC. Detection of changes in cartilage water content using MRI T2-mapping in vivo. Osteoarthritis Cartilage. 2002;10(12):907–13.
63. Dardzinski BJ, Mosher TJ, Li S, Van Slyke MA, Smith MB. Spatial variation of T2 in human articular cartilage. Radiology. 1997;205(2):546–50.
64. Regatte RR, Akella SV, Wheaton AJ, Lech G, Borthakur A, Kneeland JB, et al. 3D-T1rho-relaxation mapping of articular cartilage: in vivo assessment of early degenerative changes in symptomatic osteoarthritic subjects. Acad Radiol. 2004;11(7):741–9.
65. Regatte RR, Akella SV, Borthakur A, Kneeland JB, Reddy R. In vivo proton MR three-dimensional T1rho mapping of human articular cartilage: initial experience. Radiology. 2003;229(1):269–74.
66. Bolbos RI, Link TM, Ma CB, Majumdar S, Li X. T1rho relaxation time of the meniscus and its relationship with T1rho of adjacent cartilage in knees with acute ACL injuries at 3 T. Osteoarthritis Cartilage. 2009;17(1):12–8.
67. Li X, Ma CB, Link TM, Castillo DD, Blumenkrantz G, Lozano J, et al. In vivoT(1rho) and T(2) mapping of articular cartilage in osteoarthritis of the knee using 3T MRI. Osteoarthritis Cartilage. 2007;15:789–97.
68. Stahl R, Luke A, Li X, Carballido-Gamio J, Ma CB, Majumdar S, et al. T1rho, T(2) and focal knee cartilage abnormalities in physically active and sedentary healthy subjects versus early OA patients-a 3.0-Tesla MRI study. Eur Radiol. 2009;19:132–43.
69. Potter HG, Schachar J. High resolution noncontrast MRI of the hip. J Magn Reson Imaging. 2010;31(2):268–78.
70. Carballido-Gamio J, Link TM, Li X, Han ET, Krug R, Ries MD, et al. Feasibility and reproducibility of relaxometry, morphometric, and geometrical measurements of the hip joint with magnetic resonance imaging at 3T. J Magn Reson Imaging. 2008;28(1):227–35.
71. Domayer S, Mamisch T, Kress I, Chan J, Kim Y. Radial dGEMRIC in developmental dysplasia of the hip and in femoroacetabular impingement: preliminary results. Osteoarthritis Cartilage. 2010;18(11):1421–8.
72. Li W, Abram F, Beaudoin G, Berthiaume MJ, Pelletier JP, Martel-Pelletier J. Human hip joint cartilage: MRI quantitative thickness and volume measurements discriminating acetabulum and femoral head. IEEE Trans Biomed Eng. 2008;55(12):2731–40.
73. Domayer SE, Trattnig S, Stelzeneder D, Hirschfeld C, Quirbach S, Dorotka R, et al. Delayed gadolinium-enhanced MRI of cartilage in the ankle at 3 T: feasibility and preliminary results after matrix-associated autologous chondrocyte implantation. J Magn Reson Imaging. 2010;31(3):732–9.
74. Draper CE, Besier TF, Santos JM, Jennings F, Fredericson M, Gold GE, et al. Using real-time MRI to quantify altered joint kinematics in subjects with patellofemoral pain and to evaluate the effects of a patellar brace or sleeve on joint motion. J Orthop Res. 2009;27(5):571–7.
75. Nishii T, Kuroda K, Matsuoka Y, Sahara T, Yoshikawa H. Change in knee cartilage T2 in response to mechanical loading. J Magn Reson Imaging. 2008;28(1):175–80.

76. Mayerhoefer ME, Welsch GH, Mamisch TC, Kainberger F, Weber M, Nemec S, et al. The in vivo effects of unloading and compression on T1-Gd (dGEMRIC) relaxation times in healthy articular knee cartilage at 3.0 Tesla. Eur Radiol. 2010;20(2): 443–9.
77. Souza R, Bolbos R, Wyman B, Hellio M, Link T, Li X, et al. Changes in T1rho and T2 relaxation times of tibiofemoral articular cartilage with acute loading. Proceedings from the International Society for Magnetic Resonance in Medicine Annual Meeting 2009. Honolulu, HI; 2009.
78. Souza R, Stehling C, Wyman B, Le Graverand M, Li X, Link T, et al. The effects of acute loading on T1rho and T2 relaxation times of tibiofemoral articular cartilage. Osteoarthritis Cartilage. 2010; 18(12):1557–63.

Index

T.M. Link (ed.), *Cartilage Imaging: Significance, Techniques, and New Developments*,
DOI 10.1007/978-1-4419-8438-8, © Springer Science+Business Media, LLC 2011

MIX
Papier aus verantwortungsvollen Quellen
Paper from responsible sources
FSC® C105338

If you have any concerns about our products,
you can contact us on
ProductSafety@springernature.com

In case Publisher is established outside the EU,
the EU authorized representative is:
Springer Nature Customer Service Center GmbH
Europaplatz 3, 69115 Heidelberg, Germany

Printed by Libri Plureos GmbH
in Hamburg, Germany